Fundamentals of Body CT

FIFTH EDITION

W. RICHARD WEBB, MD
Professor Emeritus of Radiology and Biomedical Imaging
Emeritus Member, Haile Debas Academy of Medical Educators
University of California, San Francisco
San Francisco, California

WILLIAM E. BRANT, MD, FACR
Professor Emeritus
Department of Radiology and Medical Imaging
University of Virginia Health System
Charlottesville, Virginia

NANCY M. MAJOR, MD
Professor of Radiology and Orthopedics
University of Colorado School of Medicine
Aurora, Colorado

ELSEVIER

ELSEVIER

3251 Riverport Lane
St. Louis, Missouri 63043

FUNDAMENTALS OF BODY CT, FIFTH EDITION   ISBN: 978-0-323-60832-9

Notices

Practitioners and researchers must always rely on their own experience and knowledge in evaluating and using any information, methods, compounds or experiments described herein. Because of rapid advances in the medical sciences, in particular, independent verification of diagnoses and drug dosages should be made. To the fullest extent of the law, no responsibility is assumed by Elsevier, authors, editors or contributors for any injury and/or damage to persons or property as a matter of products liability, negligence or otherwise, or from any use or operation of any methods, products, instructions, or ideas contained in the material herein.

Library of Congress Control Number: 2018964895

Content Strategist: Russell Gabbedy
Content Development Specialist: Angie Breckon
Content Development Manager: Kathryn DeFrancesco
Publishing Services Manager: Shereen Jameel
Senior Project Manager: Umarani Natarajan
Design Direction: Bridget Hoette

Printed in India

Last digit is the print number: 9   8   7   6

Preface

Despite the fact that we concentrate on "fundamentals" in this book (that has always been our goal), the fundamentals keep changing and evolving, along with advances in CT techniques, our improved understanding of diseases, and changes in medical practice and disease evaluation. This new edition gives us the chance to update important topics and add new material, including a number of high-quality, state-of-the-art images.

In the chest section, this includes updates in the classification of adenocarcinoma, lung cancer screening (using lung reporting and data system; Lung-RADS), lung cancer staging, and classification and diagnosis of interstitial lung diseases using high-resolution CT.

Additions to the abdominal section include a review of the liver imaging reporting and data system (Li-RADS) for imaging and reporting small hepatocellular carcinoma, and reviews of the Atlanta classification of acute pancreatitis, the revised classification of cystic neoplasms of the pancreas, and an improved description of CT findings of histologic subtypes of renal cell carcinoma.

In the musculoskeletal (MSK) section, an emphasis has been placed on the diagnosis of abnormalities, often incidental, detected on chest and abdominal CT scans obtained for non-MSK indications.

The half-dozen or so years since the third edition was published have seen continued advances in helical CT techniques. In this edition, we review the various spiral/helical CT protocols currently used in clinical practice for the diagnosis of chest, abdominal, and musculoskeletal abnormalities, including discussions of high-resolution CT, lung nodule assessment and lung cancer screening, CT pulmonary embolism diagnosis, CT enterography, CT enteroclysis, CT colonography, and optimizing CT techniques in musculoskeletal diagnosis.

New topics, discussions of additonal diseases (too numerous to mention here), and new images have been added to all chapters, including updated descriptions and illustrations of normal anatomy and incidental findings. Disease classifications, including those for pulmonary adenocarcinoma, diffuse lung diseases, and pancreatic lesions, have been updated where appropriate.

We hope you enjoy and profit from our efforts.

W. Richard Webb
William E. Brant
Nancy M. Major

Contents

CHAPTER 1

Introduction to CT of the Thorax: Chest CT Techniques

W. RICHARD WEBB

Spiral (helical) computed tomography (CT) allows the entire chest to be imaged in a few seconds or less (i.e., during a single breath hold), with volumetric acquisition of scan data. Two- and three-dimensional reformations may be performed if desired. Because scanning is rapid, contrast agents can be injected quickly, excellent vascular opacification can be achieved, and reduced volumes of contrast agent can be used.

Multidetector CT (MDCT) scanners have multiple parallel rows of X-ray detectors (an ever-increasing number, now exceeding 250 in some scanners, and capable of reconstructing more than 500 slices at a time). With MDCT, each of the detector rows records data independently as the gantry rotates; consequently, a volume of the patient (e.g., up to 16 cm along the longitudinal axis, or z-axis, with a 256-detector scanner) is imaged with each gantry rotation. With large-area detector scanners, scanning of a volume may be performed without table motion; this is most useful for cardiac imaging. The gantry rotation time is 0.5 seconds or less.

SPIRAL CHEST CT: GENERAL PRINCIPLES

The specific protocols used for chest CT depend on the scanner used, the scanner manufacturer, and the reason for the study. However, several general principles apply to all chest scans (Table 1.1).

Scan Levels

Chest CT is usually performed from a level just above the lung apices (near the suprasternal notch) to the level of the posterior costophrenic angles; these scans also encompass the diaphragm and the upper abdomen. The distance (or volume) needed to cover the thorax (usually 25–30 cm) is determined by a preliminary projection scan (e.g., a "scout view").

Patient Position

Routinely, patients are scanned supine. Prone scans may be obtained for high-resolution CT (HRCT) or to assess movement of pleural fluid collections. The patient may also be positioned prone for biopsy of posterior lung lesions or drainage of pleural fluid collections.

Lung Volume

Scans are routinely obtained after a full inspiration (i.e., at total lung capacity) and during suspended respiration. Postexpiratory scans may be performed in some cases (particularly on HRCT) to assess air trapping.

Detector Row and Slice Thickness

Scan data are usually acquired with the thinnest detector width available on the scanner (detector rows on most scanners range from 0.25 to 0.625 mm), and the reconstructed slice thickness used for scan interpretation is determined by the indication for the scan. For example, if data are recorded with 0.625-mm detectors, slices can be reconstructed at any thickness from 0.625 to 5 mm for viewing. Thin slices are required for some specific indications, whereas thicker slices are quicker to interpret and do not occupy as much memory when they are stored.

Most chest scans are reconstructed with a 1- to 1.25-mm thickness. When one is viewing a study reconstructed with 2.5- or 5-mm-thick slices, if the scan data were collected using thinner detectors, and if the scan data are still available (they are usually preserved on the scanner disk for a day or two), you can have thinner slices reconstructed at a later time.

Usually slices are reconstructed at an interval equal to the slice thickness (e.g., 1.25 mm) to provide a volumetric data set. On occasion, scans are reconstructed at overlapping levels (e.g., 1.25-mm slices reconstructed at 0.625-mm intervals), although this is not generally necessary.

TABLE 1.1
Chest CT: General Principles

Scan levels: Lung apices to the posterior costophrenic angles

Patient position: Supine; prone scans sometimes used for diagnosis of lung disease of pleural effusions

Lung volume: Full inspiration, single breath hold; expiratory scans sometimes used to diagnose air trapping or bronchial abnormalities

Gantry rotation time 0.5 seconds or less in most instances

Scan duration: 2.5 seconds or less for the thorax, with use of multiple-detector CT and fast scanning

Detector width: Usually the thinnest detectors (e.g., 0.625 mm or less) for image acquisition

Pitch (table excursion): Depends on tolerable image noise; increased if noise is OK; decreased if there is a desire for high resolution

Reconstruction algorithm: High-resolution algorithm used for most studies; standard or soft-tissue algorithm usually used for vascular studies

Two- or three-dimensional reconstructions: Not routine; occasionally useful for lung, airway, or vascular studies

Contrast agents: Intravenous contrast agent injection in some cases; oral contrast agents only for gastrointestinal abnormalities

Pitch (Table Excursion)

The term *pitch* refers to the distance the table travels during a complete gantry rotation divided by the width of all the detectors used (e.g., table excursion/detector width × number of detector rows). With MDCT, pitch usually ranges from 1 to 2. The higher the pitch, the faster the scan, but images are generally noisier, spatial resolution is reduced somewhat, and the effective slice thickness (the thickness of the patient that is actually imaged) is increased.

Keep in mind that with the spiral technique the actual thickness of the slice you view (i.e., "effective slice thickness") may be greater than the slice thickness you select (e.g., 1.25 mm), depending on the pitch or table excursion during gantry rotation; the greater the pitch, the greater the effective slice thickness. Thus there is a trade-off; with a higher pitch, the study is quicker but the scans are not quite as good.

Scan Duration

MDCT of the chest can be easily performed during a single breath hold (2.5 seconds or less), generally avoiding respiratory motion artifacts, except in very dyspneic or uncooperative patients.

Reconstruction Algorithm

Once the scans have been performed, the scan data are reconstructed using an algorithm that determines some characteristics of the resulting image. For routine chest imaging, a *high-resolution algorithm* is often used to optimize detail, but this makes the image somewhat noisy in appearance. A standard or *soft-tissue algorithm*, which produces a smoother image, is better for assessing thoracic vascular structures (e.g., studies performed for diagnosis of pulmonary embolism, aneurysm, or aortic dissection) but is not optimal for other chest imaging. This algorithm is often used for abdominal imaging.

Two- and Three-Dimensional Reconstruction

Because the scan data are acquired continuously and volumetrically by spiral CT, scans may be reconstructed in any plane desired. A variety of display techniques have been used for imaging the thorax. These include multiplanar reconstructions, three-dimensional shaded surface display or volume rendering from an external perspective, or shaded surface or volume rendering from an internal (i.e., endoluminal) perspective, also known as *virtual bronchoscopy*.

Multiplanar, two-dimensional reconstructions offer the advantage of being quickly performed and are sufficient for diagnosis in most cases in which a reformation is considered desirable. Subsequent chapters provide a number of examples of two-dimensional reconstructions. Three-dimensional techniques, such as shaded surface display and volume rendering, can be valuable in selected cases, but they are time-consuming and require operator experience. These techniques are not commonly used in day-to-day clinical chest imaging.

Maximum- or minimum-intensity projection images representing a slab of three-dimensional data reconstructed from a volumetric data set may sometimes be useful in imaging pulmonary, airway, or vascular abnormalities.

Window Settings

For chest CT, scans must be viewed with at least three different window settings. Scans are usually viewed with a workstation having preset windows available. The presets used when one is reading chest CT scans are generally termed *lung*, *soft-tissue* (or *mediastinal*), and *bone* windows, names that also describe their primary use. These preset windows are often adjusted by the viewer during scan interpretation to optimize visibility of certain structures or abnormalities of interest.

Lung windows typically have a window mean of approximately -600 to -700 Hounsfield units (HU) and a window width of 1000 to 1500 HU. Lung windows best demonstrate lung anatomy and disease, contrasting soft-tissue structures with surrounding air-filled lung parenchyma.

Mediastinal or *soft-tissue windows* (window mean 20–40 HU; window width 450–500 HU) demonstrate soft-tissue anatomy in the mediastinum and in other areas of the thorax, allowing the differentiation of fat, fluid, tissue, calcium, and contrast-opacified vessels. This window is also of value in providing information about consolidated lung, the hila, pleural disease, and structures of the chest wall. Subsequent chapters discuss more specific uses of these two windows. In the assessment of vascular structures (e.g., for pulmonary embolism or dissection diagnosis), a wider window or higher window mean than that used for a routine mediastinal window is often selected by the radiologist to better see detail within the dense contrast column.

Bone windows typically have a window mean of approximately 300 to 500 HU and a window width of 2000 HU. They best demonstrate skeletal structures or very dense objects. This window is sometimes valuable in looking at densely opacified vascular structures.

SPIRAL CHEST CT: PROTOCOLS

In most patients, chest CT is performed with a routine protocol. This technique is designed to provide useful information about the lung, mediastinum, hila, pleura, and chest wall. It is valuable in the diagnosis of a variety of diseases and types of abnormalities. Modified CT techniques are used in specific clinical settings or to look for specific abnormalities (e.g., pulmonary embolism, aortic dissection, and diffuse lung disease). Subsequent chapters provide detailed reviews of some specific protocols.

With current scanners having a large number of detector rows (e.g., 128), protocols for evaluation of different types of thoracic abnormalities have become similar, because scanning with thin slices and with excellent contrast opacification can easily be obtained during a single breath hold regardless of why the scan is being done. A general understanding of the principles involved in obtaining CT scans for specific indications is much more important than knowing detailed specific protocols because these differ with different scanners and manufacturers, and among different institutions.

Use of Contrast Agents

Chest CT can be performed with or without the administration of an intravenous contrast agent, depending on the indication for the study. Scans obtained to rule out pulmonary metastases or to assess lung disease, generally do not require the use of contrast agent. Contrast agent should be used in patients with suspected hilar, mediastinal, or pleural abnormalities and in patients with possible vascular abnormalities. If you are unsure of the indication for the scan, the use of a contrast agent is generally appropriate.

With MDCT, injection of contrast agent at 3 to 5 mL per second, 10 to 30 seconds before scanning begins and for the duration of the scan series, provides excellent opacification of vascular structures. For routine indications, injection of contrast agent at 3 mL per second is generally sufficient. When a vascular abnormality is suspected, injection at 5 mL per second is usually used. The rate of contrast agent injection and the scan delay (the time between the start of contrast agent injection and the start of scanning) differ depending on the reason for the study.

Scanning is begun when the vessels of interest are opacified. For pulmonary embolism diagnosis, the pulmonary arteries need to be opacified; this usually requires a 10- to 15-second delay, although timing the scan to the aorta or left atrium may be beneficial. For diagnosis of aortic abnormalities, a delay of usually 20 to 30 seconds is needed. The delay differs in individual patients according to a number of factors. Timing the scan delay is usually done with a timing bolus or software available on the scanner, which shows vascular opacification during the injection, and begins scanning when contrast agent appears in the target vessel. The use of an oral contrast agent for opacification of the esophagus and gastrointestinal tract is not necessary unless a specific gastrointestinal (i.e., esophageal) abnormality is suspected.

Routine Chest CT

With an MDCT scanner, I routinely scan the chest with 0.625-mm detectors, with reconstruction of 1.25-mm slices at 1.25-mm intervals. This allows the entire thorax to be scanned in 2.5 seconds or less. Depending on the indication for the study, a high-resolution algorithm or smooth algorithm may be chosen for image reconstruction, and intravenous or oral contrast agents may be used (see earlier). Generally speaking, with the exception of vascular imaging protocols, a high-resolution reconstruction algorithm will be chosen for reconstruction of most chest CT studies. This routine protocol is used for evaluation in most patients not being assessed for a specific vascular abnormality, such as pulmonary embolism or possible aortic disease, or in patients being evaluated for a diffuse lung disease, which would require a high-resolution CT protocol.

Vascular Imaging Protocols

In some patients, chest CT is performed primarily for the diagnosis of a vascular abnormality suspected on the basis of clinical symptoms or radiographic findings. Common thoracic vascular abnormalities assessed with CT include pulmonary embolism, aortic dissection or aneurysm, and traumatic aortic rupture. Although the protocols for each indication differ among institutions and with different scanners, some general principles apply.

Vascular protocols attempt to optimize the degree of contrast enhancement of the vessels of interest and image resolution, while keeping the length of breath hold and the amount of contrast agent injected at a reasonable value. In general, a relatively smooth reconstruction algorithm is preferred for vascular imaging. Reduced image noise with smooth reconstruction makes it easier to see small filling defects (i.e., pulmonary emboli) and subtle differences in contrast enhancement.

Pulmonary Embolism

For the diagnosis of pulmonary embolism by MDCT, slices 1.25 mm thick at 1.25-mm intervals are sufficient for diagnosis, although scanning is usually performed with the thinnest detectors available (e.g., 0.625 mm). A smooth reconstruction algorithm is generally used. Intravenous contrast agent is injected rapidly (e.g., 5 mL per second). Scanning is begun when the scanner shows the pulmonary arteries or left atrium to be opacified. The delay between the start of contrast agent injection and scanning differs, but it averages about 10 to 15 seconds if pulmonary artery opacification is desired and is somewhat longer for opacification of the left atrium. In large patients, scan noise may make interpretation difficult. In such patients, reconstructing slices 2.5 mm thick may reduce noise and increase accuracy.

Aortic Disease

Aortic abnormalities assessed by CT include dissection, aneurysm, intramural hematoma, penetrating ulcer, and traumatic aortic rupture. A scan series through the thorax with relatively thick (2.5- or 5-mm) slices often precedes contrast agent injection (to look for a high-attenuation intramural hematoma; see Chapter 3). If only the thoracic aorta is being examined, scans through the thorax may be obtained with a protocol

similar to that used for pulmonary embolism diagnosis (1.25-mm slices reconstructed at 1.25-mm intervals). Intravenous contrast agent is injected rapidly (e.g., 5 mL per second), and scanning is begun when the scanner shows the left atrium or aorta to be opacified. The scan delay may range from 15 to 30 seconds, depending on the patient. If imaging of the abdominal aorta is also required (e.g., for aortic dissection), scans continue through the abdomen. Quiet breathing during the abdominal portion of the scan is usually allowed if the patient cannot hold his or her breath for the duration of the study.

High-Resolution Lung CT

HRCT is used to diagnose diffuse lung diseases, emphysema, bronchiectasis, and some focal lung lesions (e.g., a solitary nodule). HRCT requires thin slices (e.g., 0.625–1.25 mm) and image reconstruction with a sharp (high-resolution) algorithm, which reduces image smoothing and increases spatial resolution. Although use of a sharp algorithm also increases image noise, this is not usually a problem in the interpretation of lung images. Injection of contrast agent is not necessary for HRCT but may be used on occasion if pulmonary embolism is also a consideration.

Scans performed with the patient supine and prone, and following expiration, are often obtained, at least for the patient's initial examination. *Prone scans* are used to detect subtle posterior lung abnormalities; *expiratory scans* are used to detect air trapping because of airway obstruction.

HRCT can be performed in three different ways:
- *Spaced axial imaging.* Thin slices (e.g., 0.625–1.25 mm) are performed at spaced intervals (e.g., 1–2 cm) without table movement to optimize spatial resolution. Because of the spaced images, the radiation dose is reduced.
- *Volumetric HRCT* using the spiral technique, thin detectors, and 1- to 1.25-mm slice thickness reconstruction. This results in an increased radiation dose and slightly decreased resolution, but the entire thorax is imaged and two- or three-dimensional reconstruction and assessment of other abnormalities (e.g., pulmonary embolism) is also possible. If desired, the scans can be reconstructed with both a high-resolution algorithm (for diagnosis of lung abnormalities) and a smooth algorithm (for diagnosis of vascular abnormalities).
- *Combined volumetric and axial imaging.* In some patients, volumetric imaging is obtained for supine scans, with spaced axial imaging for prone and expiratory images. This optimizes the volume imaged, but with a reduced radiation dose.

Dynamic CT Techniques

The term *dynamic CT* means that a number of scans are performed in sequence. Because spiral scanning is continuous, it is a dynamic technique, but dynamic scanning can also be performed without a spiral technique (i.e., without table and patient motion during the acquisition of scans). Dynamic scanning may be performed at a single level during expiration to detect air trapping or to assess tracheal or bronchial collapse in patients with tracheomalacia or airway disease. Dynamic scanning may also be performed to assess some vascular abnormalities.

Low-Dose CT

Reducing the radiation dose is desirable whenever possible, but generally results in decreased image quality because of increased noise. The term *low-dose CT* usually implies the use of a reduced tube current (milliamperes) during the scan. Low-dose chest CT is usually used in children, for screening of patients (i.e., lung cancer screening), or if multiple follow-up examinations will be necessary in a given patient.

With current MDCT scanners, the tube current can be varied or *modulated* at different levels as the patient is scanned on the basis of the chest wall thickness or amount of soft tissue within the volume being scanned. Because the lungs are not very dense, not as much radiation is needed when the lungs (instead of the shoulders or liver) are being scanned. This technique can significantly reduce the tube current and patient dose, without much loss in scan quality, and is usually used for routine studies. A fixed, higher tube current is sometimes used when high resolution and detail is needed. *Iterative reconstruction* is another technique commonly used to reduce the radiation dose.

RADIATION DOSE WITH CHEST CT

Although the patient risk from radiation exposure during diagnostic CT is small and difficult to determine, medical radiation does result in a finite risk. In clinical practice the patient's potential benefits from a CT study need to be balanced against the small radiation risk. In general, if the study has well-defined clinical utility, it is indicated. Nonetheless, it is important for the radiologist to reduce radiation exposure during diagnostic CT, as long as important diagnostic information is not compromised as a result.

Radiation dose and the associated risk to the patient can be calculated by different methods and measurements, none of which are ideal or necessarily predictive

TABLE 1.2
Radiation Dose for Chest CT Protocols

	Radiation Dose (mSv)
Normal yearly background radiation	2.5–3.2
Chest radiograph (single view)	0.05
Routine chest CT (300 mA)	5–7
Routine chest CT (modulated tube current approximately 100–150 mA)	1.5–2
High-resolution CT with volumetric imaging (supine, expiratory; modulated tube current of approximately 100–150 mA)	1.5–2
High-resolution CT with spaced axial images (supine, prone, expiratory)	1
Low-dose volumetric CT (40 mA)	<0.5–1

of outcome. The calculation most typically used is effective dose (measured in sieverts or more typically millisieverts), which is determined by summing the absorbed doses to individual organs weighted for their radiation sensitivity. However, because an accurate measurement of all organ doses is difficult to obtain during a clinical examination, as are the risk coefficients specific to age, sex, and the organ being irradiated, the estimated dose is calculated for an idealized 70-kg, 30-year-old patient. Although limited in accuracy and predictive value, the effective dose expressed in millisieverts is the most widely used method for quantification of the radiation dose and comparison of radiologic procedures. Approximate doses for background radiation and thoracic imaging procedures are listed in Table 1.2.

SUGGESTED READING

Bankier, A. A., & Tack, D. (2010). Dose reduction strategies for thoracic multidetector computed tomography: Background, current Issues, and recommendations. *Journal of Thoracic Imaging, 25*, 278–288.

Boiselle, P. M., Hurwitz, L. M., Mayo, J. R., et al. (2011). Expert opinion: Radiation dose management in cardiopulmonary imaging. *Journal of Thoracic Imaging, 26*, 3.

Lawler, L. P., & Fishman, E. K. (2001). Multi-detector row CT of thoracic disease with emphasis on 3D volume rendering and CT angiography. *Radiographics, 21*, 1257–1273.

Lee, C. H., Goo, J. M., Lee, H. J., et al. (2008). Radiation dose modulation techniques in the multidetector CT era: From basics to practice. *Radiographics, 28*, 1451–1459.

Mayo, J. R. (2009). CT evaluation of diffuse infiltrative lung disease: Dose considerations and optimal technique. *Journal of Thoracic Imaging, 24*, 252–259.

CHAPTER 2

Mediastinum: Introduction and Normal Anatomy

W. RICHARD WEBB

Computed tomography (CT) is commonly used in patients suspected of having a mediastinal mass or vascular abnormality (e.g., an aortic aneurysm). In general, CT is performed in two situations.

First, in patients with a mediastinal abnormality visible on plain radiographs, CT is almost always the preferred imaging procedure. CT is used to confirm the presence of a significant lesion, determine its location and relationship to vascular or nonvascular structures, and characterize the mass as solid, cystic, vascular, enhancing, calcified, inhomogeneous, or fatty.

Second, CT is often used in patients in whom there is clinical suspicion of mediastinal disease, regardless of plain radiograph findings. As an example, patients with lung cancer often have mediastinal lymph node enlargement (i.e., metastases) visible on CT when chest radiographs are normal.

NORMAL MEDIASTINAL ANATOMY

The *mediastinum* is the compartment situated between the lungs, marginated on each side by the mediastinal pleura, anteriorly by the sternum and chest wall, and posteriorly by the spine and chest wall. It contains the heart, great vessels, trachea, esophagus, thymus, considerable fat, and a number of lymph nodes. Many of these structures can be reliably identified on CT by their location, appearance, and attenuation.

For the purpose of CT interpretation, the mediastinum can be thought of as consisting of three almost equal divisions along the longitudinal axis of the patient, the first beginning at the thoracic inlet and the third ending at the diaphragm. In adults, each of these divisions is about 7 to 8 cm long and is thus made up of about 15 contiguous 5-mm slices. These can be remembered as follows:
- the *supra-aortic mediastinum*: from the thoracic inlet to the top of the aortic arch;
- the *subaortic mediastinum*: from the aortic arch to the superior aspect of the heart;
- the *paracardiac mediastinum*: from the heart to the diaphragm.

In each of these compartments, specific structures are consistently seen and need to be evaluated in every patient. The following description of normal anatomy is not comprehensive but is limited to the most important mediastinal structures.

Supra-Aortic Mediastinum

When one is evaluating a CT scan of this part of the mediastinum, it is a good idea to localize the *trachea* before doing anything else (Fig. 2.1A). The trachea is easy to recognize because it contains air, is seen in cross section, and has a reasonably consistent round or oval shape. It is relatively central in the mediastinum, from front to back and from right to left, and it serves as an excellent reference point. Many other mediastinal structures maintain a consistent relation to it.

At or near the thoracic inlet, the mediastinum is relatively narrow from front to back. The *esophagus* lies posterior to the trachea at this level (Fig. 2.1), but depending on the position of the trachea relative to the spine, the esophagus can be displaced to one side or the other, usually to the left. It is usually collapsed and appears as a flattened structure of soft-tissue attenuation, but small amounts of air or air and fluid are often seen in its lumen.

In the supra-aortic mediastinum, the great arterial branches of the aortic arch and the great veins are the most recognizable structures. At or near the thoracic inlet, the *brachiocephalic veins* are the most anterior and lateral vascular branches visible, lying immediately behind the clavicular heads (Fig. 2.1A and B). Although they differ in size, their positions are relatively constant. The great arterial branches (innominate, left carotid, and left subclavian arteries) are posterior to the veins and lie adjacent to the anterior and lateral walls of the trachea. They can be reliably identified by their relative positions, but variations are common.

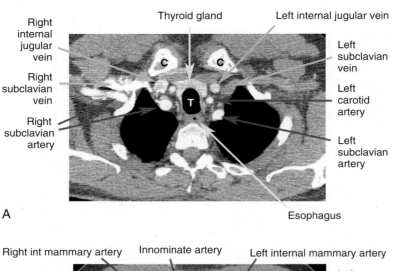

Right internal jugular vein

Thyroid gland

Left internal jugular vein

Left subclavian vein

Right subclavian vein

Left carotid artery

Right subclavian artery

Left subclavian artery

A

Esophagus

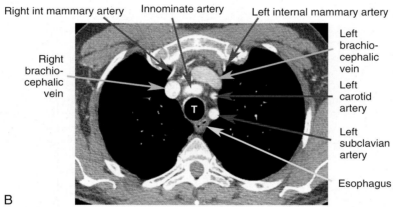

Right int mammary artery

Innominate artery

Left internal mammary artery

Right brachio-cephalic vein

Left brachio-cephalic vein

Left carotid artery

Left subclavian artery

B

Esophagus

FIG. 2.1 **Supra-aortic mediastinum.** Contrast-enhanced CT with 1.25-mm slices. (A) Near the thoracic inlet, the trachea *(T)* is clearly seen, with the air-filled esophagus posterior and slightly to the left of it. The right and left subclavian and internal jugular veins are anterior and lateral and can be seen behind the clavicular heads *(C)* and clavicles. The great arterial branches (right carotid, right subclavian, left carotid, and left subclavian arteries) are visible on each side of the trachea. The thyroid gland is anterior and lateral to the trachea. Because of its iodine content, it appears denser than other soft tissue. (B) Just below (A) the brachiocephalic veins are visible anteriorly. The large arterial branches of the aorta lie posterior to the left brachiocephalic vein. The left subclavian artery is most posterior and is situated lateral to the left tracheal wall, at the three or four o'clock position relative to the tracheal lumen and contacting the mediastinal pleura. The left carotid artery is anterior to the left subclavian artery, at about the two o'clock position, and is somewhat variable in position. The innominate artery is usually anterior and slightly to the right of the tracheal midline. The internal *(int)* mammary arteries are visible bilaterally. (C) At a level below (B) the left *(Lt)* brachiocephalic vein is visible crossing the mediastinum from left to right. The subclavian, carotid, and innominate arteries maintain the same relative positions as in (B). The right *(Rt)* internal mammary *(mamm)* vein is visible arising from the right brachiocephalic vein. The densely opacified internal mammary *(int mamm)* arteries are visible bilaterally, lateral to the internal mammary veins. The esophagus contains a small amount of air in its lumen. (D) At a level below (C) the left brachiocephalic vein joins the right brachiocephalic vein, forming the superior vena cava. The major aortic branches are again clearly seen. The fat-filled pretracheal space is anterior to the trachea and posterior and medial to the arteries and veins. (E) The supra-aortic anatomy near the level of (D). The location of the pretracheal lymph nodes is shown, although these are not visible in (D). The location of the thymic remnant, although not seen well in (D), is also indicated. The approximate level of the scan in (D) is indicated by horizontal lines.

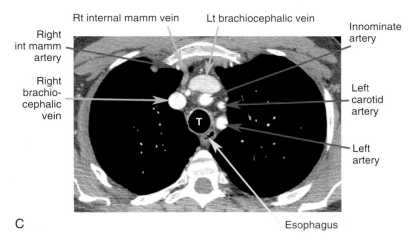

C

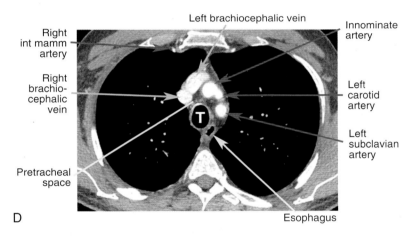

D

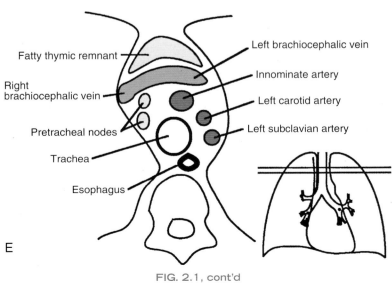

E

FIG. 2.1, cont'd

Below the thoracic inlet, anterior to the arterial branches of the aorta, the left brachiocephalic vein crosses the mediastinum from left to right (Fig. 2.1C) to join the right brachiocephalic vein, thus forming the *superior vena cava* (Fig. 2.1C–E). The *left subclavian artery* is most posterior and is situated adjacent to the left side of the trachea, at the three or four o'clock position relative to the tracheal lumen. The *left carotid artery* is anterior to the left subclavian artery, at the one or two o'clock position, and is somewhat variable in position. The *innominate artery* is usually anterior and somewhat to the right of the tracheal midline (11 or 12 o'clock position), but it is the most variable of all the great vessels and can have a number of different appearances in various patients or in the same patient at different levels.

Near its origin from the aortic arch, the innominate artery is usually oval and is somewhat larger than the other aortic branches. As it ascends toward the thoracic outlet, it may appear oval or elliptic because of its orientation or because of its bifurcation into the right subclavian and carotid arteries. This vessel can also be quite tortuous and can appear double if both limbs of a U-shaped part of the vessel are imaged in the same slice. Usually these vessels can be traced from their origin at the aortic arch to the point where they leave the chest, if there is any doubt as to what they represent.

Other than the great vessels, trachea, and esophagus, little is usually seen in the supra-aortic mediastinum. A few lymph nodes are normally visible. Small vascular branches, particularly the *internal mammary veins*, can be seen in this part of the mediastinum. In some patients the *thyroid gland* may extend into this portion of the mediastinum, and the right and left thyroid lobes may be visible on each side of the trachea. This appearance is not abnormal and does not imply thyroid enlargement. On CT the thyroid can be distinguished from other tissues or masses because its attenuation is greater than that of soft tissue (because of its iodine content). The *thymus* is sometime visible at this level anterior to the large vessels described earlier, within the *prevascular space* (described further later).

Subaortic Mediastinum

The subaortic mediastinum extends inferiorly from the top of the aortic arch to the upper portion of the heart (Fig. 2.2). Whereas the supra-aortic region largely contains arterial and venous branches of the aorta and vena cava, this compartment contains many of the undivided mediastinal great vessels (the aorta, superior vena cava, and pulmonary arteries). This compartment also contains most of the important mediastinal lymph node groups. A few key levels in this part of the mediastinum will be discussed in detail.

Aortic Arch Level

In the upper portion of the subaortic mediastinum, the *aortic arch* is easily seen and has a characteristic but somewhat variable appearance (Fig. 2.2A). The aortic arch is seen anterior and to the left of the trachea, with the posterior arch lying anterior and lateral to the spine. Usually the aortic arch is about the same diameter in its anterior and mid portions, although the posterior arch is typically somewhat smaller. The position of the anterior and posterior aspects of the arch can vary in the presence of atherosclerosis and aortic tortuosity; in patients with a tortuous aorta, the anterior arch is displaced to the right, whereas the posterior aortic arch is displaced laterally and posteriorly, to a position to the left of the spine.

At this level the *superior vena cava* is visible anterior and to the right of the trachea and is usually oval (Fig. 2.2A–C). The *esophagus* appears the same as at higher levels and is variable in position. It is posterior to the trachea and often lies to the left of the tracheal midline.

A somewhat triangular region, with the apex of the triangle directed anteriorly, marginated by the aortic arch on the left, the superior vena cava and mediastinal pleura on the right, and the trachea posteriorly, represents the *pretracheal* or *anterior paratracheal* space (Fig. 2.2A and C). This fat-filled space is important because it contains middle mediastinal lymph nodes in the paratracheal chain, which are commonly involved in various lymph node diseases. Whenever the mediastinum is being viewed for diagnosis of lymphadenopathy, you should look here first. Other mediastinal node groups are closely related pretracheal nodes, both spatially and in regard to lymphatic drainage. It is not uncommon to see a few normal-sized lymph nodes (short-axis or least diameter less than 1 cm) in the pretracheal space (see the review of mediastinal lymphadenopathy in Chapter 4 for a detailed discussion of this topic).

Anterior to the great vessels (aorta and superior vena cava) is another roughly triangular space called the *prevascular space* (Fig. 2.2A–C). This compartment constitutes part of the anterior mediastinum and primarily contains the thymus, lymph nodes, and fat. The apex of this triangular space represents the anterior junction line, which is sometimes visible on chest radiographs.

In young patients (generally up to 30 years of age), CT shows the *thymus* to be of soft-tissue attenuation and bilobed or arrowhead shaped, with each of the

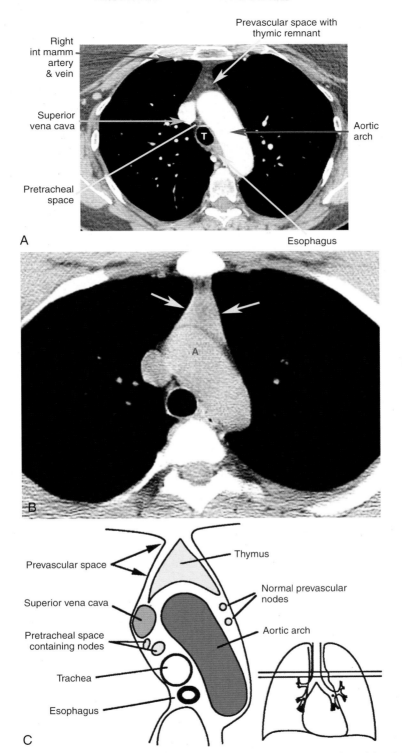

FIG. 2.2 Subaortic mediastinum. Contrast-enhanced CT with 1.25-mm slices. At the aortic arch level, (A) the aortic arch extends from a position anterior to the trachea *(T)* to the left, with the posterior part of the arch usually lying anterior and lateral to the spine. The superior vena cava contacts the right mediastinal pleura and together with the aortic arch delineates the pretracheal space. The prevascular space is anterior to the great vessels and contains the thymus, which is largely replaced by fat in this patient. (B) In a 21-year-old patient a large normal thymus with soft-tissue attenuation *(arrows)* occupies most of the prevascular space. It is separated from the aortic arch *(A)* by a fat plane. (C) The mediastinal anatomy at the aortic arch level.

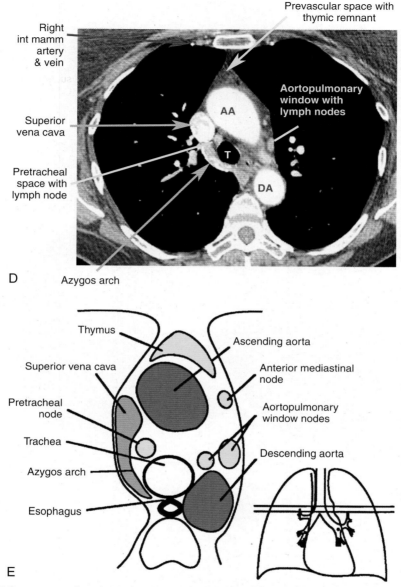

Right
int mamm
artery
& vein

Prevascular space with
thymic remnant

AA

Aortopulmonary
window with
lymph nodes

Superior
vena cava

T

Pretracheal
space with
lymph node

DA

D   Azygos arch

Thymus

Ascending aorta

Superior vena cava

Anterior mediastinal
node

Pretracheal
node

Aortopulmonary
window nodes

Trachea

Azygos arch

Descending aorta

Esophagus

E

FIG. 2.2, cont'd At the azygos arch and aortopulmonary window level, (D) the azygos arch is usually visible arising from the posterior aspect of the superior vena cava, contacting the right mediastinal pleura, and forming the lateral margin of the node bearing pretracheal space. Fat visible under the aortic arch but above the pulmonary artery is in the aortopulmonary window, which also contains lymph nodes. (E) The mediastinal anatomy at the azygos arch and aortopulmonary window level.

two lobes (right and left) contacting the mediastinal pleura and occupying most of the prevascular space. Each lobe is usually 1 to 2 cm thick (measured perpendicular to the pleura), but this differs (Fig. 2.2B). In later adulthood the thymus involutes, with soft tissue being replaced by fat. In patients older than 30 years the prevascular space appears fat filled, with thin wisps of tissue passing through the fat. Most of this, including the fat, represents the thymus. At higher levels the thymus is sometimes visible anterior to the brachiocephalic arteries and veins, also within the prevascular space.

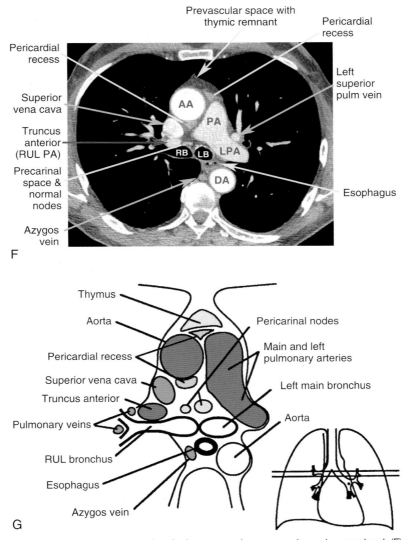

FIG. 2.2, cont'd At the main pulmonary artery, subcarinal space, and azygoesophageal recess level, (F) at the tracheal carina, the right main bronchus *(RB)* and left main bronchus *(LB)* are visible as separate branches. The main pulmonary artery *(PA)* is contiguous with the left pulmonary artery *(LPA)* more posteriorly. The truncus anterior (pulmonary artery supplying most of the right upper lobe, *RUL*) is visible as an oval structure anterior to the right main bronchus. Normal pericardial recesses containing fluid are visible posterior to the ascending aorta *(AA)* and between the anterior aorta and the main pulmonary artery. These are relatively low in attenuation and should not be confused with abnormal lymph nodes. The precarinal space containing lymph nodes is contiguous with the pretracheal space. (G) The mediastinal anatomy at this level.

Continued

Azygos Arch and Aortopulmonary Window Level

At a level slightly below the aortic arch, the ascending aorta and descending aorta are visible as separate structures. Characteristically the ascending aorta (25–35 mm in diameter) is slightly larger than the descending aorta (20–30 mm).

On the right side, the arch of the *azygos vein* (*azygos* means *unpaired*) arises from the posterior wall of the superior vena cava, passes over the right main bronchus (thus it is seen at a higher level than the bronchus itself), and continues posteriorly along the mediastinum, to lie to the right of and anterior to the spine (Fig. 2.2D and E). Below the level of the azygos arch,

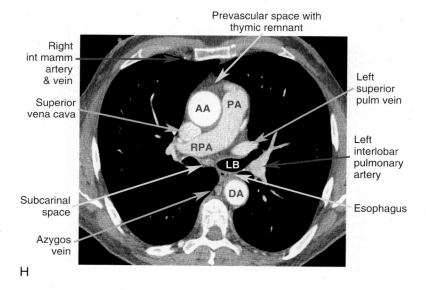

Prevascular space with
thymic remnant

Right
int mamm
artery
& vein

Superior
vena cava

Subcarinal
space

Azygos
vein

AA PA

RPA

LB

DA

Left
superior
pulm vein

Left
interlobar
pulmonary
artery

Esophagus

H

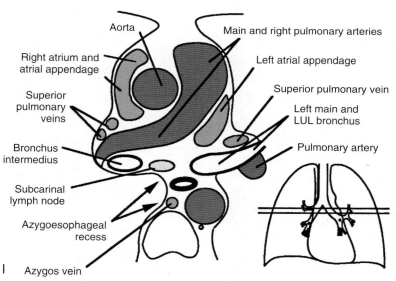

Aorta

Right atrium and
atrial appendage

Superior
pulmonary
veins

Bronchus
intermedius

Subcarinal
lymph node

Azygoesophageal
recess

Main and right pulmonary arteries

Left atrial appendage

Superior pulmonary vein

Left main and
LUL bronchus

Pulmonary artery

I   Azygos vein

FIG. 2.2, cont'd (H) Scan and (I) diagram below the tracheal carina, at the level of the right pulmonary artery and azygoe-sophageal recess. The right pulmonary artery (RPA) is visible crossing the mediastinum, filling the pretracheal and precarinal space. A small amount of fat and a normal lymph node are visible in the subcarinal space, slightly anterior to the esophagus, azygos vein, and azygoesophageal recess. The recess appears concave laterally, with the mediastinal pleura closely related to the azygos vein and esophagus. AA, Ascending aorta; DA, descending aorta; int mamm, internal mammary; LB, left bron-chus; LUL, left upper lobe; PA, pulmonary artery; pulm, pulmonary; RUL, right upper lobe; T, trachea.

the azygos vein remains visible in this position. The azygos arch is often visible on one or two adjacent slices and sometimes appears nodular. However, its characteristic location is usually sufficient to correctly identify this structure. When the azygos arch is visible, it marginates the right border of the pretracheal space.

On the left side of the mediastinum, under the aor-tic arch but above the main pulmonary artery, is the region termed the *aortopulmonary* (or *aorticopulmo-nary*) *window*. The aortopulmonary window contains fat, lymph nodes (middle mediastinal), the recur-rent laryngeal nerve, and the ligamentum arteriosum (the latter two are usually invisible, although a calcified ligamentum is sometimes seen; Fig. 2.2D and E). *Aortopulmonary window lymph nodes* freely communicate with those in the pretracheal space, and it may be difficult to distinguish nodes in the medial aortopulmonary window from those in the left part of the pretracheal space. In some patients the aortopulmonary window is not clearly visible, with the main pulmonary artery lying immediately below the aortic arch. In such patients it is difficult to distinguish lymph nodes from volume averaging of the adjacent aorta and pulmonary artery, unless thin slices are obtained.

Main Pulmonary Arteries, Subcarinal Space, and Azygoesophageal Recess Level

At or slightly below the aortopulmonary window, at the level the *ascending aorta* is first seen in cross section (i.e., it is round or nearly round), a portion of the pericardium, usually containing a small amount of pericardial fluid, extends up from below into the pretracheal space, lying immediately behind the ascending aorta. This is termed the *superior pericardial recess* (Fig. 2.2F and G). Although it can sometimes be confused with a lymph node, its typical location, immediately behind and hugging the aortic wall, its oval or crescentic shape, and its relatively low (water) attenuation allow it to be distinguished from a significant abnormality. Another part of the pericardial recess can sometimes be seen anterior to the ascending aorta and pulmonary artery (Fig. 2.2F and G).

At or near this level the trachea bifurcates into the right and left main bronchi. The *carina* itself is usually visible on CT (Fig. 2.2F).

Below the level of the carina and azygos arch (Fig. 2.2F–I), the medial aspect of the right lung tucks into the posterior portion of the middle mediastinum, adjacent to the azygos vein and esophagus. This part of the mediastinum, reasonably termed the *azygoesophageal recess*, is important because of its close relationship to the esophagus, the main bronchi, and the subcarinal space containing lymph nodes. The azygoesophageal recess appears concave laterally in most normal individuals. A convexity in this region may be attributed to the esophagus, azygos vein, enlarged lymph nodes, or a mass.

In many people, the azygoesophageal recess is somewhat posterior to the node-bearing *subcarinal space*, which lies between the main bronchi. Normal nodes are commonly visible in this space, because they are larger than normal nodes in other parts of the mediastinum and up to 1.5 cm in short-axis diameter. The esophagus is usually seen immediately behind the subcarinal space, and distinguishing nodes and the esophagus may be difficult unless the esophagus contains air or contrast material, or its course can be traced on adjacent slices. At levels below the subcarinal space, the appearance of the azygoesophageal recess is relatively constant, although it narrows in the retrocardiac region.

Also at or near this level the *main pulmonary artery* divides into its right and left branches. The *left pulmonary artery* (Fig. 2.2F–I) is somewhat higher than the right, usually seen 1 cm above it, and appears to be the continuation of the main pulmonary artery, directed posterolaterally and to the left. The *right pulmonary artery* arises at an angle of nearly 90 degrees to the main and left pulmonary arteries and crosses the mediastinum, anterior to the carina or the main bronchi. In this location the right pulmonary artery effectively fills in the pretracheal space. At the point the main bronchi and pulmonary arteries exit the mediastinum, the pulmonary hila are visible (see Chapter 5).

Paracardiac Mediastinum

On progression caudally through the mediastinum, the origins of the great vessels from the cardiac chambers can be seen to a variable degree. Although CT is not commonly used to diagnose cardiac abnormalities (echocardiography or magnetic resonance imaging is usually preferred), a simple understanding of cardiac anatomy on CT can be helpful in diagnosis, and its use is increasing with gated multidetector techniques.

The *main pulmonary artery* or pulmonary outflow tract is most anterior and is continuous with the right ventricle, which can be seen at lower levels as anterior and to the right of the ascending aorta or left ventricle (Fig. 2-3A–C). The superior vena cava joins the right atrium, which is elliptic or crescentic. The *right atrial appendage* extends anteriorly from the upper atrium, bordering the right mediastinal pleura.

Between the right atrium and the main pulmonary artery or pulmonary outflow tract, the *aortic root* enters the left ventricle. At this level it is common in adults to see some coronary artery calcification (Fig. 2.3A–C), and often, uncalcified *coronary arteries* (left main coronary artery, left anterior descending coronary artery, circumflex coronary artery, and right coronary artery) are visible surrounded by mediastinal fat. Coronary artery anatomy is discussed further in Chapter 3.

The *left atrium* is posteriorly located, usually appearing larger than the right. The *left atrial appendage* extends anteriorly and to the left and is visible below the left pulmonary artery, bordering the pleura. On each side the *superior and inferior pulmonary veins* can be seen entering the left atrium (Fig. 2.3A–E; see Chapter 5 for further discussion).

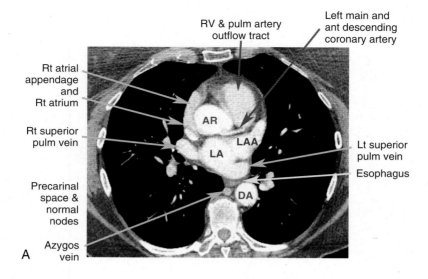

Rt atrial appendage and Rt atrium

RV & pulm artery outflow tract

Left main and ant descending coronary artery

Rt superior pulm vein

Lt superior pulm vein

Esophagus

Precarinal space & normal nodes

Azygos vein

AR

LAA

LA

DA

A

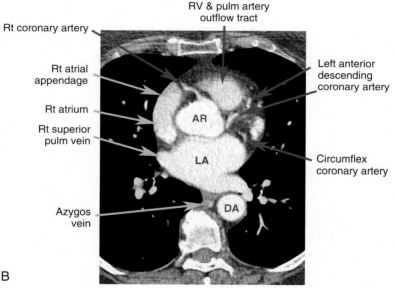

Rt coronary artery

RV & pulm artery outflow tract

Rt atrial appendage

Left anterior descending coronary artery

Rt atrium

Rt superior pulm vein

AR

LA

Circumflex coronary artery

Azygos vein

DA

B

FIG. 2.3 Paracardiac mediastinum. Contrast-enhanced 1.25-mm-slice spiral CT. (A) Most cephalad, the origins of the aorta and pulmonary artery are visible, with the aortic root *(AR)* in a central position. The right ventricular *(RV)* or pulmonary *(pulm)* outflow tract or main pulmonary artery is anterior and to the left of the aortic root at this level. The right atrium, with its appendage extending anteriorly, borders the right mediastinal pleura. The superior pulmonary veins usually enter the upper aspect of the left atrium *(LA)* at this level. The left atrial appendage *(LAA)* is also seen. The origin of the left main coronary artery (which is short) is visible at this level and is continuous with the anterior *(ant)* descending coronary artery. (B) A slice slightly below (A) showing the origin of the right coronary artery and the left anterior descending and circumflex branches of the left coronary artery.

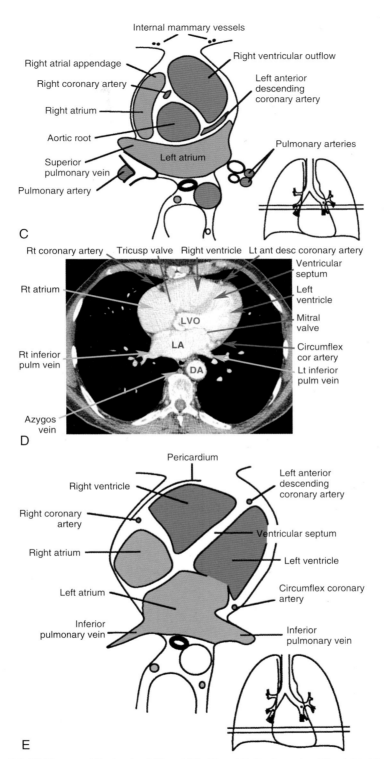

C

D

E

FIG. 2.3, cont'd (C) Diagram at the levels of (A) and (B). (D and E) At a lower level the right atrium, left atrium *(LA)*, and right and left ventricles are visible. The right ventricle is located anterior and to the right of the left ventricle. The ventricular septum and left ventricular walls are thicker than the right ventricular wall. The locations of the tricuspid *(tricusp)* and mitral valves can be identified. The left ventricular outflow *(LVO)* is visible on the scan.

Continued

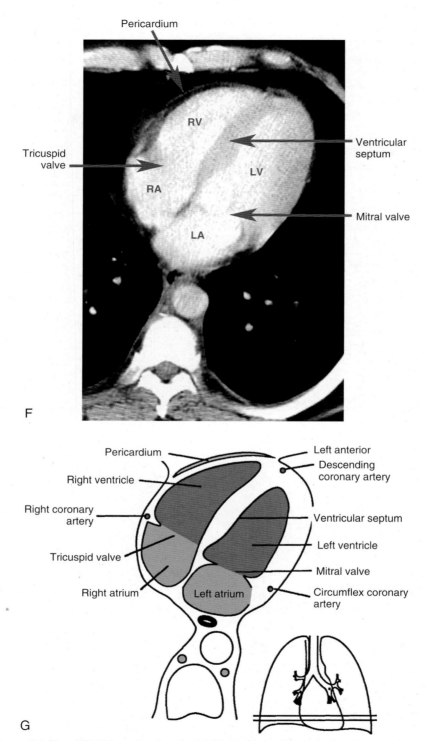

FIG. 2.3, cont'd (F and G) All four chambers are visible at this level, and the locations of the tricuspid and mitral valves can be identified. The interventricular septum and free wall of the left ventricle *(LV)* are considerably thicker than the wall of the right ventricle *(RV)*. The pericardium is visible as a thin white line surrounded by mediastinal fat. It should appear to be 1 to 2 mm thick.

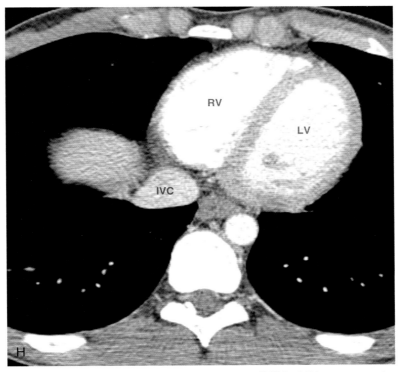

FIG. 2.3, cont'd (H) Near the diaphragm, the inferior vena cava *(IVC)* is visible as a separate structure, below the level of the right atrium. The right ventricle *(RV)* and the left ventricle *(LV)* remain visible. *ant,* Anterior; *cor,* coronary; *DA,* descending aorta; *desc,* descending; *LA,* left atrium; *Lt,* left; *pulm,* pulmonary; *RA,* right atrium; *Rt,* right; *RV,* right ventricular.

Near the level of the *diaphragm,* the *inferior vena cava* is visible as an oval structure extending caudad from the posterior right atrium (Fig. 2.3H) and is easily identifiable.

The only other structures of consequence at this level that need to be mentioned are the esophagus, which lies in a retrocardiac location; the azygos vein, which is often still visible in the same relative position as at higher levels, and the hemiazygos vein, which is usually smaller than the azygos vein and on the opposite side, behind the descending aorta. Paravertebral nodes lie in association with the azygos and hemiazygos veins but are not normally visible.

NORMAL CARDIAC ANATOMY

Without injection of contrast material, little cardiac anatomy is discernible on CT, but some differentiation of cardiac chambers is possible because of the presence of epicardial fat collections. With contrast enhancement, additional features of cardiac anatomy are visible.

The myocardium opacifies following contrast material infusion, but is often visible as a relatively low-attenuation band relative to the denser blood within the cardiac chambers. The interventricular septum is typically oriented at an angle at about the two o'clock position relative to the vertical and is convex anteriorly because of the greater left ventricular pressure (Fig. 2.3F–H). The lateral or "free" left ventricular wall is about three times thicker (approximately 1 cm thick) than the right ventricular wall (<4 mm thick).

Cardiac anatomy is easiest to understand if a scan near the cardiac apex (and diaphragm) is first considered. At this level the *left ventricle* is elliptic, with its long axis directed laterally and anteriorly (Fig. 2.3F–H). As the highest-pressure chamber, it dominates cardiac anatomy, and the other cardiac chambers mold themselves to its shape. The *right ventricle,* which is anterior and to the right, is more triangular, with the ventricular septum bowing toward it. On scans at this level or slightly above, the plane of the interventricular septum, if continued posteriorly and to the right, separates the lower *right atrium* anteriorly and laterally (and in contiguity with the right ventricle) from the lower *left atrium* posteriorly. The *mitral and tricuspid valves* are located at or near this level and can be seen if there is good contrast opacification of the cardiac chambers.

At higher levels (Fig. 2.3A–D) the *left ventricular outflow tract* and *aortic valve* are centrally located within the heart. The right ventricular outflow tract is directed toward the left and is visible anterior or to the left of the left ventricular outflow tract. That is, because of twisting of the heart during development, the left ventricular outflow tract is directed rightward and the right ventricular outflow tract is directed leftward. This accounts for the location of the aorta on the right and the pulmonary artery on the left. The aortic and pulmonic valves are located near this level and are sometimes visible in normal individuals.

THE PERICARDIUM

The normal *pericardium* (the visceral and parietal pericardium and pericardial contents) is visible as a 1- to 2-mm stripe of soft-tissue attenuation parallel to the heart and outlined by mediastinal fat (outside the pericardial sac) and epicardial fat. It is best seen near the diaphragm, along the anterior and lateral aspects of the heart, where the fat layers are thickest (Fig. 2.3F and G). As stated earlier, extensions of the pericardium into the upper mediastinum can also be seen in healthy persons.

THE RETROSTERNAL SPACE

In a retrosternal location the *internal mammary arteries and veins* are normally visible 1 or 2 cm lateral to the edge of the sternum on good CT scans (Fig. 2.2H); up to three vessels can be seen on each side (one artery and two veins). These vessels are not of much diagnostic significance, although the veins are commonly enlarged in patients with superior vena cava obstruction, but they are important because they serve to localize the *internal mammary lymph nodes.* Although normal nodes can be seen in several areas of the mediastinum (most notably the pretracheal space, aortopulmonary window, and subcarinal space), normal internal mammary nodes are not large enough to be recognized. A lymph node in this region that is large enough to be visible should be regarded as abnormal. Internal mammary node enlargement is most common in patients with breast cancer or lymphoma.

SUGGESTED READING

Aronberg, D. J., Peterson, R. R., Glazer, H. S., & Sagel, S. S. (1984). The superior sinus of the pericardium: CT appearance. *Radiology, 153,* 489–492.

Francis, I., Glazer, G. M., Bookstein, F. L., & Gross, B. H. (1985). The thymus: Reexamination of age-related changes in size and shape. *AJR American Journal of Roentgenology, 145,* 249–254.

Glazer, H. S., Aronberg, D. J., & Sagel, S. S. (1985). Pitfalls in CT recognition of mediastinal lymphadenopathy. *AJR American Journal of Roentgenology, 144,* 267–274.

Kiyono, K., Sone, S., Sakai, F., et al. (1988). The number and size of normal mediastinal lymph nodes: A postmortem study. *AJR American Journal of Roentgenology, 150,* 771–776.

Müller, N. L., Webb, W. R., & Gamsu, G. (1985). Paratracheal lymphadenopathy: Radiographic findings and correlation with CT. *Radiology, 156,* 761–765.

Müller, N. L., Webb, W. R., & Gamsu, G. (1985). Subcarinal lymph node enlargement: Radiographic findings and CT correlation. *AJR American Journal of Roentgenology, 145,* 15–19.

O'Brien, J. P., Srichai, M. B., Hecht, E. M., et al. (2007). Anatomy of the heart at multidetector CT: What the radiologist needs to know. *Radiographics, 27,* 1569–1582.

Tecce, P. M., Fishman, E. K., & Kuhlman, J. E. (1994). CT evaluation of the anterior mediastinum: Spectrum of disease. *Radiographics, 14,* 973–990.

Zylak, C. J., Pallie, W., Pirani, M., et al. (1983). Anatomy and computed tomography: A correlative module on the cervicothoracic junction. *Radiographics, 3,* 478–530.

CHAPTER 3

Mediastinum: Vascular Abnormalities and Pulmonary Embolism

W. RICHARD WEBB

AORTIC ABNORMALITIES

Computed tomography (CT) is commonly used to diagnose abnormalities of the aorta or its branches when they are suspected clinically or because of radiographic abnormalities.

Congenital Anomalies

Congenital abnormalities of the aorta and its branches are readily diagnosed with CT, and no other study is usually needed unless the anomaly is complex or is associated with congenital heart disease.

Aberrant Right Subclavian Artery

Aberrant right subclavian artery is a relatively common anomaly (1 in 100 patients). It does not usually produce a recognizable abnormality on chest radiographs and is usually detected incidentally on CT.

In patients with this anomaly the aortic arch is often higher than normal. The aberrant right subclavian artery arises from the medial wall of the descending aorta, as its last branch (Fig. 3.1), passes to the right, behind the esophagus, and ascends on the right toward the thoracic inlet. It lies more posteriorly than is normal for the subclavian artery, often anterolateral to the spine. At its point of origin the artery may be dilated, or, thinking of it in a more complicated way, the artery may arise from an *aortic diverticulum* (termed *diverticulum of Kommerell*). This may cause compression of the esophagus and symptoms of dysphagia. In some patients the diverticulum or the anomalous artery becomes aneurysmal (Fig. 3.2).

Right Aortic Arch

There are two primary types of right aortic arch: right arch associated with aberrant left subclavian artery and mirror-image right arch. *Right arch with an aberrant left subclavian artery* is most common and is present in about 1 in 1000 people. It is the reverse of a left arch with an aberrant right subclavian artery (Fig. 3.3). However,

an associated aortic diverticulum is more common in the presence of a right arch. With this anomaly, there is a low frequency (5%–10%) of associated congenital heart lesions, usually simple anomalies, such as an atrial septal defect. *Mirror-image right arch* is relatively uncommon and is almost always (98%) associated with congenital heart disease (usually complex anomalies such as tetralogy of Fallot). The CT appearance of a mirror-image arch is well described by its name; it is the mirror image of a normal left arch, with a left innominate artery present. With both types of right arch the descending aorta is usually left-sided, crossing from right to left in the lower mediastinum.

Double Aortic Arch

Double aortic arch is relatively uncommon, but because a plain radiograph shows a mediastinal abnormality (representing the right arch), it is often evaluated with CT. This anomaly is uncommonly associated with congenital heart disease, but because a complete vascular ring is present, symptoms of dysphagia are common. In this anomaly the ascending aorta splits into right and left arches. The right arch, which is usually higher and larger than the left, passes to the right of the trachea and esophagus, crosses behind these structures, and rejoins the left arch, which occupies a relatively normal position (Fig. 3.4). Each arch is smaller than normal and smaller than the descending aorta. Each arch also gives rise to a subclavian artery and a carotid artery, and no innominate artery is present. This results in a symmetric appearance of the great vessels in the supra-aortic mediastinum that is highly suggestive of the diagnosis.

Aortic Coarctation and Pseudocoarctation

Coarctation, and its rare variant pseudocoarctation, can be readily diagnosed with CT, but catheterization is usually necessary to measure intra-arterial pressures and thus the significance of the vascular obstruction.

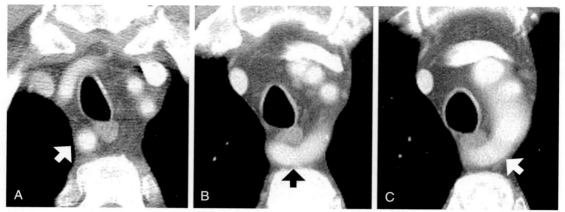

FIG. 3.1 **Aberrant right subclavian artery.** (A) An aberrant right subclavian artery *(arrow)* is located posteriorly in the right superior mediastinum. (B) At a level 7 mm below (A) the anomalous artery *(arrow)* passes posterior to the esophagus. (C) Seven millimeters below (B) the origin *(arrow)* of the anomalous artery from the posterior superior aortic arch is visible.

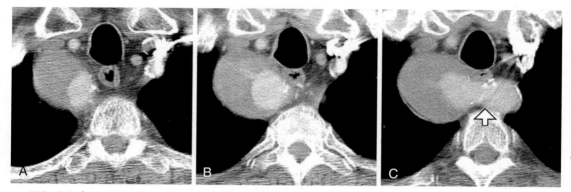

FIG. 3.2 **Aneurysm of an aberrant right subclavian artery.** (A) As in Fig. 3.1A, an aberrant right subclavian artery is situated in the right mediastinum. It is dilated, and its lumen is partially filled with a clot. (B and C) At lower levels the aberrant artery is located posterior to the esophagus, and its origin *(arrow)* from the posterior superior aortic arch is visible.

The site of narrowing in coarctation is generally at the aortic isthmus, distal to the origin of the left subclavian artery and near the ligamentum arteriosum (*juxtaductal coarctation*). On CT the narrowed segment is often visible because it is decidedly smaller than the aorta above and below this level (Fig. 3.5). This size difference reflects not only the narrowed segment at the coarctation but also some dilatation of the prestenotic and poststenotic aorta. A lengthy narrowing of the aortic arch (hypoplasia) is less common.

Images reconstructed in the plane of the aortic arch can show coarctation to best advantage. One word of caution: the degree of narrowing at the site of coarctation may be overestimated if the reformatted plane is slightly off the sagittal plane of the aorta. Dilatation of internal mammary arteries or intercostal arteries (usually the third through eighth) acting as collateral pathways can be seen.

In pseudocoarctation the aortic arch is kinked anteriorly and its lumen is somewhat narrowed, but a significant pressure gradient across the kink and collateral vessels are not present. The aortic arch is higher than normal and initially descends in an abnormally anterior position, well in front of the spine. At a level near the carina, however, the aorta again angles posteriorly, forming a second arch, and assumes its normal position

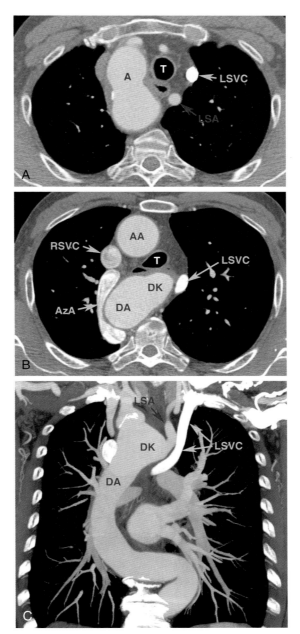

FIG. 3.3 Right aortic arch with an aberrant left subclavian artery and diverticulum of kommerell.
(A) In a patient with no evidence of congenital heart disease and with a right aortic arch *(A)*, an aberrant left subclavian artery *(LSA)* is visible in the left mediastinum. This patient also has a persistent left superior vena cava *(LSVC)*. (B) At a lower level the ascending aorta *(AA)* and descending aorta *(DA)* are visible; a retroesophageal diverticulum of Kommerell *(DK)* gives rise to the left subclavian artery seen at higher levels. The left superior vena cava *(LSVC)*, right superior vena cava *(RSVC)*, and a dilated azygos arch *(AzA)* are also visible at this level. In this patient the left superior vena cava drained into the azygos vein. (C) A thick coronal maximum-intensity projection reconstruction through the descending aorta shows the descending aorta *(DA)* and diverticulum of Kommerell *(DK)* giving rise to the aberrant left subclavian artery *(LSA)*. *LSVC*, Left superior vena cava; *T*, trachea.

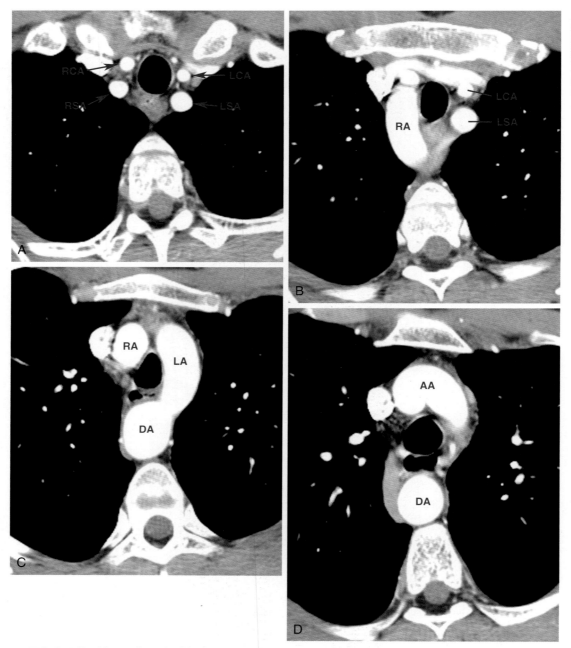

FIG. 3.4 **Double aortic arch.** (A) In the upper mediastinum the subclavian and carotid arteries appear bilaterally symmetric. (B) At a level below (A) the right arch *(RA)* is visible to the right of the trachea. On the left side of the mediastinum the left carotid artery *(LCA)* and the left subclavian artery *(LSA)*, which arise from the left arch, are visible. The right arch is characteristically higher and larger than the left arch. (C) At a level below (B) the left arch *(LA)* is now visible. The anterior right arch *(RA)* and descending aorta *(DA)* are also visible at this level. (D) At a level below (C) the ascending aorta *(AA)* and descending aorta *(DA)* are both visible. The ascending aorta has a double-barreled appearance. *LCA,* Left carotid artery; *LSA,* left subclavian artery; *RCA,* right carotid artery; *RSA,* right subclavian artery.

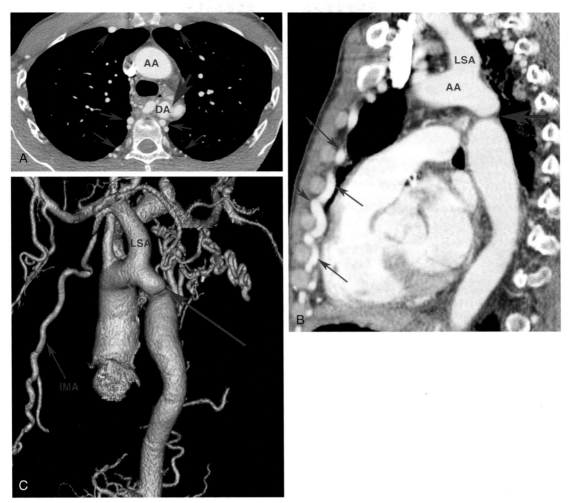

FIG. 3.5 **Aortic coarctation.** Multidetector CT with contrast enhancement in a patient with coarctation. (A) The descending aorta *(DA)*, at the level of the coarctation *(large arrow)*, is significantly smaller than the ascending aorta *(AA)*. The internal mammary and intercostal arteries *(arrows)* are dilated, serving as collateral pathways. (B) Sagittal reconstruction along the plane of the aorta shows marked narrowing at the site of the coarctation *(large arrow)*. The left subclavian artery *(LSA)* is large because it serves as a collateral pathway, reconstituting flow in the descending aorta. The dilated left internal mammary artery is visible anteriorly *(small arrows)*. (C) Three-dimensional reconstruction of the aorta and its branches showing the coarctation *(large arrow)*. The left subclavian artery *(LSA)* giving rise to the dilated left internal mammary artery *(IMA)* can also be seen. *AA,* Aortic arch.

anterolateral to the spine. This anomaly is usually not associated with symptoms.

Both coarctation and pseudocoarctation are associated with congenital bicuspid aortic valve (30%–85% of patients with coarctation); this may result in aortic stenosis. In some patients, CT shows aortic valve calcification, allowing this diagnosis to be suggested.

Aortic Aneurysm

If the ascending aorta measures more than 4 cm in diameter, it is usually referred to as *dilated* or *ectatic*. Although a diagnosis of "aortic dilatation" as opposed to "aortic aneurysm" is somewhat arbitrary, this chapter uses *aortic dilatation* or *ectasia* to refer to a generalized dilatation of relatively mild degree (4 cm), with

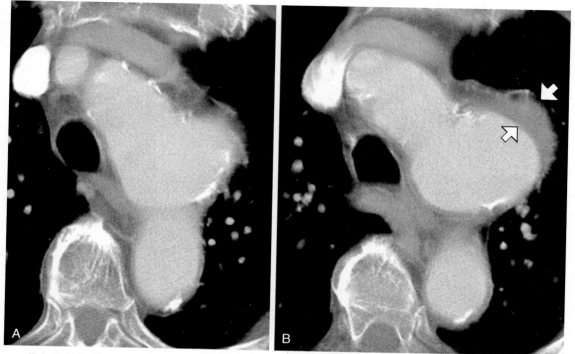

FIG. 3.6 Aortic aneurysm. (A and B) A focal, saccular aneurysm of the aortic arch shows some clot lining its lumen *(arrows)*.

the implication that it is not necessarily a serious problem. *Aneurysm*, in contrast, refers to a more focal abnormality or more severe dilatation of the entire aorta (≥5 cm). At the risk of oversimplification, for the ascending aorta, a diameter of 4 cm corresponds to aortic dilatation, 5 cm corresponds to aortic aneurysm, and 6 cm corresponds to increased risk of rupture. Surgery or insertion of an endovascular stent graft is generally recommended with an aortic diameter of 5.5 cm.

With atherosclerotic aneurysms the aortic wall is often thickened and calcified. On unenhanced CT the diagnosis can sometimes be made because of visible peripheral calcification, and thrombus within the aneurysm or adjacent hematoma may appear higher in attenuation than aortic blood.

With contrast medium infusion, the lumen of the aorta, the diameter of the aneurysm, and the thickness of the aortic wall can be defined (Fig. 3.6). There may be visible areas of plaque or thrombus within the lumen of the aneurysm (Fig. 3.7); these may also be calcified. Plaque often appears low in attenuation relative to the aortic wall because of its fat content,

or because of some opacification of the aortic wall itself. Plaque can also be seen in patients with atherosclerosis who do not have aortic dilatation. Focal ulceration of a plaque or thrombus (Fig. 3.7) may occur and should be distinguished from a penetrating atherosclerotic ulcer (PAU), if possible (see later discussion).

Aneurysms are often described as fusiform or saccular, depending on their appearance. The differential diagnosis of an aneurysm varies with its location. An *ascending aortic aneurysm* may occur with atherosclerosis, Marfan syndrome, cystic medial necrosis, syphilis, or aortic valvular disease. An *aneurysm near the ligamentum arteriosum* may be atherosclerotic in origin, a ductus aneurysm (aneurysm at the site of the ductus arteriosus or a ductus diverticulum), mycotic, related to coarctation, or posttraumatic (i.e., a pseudoaneurysm). *Mycotic aneurysms* are usually focal, and they may be associated with periaortic inflammation (visible as edema of periaortic fat) or abscess (with localized fluid collections); gas bubbles may be seen within soft tissues. A *descending aortic aneurysm* is usually atherosclerotic.

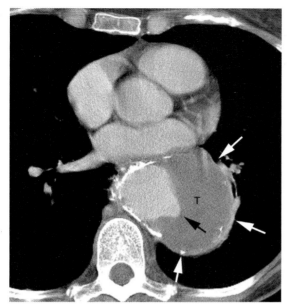

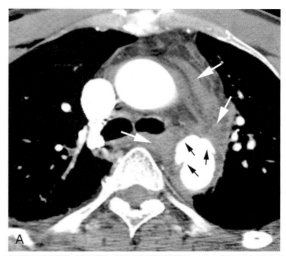

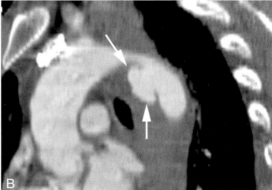

FIG. 3.7 **Aortic aneurysm containing a thrombus.** A focal, saccular aneurysm of the descending aorta *(white arrows)* shows calcification of its wall. The aneurysm contains a large thrombus *(T)* with focal ulceration *(black arrow).*

Aortic Trauma

Spiral CT has assumed an important role in the diagnosis of aortic injuries, usually associated with a fall or automobile accident. Traumatic aortic laceration, rupture, or pseudoaneurysm occurs most commonly in the following areas: (1) at the aortic root, (2) at the level of the ligamentum arteriosum, or (3) at the diaphragm and aortic hiatus. Patients with aortic root injury often die at the scene of injury; in patients who reach the hospital, injuries at the level of the ligamentum are most common (Fig. 3.8).

Mediastinal hematoma (fluid with an attenuation of about 50 Hounsfield units [HU]) contiguous with the aorta is invariably visible on CT in patients with aortic laceration or rupture (Fig. 3.8); the absence of hematoma effectively excludes this diagnosis. The presence of hematoma at the location of a sternal or vertebral fracture does not predict aortic injury.

Contrast-enhanced multidetector CT (MDCT) with thin slices (e.g., 1.25 mm) is highly accurate in diagnosing acute aortic laceration or rupture, with a sensitivity of nearly 100%. The site of rupture or tear may have the appearance of an aortic wall irregularity, dissection, or focal aneurysm (Fig. 3.8); extravasation of contrast medium is rarely seen, and if present requires immediate attention. It has been suggested that aortography is

FIG. 3.8 **Acute traumatic aortic rupture with a pseudoaneurysm.** (A) In a patient who had been involved in a motor vehicle accident, contrast-enhanced CT shows mediastinal hematoma *(white arrows)* contiguous with the aorta. There is irregularity of the proximal descending aorta, with a pseudoaneurysm anteriorly *(black arrows).* (B) A sagittal reconstruction along the aorta shows a pseudoaneurysm *(arrows)* involving the proximal descending aorta. This location is most common.

not needed if a mediastinal hematoma is not visible, or there is no recognizable aortic abnormality in patients with a mediastinal hematoma. Aortography may be necessary in some patients with inadequate CT studies or questionable CT findings, or may be performed at the time a stent graft is placed for treatment.

Chronic posttraumatic pseudoaneurysm is usually located in the region of the aortopulmonary window, below the takeoff of the left subclavian artery and near the ligamentum arteriosum (Fig. 3.9).

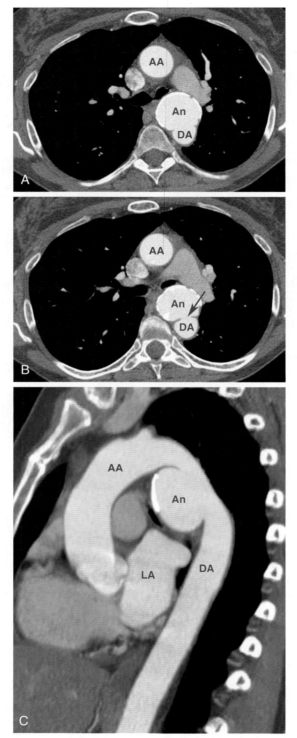

FIG. 3.9 **Chronic posttraumatic pseudoaneurysm.** Contrast-enhanced CT in a patient who had been in a motor vehicle accident. (A) A focal pseudoaneurysm *(An)* extends anteriorly from the proximal descending aorta *(DA)*, with dense calcification of its wall. (B) At a slightly lower level a defect *(arrow)* in the anterior wall of the descending aorta *(DA)* represents the site of rupture. (C) A sagittal reconstruction in the plane of the aortic arch shows the pseudoaneurysm *(An)* in a typical location. *AA,* Ascending aorta; *An,* pseudoaneurysm; *DA,* descending aorta; *LA,* left atrium.

Calcification of the wall of the pseudoaneurysm may be present.

Acute Aortic Syndromes

Acute aortic syndrome is a term used to describe several aortic abnormalities that present with acute chest pain and are often associated with similar predisposing conditions. These include *aortic dissection, intramural hematoma* (IMH), and *penetrating atherosclerotic ulcer* (PAU). They have in common the presence of penetration of the aortic intima or disruption of the media.

Aortic Dissection

Aortic dissection is often associated with hypertension, weakness of the aortic wall (e.g., Marfan syndrome or cystic medial necrosis), or trauma. Patients usually have acute chest pain. The goal in diagnosing dissection is the demonstration of an intimal flap, displaced inward from the edge of the aorta, separating the true and false channels. CT is ideally suited to this because of its cross-sectional format.

Two schemes for the classification of aortic dissections have been proposed by DeBakey and Daily. Daily's classification, commonly known as the *Stanford classification*, is most frequently used because of its simplicity and relevance to treatment.

With use of the Stanford classification, aortic dissections are divided into types A and B. *Type A* dissections involve the ascending aorta (Fig. 3.10); approximately two-thirds of acute dissections are type A. Because of the possibility of retrograde dissection and rupture into the pericardium (resulting in tamponade) or occlusion of the coronary or carotid arteries, these dissections are usually treated surgically with grafting or stent graft placement in the region of the tear. Electrocardiogram (ECG)-gated MDCT can provide exceptional detail in patients with a type A dissection (Fig. 3.11). *Type B* dissections do not involve the aortic arch but typically arise distal to the left subclavian artery (Fig. 3.12). These are generally treated medically (by normalization of blood pressure). Placement of an endovascular stent graft is also used for treatment of some type B dissections (Fig. 3.20).

CT is highly sensitive and specific (>95%) in diagnosing dissection and in determining its location and type and the aortic branches involved; consequently it is an excellent diagnostic procedure in patients with a suggestive clinical presentation. Transesophageal echocardiography may be performed in some patients with suspected acute dissection; it is highly sensitive but has lower specificity (70%). The accuracy of magnetic resonance imaging is similar to that of CT, and magnetic resonance imaging may be performed in patients unable to have radiographic contrast agents; it may also be performed before surgery in patients shown to have a type A dissection. CT or magnetic resonance imaging can be used to follow up patients with dissection after treatment to watch for redissection or extension of the dissection.

In patients with suspected dissection, CT should be performed with rapid contrast medium infusion. With use of a spiral technique, it is easy to scan through the great vessels, aortic arch, and descending aorta (1.25- or 2.5-mm detector width for MDCT) during rapid contrast medium infusion (at 2.5–3.5 mL per second) and to continue the scans to the level of the aortic bifurcation in the abdomen. A scanning delay of approximately 20 to 30 seconds should be used after the start of injection, or scanning should be timed by the scanner to show aortic enhancement. Contrast-enhanced scans are usually preceded by unenhanced scans through the thorax to look for IMH (see later discussion).

In a patient with dissection the intimal flap is usually delineated by contrast medium filling both the true channel and the false channel. A fenestration in the aortic intima may be visible at the site of origin of the dissection (Fig. 3.12). The true and false channels can often be distinguished on the basis of the following CT findings (Figs. 3.10A, 3.11, and 3.12), although this may be difficult or impossible in some cases:

- If the aortic root or ascending aorta is normal in appearance, trace the opacified aortic lumen on adjacent slices to see which of the distal channels it communicates with. This represents the true channel.
- The false channel tends to be located lateral to the true channel at the level of the aortic arch and spirals posteriorly in the descending aorta. Because of this characteristic location, the left renal artery is the abdominal branch most likely to arise from the false channel.
- The true lumen is usually smaller.
- The false channel is usually more irregular in contour, and it may contain strands of tissue termed *cobwebs* within the contrast medium stream.
- The false channel is more likely to contain a thrombus.
- Blood flow is slower and opacification is often delayed in the false channel.
- Aortic wall calcification may be seen lateral to the true channel; it is usually displaced inward from the wall of the false channel.

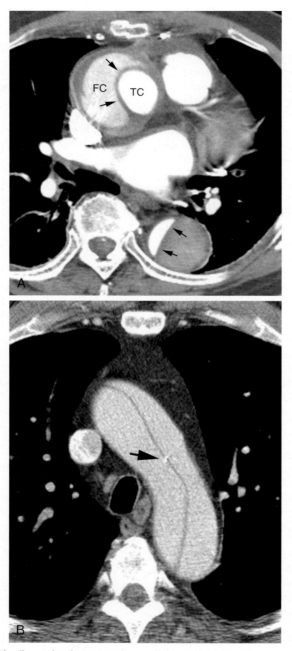

FIG. 3.10 Type A aortic dissection in two patients. (A) A patient with acute chest pain shows a type A dissection involving both the ascending aorta and the descending aorta. The intimal flap *(black arrows)* is lower in attenuation than contrast-opacified blood. In the ascending aorta the true channel *(TC)* is smaller and more densely opacified than the false channel *(FC)*. Also the false channel is more irregular in appearance and contains some thrombus. In the descending aorta the true channel is more densely opacified, and the false channel is located laterally and posteriorly. (B) In a different patient with a type A dissection, the intimal flap is visible in the aortic arch, and calcification of the intima *(arrow)* is visible.

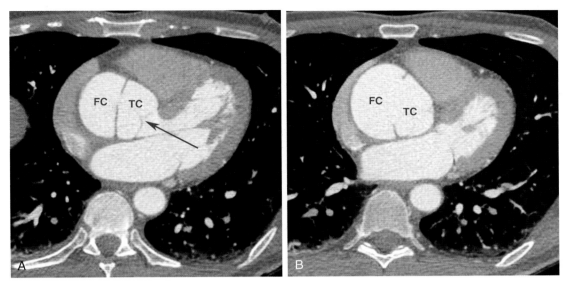

FIG. 3.11 **Type A aortic dissection.** Electrocardiogram-gated multidetector CT shows a type A dissection involving the aortic root. (A) At the level of the left ventricular outflow tract and aortic valve *(arrow)*, the true channel *(TC)* or lumen and false channel *(FC)* are identified, with the intimal fenestration at the site of origin of the dissection seen as a hole or defect in the intimal flap. The aorta is dilated. (B) At a higher level, a large fenestration in the intimal flap is visible. *FC*, False channel; *TC*, true channel.

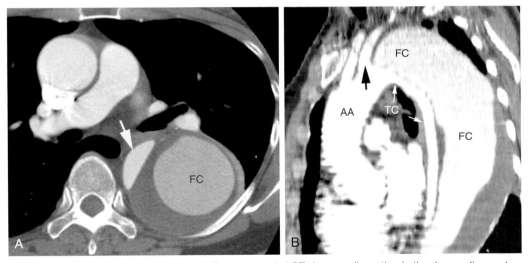

FIG. 3.12 **Type B aortic dissection.** (A) Enhanced spiral CT shows a dissection in the descending aorta. The false channel *(FC)* is larger, located posterolaterally, less opacified, and lined by a thrombus. The true channel *(arrow)* is compressed. The ascending aorta is normal in appearance. (B) A sagittal reconstruction shows the large false channel *(FC)* originating distal to the left subclavian artery *(black arrow)*. The true channel *(TC)* is small and more densely opacified; it is evident that it communicates directly with the normal ascending aorta *(AA)*. The intimal flap separating the true and false channels is visible.

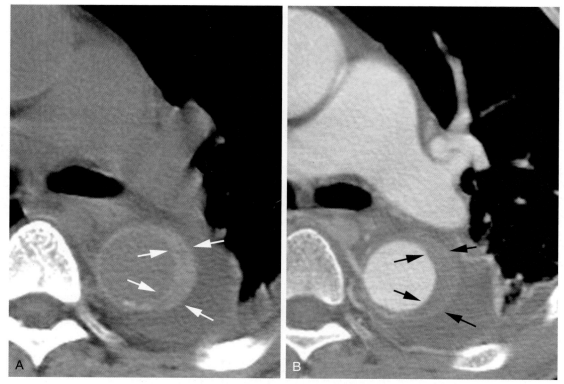

FIG. 3.13 Intramural hematoma (Type B). (A) In a man with acute chest pain, unenhanced CT shows crescentic thickening of the aortic wall *(arrows)*. This is higher in attenuation than blood in the aortic lumen. (B) Contrast-enhanced CT shows crescentic thickening of the aortic wall *(arrows)*. On the enhanced scan the high attenuation of the hematoma is difficult to appreciate. An intramural hematoma is typically crescentic, a finding that helps distinguish it from a dissection filled with thrombus.

The false channel may be opacified or thrombosed. Thrombosis of the false channel is associated with better prognosis. The false channel may dilate and sometimes ruptures. Overall, the aortic diameter may be increased at the site of a dissection because of dilatation of the false channel.

Artifacts, arising because of cardiac motion or vascular pulsations during the scan, may mimic an intimal flap. They are commonly seen at the level of the aortic root and in the descending aorta, adjacent to the border of the left side of the heart. Typically, they are less sharply defined than a true intimal flap, may extend beyond the edges of the aorta, or are inconsistently seen from one level to the next.

Two other abnormalities may closely mimic the clinical presentation of dissection. Consequently, these may be seen on CT scans obtained to evaluate possible dissection in patients with acute aortic syndrome. These are IMH and PAU. The appearances of dissection,

IMH, and PAU may overlap, with features of each being seen in a single case.

Intramural Hematoma

IMH results from hemorrhage into the aortic wall. Acute IMH may closely mimic the presentation of dissection (acute chest pain in a patient with hypertension). It is thought to occur because of bleeding from the vasa vasorum, although in some cases it may represent a sealed-off dissection.

On contrast-enhanced scans, the IMH appears as a smooth and crescentic or, less commonly, concentric thickening of the aortic wall (Figs. 3.13 and 3.14). On unenhanced scans the IMH appears denser than unenhanced blood in the aortic lumen; because of this characteristic appearance, CT in a patient with suspected dissection should be preceded by unenhanced scans through the thorax. If unenhanced scans are not obtained prospectively,

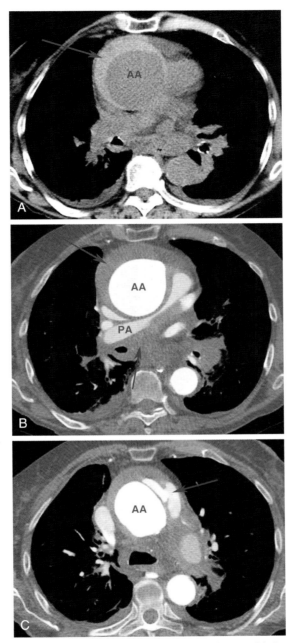

FIG. 3.14 Intramural hematoma (Type A) with aortic rupture. (A) In an elderly woman with acute chest pain, the ascending aorta *(AA)* is dilated and an intramural hematoma *(arrow)* is visible because of its high attenuation. (B) At a higher level the ascending aorta *(AA)* is dilated and high-attenuation blood *(arrows)* is seen in relation to the intramural hematoma and free in the mediastinum. The right pulmonary artery *(PA)* is markedly compressed by the dilated aorta and mediastinal hematoma. (C) Cephalad to (B), contrast opacification of a portion of the intramural hematoma is seen, as well as leakage into the mediastinum. High-attenuation blood is visible throughout the mediastinum. This patient died shortly after CT had been performed. *AA*, Ascending aorta.

delayed unenhanced scans may be obtained. Inward displacement of intimal calcification can also be seen on unenhanced scans.

It should be remembered that the normal aortic wall is a few millimeters thick. On unenhanced scans, it appears to have the same density as blood in the aortic lumen in healthy individuals. In patients with anemia (hematocrit <35%), the normal aortic wall may appear denser than blood. This should not be confused with IMH. As a rough rule, the CT density of unenhanced blood in the aortic lumen or left ventricle (in HU) is about the same as the hematocrit.

The smooth crescentic or concentric wall thickening seen with IMH is usually different in appearance from dissection with a thrombosed channel. A thrombosed dissection uncommonly appears crescentic or concentric in shape. Thrombus lining an aneurysm can also mimic IMH, but it is usually more irregular in contour. The presence of acute chest pain as a presenting symptom also suggests an acute IMH

rather than a thrombus within a chronic dissection or aneurysm.

An IMH may rupture, progress to frank dissection (by rupture into the aortic lumen), result in an aneurysm, or resolve. Treatment is similar to that for dissection occurring in the same location (i.e., type A or B), and IMH is often classified as type A or type B, as is dissection (Figs. 3.13 and 3.14). A type A IMH is treated surgically because of potential complications (Fig. 3.14).

Penetrating Atherosclerotic Ulcer

In patients with atherosclerosis, ulceration of an atherosclerotic plaque may, over time, penetrate the aortic wall, resulting in PAU. The descending aorta is most often involved, because atherosclerosis is most common there. PAU may lead to chest pain similar to that for dissection or IMH.

True PAU penetrates the intima and extends into (or through) the aortic wall (Fig. 3.15); its

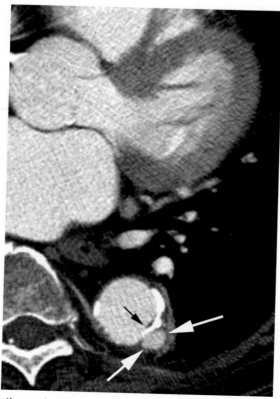

FIG. 3.15 **Penetrating atherosclerotic ulcer.** Enhanced CT in a man with chest pain shows contrast opacification of a focal ulceration extending into the aortic wall (white arrows). Calcification (black arrow) shows the location of the intima.

appearance is similar to that of a penetrating gastric ulcer (Fig. 3.16). Calcification of the aortic wall or enhancement of the wall after contrast medium infusion may help in diagnosing wall penetration. PAU may result in localized IMH (Fig. 3.17), dissection (which is usually localized), pseudoaneurysm, or, sometimes, rupture. Surgical treatment may be necessary in some cases, particularly in patients presenting with chest pain, even if the PAU is limited to the descending aorta. Incidental PAU may not require treatment.

Ulceration of an atheroma or thrombus (Figs. 3.7 and 3.18) may mimic the appearance of PAU, but it is more superficial and does not involve the aortic wall itself.

Aortic Stent Graft Treatment of Aortic Abnormalities

In recent years, catheter placement of an *endovascular stent graft* has become an important option in the treatment of acute or chronic aortic abnormalities, such as aneurysm (Fig 3.19), dissection (Fig 3.20), PAU, aortic rupture, and some congenital abnormalities, obviating surgery in many cases. CT has proven crucial in planning stent graft placement and for the evaluation of potential postprocedure complications, such as endoleak (Fig 3.19), stent migration or kinking, pseudoaneurysm or dissection, aortic perforation, thrombosis, and coverage of vital branch vessels. Evaluation of stent grafts is too complicated for this chapter but is reviewed in a reference in Suggested Reading.

SUPERIOR VENA CAVA AND GREAT VEINS
Congenital Abnormalities
Azygos Lobe
An azygos lobe is a common anomaly and is present in about 1 in 200 patients. It results in a typical appearance on plain radiographs and CT that is easily recognized and produces a characteristic alteration in normal mediastinal anatomy. In patients with this anomaly, the azygos arch is located more cephalad than normal, at, near, or above the junction of the brachiocephalic veins. Above this level the azygos fissure is visible within the lung, marginating the azygos lobe (Fig. 3.21).

Persistent Left Superior Vena Cava
The only other frequent venous anomaly is persistent left superior vena cava (LSVC), which represents failure of the embryonic left anterior cardinal vein to regress. This anomaly is difficult to recognize on plain radiography; however, in some patients, there is a slight prominence of the left superior mediastinum, or a left-sided venous catheter may be inadvertently placed in the LSVC. It is present in about 0.3% of healthy individuals, at approximately the same frequency as for an azygos lobe; it is usually unassociated with symptoms or other abnormalities but is more frequent (about 5%) in patients with congenital heart disease.

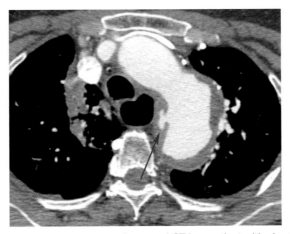

FIG. 3.16 **Penetrating atherosclerotic ulcer.** Enhanced CT in a patient with chest pain shows contrast opacification of a focal ulceration of the medial wall of the aortic arch *(arrow)*. On an unenhanced image this was associated with a focal intramural hematoma.

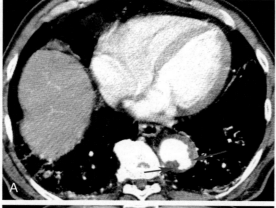

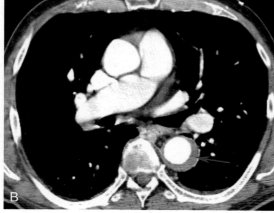

FIG. 3.17 **Penetrating atherosclerotic ulcer associated with an intramural hematoma.** (A) Enhanced CT in a patient with chest pain shows a focal ulceration in the descending aorta *(arrows)*. On this single image, this could represent an ulcerated thrombus, although when associated with chest pain, a penetrating atherosclerotic ulcer should be suspected. (B) At a higher level an intramural hematoma *(arrow)* results in crescentic thickening of the aortic wall.

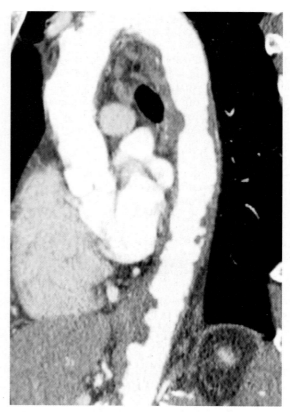

FIG. 3.18 **Ulceration of an atheromatous plaque.** A sagittal reconstruction through the aortic arch and descending aorta shows extensive ulceration of atheromatous plaque. None of the ulcers project through the aortic wall. This patient was asymptomatic.

On CT in patients with this anomaly, the LSVC is positioned lateral to the left common carotid artery in the supra-aortic mediastinum (Fig. 3.3). It descends along the left mediastinum, passing downward, anterior to the left hilum, and usually enters the coronary sinus posterior to the left atrium. In 65% of patients the left brachiocephalic vein is absent, a right vena cava is also present, and the two vessels are about the same size and in the same relative position on opposite sides of the mediastinum. If the left brachiocephalic vein is also present, joining the right superior vena cava (SVC) and the LSVC, the right SVC will be larger than the LSVC.

An LSVC will exhibit dense opacification after contrast medium injection into the left arm. If contrast medium is injected on the right and the vein is not opacified, its tubular shape and characteristic position are usually enough for a definite diagnosis.

Azygos or Hemiazygos Continuation of the Inferior Vena Cava

Embryogenesis of the inferior vena cava is complicated. During fetal development the vessels that form the azygos and hemiazygos veins normally communicate with the suprarenal inferior vena cava, but this communication normally breaks down. If it persists, then azygos or hemiazygos continuation of the inferior vena cava is said to be present.

These lesions may be associated with other congenital anomalies, including polysplenia (in patients

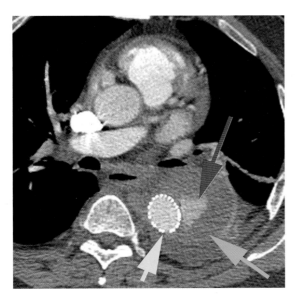

FIG. 3.19 Aortic stent graft placement with endoleak visible on contrast-enhanced CT. A patient with an aortic aneurysm has had an endovascular stent graft *(yellow arrow)* placed for treatment. A collection of contrast medium *(red arrow)* is visible outside the graft, in relation to thrombus *(green arrow)* within the aneurysm. This is abnormal and represents an endoleak, a leak through or around the graft, or occurring because of retrograde flow through an aortic branch. Endoleak may result in aneurysm enlargement.

with hemiazygos communication) or asplenia (with azygos communication), or they may be isolated abnormalities. Typical findings include marked dilatation of the azygos arch and posterior azygos vein (Fig. 3.22). If hemiazygos continuation is present, the dilated azygos vein will be seen to cross the mediastinum, from right to left, behind the descending aorta, to communicate with a dilated hemiazygos vein. A normal-appearing inferior vena cava is often visible at the level of the heart and diaphragm, draining the hepatic veins. Either anomaly may be associated with duplication of the abdominal inferior vena cava. Rarely, a dilated hemiazygos vein drains into the left brachiocephalic vein instead of joining the azygos vein.

Superior Vena Cava Syndrome

Obstruction of the SVC, or either of the brachiocephalic veins, is a common clinical occurrence, and symptoms of venous obstruction may require CT. In some patients undergoing CT for diagnosis of a mediastinal mass or

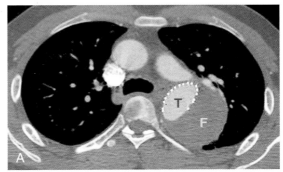

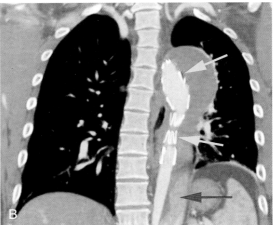

FIG. 3.20 Aortic stent graft placement in a patient with type b aortic dissection. (A) Contrast-enhanced CT shows a type B dissection with a stent graft within the true lumen *(T)*. Stent graft was placed because of marked dilatation of the false lumen *(F)*, which is not opacified at this level. (B) Coronal reconstruction shows the stent graft *(yellow arrows)* in the true lumen. Some opacification of the distal false lumen *(red arrow)* results from retrograde filling from an abdominal fenestration.

lung cancer, CT will also show findings of vena cava obstruction.

SVC obstruction can be seen in a variety of diseases, most commonly bronchogenic carcinoma, although in some parts of the United States granulomatous mediastinitis as a result of histoplasmosis is a common cause. Other causes of SVC obstruction include sarcoidosis, fibrosing mediastinitis, tuberculosis, and mediastinal radiation for neoplasm. Because of the frequent use of subclavian catheters, venous thrombosis resulting in obstruction is not uncommon.

On CT in patients with SVC obstruction (Figs. 3.23 and 3.24), a number of characteristic findings are present. Beginning peripherally, as the contrast medium

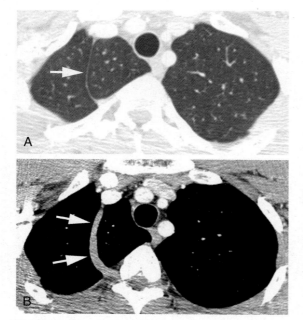

FIG. 3.21 **Azygos lobe.** (A) Within the upper lung the azygos fissure *(arrow)* distinguishes the azygos lobe medially from the remainder of the upper lobe. (B) At a lower level the azygos arch *(arrows)* passes from an anterior to a posterior position. In this patient, it arises from the right brachiocephalic vein.

bolus is injected, it is common to see opacification of a number of small venous collateral vessels in the shoulder, axilla, upper chest wall, and upper mediastinum. However, it should be remembered that some filling of small veins in the chest wall and axilla can be seen in the absence of a venous abnormality (perhaps because of poor positioning of the patient's arm for injection). Unless other findings of venous obstruction (e.g., large collateral veins) are present, this finding should not be of great concern.

In patients with obstruction of the SVC, flow of contrast medium from the arm is delayed and the scan sequence must be delayed accordingly or mediastinal vascular opacification will be poor. Collateral vessels, which are characteristically dilated in patients with obstruction of the SVC, include the intercostal veins, the internal mammary veins, the left superior intercostal vein (which results in the "aortic nipple" sometimes visible on chest radiographs), and the hemiazygos vein. The azygos vein and azygos arch usually form the final common pathway for venous return from all these collateral vessels, bypassing the area of obstruction and draining blood into the lower SVC, just above the right atrium.

In patients with thrombosis of the SVC or brachiocephalic veins, a thrombus is sometimes visible in the vessel lumen, outlined by contrast medium. One word of caution, however: if contrast medium is injected into only one arm, as is typical, streaming of unopacified blood from one brachiocephalic vein into the SVC can mimic the appearance of an SVC clot.

PULMONARY ARTERIES
Pulmonary Artery Dilatation

Dilatation of the main pulmonary artery can be seen as a result of pulmonic stenosis, a left-to-right shunt, or most often, pulmonary hypertension. A main pulmonary artery diameter of 3.5 cm or more (lateral to the ascending aorta) or exceeding the diameter of the ascending aorta suggests abnormal dilatation (Fig. 3.25A) but is not always associated with a significant abnormality. Associated right ventricular dilatation or hypertrophy may be observed (Fig. 3.25B), along with straightening of the ventricular septum. With pulmonic stenosis the main and left pulmonary arteries are dilated, whereas the right pulmonary artery is relatively normal in size. With shunts or pulmonary hypertension, both left and right pulmonary arteries are large.

Pulmonary artery aneurysms are rare; they may be mycotic or caused by catheter-related complications, Takayasu arteritis, Williams syndrome, prenatal varicella, or Behçet syndrome.

Pulmonary Embolism

Contrast-enhanced CT is commonly used to diagnose pulmonary embolism (PE) because of its accuracy and ready availability. However, it has been suggested that CT for PE diagnosis is being overused; only about 5% of patients undergoing CT for clinically suspected PE actually have PE as a cause of their symptoms. Recent clinical guidelines recommend appropriate use of clinical screening criteria (e.g., Wells score), for determining the pretest likelihood of PE, and D-dimer testing before imaging is requested.

With spiral CT an appropriate CT technique for PE diagnosis involves (1) thin slices (e.g., 1.25 mm), (2) a single breath hold of less than 5 seconds, (3) coverage of the entire thorax (approximately 25 cm), (4) contrast medium injection at a rate of 5 mL per second, and (5) scanning after an interval determined with a timing bolus, or timed by the scanner, to show opacification of the pulmonary artery (if PE alone is suspected) or the aorta (if it also needs to be evaluated).

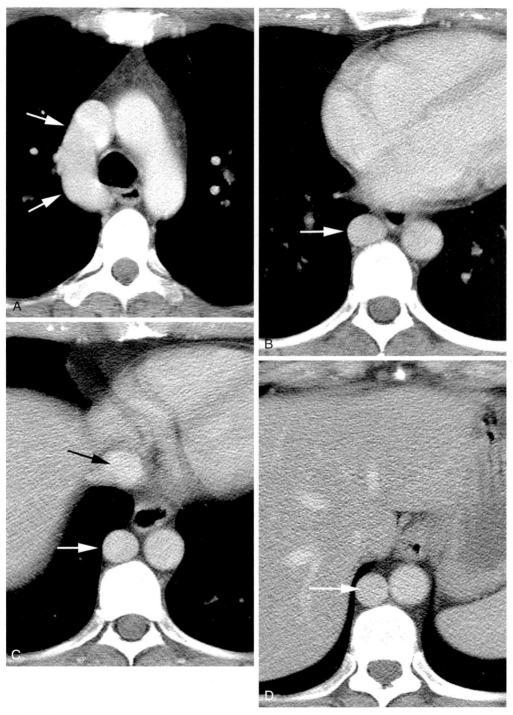

FIG. 3.22 Azygos continuation of the inferior vena cava. The azygos arch (A, *white arrows*) and the posterior azygos vein (B–D, *white arrow*) are markedly dilated. A normal-appearing inferior vena cava is visible at the level of the heart and diaphragm (C, *black arrow*), draining the hepatic veins, but it is not seen below this level.

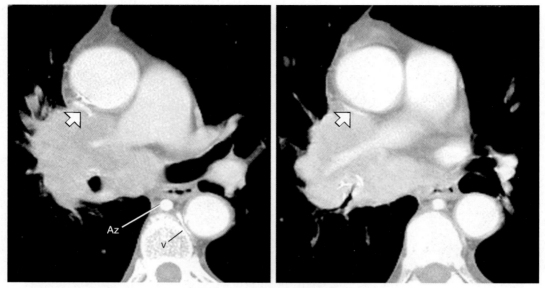

FIG. 3.23 **(A and B) Superior vena cava obstruction in bronchogenic carcinoma.** In a patient with a large right hilar mass and mediastinal invasion, the superior vena cava *(arrows)* is nearly obstructed. The azygos vein *(Az)* and a left intercostal vein *(V)* are opacified because they are serving as collateral pathways to bypass the obstruction.

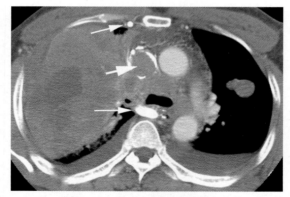

FIG. 3.24 **Superior vena cava syndrome in metastatic carcinoma.** CT with contrast enhancement in a patient with metastatic carcinoma and symptoms of superior vena cava syndrome. The superior vena cava contains a large tumor thrombus *(large arrow)*. The internal mammary vein and azygos vein *(small arrows)* are opacified because they are serving as collateral pathways. The right upper lobe is consolidated because of postobstructive pneumonia. Pleural effusions are present.

Acute Pulmonary Embolism

A filling defect visible within a pulmonary artery is usually diagnostic of PE (Figs. 3.26 and 3.27). An acute PE is typically centered in the lumen of the artery, outlined by contrast agent (Figs. 3.26 and 3.27). If the vessel is seen in cross section, this appearance is termed the *doughnut sign*. If the vessel is visible along its length, it is termed the *railroad track sign*. Some clots may completely obstruct an artery; if this is the case, the vessel may appear expanded at the point of obstruction *(the fat-vessel sign)*, with smaller or unopacified vessels downstream. Clot usually measures 60 HU or less in attenuation; the opacified blood outlining it measures considerably more (e.g., 200 HU). Acute PE usually resolves in 1 week or so.

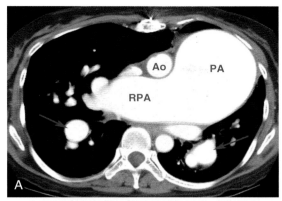

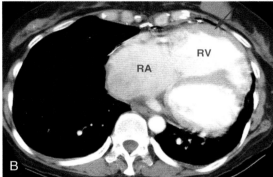

FIG. 3.25 **Marked dilation of the pulmonary artery in a patient with eisenmenger syndrome and pulmonary hypertension.** (A) The main pulmonary artery *(PA)* greatly exceeds the diameter of the ascending aorta *(Ao)*, indicating the presence of pulmonary hypertension. The right pulmonary artery *(RPA)* and interlobar pulmonary arteries *(arrows)* are also dilated. (B) CT at a lower level shows dilatation of the right ventricle *(RV)* and right atrium *(RA)*. The right ventricular wall *(arrow)* is markedly hypertrophied (thickened) because of pulmonary hypertension. This is an extreme example of pulmonary artery dilatation.

The large majority of patients undergoing CT for diagnosis of suspected PE associated with acute chest pain, dyspnea, or hypoxemia actually have another abnormality diagnosed. Other common diagnoses include atelectasis, pneumonia, pulmonary edema, pleural effusions, cancer, and diffuse lung diseases.

Chronic Pulmonary Embolism

A chronic or unresolved PE is usually adherent to the vessel wall and is located peripherally within an artery, while contrast medium is visible in the center of its lumen (Fig. 3.28). This is the opposite of what is seen with acute PE. *Pulmonary artery webs* (wispy or thin linear filling defects) can indicate a chronic embolism or

may be seen as an acute clot is resolving. Calcification of the clot or artery wall may be seen in chronic PE. Enlargement of the main pulmonary artery because of pulmonary hypertension can be seen with chronic PE, as may right ventricular dilatation, mosaic perfusion, vessel obstruction, decreased size of peripheral arteries, and an increase in systemic vascular supply to lung.

Artifacts Mimicking Pulmonary Embolism

A number of artifacts can simulate PE. These may be related to several factors:

- technical: streak artifacts, patient motion, use of an edge-enhancing algorithm, volume averaging of a vessel with a bronchus, bolus timing problems or contrast medium streaming, breathing, cardiac pulsation;
- anatomic confusion: hilar or intrapulmonary lymph nodes, mucous plugs;
- intravascular PE mimics: intravascular tumor embolism, primary sarcoma, embolism of foreign material (e.g., intravenous catheter, detachable balloon).

Pulmonary emboli are usually long or "wormshaped" and are usually visible on a number of scans when oriented perpendicular to the scan plane (i.e., the vessel is seen in cross section) or are seen along their length if the artery lies in the scan plane. An apparent filling defect visible on only one or two scans (for a vessel seen in cross section) is likely an artifact. It may be related to streak artifacts, breathing, cardiac pulsation, or patient motion.

Contrast medium streaming artifacts in patients with slow blood flow or poor opacification can result in apparent central filling defects, but the "filling defect" will usually be ill-defined and have an attenuation higher than that of a clot (Fig. 3.29). Generally speaking, if an apparent filling defect appears brighter than muscle on the same scan, it is a flow artifact rather than a PE. Measuring the attenuation of an apparent filling defect can also help in deciding if it is an artifact; flow artifacts measure greater than 100 HU.

Rarely, large filling defects mimicking clot can be seen in patients with intraluminal pulmonary artery masses (primary pulmonary artery intimal sarcoma or intravascular metastasis, occurring in patients with sarcoma, hepatocellular carcinoma [Fig. 3.30], and renal cell carcinoma). Intraluminal tumor may be seen to enhance following contrast medium infusion; emboli are not. Iatrogenic emboli (catheter fragments, glue used for vertebroplasty, radiation seeds, etc.) are occasionally seen.

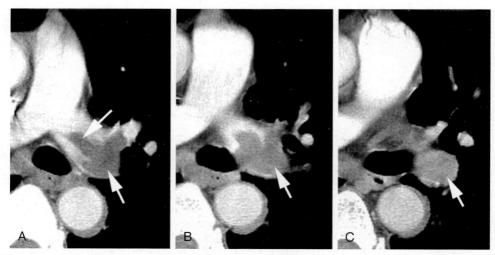

FIG. 3.26 **Acute pulmonary embolism in the left main pulmonary artery.** (A, B, and C) A clot fills the left main and interlobar pulmonary artery *(arrows)* and is outlined by contrast medium in (A).

Accuracy of CT for Pulmonary Embolism Diagnosis

The sensitivity and specificity of spiral CT in diagnosing acute PE involving the main pulmonary artery branches is 100%, and its overall sensitivity and specificity exceed 90% for segmental emboli.

It is important to recognize that regardless of its sensitivity, CT is as good as it needs to be. A number of studies have shown that if CT for PE diagnosis (even when single-detector CT with 3-mm-thick slices is used) is read as showing "no PE," patient outcome is excellent without treatment, and is just as good as when other modalities are used for diagnosis; the 3-month survival rate without recurrent PE is 99% or greater.

MDCT is much more sensitive in detecting small (subsegmental) clots than other imaging modalities, and there is now some concern that it is *too sensitive* and likely to overdiagnose PE (i.e., detect subsegmental clots that are clinically insignificant and do not require treatment). Incidental (asymptomatic) subsegmental PE is commonly seen on MDCT performed for other reasons (Fig. 3.31). Approximately 15% of patients in whom PE is diagnosed with MDCT have clots limited to subsegmental arteries.

It is unclear whether treating isolated subsegmental PE is necessary in all patients; in stable patients without other significant abnormalities, anticoagulation may not be required. However, specific guidelines are lacking and await further investigation. At present, most clinicians treat patients with isolated subsegmental clots if they have other risk factors for PE (e.g., deep vein thrombosis, malignancy) or other medical problems, such as borderline cardiac or pulmonary function or atrial fibrillation.

THE HEART AND PERICARDIUM

CT is not commonly used for evaluation of cardiac abnormalities, but some knowledge of cardiac anatomy on CT is necessary for proper interpretation of scans and identification of paracardiac abnormalities or masses and the effect they have on the heart. Occasionally, incidental cardiac abnormalities are detected on CT. Coronary artery calcification (CAC) or coronary artery stenosis can be assessed by CT, and CT is excellent for evaluating pericardial abnormalities.

Cardiac Abnormalities

With the development of rapid MDCT techniques, the use of CT in evaluating cardiac abnormalities has increased. However, echocardiography, magnetic resonance imaging, and angiography remain the modalities of choice in most patients with suspected cardiac disease.

In patients with an acute *myocardial infarction*, after bolus injection of contrast medium, infarcted myocardium can show less opacification than normal myocardium and, to some degree, infarct size can be quantitated. Ventricular thrombus can also be shown in patients with an acute myocardial infarction.

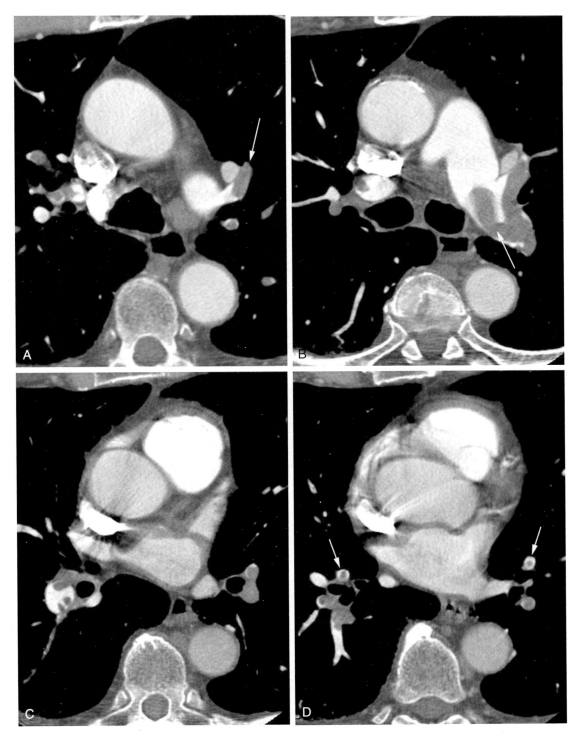

FIG. 3.27 **Multidetector CT (1.25-mm slices) in acute pulmonary embolism.** (A–D) Multiple clots *(arrows)* are visible within large central, lobar, segmental, and subsegmental pulmonary artery branches. They are outlined by contrast medium, showing examples of the "railroad track sign" (B, *arrow*) and "doughnut sign" (D, *arrows*). Some vessels are completely obstructed (A, *arrow*).

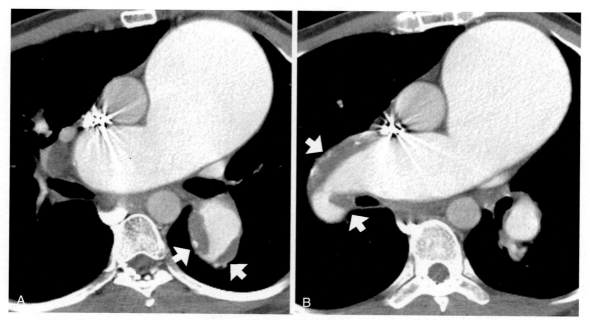

FIG. 3.28 Chronic pulmonary embolism and pulmonary hypertension in a patient with marfan syndrome. (A and B) The main pulmonary artery is dilated because of pulmonary hypertension. A thrombus *(arrows)* is adherent to the vessel wall. Some calcification of the vessel wall or clot is also seen.

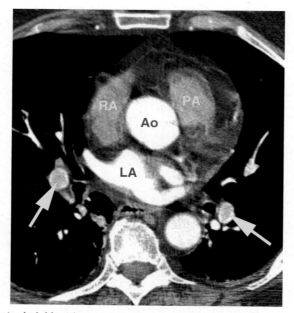

FIG. 3.29 Flow artifact mimicking the appearance of pulmonary embolism. Low attenuation in the interlobar pulmonary arteries *(arrows)* mimics the "doughnut sign" of pulmonary embolism but represents a flow artifact related to contrast streaming. Notice that contrast medium has washed out of the right atrium *(RA)* and main pulmonary artery *(PA)* because of a mistimed injection, but the left atrium *(LA)* and aorta *(Ao)* are densely opacified. Contrast medium has washed out of the central pulmonary arteries because flow is most rapid in the center of vessels, but blood remains opacified adjacent to the artery walls. The attenuation of the low-attenuation flow artifact measured 150 Hounsfield units, much higher than clot.

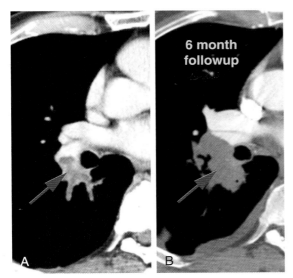

FIG. 3.30 Intravascular tumor embolism in a patient with hepatocellular carcinoma. (A) CT shows a branching filling defect *(arrow)* in the right interlobar pulmonary artery and its branches that mimics pulmonary embolism. (B) Six-month follow-up CT shows increased size of the filling defect, which now obstructs and expands the artery.

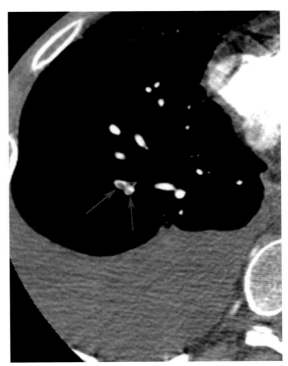

FIG. 3.31 Isolated subsegmental pulmonary embolism, likely incidental and clinically insignificant. Multidetector CT in a patient with chest pain and shortness of breath shows a small clot *(arrows)* draped over both limbs of a branching subsegmental artery. This was the only clot visible. This small pulmonary embolism is likely insignificant. The patient's symptoms were undoubtedly related to his pleural effusion.

In patients with a prior infarction, CT can be valuable in showing ventricular aneurysm, thinning of the myocardium, subendocardial fat or calcification, and ventricular thrombus (Fig. 3.32). A warning: normal papillary muscle, which appears as a left ventricular filling defect (Fig. 3.33), should not be confused with clot. Myocardial wall thickening can be seen in patients with *ventricular hypertrophy* (Figs. 3.25B and 3.33) and patients with hypertrophic cardiomyopathy.

CT is sensitive in detecting *valve and annular calcification* (Fig. 3.33). Aortic valve calcification correlates with the presence of aortic stenosis, and the more severe the calcification, the more severe the stenosis. Calcification of the mitral annulus is a common degenerative condition, which increases with age; it is unassociated with symptoms or disease. Mitral valve calcification is abnormal and associated with mitral stenosis; it is uncommon.

Intracardiac tumors can be shown with contrast-enhanced CT but are uncommon and are usually evaluated by other techniques. Metastases are much more common than primary cardiac tumors. Lung cancer with invasion of the pulmonary vein can result in a left atrial mass.

Lipomatous hypertrophy of the atrial septum is seen on CT as an incidental finding in about 2% of cases; it appears as a fat-attenuation thickening of the septum

(Fig. 3.34) and often mimics a mass on echocardiography. It is generally without clinical significance but has been associated with atrial arrhythmia. It should not be confused with a true cardiac tumor.

Coronary Calcification and Coronary CT Arteriography

Coronary artery calcification (CAC) is commonly identified in adults on routine CT scans at and below the level of the aortic root (Fig. 3.35). The *left main coronary artery* is about 1 cm in length; it arises from the aorta at about the four o'clock position and gives rise to the *left anterior descending coronary artery* (LAD) extending anteriorly and inferiorly and the *circumflex coronary artery* (CCA) extending posteriorly and inferiorly. Calcification of the left main coronary artery is said to be present if calcium is seen proximal to its point of

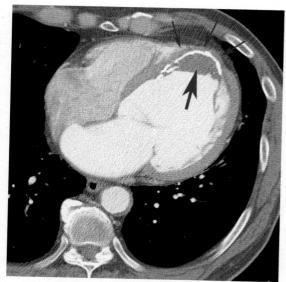

FIG. 3.32 Old myocardial infarct with a left ventricular thrombus. Multidetector CT in a patient with a prior myocardial infarct shows thinning of the septal and left ventricular myocardium *(small red arrows)*. Subendocardial calcification is present. A clot *(large red arrow)* fills the apex of the ventricle.

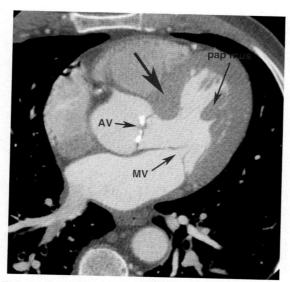

FIG. 3.33 Aortic valve calcification with focal septal hypertrophy. Multidetector CT shows dense calcification of the aortic valve *(AV)*, with focal hypertrophy (thickening) of the ventricular septum *(large arrow)*. The mitral valve *(MV)* appears normal. Normal papillary muscle *(pap mus)* should not be confused with a thrombus.

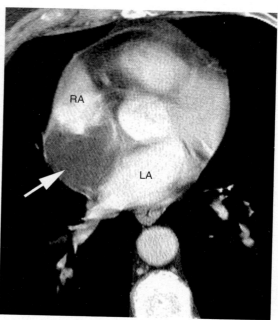

FIG. 3.34 Lipomatous hypertrophy of the atrial septum. A focal low-attenuation (fatty) mass is visible in the region of the atrial septum *(arrow)*, compressing both the right atrium *(RA)* and the left atrium *(LA)*. This abnormality is usually of no consequence, and this patient had no cardiac symptoms.

bifurcation into the left anterior descending and circumflex arteries. The *right coronary artery* arises from the anterior aorta (at about the 11 o'clock position) slightly caudal to the left main artery and extends anteriorly and inferiorly in the atrioventricular groove. Left anterior descending artery calcification almost always predominates.

The extent of CAC correlates with the presence of significant coronary artery disease and cardiac death, but also correlates with patient age and sex. Although the absence of visible coronary artery calcification does not exclude the possibility of obstructive coronary artery plaque, the risk is very low.

Dedicated ECG-gated unenhanced CT may be performed to evaluate the coronary arteries for precise quantitation of CAC. Calcification is graded with a computerized numerical scoring system (Agatston score), and the calcium score is predictive of coronary artery disease and the risk of death.

Scoring of CAC is not generally performed on routine chest CT scans, but computerized Agatston scoring may be done and correlates well with ECG-gated

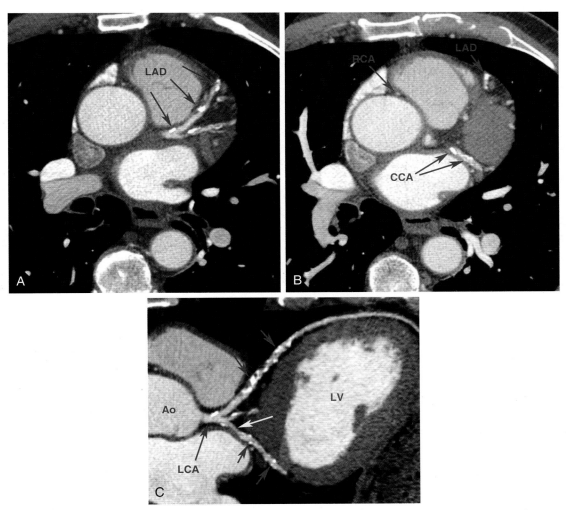

FIG. 3.35 **Coronary artery calcification and CT coronary angiography.** (A) Electrocardiogram-gated contrast-enhanced CT shows calcification of the left anterior descending coronary artery *(LAD)* and a branch. (B) At a lower level, calcification *(arrows)* of the left anterior descending coronary artery *(LAD)* and circumflex coronary artery *(CCA)* is visible. The right coronary artery *(RCA)* is noncalcified. (C) A curved reconstruction showing the left coronary artery *(LCA)* and the left anterior descending coronary artery and circumflex coronary artery along their axes. Multiple calcifications are visible *(red arrows)*. A noncalcified stenosis of the circumflex coronary artery *(yellow arrow)* is also shown. *Ao,* Aorta; *LV,* left ventricle.

CT. Simple visual estimation of CAC as absent, mild, moderate, or heavy correlates with the likelihood of coronary-related death; in a study of patients undergoing CT for lung cancer screening, the hazard ratios were 2, 3.8, and 6.9 for mild, moderate, and heavy CAC, respectively, when compared with patients without CAC. It has been recommended by some that such visual assessment be reported on unenhanced CT scans in patients aged 40 years or older.

Coronary CT angiography can be performed with ECG gating, contrast enhancement, and various reconstructions (including curved planar reconstruction) to demonstrate the coronary arteries along their length, regardless of their actual three-dimensional course (Fig. 3.35). Both calcified plaque (hard plaque) and noncalcified plaque (soft plaque) can be demonstrated, and correlation with catheter coronary arteriography is good.

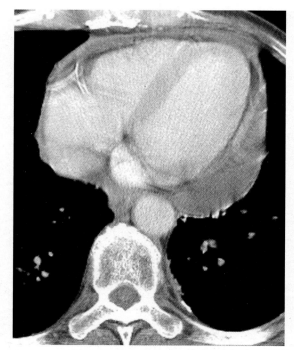

FIG. 3.36 Pericardial effusion from metastatic lung cancer. Fluid accumulates first in the dependent portions of the pericardium, posterior to the left ventricle. In this patient, most of the fluid has accumulated in this region.

Routine CT or coronary CT angiography may demonstrate coronary artery anomalies (incidence <1%). Many are innocuous, but others can be clinically significant, resulting in chest pain and the possibility of sudden death. These require surgical correction (see Suggested Reading).

Pericardial Effusion, Thickening, and Fibrosis

Pericardial effusion results in thickening of the normal pericardial stripe. Fluid first accumulates in the dependent portions of the pericardium, typically posterior to the left ventricle (Fig. 3.36). As the effusion increases in size, it is visible lateral and anterior to the right atrium and right ventricle; when it is large, it appears as a concentric opacity surrounding the heart. Large effusions can also extend into the superior pericardial recess. Exudative effusions are higher in attenuation than transudative effusions.

The presence of *cardiac tamponade*, associated with pericardial effusion, may be more directly related to the speed at which the fluid accumulates and the distensibility of the pericardium than the size of the effusion

alone. CT findings sometimes associated with cardiac tamponade include dilatation of the SVC or inferior vena cava, hepatic veins, and reflux of contrast medium into the azygos vein or inferior vena cava. None of these findings are specific.

The pericardium is normally 2 mm or less in thickness. Pericardial thickening or fibrosis is usually the result of inflammation. With contrast medium infusion, enhancement of the thickened pericardium may be seen. Pericardial thickening may also be denser than pericardial fluid, even without contrast medium infusion. Thickening may be smooth, irregular, or focal and nodular. Calcification can occur, particularly as a result of tuberculosis, purulent pericarditis, or hemopericardium.

In the presence of symptoms of *constrictive pericarditis* the CT appearance of a normal pericardium rules out the diagnosis, whereas a thickened pericardium (>4 mm) allows a presumptive diagnosis of constriction to be made, and a thickened pericardium of more than 5 to 6 mm is specific. Calcification is also helpful in making the diagnosis. In some patients the pericardium appears normal. Flattening of underlying cardiac chambers, particularly the right ventricle, may be seen.

In the presence of *pericardial metastases*, CT can show an effusion (Fig. 3.36) or nodular masses may be visible, particularly after contrast medium infusion.

SUGGESTED READING

Agarwal, P. P., Chughtai, A., Matzinger, F. R. K., & Kazerooni, E. A. (2009). Multidetector CT of thoracic aortic aneurysms. *Radiographics, 29,* 537–552.

Albrecht, M. H., Bickford, M. W., Nance, J. W., et al. (2017). State-of-the-art pulmonary CT angiography for acute pulmonary embolism. *AJR American Journal of Roentgenology, 208,* 1–10.

Bastarrika, G., Lee, Y. S., Huda, W., et al. (2009). CT of coronary artery disease. *Radiology, 253,* 317–337.

Batra, P., Bigoni, B., Manning, J., et al. (2000). Pitfalls in the diagnosis of thoracic aortic dissection at CT angiography. *Radiographics, 20,* 309–320.

Bean, M. J., Johnson, P. T., Roseborough, G. S., et al. (2008). Thoracic aortic stent-grafts: Utility of multidetector CT for pre- and postprocedure evaluation. *Radiographics, 28,* 1835–1851.

Bogaert, J., & Francone, M. (2013). Pericardial disease: Value of CT and MR imaging. *Radiology, 267,* 340–356.

Castañer, E., Andreu, M., Gallardo, X., et al. (2003). CT in nontraumatic acute thoracic aortic disease: Typical and atypical features and complications. *Radiographics, 23,* S93–S110.

Castañer, E., Gallardo, X., Ballesteros, E., et al. (2009). CT diagnosis of chronic pulmonary thromboembolism. *Radiographics, 29,* 31–53.

Chiles, C., Duan, F., Gladish, G. W., et al. (2015). Association of coronary artery calcification and mortality in the National Lung Screening Trial: A comparison of three scoring methods. *Radiology, 76*, 82–90.

Chiu, V., & O'Connell, C. (2017). Management of the incidental pulmonary embolism. *AJR American Journal of Roentgenology, 208*, 485–488.

Grosse, C., & Grosse, A. (2010). CT findings in diseases associated with pulmonary hypertension: A current review. *Radiographics, 30*, 1753–1777.

Hanneman, K., Newman, B., & Chan, F. (2017). Congenital variants and anomalies of the aortic arch. *Radiographics, 37*, 32–51.

Hecht, H. S., Cronin, P., Blaha, M. J., et al. (2017). 2016 SCCT/STR guidelines for coronary artery calcium scoring of noncontrast noncardiac chest CT scans: A report of the Society of Cardiovascular Computed Tomography and Society of Thoracic Radiology. *Journal of Cardiovascular Computed Tomography, 11*, 74–84.

Kim, S. Y., Seo, J. B., Do, K. H., et al. (2006). Coronary artery anomalies: Classification and ECG-gated multi–detector row CT findings with angiographic correlation. *Radiographics, 26*, 317–334.

Moores, L. K., Jackson, W. L., Jr., Shorr, A. F., & Jackson, J. L. (2004). Meta-analysis: outcomes in patients with suspected pulmonary embolism managed with computed tomographic pulmonary angiography. *Annals of Internal Medicine, 141*, 866–874.

Raja, A. S., Greenberg, J. O., Qaseem, A., et al. (2015). Evaluation of patients with suspected acute pulmonary embolism: Best practice advice from the clinical guidelines committee of the American College of Physicians. *Annals of Internal Medicine, 163*, 701–711.

Sonavane, S. K., Milner, D. M., Singh, S. P., et al. (2015). Comprehensive imaging review of the superior vena cava. *Radiographics, 35*, 1873–1892.

Yan, Z., Ip, I. K., Raja, A. S., et al. (2017). Yield of CT pulmonary angiography in the emergency department when providers override evidence-based clinical decision support. *Radiology, 282*, 717–725.

CHAPTER 4

Mediastinum: Lymph Node Abnormalities and Masses

W. RICHARD WEBB

LYMPH NODE GROUPS

Mediastinal lymph nodes are generally classified by location. Most descriptive systems are based on a modification of Rouvière's classification of lymph node groups. The names used in describing lymph nodes groups for the purpose of lung cancer staging may differ and are reviewed in Table 4.1.

Anterior Mediastinal Nodes

Internal mammary nodes are located in a retrosternal location near the internal mammary artery and veins (Fig. 4.1). They drain the anterior chest wall, anterior diaphragm, and medial breasts.

Paracardiac nodes (diaphragmatic, epiphrenic, and pericardial) surround the heart on the surface of the diaphragm and communicate with the lower internal mammary chain (Fig. 4.2). Like internal mammary nodes, they are most commonly enlarged in patients with lymphoma and metastatic carcinoma, particularly breast cancer.

Prevascular nodes lie anterior to the great vessels (Figs. 4.1, 4.3, and 4.4A). They may be involved in a variety of diseases, notably lymphoma, but their involvement in lung cancer is less common.

Middle Mediastinal Nodes

Lung diseases (e.g., lung cancer, sarcoidosis, tuberculosis, and fungal infections) that secondarily involve lymph nodes typically involve middle mediastinal lymph nodes.

Pretracheal or *paratracheal nodes* occupy the pretracheal (or anterior paratracheal) space (Figs. 4.1, 4.3, and 4.4A). These nodes form the final pathway for lymphatic drainage from most of both lungs (except the left upper lobe). Because of this, they are commonly abnormal regardless of the location of lung disease.

Aortopulmonary nodes are considered by Rouvière to be in the anterior mediastinal group, but they serve the same function as right paratracheal nodes (Figs. 4.3C and 4.4B and C). The left upper lobe is drained by this node group.

Subcarinal nodes are located in the subcarinal space, between the main bronchi (Fig. 4.4B–D), and drain the inferior hila and both lower lobes. They communicate in turn with the right paratracheal chain.

Peribronchial nodes surround the main bronchi on each side (Fig. 4.4B and C). They communicate with bronchopulmonary (hilar; Fig. 4.4C and D), subcarinal, and paratracheal nodes.

Posterior Mediastinal Nodes

Paraesophageal nodes lie posterior to the trachea or are associated with the esophagus, or both (Fig. 4.5). Subcarinal nodes are not included in this group.

Inferior pulmonary ligament nodes are located below the pulmonary hila, medial to the inferior pulmonary ligament. On CT, they are usually seen adjacent to the esophagus on the right and the descending aorta on the left. Below the hila, they are difficult to distinguish from paraesophageal nodes. Together with the paraesophageal nodes, they drain the medial lower lobes, esophagus, pericardium, and posterior diaphragm.

Paravertebral nodes lie lateral to the vertebral bodies, posterior to the aorta on the left (Fig. 4.5). They drain the posterior chest wall and pleura. They are most commonly involved, together with the retrocrural or retroperitoneal abdominal nodes, in patients with lymphoma or metastatic carcinoma.

Lymph Node Stations

Several numerical systems have been proposed for identifying the specific locations of intrathoracic lymph nodes (i.e., *lymph node stations*), primarily for the purpose of lung cancer staging. In 1997 the American Thoracic Society (ATS) published a classification of 14 lymph node stations, with precise anatomic and

TABLE 4.1
Relationship of the International Association for the Study of Lung Cancer Lymph Node Zones to the American Thoracic Society Lymph Node Stations

IASLC Nodal Zones	ATS Description	ATS Station
Mediastinal zone		
Upper zone	Right upper paratracheal	2R
	Left upper paratracheal	2L
	Prevascular	3
	Right lower paratracheal	4R
	Left lower paratracheal	4L
Aortopulmonary zone	Subaortic	5
	Paraaortic	6
Subcarinal zone	Subcarinal	7
Lower zone	Paraesophageal	8
	Pulmonary ligament	9
Hilar/interlobar zone	Hilar	10
	Interlobar	11
Peripheral zone	Lobar	12
	Segmental	13
	Subsegmental	14

ATS, American Thoracic Society; *IASLC*, International Association for the Study of Lung Cancer.

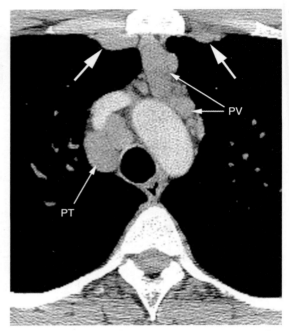

FIG. 4.1 **Internal mammary lymph node enlargement in sarcoidosis.** Bilateral internal mammary nodes *(large arrows)* are enlarged, as are pretracheal *(PT)* and prevascular *(PV)* nodes.

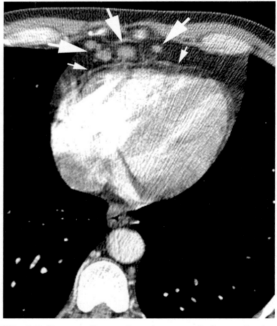

FIG. 4.2 **Paracardiac node enlargement.** In a patient with Hodgkin lymphoma, enlargement of the paracardiac nodes *(large arrows)* is visible. These lie anterior to the pericardium *(small arrows).*

CT criteria, which has been in common usage since its description, for the localization of lymph node abnormalities in a variety of diseases.

In 2009 the International Association for the Study of Lung Cancer (IASLC) introduced a simplified system for classifying lymph nodes, based on lung cancer survival statistics, for use in lung cancer staging (Table 4.1). This system classifies mediastinal nodes into four groups or *zones* known as (1) the *upper zone* (paratracheal and prevascular nodes), (2) the *aortopulmonary zone* (aortopulmonary window nodes), (3) the *subcarinal zone* (subcarinal nodes), and (4) the *lower zone* (paraesophageal and inferior pulmonary ligament nodes). In addition, the IASLC system includes the *supraclavicular zone* (right and left supraclavicular lymph nodes), the *hilar/interlobar zone* (hilar lymph

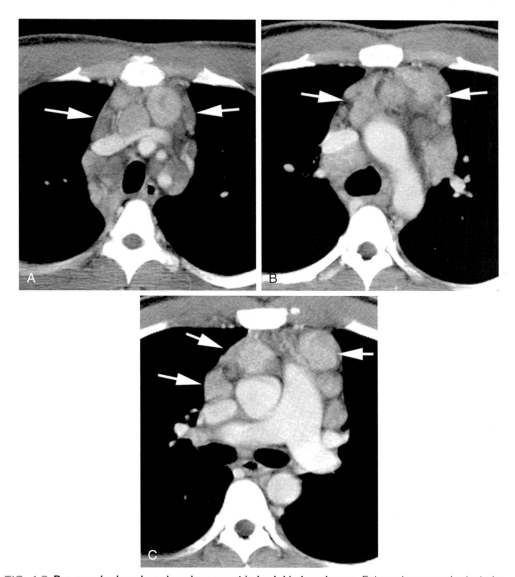

FIG. 4.3 **Prevascular lymph node enlargement in hodgkin lymphoma.** Enlarged prevascular (anterior mediastinal) lymph nodes *(arrows)* are seen anterior to the brachiocephalic veins and aortic branches (A), anterior to the aortic arch and superior vena cava (B), and anterior to the superior vena cava, aortic root, and main pulmonary artery (C). Enlarged pretracheal lymph nodes are also visible in (A) and (B). Some nodes appear low in attenuation and are probably necrotic.

nodes), and the *peripheral zone* (lobar, segmental and subsegmental nodes). Table 4.1 provides a comparison of IASLC zones and ATS lymph node stations, and Fig. 4.6 shows a diagrammatic representation of ATS lymph node stations and comparable IASLC lymph node zones. Detailed knowledge of these lymph node stations and zones is not necessary in routine clinical practice.

CT APPEARANCE OF LYMPH NODES

Lymph nodes are generally visible as discrete opacities, round or elliptical in shape, of soft-tissue attenuation, surrounded by mediastinal fat, and distinguishable from vessels by their location. They often occur in clusters (Fig. 4.7). In some locations, nodes that contact vessels may be difficult to identify without contrast medium infusion. Normal lymph nodes may show a fatty hilum (Fig. 4.7).

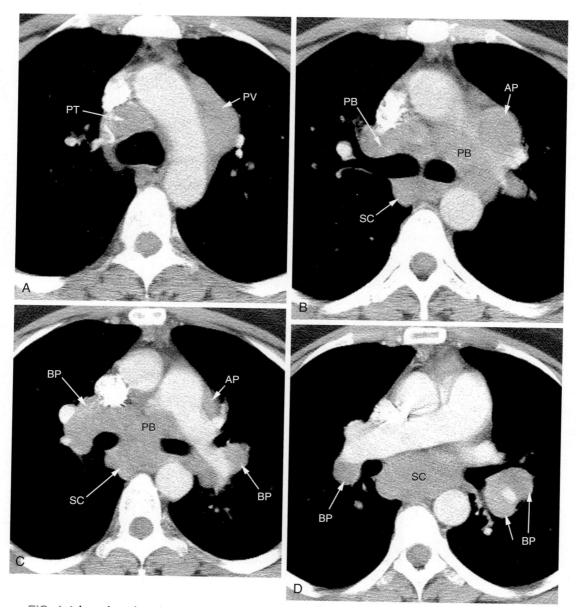

FIG. 4.4 **Lymph node enlargement in a patient with sarcoidosis.** (A) At the aortic arch level, enlarged pretracheal *(PT)* and prevascular *(PV)* nodes are visible. (B) At the level of the tracheal carina, *aortopulmonary (AP)* lymph nodes lie lateral to the left pulmonary artery. Lymph nodes adjacent to the main bronchi are termed *peribronchial (PB)*. Subcarinal *(SC)* lymph nodes are located posterior to the carina. (C) At a lower level, aortopulmonary *(AP)*, peribronchial *(PB)*, and subcarinal *(SC)* nodes are again visible. Hilar lymph nodes are termed *bronchopulmonary (BP)*. (D) Below (C) large subcarinal *(SC)* and bronchopulmonary *(BP)* nodes are again visible.

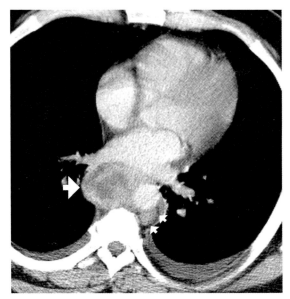

FIG. 4.5 **Paraesophageal lymph node enlargement in metastatic testicular carcinoma.** Large lymph nodes on the right *(large arrow)* can be considered paraesophageal or inferior pulmonary ligament nodes. They appear inhomogeneous and are necrotic. An enlarged left paravertebral lymph node *(small arrows)* is also visible posterior to the aorta.

Lymph Node Size

The *short-axis* or *least diameter* (i.e., the smallest node diameter seen in cross section) is generally used when one is measuring the size of a lymph node. Measuring the short-axis diameter is better than measuring the *long-axis* or *greatest diameter* because it more closely reflects the actual node diameter when nodes are obliquely oriented relative to the scan plane and shows less variation among healthy individuals.

Normal lymph nodes are commonly visible on CT. They differ in size, depending on their location. There are a few general rules:

- Subcarinal nodes can be large in healthy individuals.
- Pretracheal nodes are typically smaller than subcarinal nodes.
- Right paratracheal (pretracheal) nodes are usually larger than left-sided nodes.
- Upper mediastinum nodes are usually smaller than nodes nearer the carina.
- Internal mammary nodes, paracardiac nodes, and paravertebral nodes measure only a few millimeters.

Different values for the upper limits of normal short-axis node diameter have been found for different mediastinal node groups (Table 4.2). However, except for the subcarinal regions, a short-axis node diameter of 1 cm or less is generally considered normal for clinical purposes. In the subcarinal region, 1.5 cm is usually considered to be the upper limit of normal.

Lymph Node Enlargement

Except in the subcarinal space, lymph nodes are considered to be enlarged if they have a short-axis diameter greater than 1 cm. In most cases, abnormal nodes are outlined by fat and are visible as discrete structures (Fig. 4.3). However, in the presence of inflammation or neoplastic infiltration, abnormal nodes can be matted together, giving the appearance of a single large mass or resulting in infiltration and replacement of mediastinal fat by soft-tissue opacity.

The significance given to the presence of an enlarged lymph node must be tempered by knowledge of the patient's clinical situation. For example, if the patient is known to have lung cancer, then an enlarged lymph node has a 70% likelihood of tumor involvement. However, the same node in a patient without lung cancer is much less likely to be of clinical significance. In the absence of a known disease, an enlarged node must be regarded as likely hyperplastic or reactive.

On the other hand, the larger a node is, the more likely it is to represent a significant abnormality. Mediastinal lymph nodes larger than 2 cm are often involved by tumor, although large lymph nodes may also be seen in patients with sarcoidosis or other granulomatous diseases.

Lymph Node Calcification

Lymph node calcification can be dense, homogeneous, focal, stippled, or *eggshell* (ring-like) in appearance. The abnormal nodes are often enlarged but can also be of normal size. Multiple calcified lymph nodes are often visible, usually in contiguity.

Lymph node calcification usually indicates prior granulomatous disease, including tuberculosis, histoplasmosis and other fungal infections, and sarcoidosis (Fig. 4.8). The differential diagnosis also includes silicosis, coal workers' pneumoconiosis, treated Hodgkin disease, metastatic neoplasm, typically mutinous adenocarcinoma, thyroid carcinoma, or metastatic osteogenic sarcoma. Eggshell calcification is most often seen in patients with silicosis or coal workers' pneumoconiosis, sarcoidosis, and tuberculosis.

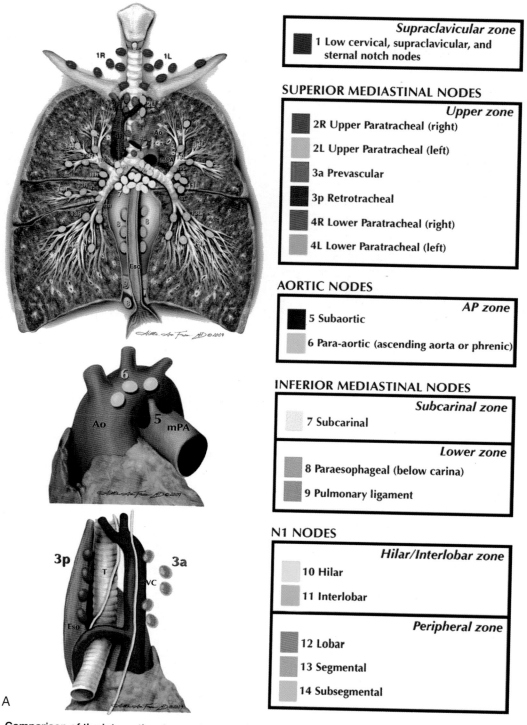

Supraclavicular zone
1 Low cervical, supraclavicular, and sternal notch nodes

SUPERIOR MEDIASTINAL NODES

Upper zone
2R Upper Paratracheal (right)
2L Upper Paratracheal (left)
3a Prevascular
3p Retrotracheal
4R Lower Paratracheal (right)
4L Lower Paratracheal (left)

AORTIC NODES

AP zone
5 Subaortic
6 Para-aortic (ascending aorta or phrenic)

INFERIOR MEDIASTINAL NODES

Subcarinal zone
7 Subcarinal

Lower zone
8 Paraesophageal (below carina)
9 Pulmonary ligament

N1 NODES

Hilar/Interlobar zone
10 Hilar
11 Interlobar

Peripheral zone
12 Lobar
13 Segmental
14 Subsegmental

FIG. 4.6 **Comparison of the international association for the study of lung cancer lymph node map and american thoracic society lymph node stations.** (A) The numbered American Thoracic Society (ATS) lymph node stations and International Association for the Study of Lung Cancer (IASLC) lymph nodes zones. Stations 3a and 3p do not appear in the ATS system, but represent terminology used by the Japan Lung Cancer Society (JLCS); ATS station 3 corresponds to JLCS 3a.

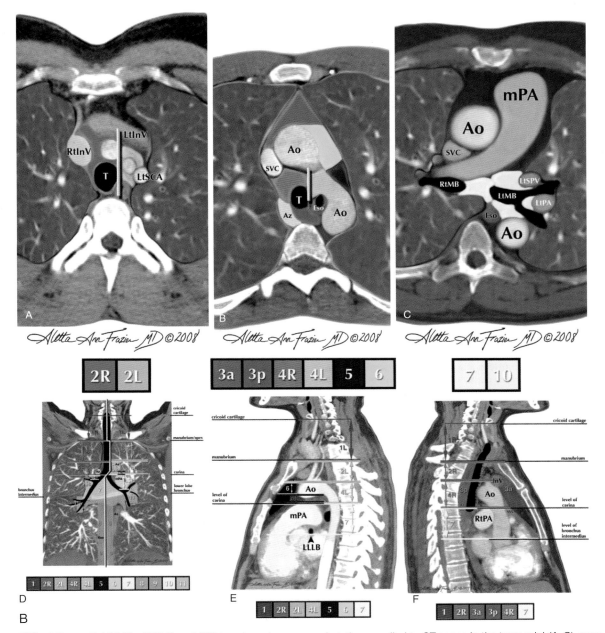

FIG. 4.6, cont'd (B) The IASLC and ATS lymph node zones and stations applied to CT scans in the transaxial *(A–C),* coronal *(D),* and sagittal *(E, F)* planes. The border between the right and left paratracheal region is shown in *A* and *B. Ao,* Aorta; *AP,* aortopulmonary; *AV,* azygos vein; *Az,* azygos arch; *Br,* bronchus; *Eso,* esophagus; *IA,* innominate artery; *InV,* innominate vein; *LLLB,* left lower lobe bronchus; *LtInV,* left innominate vein; *LtMB,* left main bronchus; *LtPA,* left pulmonary artery; *LtSCA,* left subclavian artery; *LtSPV,* left superior pulmonary vein; *mPA,* main pulmonary artery; *RtInV,* right innominate vein; *RtMB,* right main bronchus; *RtPA,* right pulmonary artery; *SCV,* superior vena cava; *T,* trachea. (Reprinted from Rusch, V. W., Asamura, H., Watanabe, H., et al. (2009). The IASLC Lung Cancer Staging Project. A proposal for a new international lymph node map in the forthcoming seventh edition of the TNM classification for lung cancer. *J Thorac Oncol,* 4, 568–577; with permission.)

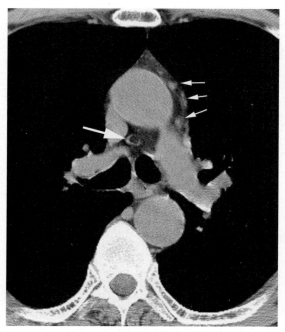

FIG. 4.7 **Normal mediastinal nodes.** Small lymph nodes are visible in the aortopulmonary window *(small arrows)* with a short-axis diameter of less than 1 cm. A normal pretracheal lymph node *(large arrow)* contains a large amount of fat.

TABLE 4.2
Upper Limits of Normal for the Short-Axis Node Diameter

Node Group	Short-Axis Node Diameter[a] (mm)
Supra-aortic paratracheal	7
Subaortic paratracheal	9
Aortopulmonary window	9
Prevascular	8
Subcarinal	12
Paraesophageal	8

[a]Mean normal node diameter plus two standard deviations.

Low-Attenuation or Necrotic Lymph Nodes

Enlarged lymph nodes may appear to be low in attenuation (Fig. 4.5), often with an enhancing rim if contrast medium has been injected. Typically, low-attenuation nodes reflect the presence of necrosis. They are commonly seen in patients with active tuberculosis, fungal infections, and neoplasms, such as metastatic carcinoma and lymphoma.

Lymph Node Enhancement

Normal lymph nodes may show some increase in attenuation after intravenous contrast medium infusion. Pathologic lymph nodes with an increased vascular supply may increase significantly in attenuation. The differential diagnosis of densely enhanced mediastinal nodes is limited and includes metastatic neoplasm (e.g., lung cancer, breast cancer, renal cell carcinoma, papillary thyroid carcinoma, sarcoma, and melanoma), Castleman disease (Fig. 4.9), infections such as tuberculosis, and sometimes sarcoidosis.

LUNG CANCER

Approximately 35% of patients in whom lung cancer has been diagnosed have mediastinal node metastases (Fig. 4.10). Lung cancer most often involves the middle mediastinal node groups. Cancers of the left upper lobe typically metastasize to aortopulmonary window nodes, whereas tumors involving the lower lobes tend to metastasize to the subcarinal and right paratracheal groups. Tumors of the right upper lobe typically involve paratracheal nodes.

Lymph Node Metastases in Lung Cancer

In patients with lung cancer the likelihood that a mediastinal node is involved by tumor is directly proportional to its size. However, although enlarged nodes are most likely to be involved by tumor (Fig. 4.10), they can be benign; similarly, although small nodes are usually normal, they can harbor metastases. Although a short-axis measurement of greater than 1 cm is used in clinical practice to identify abnormally enlarged nodes, it is important to realize that no node diameter clearly separates benign nodes from those involved by tumor.

With use of a short-axis node diameter of 1 cm as the upper limit of node size, CT will detect mediastinal lymph node enlargement in about 60% of patients with node metastases (CT sensitivity), whereas about 70% of patients with normal nodes will be classified as normal on CT (CT specificity). Although CT is not highly accurate in diagnosing node metastases, it is commonly used to guide subsequent procedures or treatment.

In contrast, if mediastinal lymph node enlargement is seen on CT, about 70% of patients will have node metastases; benign hyperplasia of mediastinal lymph nodes accounts for the other 30%. Patients with large mediastinal nodes may undergo node sampling at mediastinoscopy or by CT-guided needle biopsy before surgery.

Positron emission tomography (PET) is more accurate than CT in the assessment of mediastinal lymph node metastases in lung cancer and has assumed a significant

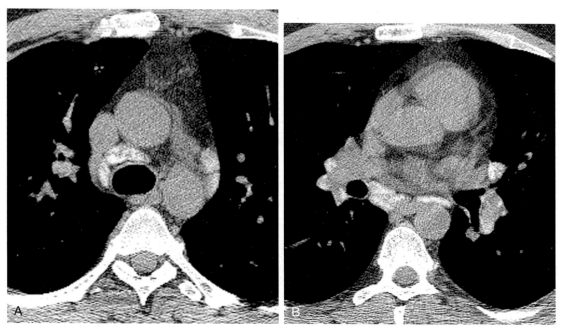

FIG. 4.8 **Lymph node calcification in sarcoidosis.** (A and B) Enlarged lymph nodes show homogeneous and stippled calcification. Pretracheal, aortopulmonary, subcarinal, and hilar lymph nodes are involved.

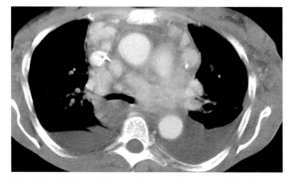

FIG. 4.9 **Multicentric castleman disease.** Extensive enhanced mediastinal lymphadenopathy in a patient with multicentric Castleman disease. The enhancement is typical of unicentric or multicentric Castleman disease. Enlarged axillary, abdominal, and inguinal lymph nodes are also visible. Bilateral pleural effusions are also present.

role in preoperative staging. PET has a sensitivity of about 80% for diagnosis of mediastinal node metastases (vs. 60% for CT) and a specificity of about 90% (compared with 70% for CT). PET is often combined with CT (PET-CT) because of the poor anatomic detail provided by PET alone. In a patient with lung cancer, PET-CT is commonly done rather than a routine CT in staging.

Lung Cancer Staging

In patients with non–small cell lung carcinoma, the genetics, cell type, and histologic characteristics of the tumor affect prognosis, but the anatomic extent of the tumor (tumor stage) is usually most important in determining the therapeutic approach and the use of chemotherapy, radiation therapy, and/or surgery. Lung cancer is staged by a TNM system, based on consideration of (1) the size, location, and extent of the primary tumor (T); (2) the presence or absence of lymph node metastases (N); and (3) the presence or absence of distant metastases (M). Tumor stage (I, II, III, or IV, with subdivisions) is based on specific groupings of T, N, and M categories and subcategories. With this classification, excellent correlations are found between tumor stage and survival after treatment.

The eighth edition of the lung cancer TNM staging system (TNM-8) has recently been published and is based on analysis of more than 75,000 lung cancer patients; the staging system was last revised in 2009 (TNM-7). A somewhat condensed and edited version of the TNM-8 categories is provided in Tables 4.3 and 4.4, and the reader is referred to Suggested Reading (Rami-Porta et al.) for a detailed review.

No changes were made in lymph node categories in TNM-8, although it has been shown that the number

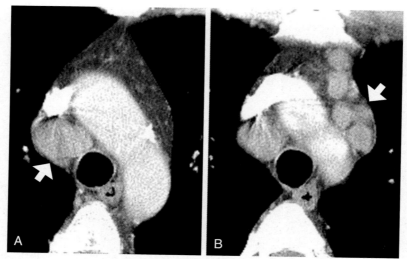

FIG. 4.10 Lymph node enlargement in a patient with a right-sided bronchogenic carcinoma. (A) Lymph node enlargement in the pretracheal space *(arrow)* is ipsilateral, N2, and potentially resectable. These nodes are large, and thus are likely involved by tumor. (B) Lymph node enlargement in the prevascular space *(arrow)* is contralateral, N3, and considered unresectable.

TABLE 4.3
TNM Classification of Lung Cancer (Eighth Edition, 2017)

T (PRIMARY TUMOR)

T0	No evidence of primary tumor
Tis	Carcinoma in situ: adenocarcinoma in situ or squamous cell carcinoma in situ
T1	A tumor that is:
	a. 3 cm or less in greatest diameter
	T1mi minimally invasive adenocarcinoma[a]
	T1a ≤1 cm[a]
	T1b >1 cm but ≤2 cm[a]
	T1c >2 cm but ≤3 cm[a]
	b. surrounded by lung or visceral pleura
	c. without invasion proximal to a lobar bronchus (i.e., not involving a main bronchus)
T2	A tumor with any of the following features:
	a. larger than 3 cm and less than or equal to 5 cm in greatest diameter[a]
	T2a >3 cm but ≤4 cm[a]
	T2b > 4 cm but ≤5 cm[a]
	b. invades the visceral pleura
	c. involves a main bronchus without involving the carina[a]
	d. associated with atelectasis or obstructive pneumonia, extending to the hilum, and involving part of or the entire lung[a]

TABLE 4.3
TNM Classification of Lung Cancer (Eighth Edition, 2017)—cont'd

T3	A tumor with any of the following features:
	a. larger than 5 cm and less than or equal to 7 cm in greatest diameter[a]
	b. associated with separate tumor nodule(s) in the same lobe
	c. invades parietal pleura, chest wall, phrenic nerve, or parietal pericardium[a]
T4	A tumor with any of the following features:
	a. more than 7 cm in greatest diameter[a]
	b. invasion of the diaphragm, mediastinum, heart, great vessels, trachea, carina, recurrent laryngeal nerve, esophagus, or vertebral body
	c. separate tumor nodule(s) in an ipsilateral lobe different from that of the primary tumor
N (REGIONAL LYMPH NODES)	
N0	No regional lymph node metastases
N1	Metastases to ipsilateral peribronchial and/or hilar and intrapulmonary nodes, including direct extension
N2	Metastases to ipsilateral mediastinal nodes and/or subcarinal nodes
N3	Metastases to contralateral hilar or mediastinal lymph nodes, or scalene or supraclavicular lymph nodes
M (DISTANT METASTASES)	
M0	Metastases absent
M1	Metastases present
	M1a intrathoracic metastases, with either
	a. tumor nodules in the contralateral lung
	b. tumor with pleural nodules or malignant pleural or pericardial effusion (pleural effusion not obviously associated with metastases has no effect on stage)
	M1b single extrathoracic metastasis; involvement of single distant lymph node[a]
	M1c multiple extrathoracic metastases in one or more organs[a]

[a]Changes from the seventh edition.
Modified from Rami-Porta, R., Asamura, A., Travis, W. D., Rusch, V. W. (2017). Lung cancer — major changes in the American Joint Committee on Cancer eighth edition cancer staging manual. *CA Cancer J Clin, 67,* 138–155.

of nodal zones or stations involved impacts prognosis. In TNM-8 (as in TNM-7) lung lymph node (N) designations are as follows:

- *N0:* absence of regional lymph node metastases;
- *N1:* metastasis to ipsilateral peribronchial and/or hilar or intrapulmonary lymph nodes;
- *N2:* metastasis to ipsilateral mediastinal and/or subcarinal lymph nodes;
- *N3:* metastasis to contralateral mediastinal or hilar nodes; or scalene or supraclavicular nodes on either side.

In routine practice a precise classification of tumor stage is not usually necessary. However, differentiation of potentially resectable stages (stage I to stage IIIa) and stages usually considered unresectable (stage IIIb to stage IV) is important (Table 4.4). Keep in mind that

the criteria for resectability are generally accepted, but are not absolute, and depend on several factors.

N0 and N1 nodes, in and of themselves, are considered resectable. N2 lymph nodes are considered potentially resectable (although this is not always the case). N3 nodes are considered unresectable (Fig. 4.10). In the absence of metastases (M1a–M1c), the following rules apply:

- N0 or N1 nodes, depending on the primary tumor, may be part of stage I, II, or IIIa.
- N2 nodes, depending on the primary tumor, may be part of stage IIIa or IIIb.
- N3 nodes are associated with stage IIIc.

A number of changes regarding primary tumor descriptors and stage classification were made in TNM-8 (Tables 4.3 and 4.4). However, a discussion of lung

TABLE 4.4
Lung Cancer Stage Based on TNM classification (Eighth Edition, 2017)

Stage	T	N	M
0	Tis	N0	M0
IA1	T1mi	N0	M0
	T1a	N0	M0
IA2	T1b	N0	M0
IA3	T1c	N0	M0
IB	T2a	N0	M0
IIA	T2b	N0	M0
IIB	T1a,b,c	N1	M0
	T2a,b	N1	M0
	T3	N0	M0
IIIA	T1a,b,c	N2	M0
	T2a,b	N2	M0
	T3	N1	M0
	T4	N0, N1	M0
IIIB	T1a,b,c	N3	M0
	T2a,b	N3	M0
	T3, T4	N2	M0
IIIC	T3, T4	N3	M0
IVA	Any T	Any N	M1a,b
IVA	Any T	Any N	M1c

Modified from Rami-Porta, R., Asamura, A., Travis, W. D., Rusch, V. W. (2017). Lung cancer — major changes in the American Joint Committee on Cancer eighth edition cancer staging manual. *CA Cancer J Clin, 67*, 138–155.

cancer staging in this chapter is limited to a review of lymph node metastases and mediastinal invasion. Other important findings in staging lung cancer are discussed in other chapters. These include hilar lymph node enlargement and hilar mass (Chapter 5), primary tumor characteristics (Chapter 6), and pleural and chest wall invasion (Chapter 7).

Mediastinal Invasion by Lung Cancer

Lung cancer can invade the mediastinum by direct extension, resulting in a mediastinal mass contiguous with the primary tumor. In TNM-8, invasions of the parietal pleura, parietal pericardium, phrenic nerve, or chest wall are termed *T3*, and in the absence of mediastinal lymph node metastases are classified as stage IIB

or IIIA (Table 4.4). Invasions of the diaphragm, mediastinum, heart, great vessels, trachea, carina, esophagus, recurrent laryngeal nerve, or vertebral body are termed *T4*, and in the absence of mediastinal lymph node metastases are classified as stage IIIA. Stage IIIA tumors are potentially resectable.

How accurate is CT in predicting mediastinal invasion? An obvious finding is that a lung mass not contacting the mediastinum is not invasive, and this is an important use of CT.

CT findings of mediastinal invasion (Fig. 4.11) include:
- replacement of mediastinal fat by tumor (i.e., soft tissue);
- compression, displacement, or obstruction of mediastinal structures;
- extensive contact of tumor with a mediastinal structure, such as the aorta or trachea (e.g., one-quarter or more of its circumference);
- obliteration of the fat planes normally seen adjacent to mediastinal structures;
- pericardial thickening associated with a mass.

LYMPHOMA, LEUKEMIA, AND LYMPHOPROLIFERATIVE DISEASES

Neoplasms of lymphoid and hematopoietic tissues, including lymphomas, leukemias, and lymphoproliferative diseases, were classified by the World Health Organization (WHO) in 2008. This complex classification, modified in 2015, consists of more than 50 entities, divided into five categories:
- mature B-cell neoplasms (85% of non-Hodgkin lymphomas)—for example, diffuse large B-cell lymphoma);
- mature T-cell neoplasms (15% of non-Hodgkin lymphomas)—for example, T-cell lymphoblastic lymphoma/leukemia;
- Hodgkin lymphoma (e.g., nodular sclerosis classic Hodgkin lymphoma);
- histiocytic and dendritic cell neoplasms (e.g., histiocytic sarcoma);
- posttransplant lymphoproliferative disorders (PTLDs), various cell types.

In this chapter, mediastinal lymphomas are considered in two groups, Hodgkin lymphoma and non-Hodgkin lymphoma, and only those specific diseases that commonly result in thoracic manifestations are reviewed. Although Hodgkin lymphoma is the less common of the two types, representing about 25% to 30% of cases, it is most common as a cause of mediastinal disease. Pulmonary lymphoma and lymphoproliferative disease are reviewed in Chapter 6.

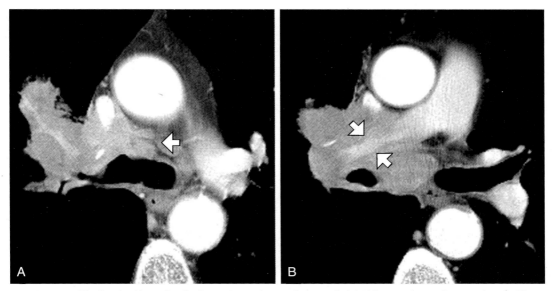

FIG. 4.11 **Mediastinal invasion by bronchogenic carcinoma.** A right hilar carcinoma is associated with extensive mediastinal invasion anterior to the carina (A, *arrow*), with tumor surrounding and narrowing the right pulmonary artery (B, *arrows*). There is extensive replacement of fat by tumor, the tumor surrounds and compresses the pulmonary artery and compresses the vena cava, and fat planes are invisible adjacent to the great vessels.

Revisions to the staging system used for lymphomas were published in 2014 as the "Lugano classification." It describes the anatomic extent of nodal disease at the time of diagnosis, both above and below the diaphragm, the presence of bulky disease, involvement of the spleen, and noncontiguous extralymphatic disease. The Lugano classification recognizes the important role of CT in staging, and the use of PET as routine in the initial evaluation and for assessment of treatment response. PET is used in Hodgkin lymphoma and fluorodeoxyglucose-avid non-Hodgkin lymphoma (almost all cell types). PET increases the accuracy of staging for both nodal and extranodal sites.

Hodgkin Lymphoma

Hodgkin lymphoma, or Hodgkin disease, has a predilection for thoracic nodal involvement. It occurs in patients of all ages but peaks in incidence in the third and fifth decades of life. It is associated with Epstein-Barr virus infection in about half of cases. It may occur in association with AIDS or may be a manifestation of PTLD.

More than 85% of patients with Hodgkin lymphoma develop intrathoracic disease, typically involving superior mediastinum (prevascular, pretracheal, and aortopulmonary lymph nodes) (Table 4.5,

TABLE 4.5
Mediastinal Lymph Node Enlargement in Hodgkin Lymphoma

Site	Abnormal (%)	Visible on CT (%)	Visible on Radiographs (%)
Pretracheal	64	64	57
Aortopulmonary window	62	62	48
Subcarinal	46	44	9
Internal mammary	38	38	4
Posterior medial	18	12	11
Paracardiac	13	10	7

Figs. 4.2, 4.3, and 4.12). An important rule is that intrathoracic lymphadenopathy not associated with superior mediastinal node enlargement is unlikely to be Hodgkin lymphoma. Also involved in Hodgkin lymphoma are subcarinal lymph nodes, internal mammary lymph nodes, and cardiophrenic angle lymph nodes. Internal mammary node enlargement

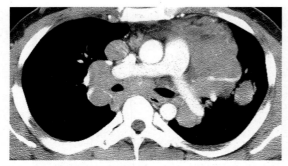

FIG. 4.12 **Hodgkin lymphoma.** Extensive enlargement of mediastinal and hilar lymph nodes is visible. A left lung nodule reflects pulmonary involvement.

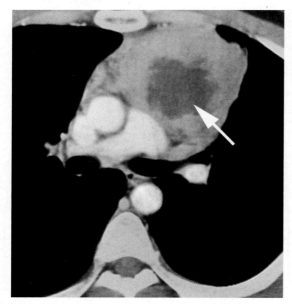

FIG. 4.13 **Anterior mediastinal hodgkin lymphoma with necrosis.** The anterior mediastinal mass contains an irregular area of cystic necrosis *(arrow).*

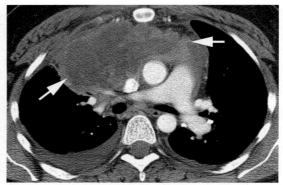

FIG. 4.14 **Lymphoblastic lymphoma involving the anterior mediastinum.** A bulky mediastinal mass *(arrows)* contains areas of low attenuation, likely caused by necrosis. Mediastinal vascular structures are displaced posteriorly. Bilateral pleural effusions are present. Involvement of a single lymph node group is common with non-Hodgkin lymphoma. Lymphoblastic non-Hodgkin lymphoma commonly presents as an anterior mediastinal mass, similar to Hodgkin disease.

with Hodgkin lymphoma can appear cystic or fluid filled on CT (Fig. 4.13). Calcification is unusual and of limited extent, except after treatment.

Non-Hodgkin Lymphoma

Non-Hodgkin lymphoma is a diverse group of diseases that differ in radiologic manifestations, clinical presentation, course, and prognosis. In comparison with Hodgkin lymphoma, these tumors generally occur in an older group of patients (40–70 years of age) and less commonly result in mediastinal abnormalities. At the time of presentation, they often involve multiple sites, and chemotherapy is most appropriate. About 40% of patients with non-Hodgkin lymphoma have intrathoracic disease and 40% of those had involvement of only one node group (Fig. 4.14).

Non-Hodgkin lymphoma may occur as a primary mediastinal mass. The most common cell types presenting in this fashion are *lymphoblastic lymphoma or leukemia* (60% of cases; Fig. 4.14) and *large B-cell lymphoma*. These resemble mediastinal Hodgkin lymphoma, with a large anterior mediastinal mass being present, and they occur in a similar age group, being most common in young patients.

Leukemia

Leukemia, particularly the lymphocytic cell types (e.g., *chronic lymphocytic leukemia*), can result in hilar or mediastinal lymph node enlargement, pleural effusion, and occasionally infiltrative lung disease. Lymphadenopathy is generally confined to the middle mediastinum,

(35% of cases) and cardiophrenic angle lymph node enlargement (10% of cases) are less common in other nodal diseases (Fig. 4.2).

Enlargement of a single node group can be seen with Hodgkin lymphoma, most commonly in the prevascular (anterior) mediastinum. This often indicates the presence of *nodular sclerosis classic Hodgkin lymphoma* histologic type, which accounts for the majority of adult Hodgkin lymphoma.

In patients with Hodgkin lymphoma, mediastinal lymph nodes may become matted, being visible as a single large mass (Fig. 4.13) rather than individual discrete nodes. Mediastinal nodes or masses in patients

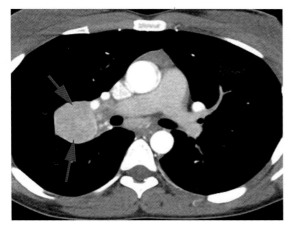

FIG. 4.15 **Unicentric castleman disease in a 19-year-old.** A smoothly marginated, round, enhancing mass *(arrows)* is visible in the right hilum

and the larger masses seen with some lymphomas generally do not occur.

Posttransplant Lymphoproliferative Disorder

Several histologic patterns of lymphocyte proliferation, known collectively as *posttransplant lymphoproliferative disorder* (PTLD), can occur after bone marrow or solid organ transplantation. The histologic patterns range from benign hyperplastic proliferation of lymphocytes to malignant lymphoma, either Hodgkin lymphoma or non-Hodgkin lymphoma.

Most cases of PTLD have been associated with Epstein-Barr virus infection. PTLD affects up to 10% of transplant recipients, most in the first year after transplantation. PTLD can manifest itself as localized or disseminated disease and has a predilection for extranodal involvement. Lung involvement may occur as part of multiorgan disease or in isolation. In 85% of cases, CT shows single or multiple pulmonary nodules, which may be small or large (0.3–5 cm); hilar or mediastinal lymphadenopathy occurs in 5% to 25% of cases.

Castleman Disease

Castleman disease is an unusual lymphoproliferative disease occurring in two primary forms. *Unicentric Castleman disease* accounts for 50% of cases. It is usually characterized by localized enlargement of middle or posterior hilar or mediastinal lymph nodes. A single smooth or lobulated mass, which can be large, is typically visible on CT, with dense opacification after contrast medium infusion (Fig. 4.15). Localized Castleman disease is of unknown cause, is usually asymptomatic, and has a benign course. It is treated surgically.

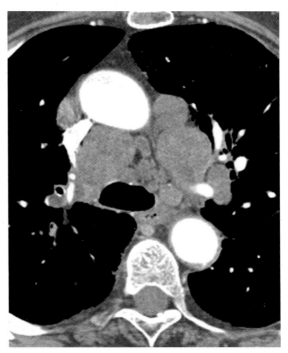

FIG. 4.16 **Extensive mediastinal lymph node metastases in colon carcinoma.** Enlarged lymph nodes are visible in the pretracheal space, prevascular space, and aortopulmonary window. Hilar lymph nodes are also enlarged.

Multicentric Castleman disease (MCD) results in generalized lymph node enlargement, usually involving mediastinal and hilar nodes, and often axillary, abdominal, and inguinal node groups. As with the localized form, marked node enhancement can be seen (Fig. 4.9). MCD is often associated with systemic symptoms and has a progressive course. It may progress to frank lymphoma in some cases. MCD is divided into two groups, each accounting for about half of cases: human herpesvirus 8 (HHV-8)-associated MCD and HHV-8-negative or idiopathic MCD. Patients with HHV-8-associated MCD are often human immunodeficiency virus (HIV) positive. MCD is treated with chemotherapy, which differs depending on the cause.

METASTASES

Extrathoracic tumors can result in mediastinal node enlargement, either with or without hilar or lung metastases (Figs. 4.5 and 4.16). Mediastinal node metastases can be present because of extension from neck masses (thyroid carcinoma and head and neck tumors), extension along lymphatic channels from below the diaphragm (testicular carcinoma, renal cell carcinoma, and gastrointestinal malignancies), or dissemination via other routes (breast carcinoma and melanoma). Middle mediastinal (paratracheal) or paravertebral mediastinal nodes are most commonly involved when the tumor is subdiaphragmatic. With breast carcinoma, internal mammary node metastases occur.

SARCOIDOSIS

Mediastinal lymph node enlargement is common in patients with sarcoidosis, occurring in 60% to 90% of cases. Typically, node enlargement is extensive, involving the hila as well as the mediastinum, and masses appear bilateral and symmetric in most patients (Figs. 4.1, 4.4, and 4.8); this distribution sometimes allows differentiation from lymphoma, which more typically produces asymmetric enlargement. In addition, lymph nodes can be quite large in patients with sarcoidosis, but large isolated masses, as seen in some patients with lymphoma, are uncommon. Paratracheal lymph nodes are typically involved. Even though it is commonly stated that sarcoidosis does not involve anterior mediastinal lymph nodes, anterior mediastinal involvement is often visible on CT; paravertebral node enlargement is visible on occasion (Table 4.6).

INFECTION

A variety of infections can cause mediastinal lymph node enlargement during the acute stage of the infection. These include a number of fungal infections (commonly histoplasmosis and coccidioidomycosis), tuberculosis, bacterial infections, and viral infections. Typically, there will be symptoms and signs of acute infection, and chest radiographs will show evidence of pneumonia.

The lymph node enlargement will often be asymmetric, involving hilar and middle mediastinal nodes. In patients with tuberculosis, enlarged nodes typically show rim enhancement and central necrosis after contrast medium injection; this appearance is nearly diagnostic in patients with an appropriate history. Lymph node calcification occurs in patients with chronic fungal or tuberculous infection.

DIAGNOSIS OF MEDIASTINAL MASSES

The location of a mediastinal mass is fundamental to its differential diagnosis. Although most mediastinal tumors can occur in different parts of the mediastinum, most have characteristic locations (Table 4.7).

Recently, the International Thymic Malignancy Interest Group introduced a new definition of mediastinal compartments, dividing the mediastinum (from the thoracic inlet to the diaphragm) into three compartments, prevascular, visceral, and paravertebral, which largely correspond, respectively, to previous definitions of anterior, middle, and posterior mediastinum. The *prevascular compartment* is defined as located posterior to the sternum and anterior to the pericardium as it surrounds the heart. The *visceral compartment* lies posterior to the prevascular compartment and anterior to a vertical line connecting a point on the thoracic vertebral bodies 1 cm posterior to the anterior margin of the spine. The *paravertebral compartment* is posterior to the visceral compartment and is marginated posterolaterally by a vertical line along the posterior margin of the chest wall at the lateral aspect of the transverse processes. Although these simple divisions are helpful in differential diagnosis, additional anatomic criteria discernable on CT aid in narrowing the differential diagnosis; these are listed in Table 4.7.

Other considerations in differential diagnosis of a mediastinal mass include its extent, whether it comprises a single localized mass or whether multifocal abnormalities are present (i.e., involving several areas of the mediastinum), the shape of the mass (round or lobulated), and additional findings, such as pleural effusion.

Attenuation of a mass (fat, fluid, soft tissue, or a combination of these, and the presence, character, and amount of calcification) is also very important in differential diagnosis (Table 4.8).

Lymph node masses, such as lymphoma, already discussed in this chapter, and abnormalities discussed in other chapters (e.g., aortic aneurysm) are not covered again but are included in Table 4.7.

TABLE 4.6
Sarcoidosis: Frequency of Enlarged Nodes Seen on CT in Patients with Nodes

Node Group	Frequency (%)
Hilar	90
Right paratracheal	100
Aortopulmonary window	90
Subcarinal	65
Anterior mediastinal	50
Posterior mediastinal	15

TABLE 4.7
Differential Diagnosis of Mediastinal Masses Based on Common Sites of Origin

PREVASCULAR COMPARTMENT (ANTERIOR MEDIASTINUM)	VISCERAL COMPARTMENT (MIDDLE MEDIASTINUM)	PARAVERTEBRAL COMPARTMENT (POSTERIOR MEDIASTINUM)

Thymic masses
 Thymoma
 Thymic carcinoma
 Thymic neuroendocrine tumor
 Thymolipoma
 Thymic cyst
 Thymic hyperplasia
 Thymic lymphoma
Germ cell tumors
 Teratoma and dermoid cyst
 Seminoma
 Nonseminomatous germ cell
  tumors
Thyroid abnormalities (goiter and
 neoplasm)
Parathyroid tumor or hyperplasia
Lymph node masses (particularly
 Hodgkin's lymphoma)
Vascular abnormalities (aorta and great
 vessels)
Mesenchymal abnormalities (e.g.,
 lipomatosis, lipoma)
Foregut cyst
Lymphangioma
Hemangioma
Anterior Cardiophrenic Angle
Masses
 Lymph node masses (particularly
  lymphoma and metastases)
 Pericardial cyst
 Fat pad
 Morgagni hernia
 Thymic masses
 Germ cell tumors
	Pretracheal Space
	Lymph node masses
	 Lung carcinoma
	 Sarcoidosis
	 Lymphoma (particularly Hodgkin's
	  disease)
	 Metastases
	 Infections (e.g., tuberculosis)
	Foregut cyst
	Tracheal tumor
	Mesenchymal masses (e.g., lipomato-
	 sis, lipoma)
	Thyroid abnormalities
	Vascular abnormalities (aorta and great
	 vessels)
	Lymphangioma and hemangioma
	Aortopulmonary Window
	Lymph node masses
	 Lung carcinoma
	 Sarcoidosis
	 Lymphoma
	 Metastases
	 Infections (e.g., tuberculosis)
	Mesenchymal masses (e.g., lipomato-
	 sis, lipoma)
	Vascular abnormalities (aorta or pul-
	 monary artery)
	Chemodectoma
	Foregut cyst
	Subcarinal Space and Azygoesoph-
	ageal Recess
	Lymph node masses
	 Lung carcinoma
	 Sarcoidosis
	 Lymphoma
	 Metastases
	 Infections (e.g., tuberculosis)
	Foregut cyst
	Dilated azygos vein
	Esophageal masses
	Varices
	Hernia
		Neurogenic tumor
		 Nerve sheath tumors
		 Sympathetic ganglia tumors
		 Paraganglioma
		Meningocele
		Foregut cyst
		Neurenteric cyst
		Thoracic spine abnormalities
		Extramedullary hematopoiesis
		Fluid collections and pseudocyst
		Vascular abnormalities
		Hernias
		Esophageal masses
		Varices
		Mesenchymal masses (e.g., lipomato-
		 sis, lipoma)
		Lymph node masses
		 Lymphoma (particularly non-
		  Hodgkin lymphoma)
		 Metastases
		Dilated azygos or hemiazygos vein
		Hernia
		Lymphangioma and hemangioma
		Thymic mass or germ cell tumor

PREVASCULAR SPACE MASSES (ANTERIOR MEDIASTINUM)

Masses in the prevascular space, when large, tend to displace the aorta and great arterial branches posteriorly (Fig. 4.14), but distinct compression or narrowing of these relatively thick-walled structures is unusual. Within the supra-aortic mediastinum, displacement, compression, or obstruction of the brachiocephalic veins is common with large masses. In the subaortic mediastinum, posterior displacement or compression of the superior vena cava is typical only with right-sided masses. On the left, compression of the main pulmonary artery can be seen.

TABLE 4.8
Attenuation Characteristics of Mediastinal Masses

Mass	Air	Fat	Water	Tissue	>Tissue*	Calcium
Thymoma	N	N	O	A	N	O
Thymolipoma	N	A	N	C	N	N
Lymphoma (thymic)	N	N	O	A	N	R
Dermoid cyst/teratoma	N	O	O	A	N	O
Germ cell tumor	N	N	R	A	N	R
Thyroid tumor	N	N	O	A	C	C
Lipoma	N	A	N	N	N	N
Hygroma	N	C	C	C	N	N
Cysts (congenital)	R	N	C	O	N	R
Hernia	O	O	N	O	N	N
Lung cancer (nodes)	N	N	O	A	N	N
Tuberculosis (nodes)	N	N	C	A	N	C
Sarcoidosis (nodes)	N	N	R	A	N	O
Castleman disease (nodes)	N	N	N	A	N	O
Neurogenic tumor	N	O	C	C	N	O
Neurenteric cyst	R	N	A	N	N	N
Meningocele	N	N	A	N	N	N
Hematopoiesis	N	O	N	A	N	N

*greater than soft tissue in attenuation, but not obviously calcified. *A*, *always*; *C*, *common*; *O*, *occasionally*; *R*, *rare*; *N*, *never* ("never" does not mean it never happens, but rather that it is so unlikely that practically the radiologist should "never" consider the diagnosis).

Although we are taught that the differential diagnosis of anterior mediastinal masses includes the "4 Ts" (thymoma, teratoma, thyroid tumor, and terrible lymphoma), the differential diagnosis should be extended to include (1) thymoma and *other thymic tumors*, (2) teratoma and *other germ cell tumors*, (3) thyroid masses, (4) lymphoma and *other lymph node masses*, and (5) parathyroid masses, cysts, fatty masses, metastases, and lymphangioma (hygroma).

Thymic Tumors

Tumors of various histologic types arise from cells of thymic origin, including thymoma, thymic carcinoma, thymic carcinoid tumor, thymolipoma, and thymic cyst. Lymphoma may arise in or involve the thymus. Thymic hyperplasia may mimic a mass.

Thymoma

Thymoma is a tumor of thymic epithelial origin and is a common cause of anterior mediastinal masses in adults. Occasionally these lesions arise in the middle or posterior mediastinum. It is difficult to determine if a thymoma is benign or malignant by histologic criteria, but the WHO has developed an alphanumeric histologic classification system (i.e., A, AB, B1–B3, C) that correlates with growth rate (i.e., doubling time) and the likelihood of invasion, metastasis, and survival.

Thymomas are often classified as *invasive* or *noninvasive* on the basis of their appearance at the time of surgery. Approximately 30% of thymomas are pathologically and surgically invasive. Invasion of mediastinal structures or the pleural space is most typical. Distant metastases are not common with invasive thymoma.

From 10% to 30% of patients with myasthenia gravis will be found to have a thymoma, whereas a larger percentage of patients with thymoma (30%–50%) have myasthenia. Other syndromes associated with thymoma include red blood cell hypoplasia and hypogammaglobulinemia.

On CT, thymomas are usually visible in the prevascular space, but they can also be seen in a paracardiac location near the diaphragm. They appear as a localized mass distorting or replacing the normally arrowhead-shaped

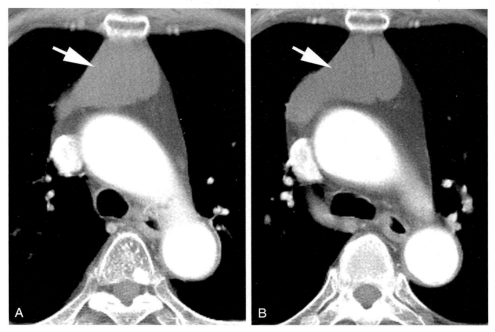

FIG. 4.17 **Noninvasive thymoma.** At two levels (A and B) a large but well-marginated mass involves the right thymic lobe *(arrows)*. A noninvasive thymoma was found during surgery. The left thymic lobe is replaced by fat.

thymus (Fig. 4.17). Often they are predominantly unilateral. Calcification and cystic degeneration can be present. On CT, bilaterality, large size, lobulated contours, poor definition of the tumor margin, obliteration of fat planes, and associated pleural effusion or nodules suggest the presence of an invasive thymoma (Fig. 4.18), but a definite diagnosis is difficult to make on CT.

In patients suspected of having thymoma because of myasthenia gravis, CT can demonstrate tumors that are invisible on plain radiographs. However, small thymic tumors may not be distinguishable from a normal or hyperplastic thymus with CT.

Thymic Carcinoma

As with thymoma, thymic carcinoma arises from thymic epithelial cells. However, unlike invasive thymoma, thymic carcinoma can be diagnosed as malignant on the basis of histology. Thymic carcinoma is classified as type C in the WHO system previously described. This tumor is aggressive and is more likely to result in distant metastases than invasive thymoma. Thymic carcinoma cannot be distinguished accurately from thymoma on CT unless metastases are visible.

Thymic Neuroendocrine Tumor

Thymic neuroendocrine tumors, which may be further classified as carcinoid, atypical carcinoid, or small cell

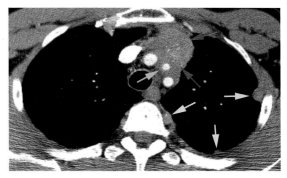

FIG. 4.18 **Invasive thymoma.** A large mass involves the left thymic lobe *(red arrows)*. Note that the mass obliterates fat planes adjacent to the great vessels and surrounds the left carotid artery *(blue arrow)*. These findings suggest invasion. Left-sided pleural nodules *(yellow arrows)* represent pleural invasion and so-called *drop metastases*.

neuroendocrine carcinoma, are usually malignant and aggressive. This type of lesion does not differ significantly from thymoma in its CT appearance, but it has a worse prognosis. Approximately 40% of patients have Cushing syndrome as a result of tumor secretion of adrenocorticotropic hormone, and nearly 20% of thymic neuroendocrine tumors have been associated with multiple endocrine neoplasia syndromes I and II.

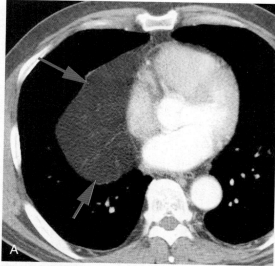

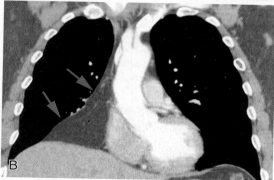

FIG. 4.19 **Thymolipoma.** (A) A large, low-attenuation, anterior mediastinal mass *(arrows)* is composed primarily of fat, but also contains some strands of soft tissue. The mass is somewhat droopy in appearance. (B) A coronal reconstruction shows the mass *(arrows)* drapes around the heart, with extensive contact with the diaphragm.

Thymolipoma

Thymolipoma is a rare, benign thymic tumor consisting primarily of fat but also containing strands or islands of thymic tissue. The tumor is generally unaccompanied by symptoms and can be large when first detected, usually on chest radiographs. Because of its fatty content and pliability, it tends to drape around and over the heart and can simulate cardiac enlargement. On CT, its fatty composition, with wisps of soft tissue within it, can permit a preoperative diagnosis (Fig. 4.19).

Thymic Cyst

Thymic cysts may be either congenital or acquired. They can be diagnosed with CT if they are thin walled and their contents have an attenuation close to that of water. In some cases a thymic cyst will be of soft-tissue attenuation. Calcification of the cyst margin can occur. Notably, thymoma can have cystic components but also demonstrates solid areas or a thick or irregular wall.

An important general rule in diagnosing mediastinal masses is that cysts can appear solid, and solid (malignant) masses can have cystic or necrotic components. A true cyst has a thin wall; a mass with cystic degeneration usually has a thick, irregular wall.

Thymic Hyperplasia and Thymic Rebound

The thymus may appear enlarged and relatively dense (containing little fat) in patients with thymic hyperplasia. In young patients the thymus may show *thymic rebound hyperplasia* 3 months to 1 year after cessation of chemotherapy for malignancy or after other types of stress. This can result in a distinctly enlarged thymus.

Thymic lymphoid follicular hyperplasia (a histologic diagnosis) may result in thymic enlargement or a focal thymic mass, or the thymus may appear normal. It may be associated with myasthenia gravis, hyperthyroidism, collagen vascular diseases, or HIV infection. When it results in a focal mass, distinction from thymoma on CT may be impossible.

Thymic Lymphoma

Anterior mediastinal lymph node enlargement (Fig. 4.3) or thymic involvement (Fig. 4.20) is present in more than half of patients with Hodgkin lymphoma and in some patients with non-Hodgkin lymphoma (particularly large B-cell lymphoma and lymphoblastic lymphoma; Fig. 4.14). In patients with thymic involvement, lymphoma can present as a single spherical or lobulated mass or with thymic enlargement. In such cases, lymphoma can be indistinguishable from thymoma or other causes of prevascular mass. However, if the abnormality is multifocal (indicating its origin from lymph nodes) or is associated with other sites of lymph node enlargement, the diagnosis is made more easily (Fig. 4.20). Cystic areas of necrosis may be visible on CT in patients with lymphoma (Fig. 4.13). Except in rare cases, calcification does not occur in the absence of radiation. Hodgkin lymphoma limited to the prevascular mediastinum is typically of the nodular sclerosis cell type.

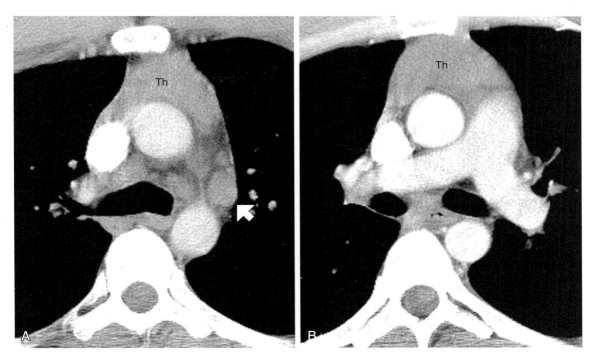

FIG. 4.20 **Hodgkin lymphoma with thymic and mediastinal lymph node enlargement.** (A and B) The thymus (*Th*) is symmetrically enlarged. This appearance could represent thymoma or another primary thymic tumor. However, enlarged lymph nodes in the aortopulmonary window (A, *arrow*) and pretracheal space are a clue to the diagnosis.

Germ Cell Tumors

Several different tumors originating from rests of primitive germ cells can occur in the anterior mediastinum. These include teratoma, dermoid cyst, seminoma, choriocarcinoma, and endodermal sinus tumor. These tumors are less common than thymoma. Germ cell tumors are usually considered in three categories: teratoma and dermoid cyst, seminoma, and nonseminomatous germ cell tumors. Approximately 80% of germ cell tumors are benign.

Teratoma and Dermoid Cyst

Teratomas can be cystic or solid and are most commonly benign. A teratoma contains tissues of ectodermal, mesodermal, and endodermal origins. A dermoid cyst is a specific type of teratoma derived primarily from epidermal tissues, although other tissues are usually present.

Teratomas are classified histologically as mature or immature. *Mature teratoma* is benign. *Immature teratoma* usually behaves in a malignant fashion in adults but may have a benign course in children. *Malignant teratoma* contains frankly malignant tissues in addition to immature or mature tissues and has a very poor prognosis.

Teratomas occur in a distribution similar to that of thymomas; they rarely originate in the posterior mediastinum. Benign lesions are often round, oval, and smooth in contour; as with thymoma, an irregular, lobulated, or ill-defined margin suggests malignancy. On average, these tumors are larger than thymomas but can be any size. Calcification can be seen (Fig. 4.21) but is nonspecific except in the unusual instance when a bone or tooth is present within the mass. They may appear cystic or contain visible fat, a finding that is of great value in differential diagnosis (Fig. 4.21). A fat-fluid level can also be seen.

Seminoma

Seminoma occurs almost entirely in young men. It is the most common malignant mediastinal germ cell tumor, accounting for 30% of such cases. On CT, seminoma presents as a large, smooth or lobulated homogeneous soft-tissue mass, although small areas of low attenuation are sometimes seen. Obliteration of fat planes is common, and pleural or pericardial

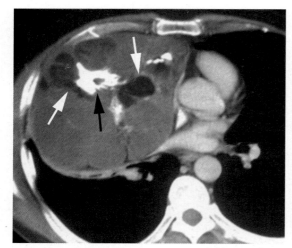

FIG. 4.21 **Mature teratoma.** A lobulated anterior mediastinal mass contains low-attenuation fat *(white arrows)*, an important finding in diagnosis, and calcium *(black arrow)*.

effusion may be present. Seminomas are radiosensitive, and the 5-year survival rate for affected patients is 50% to 75%.

Nonseminomatous Germ Cell Tumors

Nonseminomatous germ cell tumors (namely, embryonal carcinoma, endodermal sinus (yolk sac) tumor, choriocarcinoma, and mixed types) are often grouped together because of their rarity, similar appearance, and aggressive behavior. The tumors may be unresectable at the time of diagnosis because of local invasion or distant metastasis. With appropriate chemotherapy, the long-term survival rate has risen from 10% or less to 45% to 80% and is greatest for children. Surgery is reserved for those patients with radiologic evidence of persistent masses after chemotherapy, and may improve survival.

On CT, these tumors often appear heterogeneous, with ill-defined areas of low attenuation secondary to necrosis, hemorrhage, or cystic areas (Fig. 4.22). They often appear infiltrative, with obliteration of fat planes, and may be spiculated. Calcification may be seen.

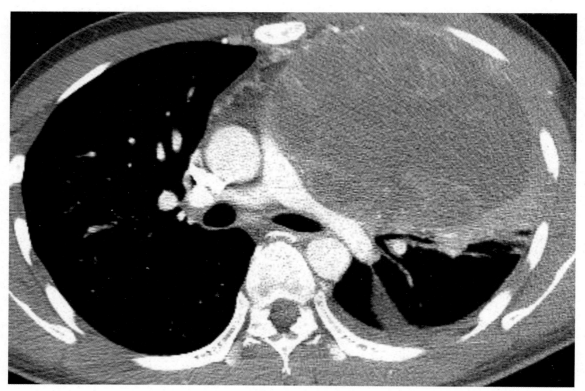

FIG. 4.22 **Nonseminomatous germ cell tumor.** A large, heterogeneous anterior mediastinal mass results in marked compression of the left pulmonary artery. A left pleural effusion is present.

Thyroid Masses

A small percentage of patients with a thyroid mass have extension of the mass into the superior mediastinum, and, rarely, a completely intrathoracic mass can arise from ectopic mediastinal thyroid tissue. In most patients such masses represent a goiter (Fig. 4.23), but other diseases (Graves disease and thyroiditis) and neoplasms can result in an intrathoracic thyroid mass. Masses are often asymmetric.

Most patients with intrathoracic goiter are asymptomatic, but symptoms of tracheal or esophageal compression can be present. CT usually shows anatomic continuity of the visible mass with the cervical thyroid gland. The location of the mass on CT is somewhat variable, and it can be anterior or posterior to the trachea. Masses anterior to the trachea splay the brachiocephalic vessels, whereas masses that are primarily posterior and lateral to the trachea displace the brachiocephalic vessels anteriorly. A location anterior to the great vessels is somewhat unusual (Fig. 4.23).

Calcification and low-attenuation cystic areas are common in patients with goiter. In addition, because of their high iodine content, the CT attenuation of goiter, Graves disease, and thyroiditis is often greater than that of soft tissue (70–85 Hounsfield units [HU]). Prolonged opacification after contrast medium injection is helpful in diagnosis. The association with lymph node enlargement suggests carcinoma.

As a rule, if a thyroid mass is suspected clinically, CT should be performed without contrast medium injection. This allows subsequent injection of radioactive iodine for diagnosis. Injection of iodinated radiographic contrast agents delays radionuclide imaging.

Mesenchymal Abnormalities
Lipomatosis and Lipoma

A diffuse accumulation of unencapsulated fat in the mediastinum, so-called *mediastinal lipomatosis*, can occur in patients with Cushing syndrome after long-term corticosteroid therapy or as a result of exogenous obesity. It produces no symptoms. CT shows a generalized increase in anterior mediastinal fat surrounding the great vessels, with some lateral bulging of the mediastinal pleural reflections. On CT, fat has a characteristic low attenuation, measuring from –50 to –100 HU.

As with other mesenchymal tumors, lipomas can occur in any part of the mediastinum but are most common anteriorly. Because of their pliability, they rarely cause symptoms. A lipoma, although of the same attenuation as lipomatosis, is localized. Most fatty masses are benign. Liposarcoma, teratoma, and thymolipoma, which are other masses that can contain fat, also contain soft-tissue elements and thus can be distinguished from lipoma or lipomatosis.

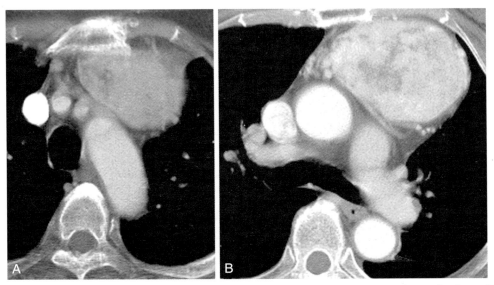

FIG. 4.23 **Mediastinal goiter.** (A) A large inhomogeneous mass is visible in the anterior mediastinum. (B) It shows enhancement after contrast medium infusion. At higher levels the mass was contiguous with the inferior aspect of the thyroid gland.

Lymphangioma (Hygroma)

Lymphangiomas are classified histologically as simple, cavernous, and cystic. *Simple lymphangioma* is composed of small, thin-walled lymphatic channels with considerable connective tissue stroma. *Cavernous lymphangioma* consists of dilated lymphatic channels, whereas *cystic lymphangioma (hygroma)* contains single or multiple cystic masses filled with serous or milky fluid and having little, if any, communication with normal lymphatic channels. Most commonly, these lesions are detected in children and may extend into the neck. However, they can be seen in adults as well. On CT, the mass can appear as a single cyst or can be multicystic or envelop, rather than displace, mediastinal structures. Discrete cysts may not be visible; calcification does not occur. Abnormal vessels that are opacified by contrast medium may be present.

Anterior Cardiophrenic Angle Masses

Although a number of the anterior mediastinal masses described so far can occur at the level of the anterior cardiophrenic angle, the differential diagnosis of lesions occurring in this location also includes several specific entities. These are pericardial cyst, large epicardial fat pad, Morgagni hernia, and enlargement of paracardiac lymph nodes (Fig. 4.2).

Pericardial Cyst

Most commonly, pericardial cysts touch the diaphragm, 60% in the anterior right cardiophrenic angle and 30% in the left cardiophrenic angle; 10% occur higher in the mediastinum. Most patients are asymptomatic. The cysts typically appear as smooth, round, homogeneous masses (Fig. 4.24). They are up to 15 cm in diameter. Although they are usually low in attenuation (i.e., near 0 HU), they may have attenuation similar to that of soft tissue.

Fat Pad

Deposition of fat in either cardiophrenic angle is not uncommon, particularly in obese patients, and can simulate a mass on plain radiographs. CT, of course, is diagnostic.

Morgagni Hernia

Hernias of abdominal contents through the anteromedial diaphragmatic foramen of Morgagni can result in a cardiophrenic angle mass; 90% of these occur on the right. The hernia usually contains fat, omentum, or liver; bowel is less common. When the hernia contains fat, CT can confirm its benign nature but does not allow its differentiation from a fat pad. When it contains liver, CT may

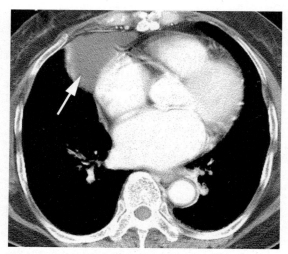

FIG. 4.24 **Pericardial cyst.** A fluid-attenuation mass (i.e., 0 Hounsfield units) is visible in the right cardiophrenic angle *(arrow)*. This appearance and location are typical of a pericardial cyst.

allow diagnosis by showing hepatic vessels or bile ducts. If bowel is present in the hernia sac, gas is usually visible.

VISCERAL COMPARTMENT MASSES (MIDDLE MEDIASTINUM)

The diagnosis, CT findings, and differential diagnosis of masses in this compartment are best considered in relation to the specific mediastinal regions (reviewed in Chapter 2) in which they arise.

Pretracheal Space Masses

Masses that occupy the pretracheal compartment characteristically replace normal pretracheal fat. Because the pretracheal space is limited by the relatively immobile aortic arch anteriorly and to the left, large pretracheal masses extend preferentially to the right, compressing the superior vena cava and displacing it anteriorly and laterally. In the presence of a pretracheal mass, the superior vena cava often appears crescentic and convex laterally. Large masses also displace the trachea posteriorly, but tracheal cartilage usually prevents significant tracheal narrowing.

Masses in this compartment are almost always of lymph node origin, but lesions more typical in other parts of the mediastinum, such as thyroid tumors, lymphangioma, and bronchogenic or pericardial cyst, may involve the pretracheal space (Table 4.7). Tracheal tumors or invasive lung cancers may extend into the pretracheal space.

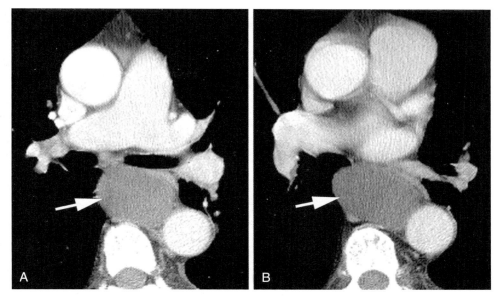

FIG. 4.25 **Bronchogenic cyst.** (A and B) A large, oval, low-attenuation cyst *(arrows)* is visible in the subcarinal region and azygoesophageal recess. This location is typical. There is no evidence of enhancement.

Aortopulmonary Window Masses

Masses in the aortopulmonary region typically replace mediastinal fat; when large, they displace the mediastinal pleural reflection laterally. Displacement or compression of the aorta, pulmonary artery, or trachea is sometimes seen.

Aortopulmonary window masses are almost always the result of lymph node enlargement (Figs. 4.3 and 4.4). Other masses occurring in this region include aortic abnormalities (aneurysm or pseudoaneurysm), lymphangioma, cysts, and chemodectoma (Table 4.7).

Subcarinal Space and Azygoesophageal Recess

Large masses in the subcarinal space can (1) produce a convexity of the azygoesophageal recess, (2) splay the carina, (3) displace the carina anteriorly, (4) displace the esophagus to the left, and/or (5) displace the right pulmonary artery anteriorly and compress its lumen. The most common abnormalities involving this compartment are lymph node masses, bronchogenic cyst, azygos vein dilatation (see Fig. 3.22), varices, hiatal hernia, and esophageal lesions such as leiomyoma (Table 4.7).

Bronchogenic and Esophageal Duplication Cysts

Congenital bronchogenic cyst results from anomalous budding of the foregut during development. Most commonly, bronchogenic cysts arise in the subcarinal space, but they can occur in any part of the mediastinum. They appear as single smooth masses that are round or elliptic (Fig. 4.25) and occasionally show calcification of their walls or contents. Air-fluid levels occurring because of communication with the trachea or bronchi are rare. When large, bronchogenic cysts can produce symptoms due to compression of mediastinal structures. A rapid increase in size can occur because of infection or hemorrhage.

Esophageal duplication cysts are indistinguishable from bronchogenic cysts but always contact the esophagus. They usually appear as well-defined solitary masses and occasionally contain an air-fluid level when they communicate with the esophagus.

CT can be of great value in diagnosing a mediastinal cyst. If a mass is thin walled and is of fluid attenuation (approximately 0 HU), it can be assumed to represent a benign cyst. However, high CT numbers (e.g., 40 HU) suggesting a solid mass can also be found in patients with foregut duplication cysts. Enhancement after contrast medium infusion does not occur. These cysts contain a thick gelatinous material or blood. In such patients, magnetic resonance imaging may be diagnostic.

Esophageal Lesions

Esophageal lesions are discussed in Chapter 17.

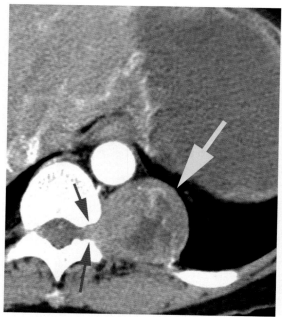

FIG. 4.26 **Schwannoma.** A spherical, sharply marginated mass is visible in a paravertebral location *(yellow arrow)*. The mass is heterogeneous in appearance, with areas of decreased attenuation and enhancement. Note enlargement of the adjacent neural foramen because of extension along the nerve root *(red arrows)*.

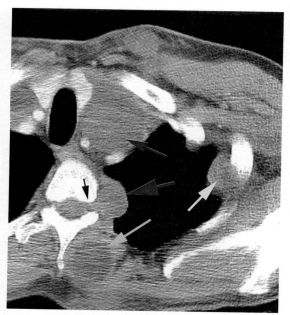

FIG. 4.27 **Multiple neurofibromas in neurofibromatosis.** A smooth, paravertebral mediastinal mass is visible *(large red arrow)*. The adjacent neural foramen is slightly enlarged *(black arrow)*. Multiple other neurofibromas are also present, involving other parts of the mediastinum *(small red arrow)*, the intercostal nerve *(yellow arrow)*, and the left paraspinous region *(blue arrow)*. The paraspinous tumor appears low in attenuation compared with surrounding muscle. A subcutaneous neurofibroma is also visible.

PARAVERTEBRAL MASSES (POSTERIOR MEDIASTINUM)

Paravertebral masses may be seen to replace paravertebral fat. On the left the normal concave mediastinal pleural reflection, posterior to the aorta, becomes convex in the presence of a significant mass. On the right a paravertebral convexity is visible in a region where little tissue normally exists (Fig. 4.5).

Neurogenic Tumors

Neurogenic tumors account for about 10% to 20% of primary mediastinal masses in adults and 30% to 35% of mediastinal tumors in children. About 75% of posterior mediastinal masses are neurogenic tumors. They are considered in three groups, depending on their sites of origin:

- from peripheral nerves or nerve sheath: neurilemmoma (schwannoma; 35% of neurogenic tumors), neurofibroma (5%–10%);
- from sympathetic ganglia: ganglioneuroma (25%), neuroblastoma (15%), ganglioneuroblastoma (10%);
- from paraganglionic cells: paraganglioma or chemodectoma (5%).

Nearly 85% of neurogenic tumors in children are of ganglionic origin, while in adults more than 75% are peripheral nerve or nerve sheath tumors. Specifically, the mean age at diagnosis is about 5 years for neuroblastoma, 10 years for ganglioneuroblastoma, 20 years for ganglioneuroma, 30 years for neurofibroma, and 40 years for neurilemmoma (also termed *schwannoma*).

Neurogenic tumors appear as well-defined round or oval soft-tissue masses, typically in a paravertebral location (Fig. 4.26). The different tumors cannot be distinguished by their appearance, but ganglioneuromas tend to be elongated and visible on multiple slices, whereas neurofibromas and neurilemmomas tend to be smaller and more spherical. Although neural tumors are frequently of soft-tissue attenuation, they can appear low in attenuation because of the presence of lipid-rich Schwann cells, fat, or cystic regions (Fig. 4.26). Heterogeneous enhancement can be seen with contrast medium injection. Neurofibroma is associated with neurofibromatosis in more than a third of cases, and patients with neurofibromatosis often have multiple neurofibromas (Fig. 4.27).

Although benign tumors tend to be sharply marginated and fairly homogeneous, and malignant tumors tend to be infiltrating and irregular, these findings are not sufficiently reliable for diagnosis. Calcification can occur, particularly in neuroblastoma; the presence of calcium does not help in distinguishing benign lesions from malignant lesions.

A neurofibroma or schwannoma arising in relation to a nerve root can extend into the neural foramen or spinal canal. In such cases the foramen may be enlarged (Figs. 4.26 and 4.27). Magnetic resonance imaging may be useful in demonstrating intraspinal extension.

Paraganglioma (chemodectoma) is a rare tumor originating from neuroectodermal cells located in relation to the autonomic nervous system, especially in the region of the aortopulmonary window and the posterior mediastinum. On unenhanced CT, paraganglioma has no characteristic features, but scanning with contrast medium infusion shows dense enhancement. About half of patients with paravertebral paraganglioma have symptoms of catecholamine secretion, but catecholamine secretion is rare in patients with aortopulmonary window tumors.

Anterior or Lateral Thoracic Meningocele

A thoracic meningocele represents anomalous herniation of the spinal meninges through an intervertebral foramen or a defect in the vertebral body. It results in a soft-tissue mass visible on chest radiographs. In most patients this abnormality is associated with neurofibromatosis; most cases are detected in adults.

Meningoceles are described as lateral or anterior, depending on their relationship to the spine. They are slightly more common on the right. Findings that suggest the diagnosis include scoliosis and/or rib and vertebral anomalies at the same level. The mass is often visible at the apex of the scoliotic curve. CT after intraspinal contrast medium injection shows filling of the meningocele (Fig. 4.28); magnetic resonance imaging is diagnostic.

Neurenteric Cyst

A neurenteric cyst, which is rare, is composed of both neural and gastrointestinal elements and is frequently attached to both the meninges and the gastrointestinal tract. It appears as a homogeneous posterior mediastinal mass and rarely contains air because of communication with the abdominal viscera. As with meningocele, it is frequently associated with a vertebral anomaly or scoliosis. As opposed to meningocele, it frequently causes pain and is generally diagnosed at a young age.

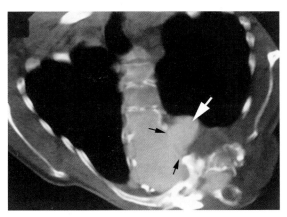

FIG. 4.28 **Lateral thoracic meningocele.** In a patient with neurofibromatosis and scoliosis, a meningocele *(white arrow)* is associated with a large foraminal defect *(black arrows)*. Myelographic contrast material opacifies the meningocele.

Diseases of the Thoracic Spine

Tumors (either benign or malignant), infectious spondylitis, or vertebral fracture with associated hemorrhage can produce a paravertebral mass. Frequently, the abnormality is bilateral and fusiform, allowing it to be distinguished from solitary masses such as a neurogenic tumor. Associated abnormalities of the vertebral bodies or disks assist in diagnosis and should be sought. Preservation of disks in association with vertebral body destruction suggests neoplasm or tuberculosis; disk destruction suggests infection other than tuberculosis.

Extramedullary Hematopoiesis

Extramedullary hematopoiesis can result in paravertebral masses in patients with severe anemia (usually thalassemia, hereditary spherocytosis, and sickle cell anemia). These masses are of unknown origin but likely arise from herniations of vertebral or rib marrow through small cortical defects. Well-marginated, lobulated paravertebral masses, usually multiple and bilateral, and caudad to the sixth thoracic vertebra, are typically seen. On CT the paravertebral masses are of homogeneous soft-tissue attenuation (30–65 HU) or may show areas of fat attenuation (–50 HU), which may increase in extent after treatment.

Fluid Collections and Pseudocyst

Occasionally, posterior pleural fluid collections can simulate a paravertebral mediastinal mass. Mediastinal extension of a pancreatic pseudocyst through the aortic or esophageal hiatus can occur but is rare.

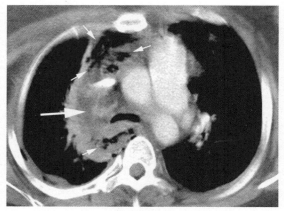

FIG. 4.29 **Acute mediastinitis caused by esophageal perforation by a car antenna.** There is mediastinal widening, increased attenuation of mediastinal fat as a result of inflammation *(large arrow)*, and multiple collections of air *(small arrows)*.

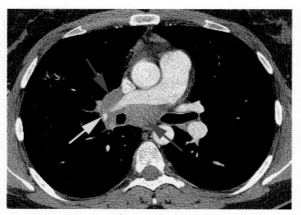

FIG. 4.30 **Fibrosing mediastinitis in a 25-year-old, proven pathologically.** A mass of fibrous tissue involves the right hilum and subcarinal space at this level *(red arrows)*. The right pulmonary artery is narrowed *(yellow arrow)*, and the right superior pulmonary vein branches are obliterated.

Vascular Abnormalities

Posteriorly located aortic aneurysms can occupy this part of the mediastinum. Azygos and hemiazygos vein dilatation also produces abnormalities in this region. Dilated azygos or hemiazygos veins, because they are visible on a number of contiguous slices, are easily distinguished from a focal mass.

DIFFUSE OR EXTENSIVE MEDIASTINAL ABNORMALITIES

Mediastinitis

Mediastinal infections (mediastinitis) can be acute or chronic.

Acute Mediastinitis

Acute mediastinitis usually results from esophageal perforation or spread of infection from adjacent tissue spaces, including the pharynx, lungs, pleura, and lymph nodes; it may occur following sternotomy. The primary symptoms are substernal chest pain and fever. CT shows mediastinal widening, replacement of normal fat by fluid attenuation, or localized fluid collections. Gas bubbles may be seen (Fig. 4.29).

Fibrosing Mediastinitis

In some patients with histoplasmosis, tuberculosis, or sarcoidosis, chronic mediastinal lymph node inflammation with surrounding fibrosis results in so-called *fibrosing mediastinitis* or *granulomatous mediastinitis*. In other patients, similar mediastinal fibrosis is associated with *IgG4-related disease*, methysergide, or Behçet disease, or may be idiopathic. IgG4-related disease is an immune-mediated fibroinflammatory condition characterized by many features previously thought to be associated with idiopathic fibrosing mediastinitis, including retroperitoneal fibrosis, Riedel thyroiditis, sclerosing cholangitis, and pseudotumor of the orbit.

In patients with fibrosing mediastinitis, a focal mass or diffuse replacement of mediastinal fat by fibrous tissue may be seen on CT. Lymph node enlargement may also be seen. Compression of mediastinal structures, such as the superior vena cava, pulmonary arteries or veins, bronchi, and esophagus is common (Fig. 4.30).

In 80% of cases, a focal pattern is visible on CT, with the fibrous mass being localized or asymmetric, and commonly involving the right paratracheal region, subcarinal region, or hila. In patients with the focal pattern, diffuse or stippled calcification is commonly present. Compression of the main bronchi (usually the left) or pulmonary arteries (usually the right) can sometimes be recognized. This pattern is most typical of histoplasmosis.

A diffuse pattern of mediastinal involvement is seen in about 20% of cases. It results in an infiltrating mass of fibrous tissue, affecting multiple mediastinal compartments, and calcification is less common than with localized disease. The diffuse pattern may be related to causes other than histoplasmosis, such as IgG4-related disease.

Mediastinal Hemorrhage

Mediastinal hemorrhage usually results from trauma such as venous or arterial laceration, from aortic rupture or dissection, or from anticoagulation (see Chapter 3). Superior mediastinal widening associated with blurring of normal mediastinal contours is usually present. Mediastinal fluid visible on CT is high in attenuation (>50 HU). Blood can dissect extrapleurally over the lung apex, resulting in a so-called apical cap. In some patients, blood will also be present in the left pleural space. Contrast-enhanced CT may be of value in diagnosing associated aortic aneurysm, dissection, or rupture.

SUGGESTED READING

Azizad, S., Sannananja, B., & Restrepo, C. S. (2016). Solid tumors of the mediastinum in adults. *Seminars in Ultrasound, CT MRI, 37*, 196–211.

Bae, Y. A., & Lee, K. S. (2008). Cross-sectional evaluation of thoracic lymphoma. *Radiologic Clinics of North America, 46*, 253–264.

Benveniste, M. F. K., Rosado-de-Christenson, M. L., Sabloff, B. S., et al. (2011). Role of imaging in the diagnosis, staging, and treatment of thymoma. *Radiographics, 31*, 1847–1861.

Camacho, J. C., Moreno, C. C., Harri, P. A., et al. (2014). Posttransplantation lymphoproliferative disease: Proposed imaging classification. *Radiographics, 34*, 2025–2038.

Campo, E., Swerdlow, S. H., Harris, N. L., et al. (2011). The 2008 WHO classification of lymphoid neoplasms and beyond: Evolving concepts and practical applications. *Blood, 117*, 5019–5032.

Carter, B. W., Benveniste, M. F., Madan, R., et al. (2017). ITMIG classification of mediastinal compartments and multidisciplinary approach to mediastinal masses. *Radiographics, 37*, 413–436.

Carter, B. W., Godoy, M. C. B., Wu, C. C., et al. (2016). Current controversies in lung cancer staging. *Journal of Thoracic Imaging, 31*, 201–214.

Cheson, B. D., Fisher, R. I., Barrington, S. F., et al. (2014). Recommendations for initial evaluation, staging, and response assessment of Hodgkin and non-Hodgkin lymphoma: The Lugano classification. *American Journal of Clinical Oncology, 32*, 3059–3068.

El-Sherief, A. H., Lau, C. T., Wu, C. C., et al. (2014). International Association for the Study of Lung Cancer (IASLC) lymph node map: Radiologic review with CT illustration. *Radiographics, 34*, 1680–1691.

Glazer, H. S., Molina, P. L., Siegel, M. J., & Sagel, S. S. (1989). Pictorial essay: Low-attenuation mediastinal masses on CT. *AJR American Journal of Roentgenology, 152*, 1173–1177.

Glazer, H. S., Siegel, M. J., & Sagel, S. S. (1991). Pictorial essay: High-attenuation mediastinal masses on unenhanced CT. *AJR American Journal of Roentgenology, 156*, 45–50.

Glazer, H. S., Wick, M. R., Anderson, D. J., et al. (1992). CT of fatty thoracic masses. *AJR American Journal of Roentgenology, 159*, 1181–1187.

Horger, M., Lamprecht, H. G., Bares, H.-G., et al. (2012). Systemic IgG4-related sclerosing disease: Spectrum of imaging findings and differential diagnosis. *AJR American Journal of Roentgenology, 199*, W276–W282.

Johnson, S. A., Kumar, A., Matasar, M. J., Schoder, H., & Rademaker, J. (2015). Imaging for staging and response assessment in lymphoma. *Radiology, 276*, 323–338.

Jolles, H., Henry, D. A., Roberson, J. P., et al. (1996). Mediastinitis following median sternotomy: CT findings. *Radiology, 201*, 463–466.

Kim, D. J., Yang, W. I., Choi, S. S., et al. (2005). Prognostic and clinical relevance of the World Health Organization schema for the classification of thymic epithelial tumors: A clinicopathologic study of 108 patients and literature review. *Chest, 127*, 755–761.

Kligerman, S. J., Auerbach, A., Franks, T. J., & Galvin, J. R. (2016). Castleman disease of the thorax: Clinical, radiologic, and pathologic correlation. *Radiographics, 36*, 1309–1332.

Ko, J. P., Drucker, E. A., Shepard, J.-A., et al. (2000). CT depiction of regional nodal stations for lung cancer staging. *AJR American Journal of Roentgenology, 174*, 775–782.

Patil, S. N., & Levin, D. L. (1999). Distribution of thoracic lymphadenopathy in sarcoidosis using computed tomography. *J Thorac Imaging, 14*, 114–117.

Quint, L. E., Glazer, G. M., Orringer, M. B., et al. (1986). Mediastinal lymph node detection and sizing at CT and autopsy. *AJR American Journal of Roentgenology, 147*, 469–472.

Rami-Porta, R., Asamura, A., Travis, W. D., & Rusch, V. W. (2017). Lung cancer — major changes in the American Joint Committee on Cancer eighth edition cancer staging manual. *CA: A Cancer Journal for Clinicians, 67*, 138–155.

Rossi, S. E., McAdams, H. P., Rosado-de-Christenson, M. L., et al. (2001). Fibrosing mediastinitis. *Radiographics, 21*, 737–757.

Sharma, A., Fidias, P., Hayman, L. A., et al. (2004). Patterns of lymphadenopathy in thoracic malignancies. *Radiographics, 24*, 419–434.

Tateishi, U., Muller, N. L., Johkoh, T., et al. (2004). Primary mediastinal lymphoma: Characteristic features of the various histological subtypes on CT. *Journal of Computer Assisted Tomography, 28*, 782–789.

Tomiyama, N., Johkoh, T., Mihara, N., et al. (2002). Using the World Health Organization classification of thymic epithelial neoplasms to describe CT findings. *AJR American Journal of Roentgenology, 179*, 881–886.

Vargas, D., Suby-Long, T., & Restrepo, C. S. (2016). Cystic lesions of the mediastinum. *Seminars in Ultrasound, CT MRI, 37*, 212–222.

CHAPTER 5

The Pulmonary Hila

W. RICHARD WEBB

CT is helpful in the diagnosis of endobronchial lesions, hilar and parahilar masses, and hilar vascular lesions.

TECHNIQUE

In most patients the hila are adequately assessed with spiral CT with a 5-mm slice thickness (it takes about 15 contiguous 5-mm slices to image the hila), but thinner slices are optimal in identifying some findings such as bronchial abnormalities, small lymph nodes, and hilar vessels. Scans with a 1.25-mm thickness are routinely obtained for most chest CT studies and are used in this chapter to illustrate normal anatomy. Contrast medium infusion is optimal for imaging the hila.

Scans are usually viewed with a mean window level of –600 to –700 Hounsfield units (HU) and a window width of 1000 or 1500 HU (lung window) for accurate assessment of hilar contours and bronchial anatomy. Scans are also viewed at a mean window level of 0 to 50 HU and a window width of 400 to 500 HU (soft-tissue or mediastinal window) to obtain information about hilar vessels, lymph nodes, and masses. Both views are necessary.

DIAGNOSIS OF HILAR MASS AND LYMPHADENOPATHY

A detailed understanding of cross-sectional hilar anatomy is needed to detect and accurately localize hilar abnormalities on CT. Contrast enhancement simplifies the identification of hilar masses and lymph node enlargement.

Lobar and segmental bronchi (Fig. 5.1) are consistently seen on CT and reliably localize successive hilar levels; their identification is key to interpretation of hilar CT. In general, hilar anatomy and contours, at the same bronchial levels, are relatively consistent from one patient to another. Bronchial anatomy and branching is less variable than the branching patterns of arteries or veins.

In some locations, normal hilar silhouettes, visible with a lung window, are consistent enough that a diagnosis of hilar adenopathy or mass can be suggested on the basis of hilar contour alone. In other locations, hilar contours vary according to the size and position of the pulmonary arteries and veins, and contrast opacification of pulmonary vessels is essential for accurate diagnosis.

A hilar mass or lymph node enlargement may be suggested by a local or generalized alteration in hilar contour; a visible mass or lymph node enlargement; bronchial narrowing, obstruction, or displacement; or thickening or obliteration of the walls of bronchi that normally contact the lungs.

As a general rule, any nonvascular (unenhancing) hilar structure larger than 5 to 10 mm (short-axis) should be regarded with suspicion and may represent an enlarged lymph node. However, normal amounts of soft tissue larger than this and representing fat and normal nodes are visible in some hilar regions. Mild lymph node enlargement is commonly present in patients with inflammatory lung disease (e.g., pneumonia), and such lymph node enlargement should not be of great concern. In patients with lung cancer, a lymph node larger than 1 cm should be considered enlarged.

NORMAL AND ABNORMAL HILAR ANATOMY

There are two ways to read hilar CT. The first way is to look at each hilum separately, identifying each important structure, and the second is to compare one side with the other at successive scan levels, looking for points of similarity and difference. It is a good idea to do both.

I suggest that as you read the next section, you first learn about right hilar anatomy, skipping what is written about the left hilum. When you finish, and are somewhat oriented, you should start over, reading about both hila, comparing their anatomy, noting what is symmetric and what is not, and learning how

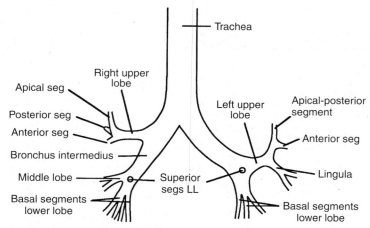

FIG. 5.1 Normal bronchial tree. All the bronchi shown are visible on CT in most patients. Those bronchi that appear horizontal (such as the right upper lobe) or nearly vertical are usually seen better than those that have an oblique course relative to the scan plane (such as the right middle lobe or lingular bronchi). *LL,* Lower lobe; *seg,* segment.

the left hilum differs from the right. Also, you should learn to trace each lobar bronchus from its origin to its segmental branches, because this should be done during interpretation of CT.

Although the hila are not symmetric, they have a number of similarities, and identifying these can be of value. These similarities are emphasized in the following descriptions. To reinforce the normal appearances and their significance, and expected alterations in anatomy occurring because of mass or node enlargement, abnormal findings are discussed for each hilar level described.

Some variation exists among patients in the relative levels of the right and left hila; therefore there is some variation in the levels at which specific right and left hilar structures are visible on CT. The right-to-left relations illustrated in Fig. 5.1 and described in the following text may not be present in individual cases, although side-to-side variation will usually be minor (1 or 2 cm).

Because recognizing lobar and segmental bronchial anatomy is fundamental to interpreting hilar CT, it is reviewed briefly in Table 5.1. Each of the segments listed is commonly, but not invariably, visible.

Five levels are reviewed, each localized by the bronchi that are usually visible. These levels are:

- upper hila and the right apical and left apical-posterior segments
- right upper lobe bronchus and left upper lobe segments
- right bronchus intermedius and left upper lobe bronchus

- right middle lobe and left lower lobe bronchi
- lower lobe bronchi and basal segmental branches

Upper Hila
Right Hilum
CT at the level of the distal trachea or carina shows the apical segmental bronchus of the right upper lobe in cross section, surrounded by several vessels of similar size (Fig. 5.2A–B). On either side a mass or lymphadenopathy is easily recognized. Anything larger than the expected pulmonary vessels is abnormal (Figs. 5.3 and 5.4). Comparison with the opposite side at this level is helpful.

Left Hilum
The apical-posterior segmental bronchus and associated arteries and veins have a similar appearance to the right side at this level (Fig. 5.2B), as does lymph node enlargement (Fig. 5.3A).

Right Upper Lobe Bronchus and Left Upper Lobe Segments
Right Hilum
Approximately 1 cm distal to the carina, the right upper lobe bronchus is usually visible along its length, with its anterior and posterior segmental branches both generally seen at the same level (Fig. 5.5A–D). The anterior segment, usually lying in or near the scan plane, is commonly seen over a length of 1 or 2 cm. The posterior segmental bronchus usually angles slightly cephalad, out of the scan plane, and may not be seen as well. If

TABLE 5.1
Lobar and Segmental Bronchial Anatomy

RIGHT LUNG			LEFT LUNG	
Upper Lobe	**Middle Lobe**	**Lower Lobe**	**Upper Lobe**	**Lower Lobe**
Apical	Medial	Superior	Apical-posterior	Superior
Posterior	Lateral	Anterior	Anterior	Anteromedial
Anterior		Medial	Superior lingula	Lateral
		Lateral	Inferior lingula	Posterior
		Posterior		

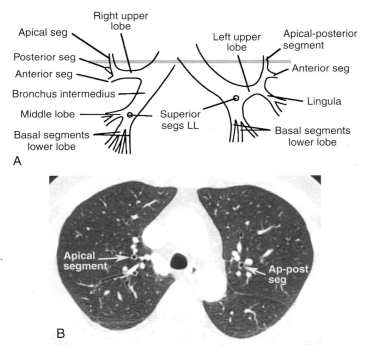

FIG. 5.2 **Upper hilar level: normal anatomy.** (A) Approximate scan level shown in (B). (B) CT with lung window settings at a level slightly above the carina shows the apical segmental bronchus of the right upper lobe in cross section, with several adjacent vessels of similar size. On the left the apical-posterior segmental bronchus *(Ap-post)* of the upper lobe of the left lung and associated arteries and veins have a similar appearance. *LL,* Lower lobe; *seg,* segment.

it is not seen at the level of the upper lobe bronchus, you should look for it at the next higher level. In some normal individuals the origin of the apical segment can be seen at this level as a round lucency, usually at the point of bifurcation (or, in this case, trifurcation) of the right upper lobe bronchus.

Anterior to the right upper lobe bronchus, the truncus anterior (pulmonary artery supplying most of the upper lobe) produces an oval opacity of variable size but often about the same size as the right main bronchus visible at the same level (Fig. 5.5D). An upper lobe vein branch (posterior vein), lying in the angle between anterior and posterior segmental branches, is present and is visible in almost all patients. The posterior wall of the right upper lobe bronchus is usually outlined by lung and appears smooth and 2 to 3 mm thick.

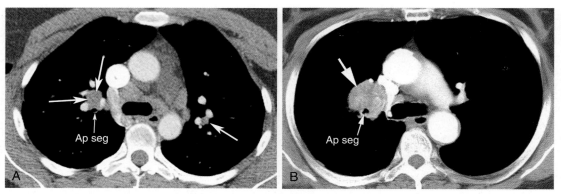

FIG. 5.3 Abnormal upper hila in two patients. (A) In a patient with sarcoidosis and bilateral hilar adenopathy, a contrast-enhanced scan through the upper hila shows lymph node enlargement *(arrows)*. On the right a large node is visible anterior to the apical segmental bronchus *(Ap seg)* of the right upper lobe lung. On the left an enlarged lymph node is visible lateral to pulmonary vessels. (B) In a patient with a carcinoma of the right upper lobe, lymph node enlargement *(arrow)* is visible anterior to the apical segmental bronchus of the right upper lobe.

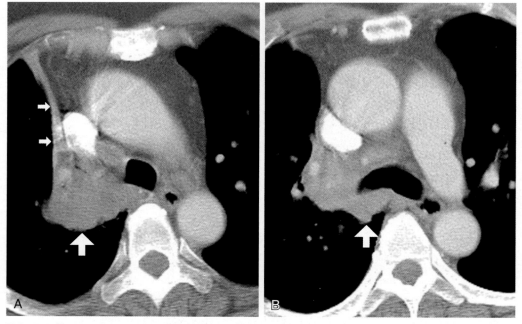

FIG. 5.4 Abnormal upper right hilum in bronchogenic carcinoma. (A) A large mass *(large arrow)* encompasses the region of the apical segmental bronchus of the right upper lobe. A thin linear opacity *(small arrows)* along the right mediastinum reflects collapse of the right upper lobe. (B) Below the level shown in (A) the mass results in obstruction of the right upper lobe bronchus. The mass *(arrow)* is also visible posterior to the right main bronchus.

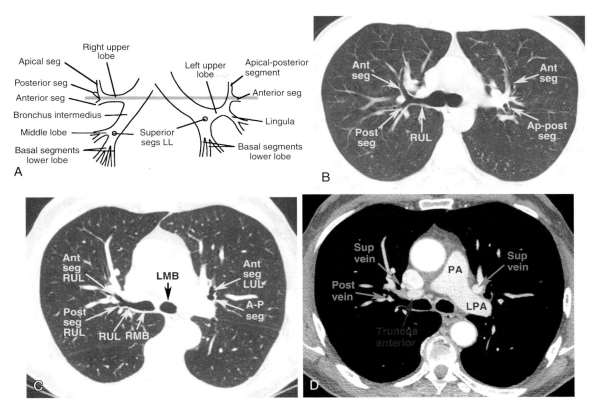

FIG. 5.5 Level of the right upper lobe bronchus and left upper lobe segments: normal anatomy.
(A) Approximate level of scans shown in (B)–(D). (B) Right hilum: CT with 2.5-mm slice thickness shows the right upper lobe bronchus *(RUL)* along its length, together with its anterior segmental branch *(Ant seg)* and posterior segmental branch *(Post seg)* arising from the right upper lobe bronchus in a Y-shaped pattern. Left hilum: On the left side, the apical-posterior segmental bronchus *(Ap-post seg)* and anterior segmental bronchus of the left upper lobe are both visible. The apical-posterior segment is seen in cross section, whereas the anterior segment is directed anteriorly. (C and D) Slices of 1.25-mm at this level in a patient different from the patient for the scan shown in (B). Right hilum: The right upper lobe bronchus *(RUL)* arises from the right main bronchus *(RMB)* just below the carina. The anterior segmental bronchus *(Ant seg)* and posterior segmental bronchus *(Post seg)* arise from the right upper lobe bronchus. The posterior wall of the right upper lobe bronchus contacts lung and is a few millimeters thick. The truncus anterior is anterior to the right upper lobe bronchus. An upper lobe vein branch *(Post vein)* lies in the angle between the anterior and posterior segmental branches. A superior vein branch *(Sup vein)* lies anteriorly. Left hilum: The left main bronchus *(LMB)* is within the mediastinum. In this patient the anterior segmental bronchus *(LUL)* is seen at the point at which it separates from the apical-posterior segment *(A-P seg)*. (D) The left upper lobe segmental bronchi lie lateral to the main branch of the left pulmonary artery *(LPA)*, which produces a convexity in the posterior hilum, and the superior pulmonary vein, which results in an anterior convexity. The artery supplying the anterior segment of the left upper lobe is seen medial to the anterior segmental bronchus and adjacent to the vein. *LL*, Lower lobe; *PA*, main pulmonary artery; *seg*, segment.

Within the anterior right hilum at this level, a mass or lymph node enlargement can be identified if a soft-tissue opacity larger than the expected size of the truncus anterior is visible (Fig. 5.6). This, of course, could be confirmed by contrast medium injection. Laterally, in the angle between the anterior and posterior segmental bronchi, anything larger than the expected vein is abnormal (Fig. 5.6). Posteriorly, thickening of the wall of the upper lobe bronchus or main bronchus (Fig. 5.7) or a focal soft-tissue opacity behind it will almost always be abnormal. An anomalous pulmonary vein branch may sometimes be seen posterior to the bronchus; it is seen at multiple adjacent levels.

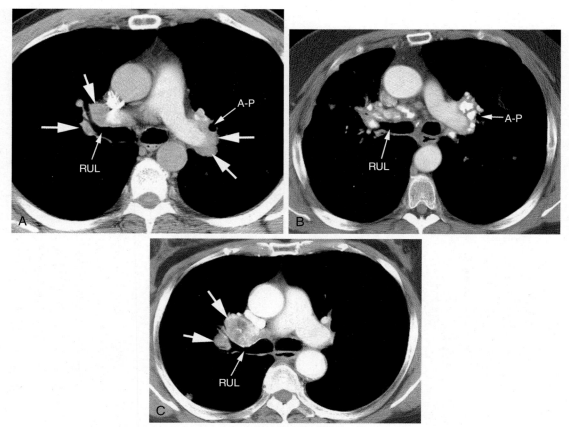

FIG. 5.6 **Hilar adenopathy in three patients shown at the same level as in fig. 5.5C and D.** (A) In a patient with sarcoidosis, there is extensive adenopathy *(arrows)* at the level of the right upper lobe bronchus *(RUL)* and the apical-posterior segmental bronchus *(A-P)* of the left upper lobe. On the right, nodes are visible as unopacified structures anteriorly and laterally. The soft-tissue opacity seen in the position of the posterior vein on the right is too large to represent a vessel. On the left side, there are enlarged nodes *(arrows)* in both the lateral and the posterior hilum, which are distinguishable from the opacified left pulmonary artery. (B) CT at the level of the right upper lobe bronchus *(RUL)* and the apical-posterior segmental bronchus *(A-P)* of the upper lobe of the left lung shows extensive lymph node calcification secondary to sarcoidosis. The calcified lymph nodes are similar in location to those shown in (A). (C) Lymph node enlargement *(arrows)* at the level of the right upper lobe bronchus *(RUL)* in the same patient as shown in Fig. 5.3B.

Left Hilum

On the left side, at or near this level, the apical-posterior and anterior segmental bronchi of the left upper lobe are usually visible (Fig. 5.5A–C). The apical-posterior segment is seen in cross section as a round lucency, whereas the anterior segment is directed anteriorly, roughly in the scan plane, at about the one o'clock position. In some individuals the anterior segmental bronchus is seen at a lower level. These bronchi lie lateral to the main branch of the left pulmonary artery, which produces a large convexity in the posterior hilum at this level, and the superior pulmonary vein, which results in an anterior convexity. In many normal individuals the artery supplying the anterior segment of the upper lobe is seen medial to the anterior segmental bronchus. Lymphadenopathy can be seen in relation to all these structures and is most easily recognized after contrast medium infusion (Fig. 5.6A and B).

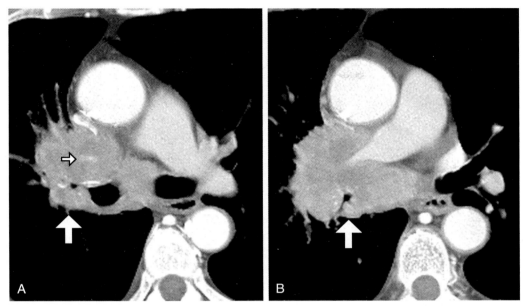

FIG. 5.7 **Bronchogenic carcinoma with a right hilar mass.** (A) A large carcinoma causes narrowing of the right upper lobe bronchus and obstruction of the anterior and posterior segmental bronchi. The truncus anterior *(small arrow)*, anterior to the bronchus, is markedly narrowed and surrounded by tumor. The posterior walls of the right upper lobe bronchus *(large arrow)* and right main bronchus are thickened. (B) At a lower level the bronchus intermedius is narrowed and its posterior wall is thickened *(arrow)*. The mass also invades the mediastinum, surrounding and narrowing the right pulmonary artery.

Right Bronchus Intermedius and Left Upper Lobe Bronchus

Right Hilum

Below the level of the right upper lobe bronchus, the bronchus intermedius is visible as an oval lucency at several adjacent levels (Fig. 5.8). Its posterior wall is sharply outlined by lung. Anterior and lateral to the bronchus, the hilar silhouette may differ in appearance, primarily because of variations in the sizes and positions of pulmonary veins. A collection of fat and normal-sized nodes, sometimes measuring more than 10 mm in diameter, is commonly seen at the level of the bifurcation of the right pulmonary artery, anterior and lateral to the bronchus intermedius (Fig. 5.8). A mass involving the posterior hilum can be readily diagnosed without contrast medium injection because of thickening of the posterior bronchial wall (Fig. 5.7); thickening of the posterior wall of the bronchus intermedius is a common finding in patients with a right hilar mass, particularly when it results from lung cancer.

Diagnosis of anterior or lateral hilar masses at this level generally requires contrast medium administration (Figs. 5.9 and 5.10). Normal soft tissue and nodes (Fig. 5.8) should not be mistaken for a hilar mass.

Left Hilum

The left upper lobe bronchus is usually visible at the level of the bronchus intermedius on the right. It is typically seen along its axis, extending anteriorly and laterally from its origin at an angle of 10 to 30 degrees (Fig. 5.8). The apical-posterior and anterior segmental bronchi of the left upper lobe usually arise from a common trunk that originates from the upper aspect of right upper lobe bronchus. The left superior pulmonary veins are anterior and medial to the left upper lobe bronchus at this level, and the descending branch of the left pulmonary artery forms an oval soft-tissue opacity posterior and lateral to it. Normal lymph nodes (<5 mm in diameter) are commonly visible medial to the artery and lateral to the bronchus. Because only the oval artery occupies the lateral hilum, lobulation of the lateral hilum (more than one convexity) indicates a mass or lymphadenopathy (Figs. 5.9–5.11).

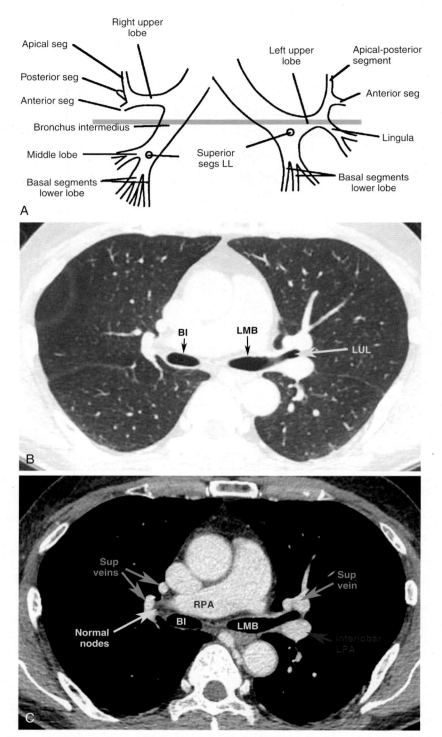

FIG. 5.8 Normal bronchus intermedius and left upper lobe bronchus level. (A) Approximate level of the scans shown in (B) and (C). (B and C) The bronchus intermedius (BI) is visible as an oval lucency with its posterior wall sharply outlined by the lung. Anterior and lateral to the bronchus, the hilum is made up of the right pulmonary artery (RPA) and superior pulmonary veins (Sup veins). Normal lymph nodes and fat are visible in the anterolateral hilum, between the opacified pulmonary artery and veins. On the left the left main bronchus (LMB) and left upper lobe bronchus (LUL) are visible. The left superior pulmonary vein is anterior to the bronchi, and the interlobar or descending branch of the left pulmonary artery (LPA) forms an oval soft-tissue opacity posterior to the left upper lobe bronchus. LL, Lower lobe; seg, segment.

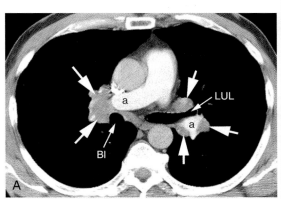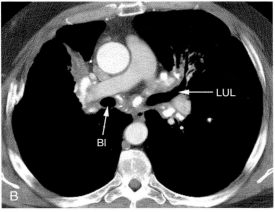

FIG. 5.9 Abnormal bronchus intermedius and left upper lobe bronchus level in two patients with sarcoidosis. (A) On the right a scan at the level of the bronchus intermedius *(BI)* shows enlargement of the normal node group *(arrows)* shown in Fig. 5.8B, situated lateral to the pulmonary artery *(a)*. On the left a scan at the level of the left upper lobe bronchus *(LUL)* shows enlarged lymph nodes *(arrows)* in the anterior hilum and surrounding the opacified pulmonary artery *(a)*. Enlarged lymph nodes are situated posterior to the left upper lobe bronchus. (B) A scan at the level of the bronchus intermedius *(BI)* and left upper lobe bronchus *(LUL)* shows multiple calcified lymph nodes.

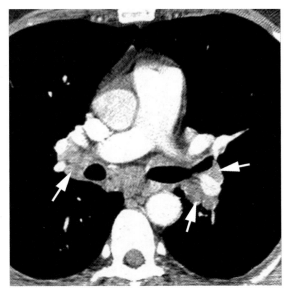

FIG. 5.10 Abnormal bronchus intermedius and left upper lobe bronchus level. In a patient with non-Hodgkin lymphoma and bilateral hilar adenopathy *(arrows)*, enlarged lymph nodes are clearly distinguished from opacified pulmonary vessels.

Although the lung contacts and sharply outlines the posterior wall of the bronchus intermedius at several levels, the left posterior bronchial wall is usually outlined by the lung only at this level; that is, at the level of the left upper lobe bronchus. In approximately 90% of individuals the lung sharply outlines the posterior wall of the left main or upper lobe bronchus, medial to the descending pulmonary artery (Figs. 5.8 and 5.12B and C); this is termed the *left retrobronchial stripe.* As on the right, the bronchial wall should measure 2 to 3 mm in thickness. Thickening of this stripe, or a focal soft-tissue opacity behind it, indicates lymph node enlargement or bronchial wall thickening (Figs. 5.9 and 5.11). In 10% of normal individuals, however, the lung does not contact the bronchial wall because the descending pulmonary artery is medially positioned against the aorta. This should not be misinterpreted as abnormal.

Usually the lingular bronchus is also seen on the left at the level of the bronchus intermedius (Fig. 5.12). The lingular bronchus is usually visible at a level near the undersurface of the left upper lobe bronchus, from which it originates; its two segments (superior and inferior) can sometimes be seen (Fig. 5.12). The superior segmental bronchus of the lower lobe is often visible at this level, arising posteriorly. The pulmonary artery and veins appear the same as at the level of the left upper lobe bronchus (Fig. 5.8). Normal lymph nodes are commonly visible medial to the artery. At this level,

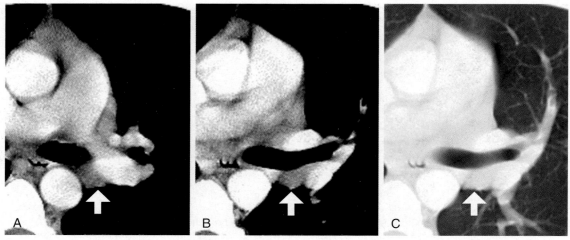

FIG. 5.11 **Left hilar adenopathy (left upper lobe bronchus level).** (A) Lymph node enlargement *(arrow)* is visible in the posterior hilum, behind the left upper lobe bronchus, and between the aorta and the left pulmonary artery. (B and C) The enlarged lymph node *(arrows)* lies posterior to the bronchus (i.e., in the region of the retrobronchial stripe) and prevents the lung from outlining its posterior wall.

significant lobulation of the lateral hilar contour indicates a mass or adenopathy (Fig. 5.13).

Right Middle Lobe Bronchus and Left Lower Lobe Bronchus
Right Hilum
On the right, at the level of the lower bronchus intermedius, the middle lobe bronchus arises anteriorly and extends anteriorly, laterally, and inferiorly at an angle of about 30 to 45 degrees (Fig. 5.14). Because of its obliquity, only a short segment of its lumen is visible at each level on CT, and this appearance should not be misinterpreted as bronchial obstruction. Often the superior segmental bronchus of the lower lobe arises posterolaterally at this level (Fig. 5.14).

At the level of the origin of the middle lobe bronchus, the superior pulmonary veins lie anterior and medial to the bronchus, whereas the descending (interlobar) branch of the right pulmonary artery lies beside and behind it (Fig. 5.12). Normal lymph nodes (<5 mm in diameter) are commonly visible lateral to the artery and bronchus. Because of this separation of the artery and veins, the lateral hilum at this level (representing the artery) is oval, without prominent lobulation. Any lobulation of significant size suggests hilar adenopathy or a mass (Figs. 5.15–5.17).

The left hilum at the level of the left upper lobe bronchus or lingular bronchus (Fig. 5.12) can appear as the mirror image of the right hilum at the level of the right middle lobe bronchus, and comparison of the two sides is common practice. However, the left upper lobe bronchus or lingular bronchus is usually visible 1 to 2 cm above the right middle lobe bronchus.

Left Hilum
At the level of the right middle lobe bronchus, the basal bronchial trunk of the left lower lobe is usually visible (Fig. 5.14), although in some patients the superior segmental bronchus of the lower lobe of the left lung or segments of the lower lobe of the left lung may be visible.

Lower Lobe Bronchi (Basal Segments)
Right and Left Hilum
At this level the hila are relatively symmetric, and comparison of one side with the other can be helpful. The main lower lobe bronchial trunk on each side (Fig. 5.14B and C), which eventually gives rise to the basal segmental bronchi, branches in a variable fashion. It is common for the lower lobe bronchial trunk on the right to divide into two basal bronchial branches or trunks at a level above the origins of the basal segmental bronchi.

At the level of the lower lobe bronchial trunk, on either side, the anterior bronchial wall is usually outlined by lung, with pulmonary artery branches lateral to the bronchus and veins posterior and medial to the bronchus (Fig. 5.14B and C). Enlarged lymph nodes can be identified anterior to the bronchus at this level.

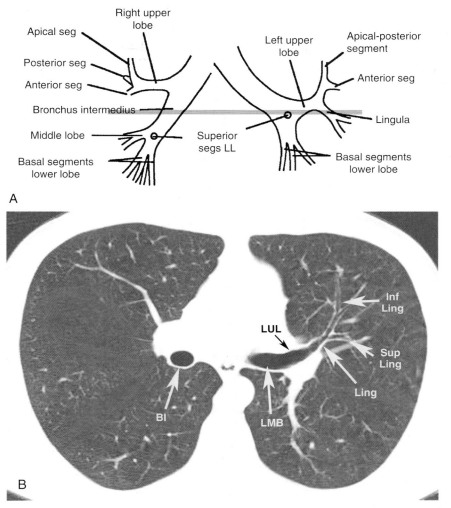

FIG. 5.12 Normal bronchus intermedius and lingular bronchus level. (A) Approximate level for scans shown in (B)–(D). (B) CT with 2.5-mm slice thickness. At a level below that in Fig. 5.8, the bronchus intermedius *(BI)* is visible as an oval lucency on the right, with its posterior wall sharply outlined by lung tissue. On the left the left upper lobe bronchus *(LUL)* is visible, extending anteriorly and laterally from the left main bronchus *(LMB)*. The left posterior bronchial wall is outlined by the lung at this level. This is termed the *left retrobronchial stripe*. The lingular bronchus *(Ling)* arises from the lower edge of the left upper lobe bronchus and divides into two branches, the superior lingular segment *(Sup Ling)* and inferior lingular segment *(Inf Ling)*. (C and D) Slices of 1.25 mm at a level slightly below that shown in (B). Right hilum: On the right the bronchus intermedius *(BI)* is visible as an oval lucency, with its posterior wall sharply outlined by the lung. The interlobar pulmonary artery *(IPA)* and superior pulmonary veins *(Sup vein)* are anterior and lateral to the bronchus. The artery branch to the superior segment of the right lower lobe *(Sup seg art)* is directed posteriorly. Left hilum: Below the level of the left upper lobe bronchus, the lingular bronchus branches into the superior and inferior lingular segments. The proximal left lower lobe bronchus *(LLL)* is visible, along with its first branch, the superior segmental bronchus *(Sup seg)*. The left superior pulmonary vein is anterior and medial to the bronchus, and the descending branch of the left interlobar pulmonary artery is posterior to the lingular bronchus and lateral to the lower lobe bronchus. The lingular artery *(Ling art)* accompanies the lingular bronchus. *Inf ling*, Inferior lingular segment; *LL*, lower lobe; *seg*, segment; *Sup ling*, superior lingular segment.

Continued

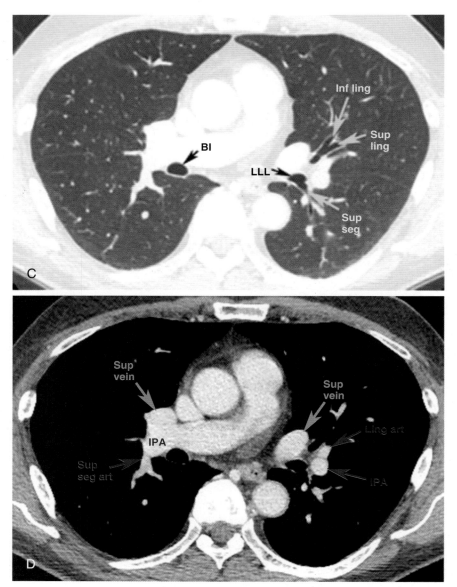

FIG. 5.12, cont'd

The basal segmental branches of the lower lobe bronchi differ in appearance, depending on their courses (Fig. 5.18). On the right the four segmental branches (medial, anterior, lateral, and posterior) are usually visible; on the left are three basal segments (anteromedial, lateral, and posterior). These segments are much better seen with thin slices. It is not unusual to have trouble identifying all specific basal lower lobe segments, but this is not generally of clinical significance.

The segmental bronchi are accompanied by pulmonary artery branches that are slightly larger than the bronchi; the bronchi and arteries are nearly perpendicular to the scan plane and thus are seen in cross section (Fig. 5.18). The inferior pulmonary veins pass behind and medial to the bronchi to enter the left atrium and, unlike the arteries, tend to be seen along their axis. Hilar masses or lymph node enlargement can be diagnosed on the basis of contour

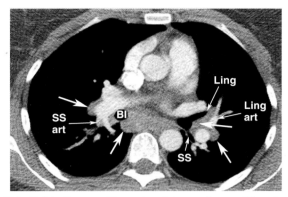

FIG. 5.13 Abnormal bronchus intermedius and lingular bronchus level in a patient with sarcoidosis. On the right, enlarged lymph nodes *(large arrows)* are visible adjacent to the bronchus intermedius *(BI)* and pulmonary artery. On the left, enlarged lymph nodes *(large arrows)* are visible medial and lateral to the interlobular pulmonary artery and posterior to the lingular bronchus *(Ling)*. *Ling art,* Lingular artery; *SS,* superior segment of the left lower lobe bronchus; *SS art,* superior segment of the right lower lobe artery.

abnormalities or asymmetries between the hila. Soft-tissue densities that seem too large to be the pulmonary artery or vein branches should be regarded with suspicion (Figs. 5.19–5.21). The largest nodes seen at this level tend to be anterior.

BRONCHIAL ABNORMALITIES

The excellent contrast and spatial resolution of CT allow accurate assessment of bronchial lesions, and CT is often performed to guide bronchoscopy in patients in whom a hilar or bronchial abnormality is suspected. Accurate indicators of bronchial disease include:

- bronchial wall thickening
- an endobronchial mass
- narrowing or obstruction of the bronchial lumen

Bronchial wall thickening is most easily assessed on CT in regions where hilar bronchi contact lung: the posterior walls of the right main bronchus and both upper lobe bronchi and the posterior wall of the bronchus intermedius. Smooth bronchial wall thickening can be caused by inflammatory disease, pulmonary edema, or tumor infiltration (Figs. 5.7 and 5.22), whereas localized or lobulated thickening usually indicates tumor infiltration or lymph node enlargement (Fig. 5.11).

An *endobronchial mass* is most easily diagnosed with thin slices. Polypoid endobronchial masses may appear

round or lobulated (Figs. 5.23 and 5.24) and in some cases tend to expand the bronchus in which they arise.

Bronchial narrowing and obstruction may be caused by an endobronchial tumor (Fig. 5.25) or compression by an extrinsic mass (Figs. 5.7 and 5.17). Abrupt changes in bronchial caliber on CT usually indicate circumferential tumor infiltration or an endobronchial mass (Fig. 5.25), but it is important to look at adjacent scans to confirm that the apparent bronchial narrowing does not reflect an oblique bronchial course, with the bronchus leaving the scan plane (as with the right middle lobe bronchus). Bronchial abnormalities that are primarily mucosal can be missed with CT because of their minimal thickness.

In general, scans viewed with a lung window setting are best for identifying normal bronchi and detecting bronchial abnormalities, but they often overestimate the degree of bronchial narrowing if thick (e.g., 5-mm) slices are used. Soft-tissue (mediastinal) window settings are more accurate for assessing bronchial abnormalities in the presence of a mass, but overestimate luminal diameter. If a bronchial lesion is suspected, an intermediate window setting is optimal. Thin scans, particularly with multidetector CT, can be of great value in identifying bronchial abnormalities.

DIFFERENTIAL DIAGNOSIS OF HILAR MASS AND HILAR BRONCHIAL ABNORMALITIES
Lung Cancer

The most common cause of a hilar mass or lymph node enlargement is lung cancer. The hilar mass can appear irregular because of local infiltration of the lung parenchyma. In patients with tumors arising centrally (usually *squamous cell carcinoma* or *small cell carcinoma*), bronchial abnormalities (narrowing or obstruction) are commonly visible on CT (Figs. 5.7, 5.17, and 5.25). *Adenocarcinoma* and *large cell carcinoma* may also present with a hilar mass, but this is less common. If the bronchial abnormality involves the tracheal carina, resection may be impossible; bronchoscopy rather than CT, however, is most accurate for making this determination.

When the carcinoma arises in the peripheral lung and the hila are abnormal because of lymph node metastases, the hilar mass or masses may be smoother and more sharply defined than when the hilar mass represents the primary tumor. However, this distinction is not always easily made. Patients with a central mass and bronchial obstruction often show peripheral

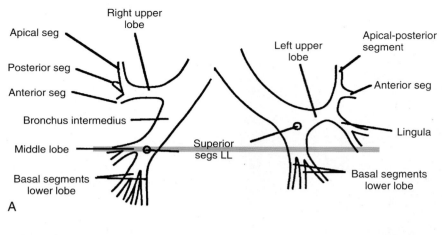

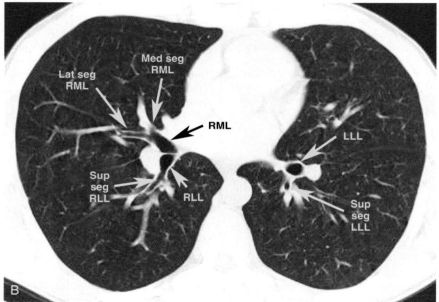

FIG. 5.14 **Normal right middle lobe and left lower lobe bronchus level.** (A) Approximate level for scans shown in (B)–(E). (B) CT with 2.5-mm slice thickness through the right middle lobe bronchus *(RML)* shows its division into its medial segmental branch *(Med seg RML)* and lateral segmental branch *(Lat seg RML)*. The middle lobe bronchus extends anteriorly and laterally at an angle of about 45 degrees. The right lower lobe bronchus *(RLL)* is also visible at this level, giving rise to its superior segmental branch *(Sup seg RLL)* posterolaterally. The interlobar pulmonary artery lies lateral to the bronchi. On the left the left lower lobe bronchus *(LLL)* is visible along with a short segment of its superior segmental branch *(Sup seg LLL)*. The lower lobe artery is lateral to the left lower lobe bronchus. (C and D) A 1.25-mm slice in a different patient. Right hilum: The right middle lobe bronchus *(RML)* is visible, but because it angles caudad, only a short segment of its lumen is visible. The right lower lobe bronchus *(RLL)* and its superior segment *(Sup seg)* are also visible, as in (B). The superior pulmonary vein *(Sup vein)* lies anterior and medial to the right lower lobe bronchus, whereas the oval descending (interlobar) branch of the right pulmonary artery *(IPA)* lies beside and behind it. The right middle lobe pulmonary artery *(RML PA)* accompanies the right middle lobe bronchus. The appearance of the right hilum at this level is quite similar to that of the left hilum at the levels of the left upper lobe and lingular bronchi. Left hilum: The left lower lobe bronchus *(LLL)* is visible below the takeoff of the superior segment. It has a double-barreled appearance as it begins to divide into the basal segments of the LLL. As on the right, the superior pulmonary vein *(Sup vein)* is anterior. The basal segmental branches *(LLL seg arteries)* of the pulmonary artery are lateral. (E) Slightly below (C) the right middle lobe medial segmental bronchus *(Med seg RML)* and lateral segmental bronchus *(Lat seg RML)* are visible. *LL,* Lower lobe; *seg,* segment.

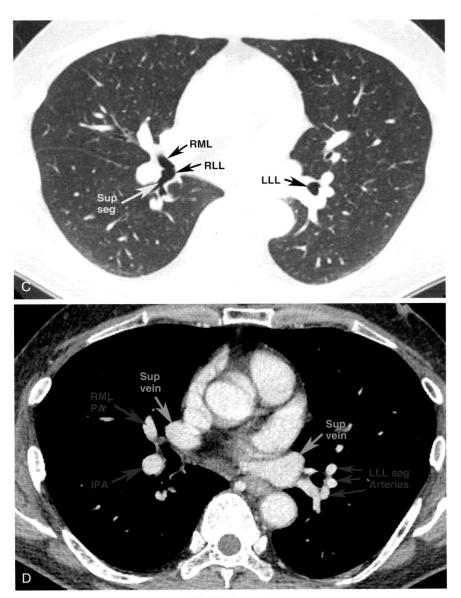

FIG. 5.14, cont'd

Continued

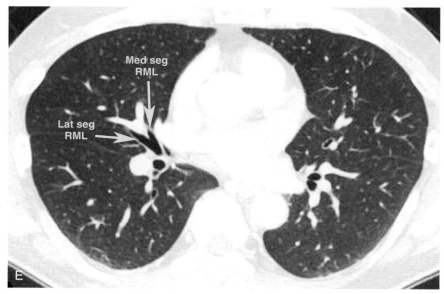

FIG. 5.14, cont'd

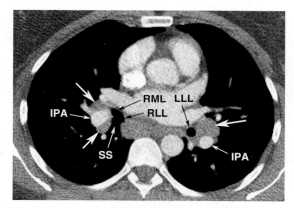

FIG. 5.15 **Abnormal right middle lobe and left lower lobe bronchus level in a patient with sarcoidosis.** On the right, enlarged lymph nodes *(large arrows)* are seen anterior and posterior to the interlobar pulmonary artery *(IPA)* and are situated lateral to the right middle lobe bronchus *(RML)*, right lower lobe bronchus *(RLL)*, and superior segmental bronchus *(SS)*. Subcarinal lymph node enlargement is also present. On the left, enlarged nodes *(large arrow)* are lateral to the lower lobe bronchus *(LLL)* and surround the interlobar pulmonary artery *(IPA)*.

parenchymal abnormalities. In patients with hilar node metastases, a bronchial abnormality seen on CT usually reflects external compression by the enlarged hilar nodes, but bronchial invasion may also be present.

Hilar node metastases are present at surgery in 15% to 40% of patients with lung cancer.

In patients with bronchogenic carcinoma, enlarged hilar nodes visible on CT may not be caused by node metastasis. Hyperplastic nodal enlargement often occurs in patients with lung cancer, particularly when there is bronchial obstruction and distal pneumonia or atelectasis. Conversely, a normal-sized hilar node can harbor microscopic metastases.

In the eighth edition of the TNM lung cancer staging system (Table 4.3), a primary tumor involving the hilum may be classified as *T1 to T4* depending on its size, involvement of main bronchus or carina, or association with atelectasis or obstructive pneumonia. Ipsilateral hilar lymph node metastases from a lung tumor are termed *N1*. Contralateral hilar lymph node metastases are classified as *N3*.

Carcinoid tumor, another cell type of lung cancer, most commonly presents as a hilar mass or bronchial abnormality. This low-grade malignant neuroendocrine tumor arises from the main, lobar, or segmental bronchi in 80% to 90% of cases (Fig. 5.23). It tends to grow slowly and is locally invasive; distant metastases occur in a small percentage of cases. A well-defined endobronchial mass or hilar mass is most common on CT, but carcinoid tumor may also present as a solid-appearing lung nodule. Carcinoid tumors are highly vascular and usually densely

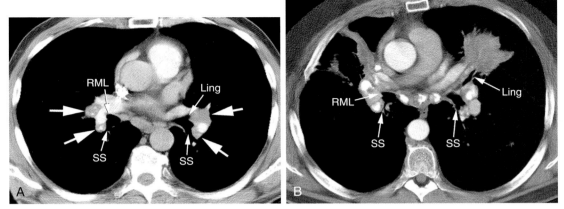

FIG. 5.16 Abnormal right middle lobe bronchus and lingular level in two patients with sarcoidosis. (A) On the right a scan at the level of the origin of the right middle lobe bronchus *(RML)* shows enlargement of nodes *(large arrows)* anterior and posterior to the pulmonary artery. Several of the nodes show calcification. On the left a scan at the level of the lingular bronchus *(Ling)* shows enlarged lymph nodes *(large arrows)* anterior and posterior to the opacified pulmonary artery (as on the right side). (B) As in (A) a scan at the level of the right middle lobe bronchus *(RML)* and lingular bronchus *(Ling)* shows lymph node enlargement (and calcification) anterior and posterior to the pulmonary artery. *SS*, Superior segment bronchus of the lower lobe.

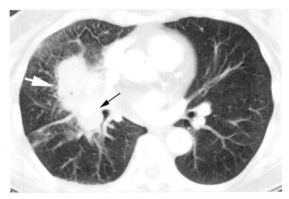

FIG. 5.17 Right hilar mass (bronchogenic carcinoma). The right middle lobe bronchus is invisible *(small black arrow)* and obstructed. A large right hilar mass *(large white arrow)* is present.

enhance after contrast medium infusion. Also, they can be densely calcified.

Adenoid cystic carcinoma (*cylindroma*) can result in a CT appearance similar to that of a carcinoid tumor, but dense enhancement is not typical. It arises in the trachea more commonly than carcinoid tumor.

Benign bronchial tumors, such as hamartoma, fibroma, chondroma, and lipoma, usually appear focal and endobronchial on CT and are not commonly

associated with an extrinsic mass. Obstruction is the primary finding on CT.

Lymphoma

Hilar adenopathy is present in 25% of patients with Hodgkin lymphoma and 10% of patients with non-Hodgkin lymphoma (Figs. 4.12 and 5.10). Hilar involvement is usually asymmetric. Multiple nodes in the hilum or mediastinum are usually involved. Endobronchial lesions can be seen, or bronchi may be compressed by enlarged nodes. However, this is much less common than with lung cancer. There are no specific features of the hilar abnormality seen in patients with lymphoma that allow a definite diagnosis.

Metastases

Metastases to hilar lymph nodes or bronchi from an extrathoracic primary tumor are not uncommon. Hilar node metastases may be unilateral or bilateral. Endobronchial metastases can also be seen (Figs. 4.16, 5.24, and 5.26) without the presence of hilar node metastases; these may appear to be focal and endobronchial or infiltrative. Head and neck carcinomas, thyroid carcinoma, genitourinary tumors (particularly renal cell and testicular carcinoma), melanoma, and breast carcinomas are most commonly responsible for hilar or endobronchial metastases.

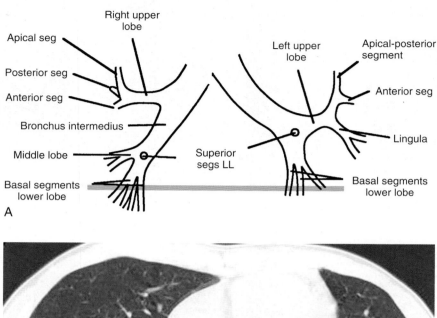

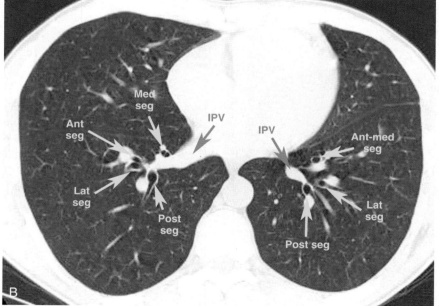

FIG. 5.18 **Normal lower lobe bronchi (basal segments).** (A) Approximate level for the scan shown in (B). (B) On the right the medial segmental bronchus *(Med seg)*, anterior segmental bronchus *(Ant seg)*, lateral segmental bronchus *(Lat seg)*, and posterior segmental bronchus *(Post seg)* of the right lower lobe are visible. The basal segmental bronchi arise in a variable fashion. The inferior pulmonary vein *(IPV)* is posterior and medial to the bronchi, and segmental pulmonary artery branches with a round appearance accompany the bronchi. On the left the anteromedial segmental branch *(Ant-med seg)*, lateral segmental branch *(Lat seg)*, and posterior segmental branch *(Post seg)* of the left lower lobe bronchus are visible. The vascular anatomy is the same as on the right. *LL,* Lower lobe; *seg,* segment.

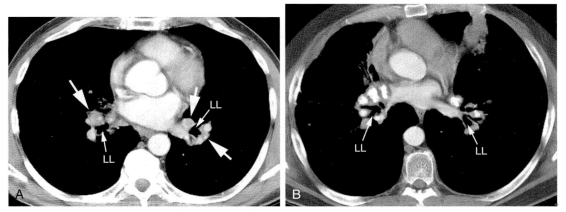

FIG. 5.19 **Abnormal lower lobe bronchial level in two patients with sarcoidosis.** (A and B) At the level of the lower lobe segments *(LL)*, abnormal lymph nodes *(arrows)* are visible anteriorly and adjacent to the vascular branches.

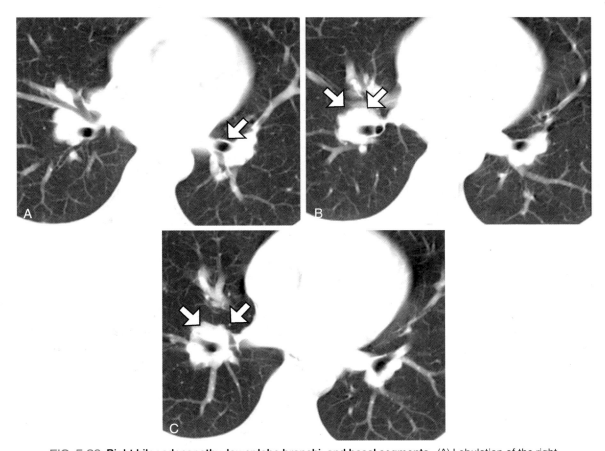

FIG. 5.20 **Right hilar adenopathy, lower lobe bronchi, and basal segments.** (A) Lobulation of the right hilum at the level of the right middle lobe bronchus indicates lymph node enlargement. The lung contacts the anterior wall of the left lower lobe bronchial trunk *(arrow)*, and arteries and veins are lateral, posterior, and medial to the bronchus. This appearance is normal. (B) The right lower lobe bronchial trunk has divided into two branches. Soft tissue anterior to these branches represents lymph node enlargement *(arrows)*. On the left the lower lobe bronchial trunk remains outlined by the lung anteriorly. (C) At the level of the basal segments, the right and left sides appear asymmetric. The right bronchial segments are surrounded by soft tissue. Nodes *(arrows)* are anterior to the bronchi.

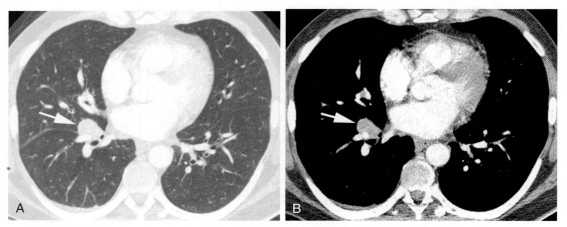

FIG. 5.21 **Right hilar adenopathy, lower lobe bronchi.** (A) Lung window. (B) Mediastinal window. In a patient with non-Hodgkin lymphoma, an enlarged lymph node *(arrow)* is visible anterior to the right lower lobe bronchial branches.

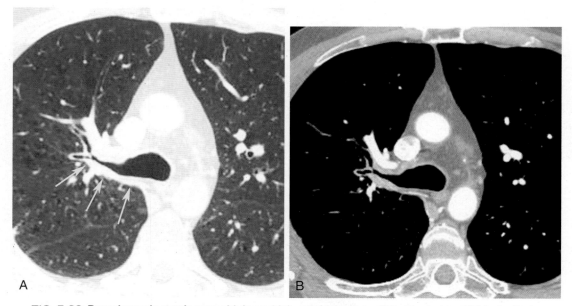

FIG. 5.22 **Bronchogenic carcinoma with bronchial wall thickening.** (A) Lung window. (B) Mediastinal window. There is thickening of the posterior wall of the right upper lobe bronchus and right main bronchus because of tumor infiltration *(arrows)*. Irregular narrowing of the lumen of the right upper lobe bronchus is also visible. The wall of the right upper lobe bronchus is normally smooth and thin.

Inflammatory Disease

Unilateral or bilateral hilar lymphadenopathy and bronchial narrowing can be seen in a number of infectious and inflammatory conditions. Primary tuberculosis usually causes unilateral hilar adenopathy. Fungal infections, most notably histoplasmosis and coccidioidomycosis, cause unilateral or bilateral adenopathy. Sarcoidosis causes bilateral and symmetric adenopathy in most patients (Fig. 5.9). Silicosis and coal workers' pneumoconiosis are also commonly associated with bilateral hilar lymph node enlargement.

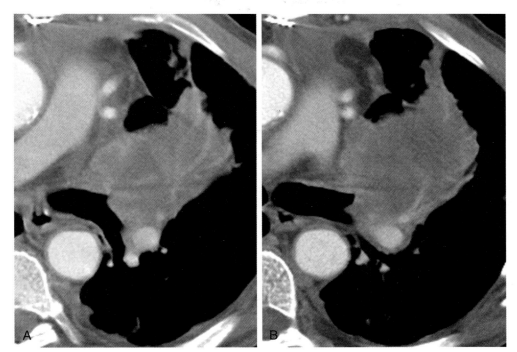

FIG. 5.23 **Bronchogenic carcinoma with left upper lobe bronchus obstruction.** (A and B) There is abrupt termination of the left upper lobe bronchus, associated with distal collapse and consolidation of the left upper lobe. This appearance strongly suggests bronchogenic carcinoma.

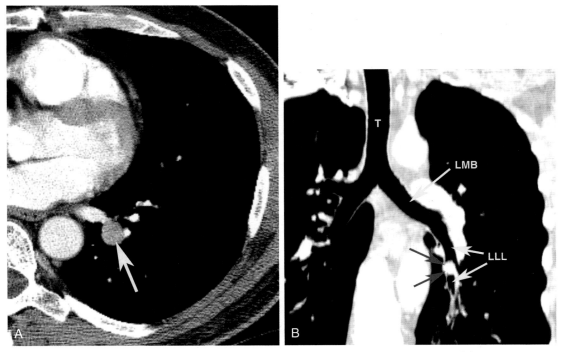

FIG. 5.24 **Endobronchial carcinoid tumor in a young patient with recurrent left lower lobe pneumonia.** (A) Spiral CT with a 1.25-mm slice shows a round mass *(arrow)* in the location of the left lower lobe bronchus. Although it might be mistaken for a vessel, it is much less dense than enhanced arteries and veins. (B) Coronal reconstruction shows a round mass *(red arrows)* within the left lower lobe bronchus *(LLL). LMB,* Left main bronchus; *T,* trachea.

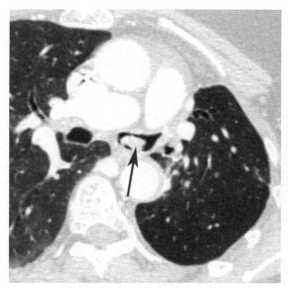

FIG. 5.25 **Endobronchial metastasis from colon carcinoma.** A focal endobronchial lesion *(arrow)* is visible within the left main bronchus. This represents an endobronchial metastasis.

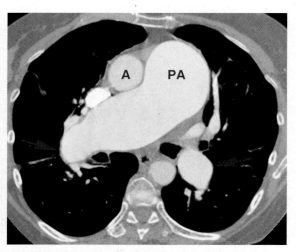

FIG. 5.27 **Pulmonary artery enlargement in pulmonary hypertension.** The main pulmonary artery *(PA)* is larger than the ascending aorta *(A)*, which is a good sign of pulmonary hypertension. Enlargement of the hilar arteries *(arrows)* is also seen.

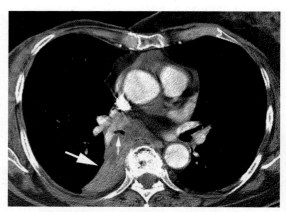

FIG. 5.26 **Endobronchial metastasis from breast carcinoma.** In a patient with a right-sided mastectomy, a focal lesion narrowing the lower lobe bronchus *(small arrow)* is associated with right lower lobe atelectasis *(large arrow)*. This represents an endobronchial metastasis.

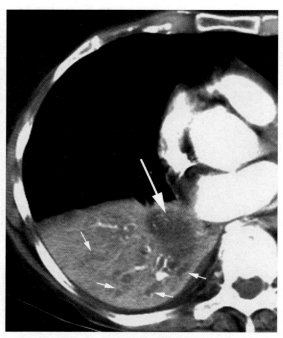

FIG. 5.28 **Hilar mass with atelectasis.** In a patient with right hilar carcinoma associated with right lower lobe atelectasis, the hilar mass can be distinguished from the collapsed lung after contrast medium infusion. The mass *(large arrow)* appears less dense than the opacified and enhancing lung tissue. Low-attenuation, mucus-filled bronchi *(small arrows)* are visible within the consolidated lung. These are associated with bronchial obstruction and are termed *mucous bronchograms.*

In patients with prior tuberculosis, histoplasmosis, sarcoidosis, or silicosis, calcified hilar nodes are commonly seen (Fig. 5.9). *Eggshell* (peripheral) calcification of lymph nodes is most commonly seen with silicosis, sarcoidosis, or tuberculosis. Calcified nodes can erode into a bronchus, causing obstruction (i.e., so-called *broncholithiasis*).

Mucus

Blobs of mucus may simulate one or more endobronchial lesions on CT; these are usually located along the posterior bronchial wall. If this diagnosis is suggested (e.g., if a focal bronchial lesion is seen when it is not expected), a repeated scan can be obtained after the patient has coughed. The abnormality will disappear if it is just mucus. Large mucus plugs can also mimic hilar masses or can be seen as a bronchial abnormality on CT.

PULMONARY VASCULAR DISEASE

CT is useful in differentiating pulmonary vascular disease from hilar adenopathy. Pulmonary hypertension with dilatation of the pulmonary arteries is relatively common and can simulate a hilar mass on plain radiographs (Fig. 5.27). CT can accurately define the size of the pulmonary arteries in patients with arterial dilatation. If the main pulmonary artery is larger than the ascending aorta (see Chapter 3; Figs. 3.25 and 3.26), it is dilated; pulmonary hypertension is the most likely cause. Rarely, in patients with chronic pulmonary hypertension, pulmonary artery calcification can be seen as a result of atherosclerosis. Other causes of pulmonary artery enlargement are reviewed in Chapter 3.

In lung cancer, involvement of the main pulmonary artery or intrapericardial portions of the right or left pulmonary artery is classified as *T4*. Encasement or compression of one of the hilar pulmonary arteries by tumor in patients with a lung carcinoma can be of value in assessing the extent of surgery that will be required for resection. For example, tumor surrounding the hilar portion of the left pulmonary artery generally indicates that pneumonectomy rather than lobectomy is required. However, caution must be exercised in making the diagnosis of artery invasion; narrowing of the pulmonary artery can reflect compression rather than encasement. Adequate assessment requires the use of intravenous contrast medium.

The CT diagnosis of pulmonary embolism is discussed in Chapter 3.

MASS VERSUS ATELECTASIS

In patients with a hilar mass and bronchial obstruction, collapse or consolidation of the distal portion of the lung can obscure the margins of the mass, making it difficult to diagnose. On plain radiographs the mass can sometimes be detected because of alterations in the shape of the collapsed or consolidated lobe or lobes (i.e., Golden's S sign). Similarly, alterations in the shape of a collapsed lobe can be seen on CT in the presence of a mass.

If contrast medium is injected, the collapsed lobe usually enhances to a greater degree than the mass causing the collapse (Fig. 5.28). Of additional value in distinguishing mass and lung consolidation are air bronchograms, which are sometimes visible despite bronchial obstruction. These indicate the presence of lung consolidation and are not usually visible with the mass itself. In some patients, low-attenuation, fluid-filled bronchi (i.e., *mucous bronchograms*) are seen within the collapsed lung.

SUGGESTED READING

El-Sherief, A. H., Lau, C. T., Wu, C. C., et al. (2014). International Association for the Study of Lung Cancer (IASLC) lymph node map: Radiologic review with CT illustration. *Radiographics, 34*, 1680–1691.

Grosse, C., & Grosse, A. (2010). CT findings in diseases associated with pulmonary hypertension: A current review. *Radiographics, 30*, 1753–1777.

Ko, J. P., Drucker, E. A., Shepard, J.-A., et al. (2000). CT depiction of regional nodal stations for lung cancer staging. *AJR American Journal of Roentgenology, 174*, 775–782.

Naidich, D. P., Khouri, N. F., Scott, W. J., et al. (1981). Computed tomography of the pulmonary hila: I. Normal anatomy. *Journal of Computer Assisted Tomography, 5*, 459–467.

Naidich, D. P., Khouri, N. F., Stitik, F. P., et al. (1981). Computed tomography of the pulmonary hila: II. Abnormal anatomy. *Journal of Computer Assisted Tomography, 5*, 468–475.

Ng, C. S., Wells, A. U., & Padley, S. P. (1999). A CT sign of chronic pulmonary arterial hypertension: The ratio of main pulmonary artery to aortic diameter. *Journal of Thoracic Imaging, 14*, 270–278.

Patil, S. N., & Levin, D. L. (1999). Distribution of thoracic lymphadenopathy in sarcoidosis using computed tomography. *Journal of Thoracic Imaging, 14*, 114–117.

Rami-Porta, R., Asamura, A., Travis, W. D., & Rusch, V. W. (2017). Lung cancer — major changes in the American Joint Committee on Cancer eighth edition cancer staging manual. *CA: A Cancer Journal for Clinicians, 67*, 138–155.

Remy-Jardin, M., Duyck, P., Remy, J., et al. (1995). Hilar lymph nodes: Identification with spiral CT and histologic correlation. *Radiology, 196*, 387–394.

Rosado de Christenson, M. L., Abbott, G. F., Kirejczyk, W. M., et al. (1999). Thoracic carcinoids: Radiologic-pathologic correlation. *Radiographics, 19*, 707–736.

Sone, S., Higashihara, T., Morimoto, S., et al. (1983). CT anatomy of hilar lymphadenopathy. *AJR American Journal of Roentgenology, 140*, 887–892.

Webb, W. R., Gamsu, G., & Glazer, G. (1981). Computed tomography of the normal pulmonary hilum. *Journal of Computer Assisted Tomography, 5*, 476–484.

Webb, W. R., Gamsu, G., & Glazer, G. (1981). Computed tomography of the abnormal pulmonary hilum. *Journal of Computer Assisted Tomography, 5*, 485–490.

CHAPTER 6

Lung Disease

W. RICHARD WEBB

On CT, normal lung varies in appearance, depending on the window settings used. With a window mean of –600 to –700 Hounsfield units (HU) and a width of 1000 to 1500 HU, the lungs appear dark, but not as black as the air visible in the trachea or bronchi. This slight difference in attenuation between lung parenchyma and air should be sought in choosing an appropriate window setting. If the lungs are viewed with too high a window mean, soft-tissue structures in the lung (vessels, bronchi, or lung nodules) are difficult to see or are underestimated in terms of their size, and any areas of lucency, such as bullae, may be missed. If too low a window mean is used, the size of soft-tissue structures in the lung will be overestimated.

The following discussion of lung diseases is divided into six parts, each part reviewing an important topic in the CT diagnosis of lung disease. Separate reading lists are provided for each part.

A: LOBAR ANATOMY, LOBAR PNEUMONIA, AND ATELECTASIS

THE FISSURES AND LOBAR ANATOMY

The lobes are delineated by the major and minor fissures (Fig. 6.1).

Major Fissures

The major fissures separate the lower lobes posteriorly from the upper lobe on the left and the middle and upper lobes on the right. They are not clearly visible on CT with 5-mm collimation but are easily seen as thin white lines on CT with thin slices (Fig. 6.1). The lung parenchyma immediately adjacent to the fissures, being peripheral, contains few visible vessels and appears relatively avascular. The major fissures are incomplete in many patients (i.e., they do not completely separate the lobes).

Within the lower thorax, the major fissures angle anterolaterally from the mediastinum, contacting the anterior third of the hemidiaphragms. In the upper thorax, the major fissures angle posterolaterally. Above the aortic arch, they contact the posterior chest wall.

Minor Fissure

The minor fissure separates the right middle lobe from the right upper lobe. Although it parallels the scan plane, and is more difficult to see than the major fissure, it is usually visible on thin slices as a white line of varying sharpness and thickness. The relatively avascular lung on both sides of the fissure is visible on CT in most patients. In some patients the minor fissure mimics the appearance of the major fissure but is seen anterior to it.

Because the minor fissure often angles caudally, the right lower, middle, and upper lobes may all be seen on a single scan. If the minor fissure is concave caudally, it can sometimes be seen in two locations or can appear ring-shaped (Fig. 6.2), with the middle lobe between the fissure lines or in the center of the ring and the upper lobe anterior to the most anterior part of the fissure.

Accessory Fissures

In patients with an azygos lobe, the four layers of the *mesoazygos*, or azygos fissure, are invariably visible above the level of the intrapulmonary azygos vein. The azygos fissure is C-shaped and convex laterally, beginning anteriorly at the right brachiocephalic vein and ending posteriorly at the right anterolateral surface of the vertebral body (Fig. 3.21). Other accessory fissures, most commonly the *inferior accessory fissure* (separating the medial basal segment of either lower lobe from the other lower lobe segments), are

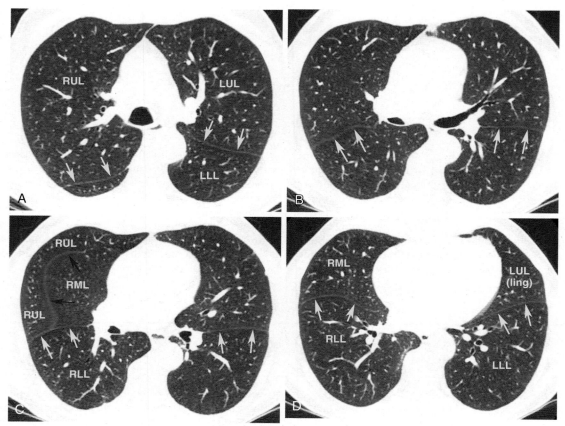

FIG. 6.1 **Normal fissures.** (A) At a level slightly below the aortic arch, the major fissures *(arrows)* are visible as thin lines. They angle posterolaterally. On the right the major fissure separates the right upper lobe *(RUL)* from the superior segment of the right lower lobe. On the left it separates the left upper lobe *(LUL)* and left lower lobe *(LLL)*. (B) Several centimeters lower the major fissures *(arrows)* are more anteriorly positioned. (C) The major fissures *(yellow arrows)* remain visible. The minor fissure *(red arrows)* separates the right middle lobe of *(RML)* medially from the right upper lobe *(RUL)* laterally and anteriorly. (D) At a lower level the major fissures angle anterolaterally *(arrows)*. Their bowed appearance is normal. The right middle lobe *(RML)* is located anterior to the right major fissure. On the left the lingular *(ling)* portion of the left upper lobe *(LUL)* is anterior to the fissure. *LLL,* left lower lobe *RLL,* right lower lobe.

occasionally seen on CT. They are not generally of diagnostic significance.

LOBAR PNEUMONIA

Pneumonia usually results in lung consolidation. The term *consolidation* is used to describe the presence of homogeneous lung opacity resulting from replacement of alveolar air by something else, with obscuration of the underlying vessels and bronchial walls; *air bronchograms* (visible air-filled bronchi) are typically visible but not invariably present. On enhanced CT, vessels with a normal appearance and course can often be seen within consolidated lung. In contrast, a mass or space-occupying lung lesion usually displaces vessels or bronchi, or they may be narrowed or invisible because of compression or invasion.

In some patients with pneumonia, consolidation involves most of a lobe or an entire lobe; this

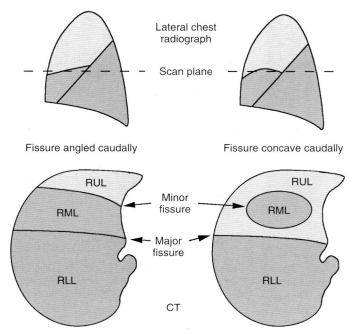

Lateral chest radiograph

Scan plane

Fissure angled caudally

Fissure concave caudally

RUL

RML

RLL

RUL

RML

RLL

Minor fissure

Major fissure

CT

FIG. 6.2 **Possible appearances for the minor fissure.** Depending on the orientation of the minor fissure, its appearance and the relations of the right lobes can vary. If the minor fissure angles downward, both the middle lobe and the upper lobe can be seen on a single scan. If the minor fissure is concave caudad, it may appear ring-shaped or curved, as in Fig. 6.1C. *RLL*, right lower lobe *RML*, right middle lobe *RUL*, right upper lobe.

is termed *lobar pneumonia*. In a patient with lobar pneumonia, the volume of the consolidated lobe is normal or sometimes increased (Fig. 6.3). Usually the infectious organisms responsible for lobar pneumonia lead to an exuberant watery exudate. The exudate easily spreads from one alveolus to another, resulting in an expanding sphere of consolidation that stops when it reaches a fissure. If lobar pneumonia is imaged early in its evolution, it may appear as a rounded, poorly marginated area of consolidation. This is sometimes referred to as *round pneumonia*. Common causes of lobar pneumonia include *Streptococcus pneumoniae, Klebsiella pneumoniae, Legionella, Mycoplasma, Mycobacterium tuberculosis*, and some viruses and fungi. In addition to pneumonia, other causes of lobar consolidation include *obstructive pneumonia* (lung consolidation associated with a central bronchial obstruction, even if uninfected), invasive mucinous adenocarcinoma, aspiration, pulmonary edema, and in rare cases, pulmonary hemorrhage or a vascular abnormality (e.g., pulmonary embolism).

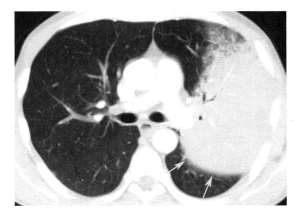

FIG. 6.3 **Lobar left upper lobe pneumonia.** Pneumococcal pneumonia results in homogeneous consolidation of the posterior left upper lobe marginated by the left major fissure. The fissure is bowed posteriorly *(yellow arrows)*. The right major fissure is also seen *(red arrows)*.

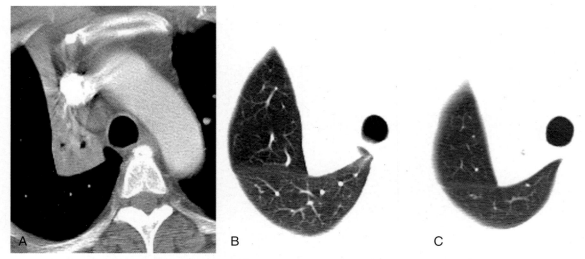

FIG. 6.4 **Right upper lobe collapse.** (A) In a patient with carcinoma obstructing the right upper lobe bronchus, air bronchograms and opacified vessels are visible within the collapsed lobe. (B and C) The upper lobe has a triangular shape. The middle lobe borders the lateral aspect of the collapsed lobe, whereas the lower lobe is posterior to it.

Pulmonary infections can also present with other CT patterns. These are discussed later in this chapter and include patchy consolidation (*bronchopneumonia* or *lobular pneumonia*); single or multiple nodules, masses, or cavities; *tree-in-bud* opacities; *centrilobular* nodules; *ground-glass* opacity (GGO); and *miliary* or *random* nodules.

ATELECTASIS: TYPES AND PATTERNS OF LOBAR COLLAPSE

Atelectasis most commonly occurs because of bronchial obstruction (*obstructive atelectasis*), pleural effusion or other pleural processes that allow the lung to collapse (*passive or relaxation atelectasis*), or lung fibrosis (*cicatrization atelectasis*). These conditions have different appearances. Generally, the signs of volume loss on CT are the same as those on chest radiographs. Mediastinal shift (particularly of the anterior mediastinum), elevation of the diaphragm, and displacement of fissures are well seen on CT.

Obstructive Atelectasis

Obstructive atelectasis often occurs because of lung cancer or other bronchial tumors, and the airways should be examined closely. Lobar atelectasis commonly results; typically, the affected lobe is partially or completely consolidated (Fig. 6.4). Air bronchograms

are usually, but not always, absent. *Mucus bronchograms* (low-density fluid or mucus within obstructed bronchi) can sometimes be seen on CT. The air- or mucus-filled bronchi can be dilated in the presence of atelectasis, simulating bronchiectasis. If contrast medium infusion is used, opacified vessels are often visible within the consolidated and collapsed lobe (a collapsed lung is not simply airless; the alveoli are usually filled with fluid). If little volume loss is present, the term *obstructive pneumonia* is often used (Fig. 6.5).

On CT, atelectasis can be diagnosed when displacement of fissures is seen. Typical patterns of lobar collapse can be identified (Figs. 6.6 and 6.7).

Right Upper Lobe Collapse

With collapse the major fissure rotates anteriorly and medially as the upper lobe progressively flattens against the mediastinum (Figs. 6.4 and 6.6). The fissure can be bowed anteriorly. In the presence of a hilar mass, an appearance similar to *Golden's S sign*, as seen on plain radiographs, is visible. In some patients the lobe assumes a triangular shape (Fig. 6.4).

Left Upper Lobe Collapse

As on the right, the major fissure rotates anteromedially. However, above the hilum the superior segment of the lower lobe may displace part of the upper lobe

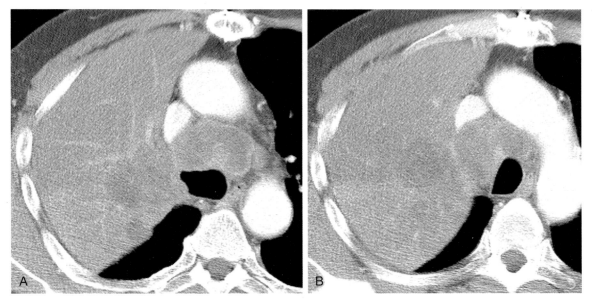

FIG. 6.5 **Lung carcinoma with obstructive pneumonia.** (A and B) The right upper lobe is consolidated, but no volume loss is present. No air bronchograms are seen, but opacified vessels are visible. Large, low-density, necrotic mediastinal lymph nodes are also present.

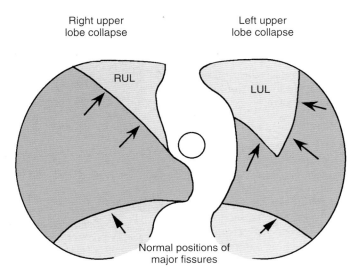

FIG. 6.6 **Typical patterns of upper lobe collapse.** The major fissures are displaced anteriorly and medially *(arrows)* from their normal positions. *LUL*, left upper lobe *RUL*, right upper lobe.

away from the mediastinum, giving the posterior margin of the collapsed lobe a V shape (Fig. 6.6). A similar appearance is sometimes seen on the right (Fig. 6.4). On chest radiographs this appearance results in the so-called *Luftsichel sign*.

Middle Lobe Collapse

As the middle lobe loses volume, the minor fissure rotates downward and medially. The collapsed lobe assumes a triangular shape, with one side of the triangle abutting the mediastinum (Fig. 6.7). The upper lobe

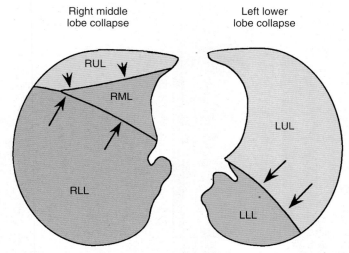

FIG. 6.7 **Typical patterns of middle and lower lobe collapse.** *LLL*, left lower lobe *LUL*, left upper lobe *RLL*, right lower lobe *RML*, right middle lobe *RUL*, right upper lobe.

can be seen anterolaterally, bordering the collapsed lobe, with the lower lobe bordering it posterolaterally. These aerated lobes usually separate the collapsed middle lobe from the lateral chest wall.

Lower Lobe Collapse

On either side the major fissure rotates posteromedially (Fig. 6.7). The collapsed lobe contacts the posterior mediastinum and posteromedial chest wall and maintains contact with the medial diaphragm.

Passive Atelectasis

In the presence of pleural effusion the lung tends to retract or collapse toward the hilum, and fluid entering the fissures allows the lobes to separate. With injection of contrast medium, the collapsed lung opacifies and is clearly distinguishable from surrounding fluid. Air bronchograms may be seen within collapsed lobes. *Rounded atelectasis* is a form of passive atelectasis. *Linear, disk, or platelike atelectasis* at the lung bases may be seen as a result of limited diaphragmatic motion.

Rounded Atelectasis

Rounded atelectasis represents focal, collapsed, and often folded lung. It is common and almost always occurs in association with pleural thickening or pleural effusion.

Rounded atelectasis is most common in the posterior paravertebral regions and may be bilateral in patients with bilateral pleural abnormalities. Areas of rounded atelectasis, which appear as a mass or

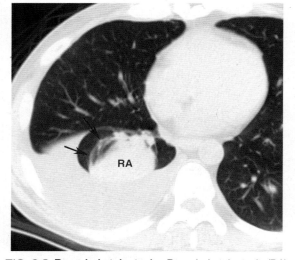

FIG. 6.8 **Rounded atelectasis.** Rounded atelectasis *(RA)* is present in a patient with a large right pleural effusion. The atelectatic lung shows vessels *(arrows)* curving into its edge, the comet-tail sign. The lesion shows extensive pleural contact, and there is posterior displacement of the major fissure, indicating lower lobe volume loss.

mass-like consolidation, are usually several centimeters in diameter. Bending or bowing of adjacent bronchi and arteries toward the edge of the area of rounded atelectasis, because of volume loss or folding of lung, is characteristic (Fig. 6.8); this finding has been termed the *comet-tail sign.* Air bronchograms can sometimes be seen within the mass. Rounded atelectasis opacifies after contrast medium infusion.

Four findings must be present to make a confident diagnosis of rounded atelectasis on CT; if these are present, follow-up is usually unnecessary (Fig. 6.8). However, if one or more of these findings is lacking, you should be cautious in making the diagnosis, and close follow-up or biopsy may be necessary. The four findings of rounded atelectasis are:
- ipsilateral pleural effusion or thickening
- significant contact between the lung lesion and the abnormal pleural surface
- the *comet-tail* sign
- volume loss in the lobe in which the opacity is seen
Rounded atelectasis may be associated with asbestos-related pleural thickening, occurring adjacent to regions of thickened pleura, but often has an atypical appearance. Areas of atelectasis or focal fibrosis in patients exposed to asbestos can be irregular, may not have extensive pleural contact, and may not be associated with the comet-tail sign.

Cicatrization Atelectasis
Cicatrization atelectasis occurs in the presence of pulmonary fibrosis and may be associated with tuberculosis (TB), radiation, or chronic bronchiectasis. In this condition, there is no evidence of bronchial obstruction. Rather, air bronchograms and bronchial dilation (bronchiectasis) are usually visible within the area of collapse. The volume loss is often severe.

SUGGESTED READING

Batra, P., Brown, K., Hayashi, K., & Mori, M. (1996). Rounded atelectasis. *J Thorac Imaging, 11*, 187–197.

Berkman, Y. M., Auh, Y. H., Davis, S. D., & Kazam, E. (1989). Anatomy of the minor fissure: Evaluation with thin-section CT. *Radiology, 170*, 647–651.

Godwin, J. D., & Tarver, R. D. (1985). Accessory fissures of the lung. *AJR. Am J Roentgenol, 144*, 39–47.

Hansell, D. M., Bankier, A. A., MacMahon, H., McLoud, T. C., Muller, N. L., & Remy, J. (2008). Fleischner society: Glossary of terms for thoracic imaging. *Radiology, 246*, 697–722.

Proto, A. V., & Ball, J. B. (1983). Computed tomography of the major and minor fissures. *AJR. Am J Roentgenol, 140*, 439–448.

Raasch, B. N., Carsky, E. W., Lane, E. J., et al. (1982). Radiographic anatomy of the interlobar fissures: A study of 100 specimens. *AJR. Am J Roentgenol, 138*, 1043.

Woodring, J. H., & Reed, J. C. (1996). Types and mechanisms of pulmonary atelectasis. *J Thorac Imaging, 11*, 92–108.

Woodring, J. H., & Reed, J. C. (1996). Radiographic manifestations of lobar atelectasis. *J Thorac Imaging, 11*, 109–144.

B: CONGENITAL LESIONS

Congenital lung lesions may result from anomalous development of bronchi, lung parenchyma, vasculature, or a combination of these. The most common or significant abnormalities are reviewed.

PULMONARY AGENESIS AND APLASIA
Pulmonary agenesis consists of the complete absence of a lung and its bronchi and vascular supply. With pulmonary aplasia, a rudimentary bronchus is present, ending in a blind pouch, but lung parenchyma and pulmonary vessels are absent (Fig. 6.9).

TRACHEAL BRONCHUS
The origin of all or part (usually the apical segment) of the right upper lobe bronchus from the trachea is termed a *tracheal bronchus* (Fig. 6.10); its incidence is less than 1%. A left-sided tracheal bronchus supplying part of the left upper lobe is much less common. Tracheal bronchus is common in cloven-hoofed animals such as pigs, sheep, goats, camels, and giraffes; it is sometimes called a *pig bronchus* or *bronchus suis*. It may be associated with recurrent infection.

BRONCHIAL ATRESIA AND CONGENITAL LOBAR OVERINFLATION
Bronchial atresia is characterized by local narrowing or obliteration of a lobar, segmental, or subsegmental bronchus. It is most common in the left upper followed by the right upper and middle lobes. Mucus commonly accumulates in dilated bronchi distal to the obstruction, resulting in a tubular, branching, or ovoid mucus plug or *mucocele*. The lung remains aerated distal to the obstruction because of collateral ventilation, but air trapping occurs, and the obstructed lobe or segments

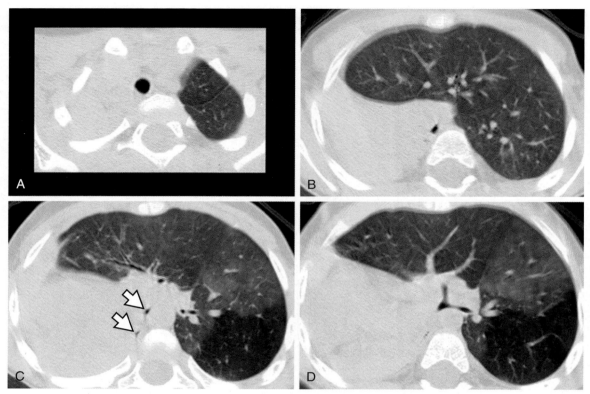

FIG. 6.9 Pulmonary aplasia in a child. (A–D) The right lung is completely absent, with mediastinal shift to the right and herniation of the left lung across the midline. The presence of rudimentary bronchi on the right (C, *arrows*) indicates that this represents aplasia rather than agenesis.

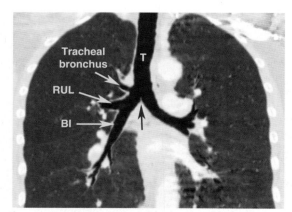

FIG. 6.10 Tracheal bronchus. Coronal reconstruction through the trachea *(T)* and bronchi. A tracheal bronchus arises from the lateral wall of the trachea above the carina *(red arrow)*. The main right upper lobe bronchus *(RUL)* is visible at a lower level. *BI*, Bronchus intermedius.

often appear hyperlucent and hypovascular. Bronchial atresia is usually diagnosed in adults. Many patients are asymptomatic although infection of obstructed lung may occur.

Congenital lobar overinflation (CLO), formerly known as *congenital lobar emphysema*, is characterized by marked overinflation of a lobe. Most cases present within the first month of life; symptoms of respiratory distress are typical. Most cases of CLO are associated with partial or complete bronchial obstruction occurring as a result of deficient cartilage, external compression, or luminal obstruction. CLO is most common in the left upper lobe (40%), middle lobe (35%), and right upper lobe (20%) (note the similarity of this distribution to that of bronchial atresia). Mediastinal shift away from the abnormal lobe usually occurs. Resection is often necessary. It is reasonable to assume that cases of CLO that go unrecognized at birth may be diagnosed years later as bronchial atresia.

Bronchogenic Cyst

The appearance of a mediastinal bronchogenic cyst is described in Chapter 4. Pulmonary bronchogenic cysts are typically well defined, round or oval, and of fluid or soft-tissue attenuation; previously infected cysts can contain air or an air-fluid level. When a cyst contains air, its wall appears very thin, although consolidation of surrounding lung may be present. Such cysts are most common in the lower lobes.

ARTERIOVENOUS MALFORMATION
Pulmonary Arteriovenous Malformation

Pulmonary arteriovenous malformation (AVM) is supplied by the pulmonary artery(s) and drained by the pulmonary vein(s). Pulmonary AVM can be single (65%) or multiple (35%) and is often associated with Osler-Weber-Rendu syndrome (65%). On CT, pulmonary AVM can appear as a single dilated vascular sac or fistula, visible as a smooth, sharply defined round or oval nodule (most common), or a tangle of dilated tortuous vessels, appearing as a lobulated or serpiginous mass. In each type the feeding pulmonary artery (or arteries) and the draining pulmonary vein (or veins) are dilated and should be easily seen on CT (Fig. 6.11).

An AVM with a single feeding artery and draining vein (*simple AVM*) is most common; a *complex AVM* with multiple supplying vessels is less frequent. In most cases the fistula is immediately subpleural in location. These characteristic findings are generally sufficient to make a specific diagnosis on scans without contrast medium infusion, even for AVMs only a few millimeters in diameter.

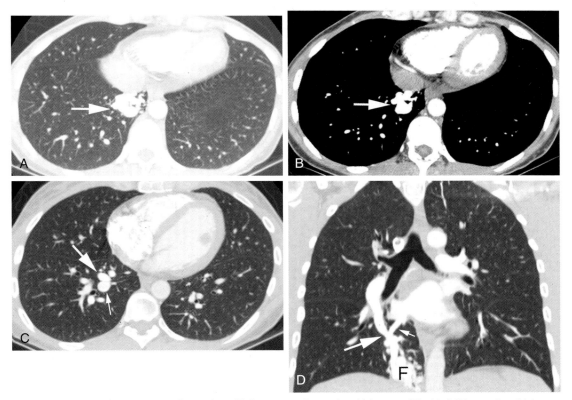

FIG. 6.11 Arteriovenous malformation. (A) Contrast-enhanced multidetector CT with 1.25-mm slice thickness (lung window) shows a lobulated and serpiginous mass at the right lung base typical of an arteriovenous malformation *(arrow)*. (B) With a soft-tissue window setting, dense enhancement is visible *(arrow)*. (C) At a more cephalad level the feeding artery *(large arrow)* and draining vein *(small arrow)* are visible. (D) A coronal reformation shows the feeding artery *(large arrow)*, draining vein *(small arrow)*, and subpleural fistula *(F)*.

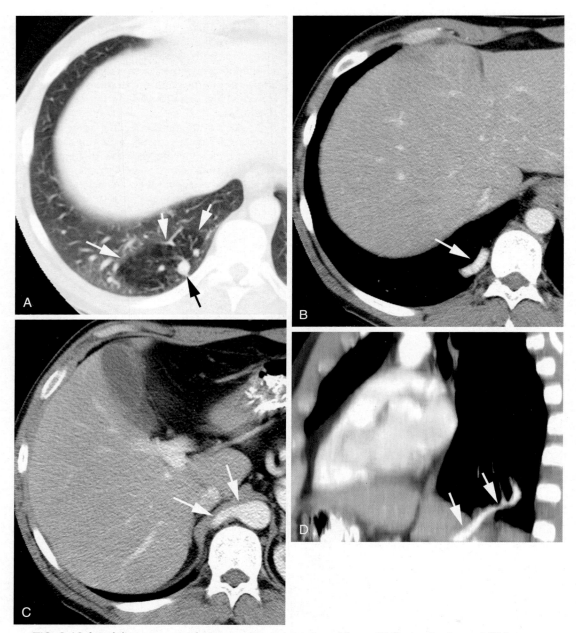

FIG. 6.12 Intralobar sequestration appearing as hyperlucent lung. (A) Contrast-enhanced CT (lung window) in a patient with intralobar sequestration shows an area of lucent lung *(white arrows)* at the right lung base. An abnormal vessel *(black arrow)* is visible within the area of lucency. (B) Soft-tissue window at a lower level shows the abnormal vessel *(arrow)*. (C) A scan near the lung base shows that the abnormal vessel arises from the aorta *(arrows)*. (D) Sagittal reformation shows the abnormal vessel *(arrows)*, originating in the abdomen, which supplies the posterior lower lobe.

Although contrast medium is not usually needed for diagnosis, a pulmonary AVM shows rapid and dense opacification after bolus contrast medium injection, followed by rapid washout of the contrast (Fig. 6.11). As would be expected, opacification occurs just after opacification of the right ventricle and pulmonary artery. For a fistula larger than 3 mm, catheter embolization is the treatment of choice. Catheter pulmonary angiography is generally performed in association with embolization.

Systemic Arteriovenous Malformation

Rarely, an anomalous systemic artery arising from the aorta or one of its branches supplies an area of otherwise normal lung. Drainage into pulmonary veins is via normal capillaries rather than through a dilated vascular sac or fistula. Systemic AVM is usually diagnosed incidentally, although hemoptysis may occur. In contrast to sequestration, described next, systemic AVM supplies normally aerated lung, containing normal bronchi (i.e., there is no sequestered lung).

PULMONARY SEQUESTRATION

Pulmonary sequestration represents a focal lung anomaly, without normal bronchial or pulmonary artery supply, fed by an anomalous systemic artery or arteries. Between 70% and 90% of sequestrations are located posteriorly and medially at the left lung base. In most cases the feeding systemic artery(s) is visible on contrast-enhanced CT (Figs. 6.12 and 6.13). There are two types.

Intralobar Sequestration

Intralobar sequestration is most common and is usually diagnosed in adults. It is contained within an otherwise normal lobe, usually the left lower lobe. Recurrent or chronic infection is common. Venous drainage is usually by means of pulmonary veins, although systemic (azygos) vein drainage can be seen. Intralobar sequestration typically contains air but can be quite variable in appearance. On CT, intralobar sequestration can appear as

- a region of hyperlucent lung (Fig. 6.12A)
- a cystic or multicystic abnormality (sometimes with air-fluid levels)
- consolidated or collapsed lung (Fig. 6.13)
- a combination of these findings

Areas of lucent lung in association with or representing part of an intralobar sequestration are common (Fig. 6.12A). Normal bronchi are not seen in the sequestration, and if the sequestration is aerated, the vascular branching pattern within it may appear abnormal.

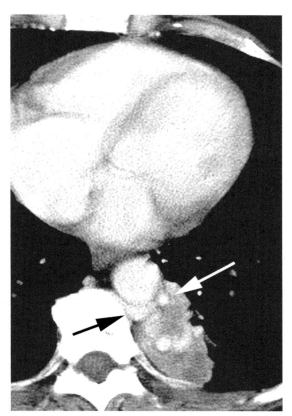

FIG. 6.13 **Intralobar sequestration appearing as consolidated lung.** Contrast-enhanced CT (soft-tissue window) in a patient with intralobar sequestration shows an area of consolidation adjacent to the aorta in the left lower lobe. An anomalous artery *(white arrow)* arises from the descending aorta and supplies the sequestration. The draining vein *(black arrow)* communicates with the hemiazygos vein.

Extralobar Sequestration

Extralobar sequestration is relatively uncommon and is usually diagnosed in infants or children. Infection is rare. It has its own pleural envelope, rarely contains air, and almost always appears as a solid mass. Venous drainage is usually by systemic veins.

CONGENITAL PULMONARY AIRWAY MALFORMATION

Congenital pulmonary airway malformation (CPAM), also known as *congenital cystic adenomatoid malformation*, consists of an intralobar mass of disorganized lung tissue, derived primarily from bronchioles, and often cystic or multicystic. About 70% present during the first week of life, but 10% are diagnosed after the first year, and some are first diagnosed in adults. Lower lobes are most often involved, but any lobe can be affected.

Five types (numbered 0–4) of CPAM have been described, on the basis on their histologic features. In adults, CPAM usually presents as an air-filled, or air- and fluid-filled cystic or multicystic mass. It may also appear as a solid mass or focal consolidation. It may mimic sequestration on CT but is less common.

HYPOGENETIC LUNG (SCIMITAR) SYNDROME

Hypogenetic lung syndrome (also known *as scimitar syndrome* and *venolobar syndrome*) is a rare anomaly

almost always occurring on the right side. The term *scimitar syndrome* derives from the scimitar-like appearance of the anomalous vein that is commonly present. It is characterized by four features that coexist in various degrees:
- hypoplasia of the lung with abnormal segmental or lobar anatomy;
- hypoplasia of the ipsilateral pulmonary artery;
- anomalous pulmonary venous return (the *scimitar vein*) from the right upper lobe or the entire right lung, usually to the vena cava or right atrium;
- anomalous systemic arterial supply to a portion of the hypoplastic lung, usually the lower lobe.

On CT the hypoplastic right lung is recognizable because of dextroposition of the heart and mediastinal shift to the right (Fig. 6.14). The hypoplastic lung may also show abnormal bronchial anatomy, deficient

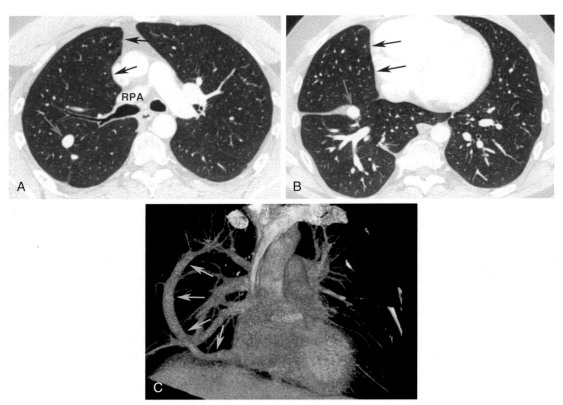

FIG. 6.14 **Hypogenetic lung syndrome.** (A) At the level of the right upper lobe bronchus, the right lung is reduced in volume and the mediastinum is shifted toward the right *(red arrows)*. The right pulmonary artery *(RPA)* appears small compared with the left pulmonary artery. The scimitar vein *(blue arrow)* is visible within the right lung. (B) At the level of the heart a rightward mediastinal shift *(red arrows)* is again seen, with the scimitar vein *(blue arrow)* visible in relation to a thickened major fissure. (C) A three-dimensional reconstruction shows the anomalous vein *(blue arrows)* draining into the right atrium. Its curved shape resembles a Turkish scimitar.

bronchial divisions, or mirror-image bronchial or pulmonary artery branching. When an anomalous (scimitar) vein is present, it is clearly visible on CT, often draining into the right atrium or inferior vena cava. Hypoplasia of the pulmonary artery is usually recognizable by the decreased size of vessels in the hypoplastic lung. This entity may be associated with congenital heart disease.

SUGGESTED READING

Biyyam, D. R., Chapman, T., Ferguson, M. R., Deutsch, G., & Dighe, M. K. (2010). Congenital lung abnormalities: Embryologic features, prenatal diagnosis, and postnatal radiologic-pathologic correlation. *Radiographics, 30*, 1721–1738.

Do, K. H., Goo, J. M., Im, J. G., et al. (2001). Systemic arterial supply to the lungs in adults: Spiral CT findings. *Radiographics, 21*, 387–402.

Ghaye, B., Szapiro, D., Fanchamps, J. M., & Dondelinger, R. F. (2001). Congenital bronchial abnormalities revisited. *Radiographics, 21*, 105–119.

Konen, E., Raviv-Zilka, L., Cohen, R. A., et al. (2003). Congenital pulmonary venolobar syndrome: Spectrum of helical CT findings with emphasis on computerized reformatting. *Radiographics, 23*, 1175–1184.

Lee, E. Y., Boiselle, P. M., & Cleveland, R. H. (2008). Multidetector CT evaluation of congenital lung abnormalities. *Radiology, 247*, 632–648.

Mata, J. M., Caceres, J., Lucaya, J., & Garcia-Conesa, J. A. (1990). CT of congenital malformations of the lung. *Radiographics, 10*, 651–674.

McAdams, H. P., Kirejczyk, W. M., Rosado-de-Christenson, M. L., & Matsumoto, S. (2000). Bronchogenic cyst: Imaging features with clinical and histopathologic correlation. *Radiology, 217*, 441–446.

Patz, E. F., Jr., Müller, N. L., Swensen, S. J., & Dodd, L. G. (1995). Congenital cystic adenomatoid malformation in adults: CT findings. *J Comput Assist Tomogr, 19*, 361–364.

Remy, J., Remy-Jardin, M., Wattinne, L., & Deffontaines, C. (1992). Pulmonary arteriovenous malformations: Evaluation with CT of the chest before and after treatment. *Radiology, 182*, 809–816.

Sener, R. N., Tugran, C., Savas, R., & Alper, H. (1993). CT findings in scimitar syndrome. *AJR. Am J Roentgenol, 160*, 1361.

Shenoy, S. S., Culver, G. J., & Pirson, H. S. (1979). Agenesis of lung in an adult. *AJR. Am J Roentgenol, 133*, 755–757.

Shimohira, M., Hara, M., Masanori, K., et al. (2007). Congenital pulmonary airway malformation: CT-pathologic correlation. *J Thorac Imaging, 22*, 149–153.

C: SOLITARY PULMONARY NODULE AND FOCAL LUNG LESIONS

CT is often used to evaluate a solitary nodule, mass, or focal lung lesion. It is used to (1) *evaluate morphology*, which can sometimes be diagnostic (e.g., pulmonary AVM), (2) *determine attenuation*, including the presence of ground-glass opacity (GGO), soft-tissue attenuation, calcium, fat, or opacification after contrast medium infusion, (3) *assess growth rate (or absence of growth)* for nonspecific lesions when a more aggressive approach is not warranted, and (4) *plan procedures*, such as percutaneous biopsy or resection or other interventions. CT is also used to detect lung nodules in patients being screened for lung cancer or being followed up for a known malignancy, and in conjunction with positron emission tomography (PET) scanning (i.e., PET-CT) to evaluate the metabolic activity of a nodule or lung lesion.

To make a semantic point, the term *nodule* is usually used to refer to a focal lung lesion 3 cm or less in diameter, which is relatively well defined, roughly spherical, and at least partially outlined by lung. *Mass* is used for a lesion larger than 3 cm. These measurements also distinguish a T1 tumor (≤3 cm) from a T2 to T4 tumor (>3 cm) in the lung cancer staging system (Table 4.3).

With multidetector CT, a 1- to 1.5-mm slice thickness is optimal, but lung cancer screening may be done with thicker slices (i.e., 2–5 mm) and a low-dose technique. A high-resolution reconstruction algorithm should generally be used for image reconstruction.

MORPHOLOGY OF FOCAL LESIONS AND LUNG NODULES

The differential diagnosis of a solitary nodule or mass is long (Table 6.1). However, lung cancers and some other focal lesions can have characteristic appearances on CT, which may be diagnostic or suggest a limited differential diagnosis.

Lung Cancer

Adenocarcinoma is the most common cell type of lung cancer (50% of cancers) and is the most common cell type presenting as a lung nodule (60%–70%), but any lung cancer cell type can present in this manner. On CT, lung cancers may appear solid, of GGO, or of mixed GGO and solid.

TABLE 6.1
Differential Diagnosis of a Solitary or Multiple Pulmonary Nodule(s)

Congenital lesions and normal variants

Arteriovenous malformation[a]

Bronchogenic cyst

Mucoid impaction (bronchial atresia)

Sequestration

Malignant neoplasm

Carcinoma[a]

Lymphoma[a]

Lymphoproliferative disease[a]

Metastatic neoplasm[a]

Lung sarcoma (e.g., chondrosarcoma, liposarcoma, fibrosarcoma)

Benign neoplasms and neoplasm-like conditions

Hamartoma

Lymphoproliferative disease[a]

Benign tumors (e.g., chondroma, lipoma, fibroma)

Infection and parasites

Angioinvasive aspergillosis[a]

Dirofilaria immitis (dog heartworm)

Echinococcus[a]

Focal (round) pneumonia[a]

Granulomatous infection or granuloma (tuberculosis, nontuberculous mycobacteria, fungus)[a]

Lung abscess[a]

Mycetoma (aspergilloma)[a]

Inflammatory (noninfectious) conditions

Organizing pneumonia[a]

Rheumatoid nodule[a]

Sarcoidosis[a]

Granulomatosis with polyangiitis (Wegener granulomatosis)[a]

Airway and inhalational disease

Mucoid impaction (mucous plug) in bronchiectasis[a]

Conglomerate mass or progressive massive fibrosis (e.g., silicosis)[a]

Lipoid pneumonia[a]

Vascular abnormalities

Hematoma

Infarction[a]

Septic embolism[a]

Miscellaneous

Amyloidosis[a]

Rounded atelectasis

[a]Also commonly presents with multiple nodules.

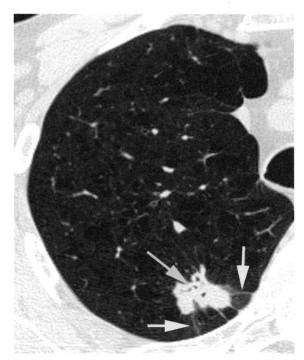

FIG. 6.15 **Spiculated invasive adenocarcinoma.** High-resolution CT in a patient with a nodule in the left lower lobe shows a lobulated and spiculated mass typical of carcinoma. Linear opacities contacting the pleural surface *(yellow arrows)* are termed *pleural tails*. The nodule contains several air bronchograms or air-filled cystic areas *(blue arrows)*.

Although a definite diagnosis of lung cancer cannot be made on CT, findings that suggest malignancy in a patient with a solitary nodule include:

- an irregular or spiculated nodule margin, usually caused by fibrosis or invasion of surrounding lung (90% of nodules with a spiculated edge are malignant; Fig. 6.15);
- a lobulated contour (Fig. 6.16);
- air bronchograms (Fig. 6.15) or cystic or "bubbly" air–containing regions within the nodule (seen in 65% of cancers but only 5% of benign lesions);
- a nodule exceeding 6 mm that is of GGO or of mixed GGO and solid attenuation (two-thirds are malignant; Fig. 6.17);
- cavitation (Fig. 6.16) with a nodular cavity wall or a wall exceeding 15 mm in greatest thickness (90% are cancers);
- an upper lobe nodule;
- a diameter exceeding 2 cm (95% are cancers);
- associated emphysema or lung fibrosis.

A spiculated edge and the presence of air bronchograms (Fig 6.15) or cystic air-containing regions are particularly common with adenocarcinoma. Lobulation of the nodule also suggests the diagnosis of carcinoma but may also be seen with other lesions, particularly hamartoma.

Both primary lung carcinomas and metastases can cavitate. Typically, a cavitary carcinoma has a thick, irregular, and nodular wall (Fig. 6.16), but some metastatic tumors, particularly sarcomas and those of squamous cell origin, can be thin walled. A cavitary nodule with a thin wall (<5 mm) is most likely (90%) benign.

Adenocarcinoma

Adenocarcinoma most commonly appears as a solid (soft-tissue attenuation) nodule. However, many adenocarcinomas present as a nodule of GGO or a nodule with both GGO and solid components (Fig. 6.17). The term *ground-glass opacity* (GGO) is used to describe hazy increased lung attenuation that does not obscure underlying vessels or bronchial walls.

The classification of pulmonary adenocarcinomas was revised in 2011 and is summarized in Table 6.2. Subtypes of adenocarcinoma include *adenocarcinoma in situ* (*AIS*), *minimally invasive adenocarcinoma* (*MIA*), and *lepidic predominant adenocarcinoma* (*LPA*).

AIS, MIA, and LPA are characterized, at least in part, by *lepidic growth*, which is defined as tumor growth along alveolar walls without invasion being present, appearing on CT as GGO. Pathologically, AIS is characterized by pure lepidic growth, MIA has lepidic growth with 5 mm or less of invasion, and LPA shows lepidic growth with more than 5 mm of invasion.

Typically, each of the newly described histologic subtypes of adenocarcinoma show some GGO on CT. AIS usually appears as a pure GGO nodule (Fig. 6.17A). MIA and LPA usually present as a nodule of mixed GGO and solid attenuation (e.g., the halo sign; Fig. 6.17B). The term *halo sign* is used to describe a nodule with a soft-tissue attenuation center surrounded by a less dense halo of GGO. These three types of adenocarcinoma have a relatively good prognosis (100% 5-year survival rate for AIS and MIA, and 75% for LPA) compared with other cell types of lung cancer. A premalignant lesion, *atypical adenomatous hyperplasia*, typically presents as a GGO nodule 5 mm or less in diameter.

So-called *invasive adenocarcinoma* has several histologic subtypes. These appear as solid nodules on CT (Figs. 6.15 and 6.16) or a predominantly solid

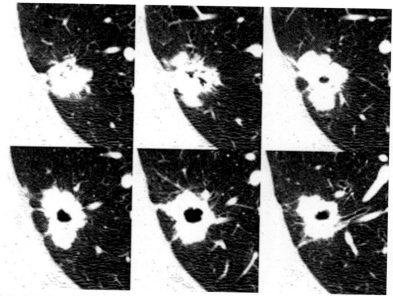

FIG. 6.16 **Spiculated invasive adenocarcinoma with an irregular cavity.** Six contiguous 1-mm scans through a speculated nodule with a lobulated contour. The nodule contains a thick-walled cavity. Pleural tails are also visible.

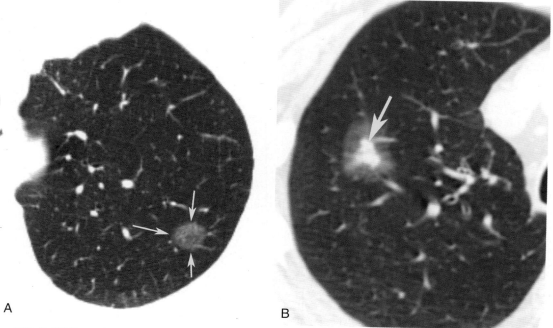

FIG. 6.17 **Two adenocarcinomas associated with ground-glass opacity.** (A) A nodule *(arrows)* consisting of pure ground-glass opacity represents an adenocarcinoma in situ. (B) A nodule with a dense center *(arrow)* surrounded by a halo of ground-glass opacity (the halo sign) represents a lepidic predominant adenocarcinoma. The soft-tissue attenuation center measures more than 5 mm.

TABLE 6.2
Classification of Pulmonary Adenocarcinoma (2011)
Premalignant
Atypical adenomatous hyperplasia
Preinvasive
Adenocarcinoma in situ
Minimally invasive adenocarcinoma
Invasive adenocarcinoma
Lepidic predominant adenocarcinoma
Invasive adenocarcinoma (various cell types)
Variants of invasive adenocarcinoma
Invasive mucinous adenocarcinoma
Various cell types

nodule with a small GGO component. Overall, the 5-year survival rate for invasive adenocarcinoma is about 50%. CT findings associated with invasive adenocarcinoma may include spiculation, lobulated borders, air bronchograms, and cavitation. *Invasive mucinous adenocarcinoma* usually presents with multiple nodules or multifocal GGO or consolidation; it is described later in this chapter and has a poor prognosis.

Although pulmonary adenocarcinoma typically presents with a solitary nodule, up to 20% of patients with adenocarcinoma have multiple synchronous cancers. These may be solid or of GGO.

Other Cell Types of Lung Cancer

Other common cell types of lung cancer include squamous cell carcinoma (15%–20% of lung cancer cases), large cell carcinoma, and small cell (neuroendocrine) carcinoma.

Large cell carcinoma typically appears as a lung nodule or mass, larger on average than adenocarcinoma, but otherwise having a similar appearance.

Squamous cell carcinoma and *small cell carcinoma* may present with a solid lung nodule resembling invasive adenocarcinoma, but more typically present with central or hilar masses resulting in bronchial obstruction. Small cell carcinoma has a very poor prognosis compared with other cell types of lung cancer.

Other cell types include *carcinoid tumor*, described in Chapter 5, and *large cell neuroendocrine carcinoma*, which resembles large cell carcinoma in appearance.

CT Diagnosis of Nodule Calcification

CT is important in the diagnosis of nodule calcification, a finding that may be very helpful in determining that the nodule is benign. About 25% to 35% of benign nodules appearing uncalcified on chest radiographs show calcification on thin-slice CT. CT with thin slices is optimum for detecting calcium, but dense calcification can also be seen with 5-mm slices. Soft-tissue window settings are best for showing that calcium is present.

When you are using CT to diagnose "benign" calcification, you must be sure that the calcification is *benign* in appearance (Fig. 6.18A). To be reasonably sure of a benign diagnosis, one of the following patterns must be present:
- diffuse calcification (Fig. 6.18B), typical of a granuloma;
- dense, central (i.e., *bull's-eye*) calcification, most typical of histoplasmosis (Fig. 6.18C);
- central and *popcorn* calcification, typical of hamartoma (Fig. 6.20B);
- concentric rings of calcification (*target* calcification; Fig. 6.18D), typical of histoplasmosis.

A caveat is that sarcomas and carcinoid tumors may be associated with dense calcification that is either homogeneous or "chunky."

About 5% to 10% of carcinomas contain some calcium, either as a result of tumor calcification or because the carcinoma has engulfed a preexisting granuloma. Calcification in malignancies is typically punctate or stippled or is eccentric within the nodule (Fig. 6.19). Although these patterns of calcification may also be seen in benign lesions, they should be considered to be indeterminate or potentially associated with malignancy.

Hamartoma

CT can be valuable in diagnosing pulmonary hamartoma. Hamartoma usually appears as a smooth and sharply marginated nodule, rounded, or with a lobulated contour. By CT with thin slices, about two-thirds of hamartomas can be correctly diagnosed because of visible fat (60%; Fig. 6.20A) that is either focal or diffuse, fat and calcification (30%), or calcification (10%). Fat is easily seen on thin-slice CT, with CT numbers ranging between –40 and –120 HU. Calcification may have a "popcorn" appearance because of calcification of nodules of cartilage (Fig. 6.20B) or may be diffuse.

Granulomas

Granulomas usually appear rounded and well defined. They may contain calcium, which may be dense and

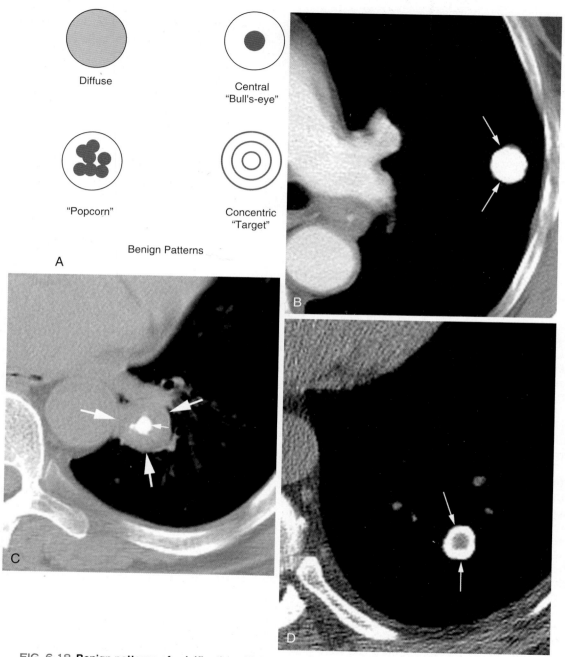

FIG. 6.18 Benign patterns of calcification. (A) Patterns of calcification typically associated with benign nodules. (B) Diffuse nodule calcification *(arrows)* in tuberculoma. (C) A nodule *(large arrows)* in the left lower lobe shows dense central (bull's-eye) calcification *(small arrow)*. (D) A concentric ring of calcification *(arrows)* outlines a lung nodule.

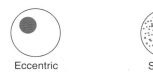

Eccentric   Stippled

Indeterminate patterns

A

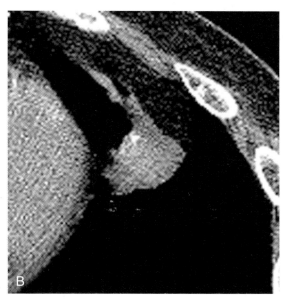

B

FIG. 6.19 **Indeterminate calcification.** (A) Patterns of calcification that may be seen in either benign or malignant nodules. (B) Thin-slice CT in a patient with an adenocarcinoma in the lingula shows a nodule with eccentric calcification. Eccentric calcification can be seen in carcinomas.

central, diffuse, or on occasion, ring-shaped (Fig. 6.18). An infection or noninfectious granulomatous lesion (e.g., sarcoidosis) presenting as a lung nodule or mass may be associated with small nodules adjacent to or surrounding it (i.e., *satellite nodules*; Fig. 6.21). In patients with sarcoidosis, this appearance has been referred to as the *galaxy sign*. Satellite nodules may also be seen with lung carcinoma, but they are evident in only a small percentage of cases.

Tuberculosis, Atypical Mycobacterial, and Fungal Infection

In most patients with TB exposure and a positive PPD skin test result, CT findings are normal. A small lung nodule, calcified or uncalcified and representing the original site of infection, is sometimes visible; associated calcified lymph nodes may be present. Small scattered nodules in the lung apex reflect the presence of

hematogenous spread at the time of the original infection. In most patients, these heal without progression.

In a small percentage of individuals, usually children and immunosuppressed patients, primary exposure to TB results in a focal pneumonia (which may involve any lobe). In half of these cases, associated hilar or mediastinal node enlargement is present. Nodes often appear to be low in attenuation on enhanced CT.

Progression of primary TB (often in patients with immune compromise) or after primary reactivation of an earlier infection (usually in the lung apices) can result in cavitation (Fig. 6.22). Cavities are usually irregular in shape and have irregular walls and multiple septations. Air-fluid levels are typically absent, although hemorrhage or superinfection may result in this finding. Cavities may be multiple and associated with satellite nodules.

The spread of infected material through the airways can result in findings of bronchopneumonia (i.e., patchy consolidation, *tree-in-bud* or *centrilobular nodules*), often in regions near the cavity or in the lower lobes (Fig. 6.22). Tree-in-bud and centrilobular nodules are described in the part of this chapter devoted to high-resolution CT (HRCT).

Infection with pathogenic atypical mycobacteria can result in identical findings. Fungal infections can result in findings indistinguishable from TB. If TB is considered in the differential diagnosis, it is generally a good idea to consider fungal infection as well.

The Halo Sign and Angioinvasive Aspergillosis

The halo sign, visible on CT, was first described in immunosuppressed patients with angioinvasive aspergillosis (Fig. 6.23). As indicated in the previous discussion, the term *halo sign* is used to describe a nodule with a soft-tissue attenuation center surrounded by a less dense halo of GGO.

In patients who are severely immunocompromised, particularly those with treated leukemia and neutropenia, this appearance is typical and highly suggestive of angioinvasive aspergillosis; often treatment is begun without confirmation of the diagnosis. In patients with angioinvasive aspergillosis, the halo sign reflects the presence of a septic infarction (the dense center) surrounded by hemorrhage (the halo).

Although suggestive of angioinvasive aspergillosis in the proper clinical setting, the halo sign is nonspecific and can be seen with other infections (e.g., TB, *Legionella* infection, nocardiosis, and cytomegalovirus infection), with some tumors (particularly adenocarcinomas,

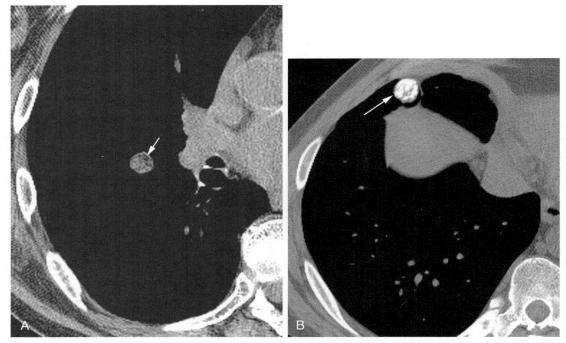

FIG. 6.20 Hamartoma: common appearances in two patients. (A) High-resolution CT with soft-tissue (mediastinal) window settings in a patient with a small lung nodule detected on plain radiographs. The nodule is round and sharply defined. It contains areas of low attenuation *(arrow)*, indicating the presence of fat. This appearance is diagnostic of hamartoma. (B) In another patient with hamartoma *(arrow)*, a rounded and sharply defined nodule shows "popcorn" calcification. This appearance is seen in some patients with hamartoma.

lymphoma, and Kaposi sarcoma), and in patients with pulmonary infarction and granulomatosis with polyangiitis (GPA), formerly termed *Wegener granulomatosis*. The histologic correlate with the halo varies with the entity. It may represent hemorrhage (e.g., aspergillosis, infarction, Kaposi sarcoma, and GPA), heterogenous consolidation in pneumonia, or lepidic growth of tumor (adenocarcinoma).

The Air-Crescent Sign and Mycetoma

The presence of a lung mass capped by a crescent of air is termed the *air-crescent sign* (Figs. 6.24 and 6.25). It usually indicates the presence of a mass within a cavity. The air-crescent sign is most typical of mycetoma, but it may also be seen in the later stages of angioinvasive aspergillosis, some bacterial infections with lung infarction, cavitary tumors, a clot or neoplasm within a cavity, and echinococcal cysts.

In patients with a preexisting pulmonary cyst or cavity, a mycetoma or fungus ball can form as a result of saprophytic infection, usually by *Aspergillus* (Fig. 6.25).

On CT a round or oval mass (the fungus ball) can be seen in a dependent location within the cavity and is typically mobile. The mass is capped by a crescent of air. Thickening of the cavity wall is common. In patients with a developing mycetoma, the fungus ball can contain multiple air collections. The same appearance can be seen in semiinvasive (chronic necrotizing) aspergillosis, in which the fungus also invades the wall of the cyst or cavity. Hemorrhage and hemoptysis are common associations. With angioinvasive aspergillosis, septic infarction of the lung can result in an air-crescent sign as the patient recovers (Fig. 6.24).

Lung Abscess and Cavities

A lung abscess can occur with a variety of bacterial, fungal, and parasitic infections. The hallmark of a lung abscess is necrosis or cavitation within an area of pneumonia or dense consolidation; the necrotic region can appear quite irregular. Necrosis is commonly visible on contrast-enhanced CT as one or more areas of low attenuation within opacified lung. Cavitation is said to

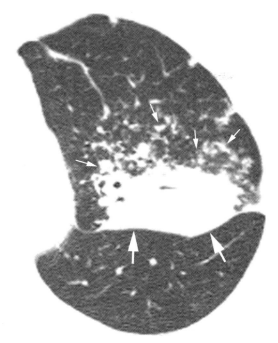

FIG. 6.21 **Satellite nodules in sarcoidosis.** High-resolution CT in a patient with sarcoidosis and a mass in the left lower lobe, marginated posteriorly by the major fissure *(large arrows)*. On high-resolution CT the mass is surrounded by a number of smaller satellite nodules *(small arrows)*. This appearance is most typical of a granulomatous process. It has also been referred to as the *galaxy sign* of sarcoidosis.

be present if air is visible within the lesion, and CT is often performed to confirm this diagnosis when a plain radiograph is suggestive. In an acute abscess the cavity wall may be irregular or thin and of uniform thickness; with healing the cavity wall is typically thin and uniform. An air-fluid level (or levels) is commonly present with bacterial infection (Fig. 6.26) and is uncommon with cavitary carcinoma, TB, or fungal infection. CT can also be helpful in distinguishing a lung abscess from empyema. Chapter 7 contrasts the CT appearances of lung abscess and empyema.

Pulmonary Infarction and Septic Embolism

Bland infarction with pulmonary embolism can result in a focal pulmonary opacity. Septic emboli are usually multiple. In either instance, opacities typically (1) are peripheral or abut a pleural surface, (2) are round or wedge-shaped, and (3) have a pulmonary artery branch leading to them (the *feeding vessel sign*). Some are associated with a halo sign because of surrounding hemorrhage. In patients with septic embolism, cavitation of lung nodules is common. Using contrast-enhanced CT, associated clots may be identified in the proximal pulmonary artery in patients with pulmonary infarction, but a visible clot is not typical of septic embolism.

Lipoid Pneumonia

Chronic aspiration of lipid (animal, vegetable, or mineral) can lead to lipoid pneumonia, with fat and variable amounts of fibrosis resulting in focal consolidations or masses. In some patients, most typically those with mineral oil aspiration, CT shows low-attenuation (−50 to −140 HU) consolidation indicative of its lipid content. When fibrosis predominates, the masses are of soft-tissue attenuation. Lipoid pneumonia differs from hamartoma, which may also contain fat, in that masses are larger and less well defined and usually appear more irregular.

Pleural (Fissural) Lesions

Small (a few millimeters) perifissural nodules are commonly seen on CT and are generally of no concern. Often they are flat or triangular. However, small rounded nodules with minimal fissural contact may represent a significant abnormality, and follow-up may be appropriate, on the basis of its size and suspicious morphology.

Occasionally, a pleural abnormality located in a fissure (e.g., a plaque, loculated effusion, or localized fibrous tumor of the pleura) may be misinterpreted as a lung nodule. Looking for the fissures on the CT will sometimes avoid this mistake.

NODULE GROWTH RATE AND CT FOLLOW-UP OF LUNG NODULES

The growth rate of a nodule, measured as the time required for doubling of volume (i.e., *doubling time,* corresponding to a 26% increase in nodule diameter), may be used to determine its likelihood of being malignant. A pulmonary nodule that doubles in volume in less than 1 month or more than 16 months is usually benign. Cancers appearing solid on CT usually have doubling times of 100 to 400 days. However, malignancy should be suspected if any growth occurs, no matter how slow. Carcinomas appearing on CT as a nodule of GGO or mixed GGO and soft tissue have slower growth rates, with doubling times usually ranging from 3 to 5 years.

Small, nonspecific pulmonary nodules are commonly seen on CT performed for other reasons

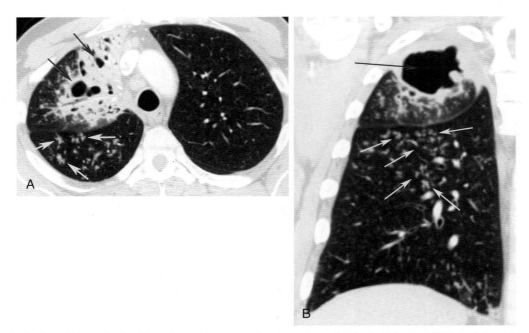

FIG. 6.22 **Tuberculosis with endobronchial spread and tree-in-bud opacity.** Thin-slice CT through the right upper lobe (A), and thin coronal reconstruction (B). In a patient with active tuberculosis, irregular cavitary lesions *(red arrows)* are visible in the right lung apex. Centrilobular nodules and branching tree-in-bud opacities *(yellow arrows)* in the adjacent lung represent endobronchial spread of infection and are common in active tuberculosis.

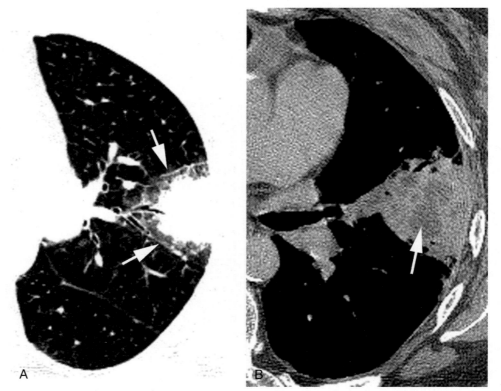

FIG. 6.23 **Invasive aspergillosis with the halo sign.** (A) In an immunosuppressed patient with leukemia, an ill-defined lung mass is surrounded by a less dense halo *(arrows)*. This finding is highly suggestive of invasive aspergillosis in a patient with the appropriate history. (B) A soft-tissue window at the same level shows central necrosis *(arrow)*.

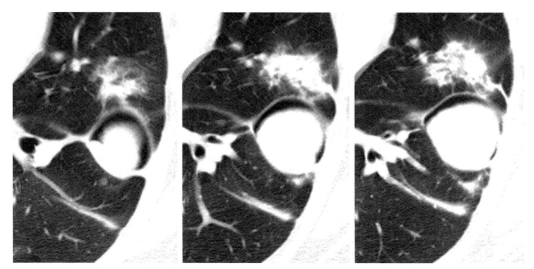

FIG. 6.24 **Invasive aspergillosis with an air-crescent sign.** A crescent of air outlines a mass within a cavity. In invasive aspergillosis the mass represents a ball of infarcted lung and the cavity represents the space the lung used to occupy. This is distinct from aspergilloma, in which an air-crescent sign reflects fungus within a preexisting cavity. Focal consolidation as a result of acute infection is visible anterior to the cavitary lesion.

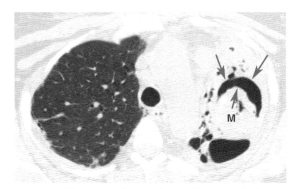

FIG. 6.25 **Mycetoma in a patient with a preexisting cavity.** A crescent of air *(arrows)* outlines a mass (mycetoma, *M*) within a cavity resulting from a prior tuberculosis infection. The mass was mobile and changed position when the patient was prone.

(i.e., an incidental lung nodule). CT is commonly used to follow a newly detected lung nodule or nodules to determine the presence or absence of growth when the nodule size or appearance or clinical factors do not indicate that a more aggressive approach is needed. It is generally agreed that a solid pulmonary nodule that does not grow over a 2-year period is very likely benign and does not require resection.

In a follow-up CT study to assess a small lung nodule or nodules for change in size, it is important to obtain scans with the same slice thickness and view them with the same window settings as in the original study. With spiral CT and volumetric imaging, nodules are not usually missed, but this is possible if the patient breathes during the study. When one is looking for or comparing nodule size, it is important to look at exactly the same levels on the two scans. Identifying and matching the pattern of branching vessels in the peripheral lung in the region of the nodule is the only way of knowing exactly what level is being viewed. If the same vessels are visible on both the original sans and the follow-up scans and the nodule looks different, then the nodule is different. If a different branching pattern is visible, then an apparent difference in nodule size may not be real.

Fleischner Society Guidelines

The Fleischner Society has published recommendations for the follow-up of incidental lung nodules detected with CT (i.e., lung nodules detected in patients not being screened for lung cancer or being followed up for a known cancer) that were widely accepted. The Fleischner Society has recently revised its recommendations for incidental lung nodules appearing solid (Table 6.3) or subsolid (entirely of GGO, or partly of GGO and partly solid; Table 6.4). Its guidelines are tailored to provide criteria that will result in follow-up of nodules with a greater than 1% chance of malignancy (approximately). It is important to emphasize

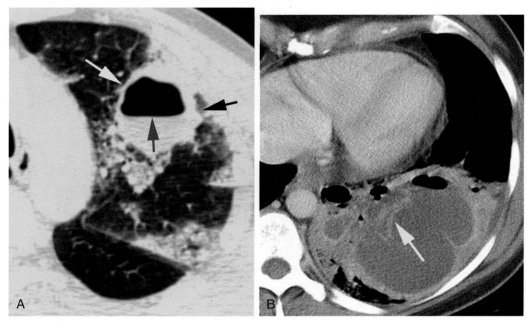

FIG. 6.26 **Two example of bacterial lung abscess.** (A) A lung abscess has a thin wall medially *(yellow arrow)*, has a thick and irregular wall laterally *(blue arrow)*, and contains an air-fluid level *(red arrow)*. Patchy consolidation is visible in the lung because of patchy pneumonia. (B) A large lung abscess has an irregular, thick wall, and contains residual strands of lung parenchyma and consists of several collections of air and fluid.

TABLE 6.3
Fleischner Society Guidelines for Management of Incidental Solid Nodules[a]

Nodule Type and Risk Factors	NODULE SIZE			Comments
	<6 mm	6–8 mm	>8 mm	
Solitary				
Low risk	No routine follow-up	CT at 6–12 months, consider CT at 18–24 months	Consider CT, PET-CT, or biopsy at 3 months	A nodule smaller than 6 mm with suspicious morphology or upper lobe location may warrant 12-month follow-up in a high-risk patient
High risk	Optional CT at 12 months	CT at 6-12 months, then CT at 18–24 months	Consider CT, PET-CT, or biopsy at 3 months	
Multiple				
Low risk	No routine follow-up	CT at 3–6 months, consider CT at 18–24 months	CT at 3–6 months, consider CT at 18–24 months	Use most suspicious nodule as a guide. Follow-up intervals may differ according to size and risk
High risk	Optional CT at 12 months	CT at 3–6 months, then CT at 18–24 months	CT at 3–6 months, then CT at 18–24 months	

[a]These recommendations do not apply to lung cancer screening, patients with immunosuppression, or patients with known primary cancer. Nodule dimensions are the average of long and short axes, rounded to the nearest millimeter.

TABLE 6.4
Fleischner Society Guidelines for Management of Incidental Subsolid Nodules[a]

Nodule Type	NODULE SIZE		Comments
	<6 mm	**≥6 mm**	
Solitary, ground-glass opacity	No routine follow-up	CT at 6–12 months; if the nodule persists, then CT every 2 years for a total of 5 years	For a suspicious ground-glass opacity nodule of 6 mm or smaller, consider follow-up at 2 and 4 years. Consider resection if it grows or develops a solid component
Solitary, part solid	No routine follow-up	CT at 3–6 months; if unchanged and solid component remains smaller than 6 mm, annual CT for 5 years	Persistent part-solid nodules with a solid component of 6 mm or larger should be considered highly suspicious
Multiple	CT at 3–6 months. If stable, consider CT at 2 and 4 years	CT at 3–6 months. Subsequent management based on the most suspicious nodule(s)	Multiple nodules smaller than 6 mm are usually benign, but consider follow-up at 2 and 4 years in selected high-risk patients

[a]These recommendations do not apply to lung cancer screening, patients with immunosuppression, or patients with known primary cancer. Nodule dimensions are the average of long and short axes, rounded to the nearest millimeter.

that these recommendations do not apply to patients younger than 35 years, in whom lung cancer is rare, immunosuppressed patients, patients with a known cancer, or patients undergoing CT for lung cancer screening. Recommendations for follow-up and management of patients undergoing CT screening (Lung-RADS) are described later.

Incidental Solid Nodules

In general, for an incidentally detected nodule (or nodules) that appears solid on CT, if the patient is at low risk of lung cancer, and the nodule is less than 6 mm in diameter, no follow-up is required (Table 6.3). Nodule diameter is determined by the average of the long and short nodule axes, rounded to the nearest millimeter. Clinical risk factors include increased age, smoking, exposure to carcinogens, family history of lung cancer, a history of emphysema or lung fibrosis, and sometimes sex and race; risk is determined by means of calculations recommended by the American College of Chest Physicians. If the patient is considered to be at high risk, then CT follow-up at 1 year is optional for a nodule smaller than nodule, and may be warranted if the nodule is suspicious on the basis of an upper lobe location or morphology.

For lung nodules of 6 to 8 mm, follow-up CT at 6 to 12 months is recommended regardless of risk, with further follow-up at 18 to 24 months if the patient is at high risk. If the nodule exceeds 8 mm, a more aggressive approach may be taken, with consideration of 3-month CT follow-up, PET-CT, or biopsy (Table 6.3).

In patients with multiple solid nodules, a different follow-up schedule is recommended (Table 6.3), and generally, management is determined by the most suspicious appearing nodule. If the patient has a known cancer, then a nodule of any size will be followed up, with the interval generally determined by clinical considerations.

Incidental Nodules Associated With Ground-Glass Opacity

For a GGO nodule or a part-solid (mixed GGO and solid attenuation) nodule smaller than 6 mm, no follow-up is required, and risk is not a consideration (Table 6.4). For a GGO nodule larger than 6 mm, 6 to 12-month follow-up is recommended to confirm that the nodule persists, with follow-up every 2 years for a total of 5 years. For a GGO nodule 6 mm or larger, consider resection if the nodule grows or a solid component develops during follow-up. Development of a solid component in a GGO nodule may indicate that invasion has occurred.

For a part-solid nodule 6 mm or larger, CT should be performed at 3 to 6 months to confirm persistence. If unchanged and solid component remains smaller than 6 mm, annual CT should be performed for 5 years. Persistent part-solid nodules with solid components 6 mm or larger should be considered highly suspicious.

TABLE 6.5
American College of Radiology Lung-RADS for Lung Cancer Screening (Abridged and Edited)

Category	Descriptor	Category Number	Findings	Management	likelihood of cancer
Negative	No nodules or definitely benign nodules	1	No lung nodules or nodules with benign type calcification or fat		
Benign appearance or behavior	Nodules with a very low likelihood of becoming a clinically active cancer because of small size or lack of growth	2	**Solid nodule(s)** <6 mm; new <4 mm **Part-solid nodule(s)** <6 mm total diameter on baseline screening **Nonsolid nodule(s) (GGN)** <20 mm or ≥20 mm and unchanged or slowly growing **Category 3 or 4 nodules** unchanged for ≥3 months	Continue with annual screening	<1%
Probably benign	Probably benign findings: short-term follow up suggested; includes nodules with a low likelihood of becoming a clinically active cancer	3	**Solid nodule(s)** ≥6 mm to <8 mm at the baseline or new 4 mm to <6 mm **Part-solid nodule(s)** ≥6 mm total diameter with solid component <6 mm or new <6 mm total diameter **Nonsolid nodule(s) (GGN)** ≥20 mm on baseline CT or new	6-month CT follow-up	1–2%
Suspicious	Findings for which additional diagnostic testing and/or tissue sampling is recommended	4A	**Solid nodule(s)** ≥8 mm to <15 mm at the baseline or growing <8 mm or new 6 mm to <8 mm **Part-solid nodule(s)** ≥6 mm with solid component, ≥6 mm to <8 mm or with a new or growing <4-mm solid component **Endobronchial nodule**	3-month CT follow-up; PET-CT may be used when there is a ≥8 mm solid component	5–15%
		4B	**Solid nodule(s)** ≥15 mm or new or growing, and ≥8 mm **Part-solid nodule(s)** with solid component ≥8 mm or new or growing ≥4 mm solid	CT with or without contrast; PET/CT and/or tissue sampling depending on the probability of malignancy and comorbidities. PET/CT may be used when there is a ≥8 mm solid component	>15%
		4X	Category 3 or 4 nodules with features that suggest malignancy		

GGN; ground glass nodule (i.e. nodule entirely GGO)

As in patients with solid nodules, in patients with multiple GGO or part-solid nodules, a different follow-up schedule is recommended (Table 6.4), and generally, follow-up and management are based on the most suspicious nodule.

Decreased Nodule Size on Follow-up

Usually a nodule that decreases in size on follow-up is benign. However, on occasion, a lung cancer can show a transient decrease in size on follow-up. A single follow-up scan showing a decrease in nodule size is not sufficient to call the nodule *benign*. A second scan showing a continued decrease in size or resolution should be obtained.

PET Scanning

PET scanning has high sensitivity (97%) and specificity (80%) in diagnosing cancers that are 1 cm or larger and appear solid on CT. Its sensitivity in the diagnosis of carcinomas appearing as a GGO nodule is low. It is not generally recommended in evaluation of a GGO nodule.

CT LUNG CANCER SCREENING

CT is used to screen patients at high risk of lung cancer because of smoking history. In comparison with screening with chest radiographs, more lung cancers, smaller lung cancers, and more early-stage (stage I) cancers are detected by CT screening. However, false positives are common (up to 70% of screened patients in some parts of the US at least one lung nodule).

In the National Lung Cancer Screening Trial, more than 52,000 high-risk patients were randomly screened with use of low-dose CT using 2- to 3-mm-thick slices or chest radiographs, and were then followed up with annual screenings for up to 5 years. On initial CT screening, 27% of participants had at least one nodule of 4 mm or larger, and about 40% had at least one nodule detected by CT during the study. CT, compared with chest radiography, was more sensitive (94% vs. 74%) and less specific (74% vs. 91%) in detecting cancer. Overall, about 1.1% of CT-screened participants were found to have lung cancer. Participants screened by CT had a 20% reduction in lung cancer mortality and a reduction in overall mortality of 6.7%.

Lung nodules detected as a result of CT lung cancer screening are reported and followed up with use of a system developed by the American College of Radiology, termed *Lung-RADS* (*Lung Imaging Reporting and Data System*) (Table 6.5). This system is designed to reduce false positives, reduce confusion in lung cancer screening CT interpretations, provide reporting and management recommendations, and facilitate outcome monitoring and development of a nationwide database.

Lung-RADS includes criteria for follow-up of solid and nonsolid nodules, but the follow-up intervals and size criteria differ somewhat from those recommended by the Fleischner Society for incidental nodules and are difficult to remember. Having a complete copy of the Lung-RADS criteria on hand (https://www.acr.org/Quality-Safety/Resources/LungRADS) is essential when one is reading lung cancer screening studies. Because patients reported with this system are being screened with yearly CT, nodules with a low likelihood of being a cancer require only yearly rescreening.

USE OF CT TO GUIDE BIOPSY

Bronchoscopy is most accurate in diagnosing central masses that have an endobronchial component, whereas needle biopsy is best for peripheral lung lesions. CT is usually used for needle aspiration biopsy of lung nodules. It allows precise localization of the needle tip within the nodule and allows the least dangerous approach to the nodule to be chosen (avoiding bullae, large vessels, etc.).

Thoracoscopic biopsy or resection of peripheral lung nodules can be assisted by CT-guided localization techniques. These may involve injection of methylene blue into lung adjacent to the nodule or placement of a hooked wire within the nodule.

SUGGESTED READING

Aberle, D. R., Adams, A. M., Berg, C. D., et al. (2011). Reduced lung-cancer mortality with low-dose computed tomographic screening. *N Engl J Med, 365*, 395–409.

Chong, S., Lee, K. S., Chung, M. J., Han, J., Kwon, O. J., & Kim, T. S. (2006). Neuroendocrine tumors of the lung: Clinical, pathologic, and imaging findings. *Radiographics, 26*, 41–57.

Church, T. R., Black, W. C., Aberle, D. R., et al. (2013). Results of initial low-dose computed tomographic screening for lung cancer. *N Engl J Med, 368*, 1980–1991.

Fintelmann, F. J., Bernheim, A., Digumarthy, S. R., et al. (2015). The 10 pillars of lung cancer screening: Rationale and logistics of a lung cancer screening program. *Radiographics, 35*, 1893–1908.

Gimenez, A., Franquet, T., Prats, R., et al. (2002). Unusual primary lung tumors: A radiologic-pathologic overview. *Radiographics, 22*, 601–619.

MacMahon, H., Naidich, D. P., Goo, J. M., et al. (2017). Guidelines for management of incidental pulmonary nodules detected on CT images: From the Fleischner Society 2017. *Radiology, 284*, 228–243.

Mahoney, M. C., Shipley, R. T., Cocoran, H. L., & Dickson, B. A. (1990). CT demonstration of calcification in carcinoma of the lung. *AJR. Am J Roentgenol, 154*, 255–258.

McWilliams, A., Tammemagi, M. C., Mayo, J. R., et al. (2013). Probability of cancer in pulmonary nodules detected on first screening CT. *N Engl J Med, 369*, 910–919.

Pinsky, P. F., Gierada, D. S., Black, W., et al. (2015). Performance of Lung-RADS in the National Lung Screening Trial: A retrospective assessment. *Ann Intern Med, 162,* 485–491.

Primack, S. L., Hartman, T. E., Lee, K. S., & Müller, N. L. (1994). Pulmonary nodules and the CT halo sign. *Radiology, 190,* 513–515.

Rosado de Christenson, M. L., Abbott, G. F., Kirejczyk, W. M., et al. (1999). Thoracic carcinoids: Radiologic-pathologic correlation. *Radiographics, 19,* 707–736.

Schultz, E. M., Sanders, G. D., Trotter, P. R., et al. (2008). Validation of two models to estimate the probability of malignancy in patients with solitary pulmonary nodules. *Thorax, 63,* 335–341.

Siegelman, S. S., Khouri, N. F., Scott, W. W., et al. (1986). Pulmonary hamartoma: CT findings. *Radiology, 160,* 313–317.

Templeton, P. A., & Zerhouni, E. A. (1991). High-resolution computed tomography of focal lung disease. *Semin Roentgenol, 26,* 143–150.

Travis, W. D., Brambilla, E., Nicholson, A. G., et al. (2015). The 2015 World Health Organization classification of lung tumors: Impact of genetic, clinical and radiologic advances since the 2004 classification. *J Thorac Oncol, 10,* 1243–1260.

Travis, W. D., Brambilla, E., Noguchi, M., et al. (2011). International Association for the Study of Lung Cancer/American Thoracic Society/European Respiratory Society international multidisciplinary classification of lung adenocarcinoma. *J Thorac Oncol, 6,* 244–285.

Truong, M. T., Ko, J. P., Rossi, S. E., et al. (2014). Update in the evaluation of the solitary pulmonary nodule. *Radiographics, 34,* 1658–1679.

Webb, W. R. (1990). Radiologic evaluation of the solitary pulmonary nodule. *AJR. Am J Roentgenol, 154,* 701–708.

Zwiebel, B. R., Austin, J. H. M., & Grines, M. M. (1991). Bronchial carcinoid tumors: Assessment with CT of location and intratumoral calcification in 31 patients. *Radiology, 179,* 483–486.

Zwirewich, C. V., Vedal, S., Miller, R. R., & Müller, N. L. (1991). Solitary pulmonary nodule: High-resolution CT and radiologic–pathologic correlation. *Radiology, 179,* 469–476.

D: MULTIPLE LUNG NODULES AND MASSES

The differential diagnosis of multiple nodules and masses includes metastases (Figs. 6.27 and 6.28); lymphoma; lung carcinoma with synchronous primary tumors; bacterial (Fig. 6.29), fungal, and sometimes viral infections; granulomatous diseases; sarcoidosis; GPA; rheumatoid lung disease (rheumatoid nodules); amyloidosis; and septic embolism. Also, many of the causes of a solitary nodule (Table 6.1) can also result in multiple nodules. Entities characteristically resulting in multiple nodules or masses are described next.

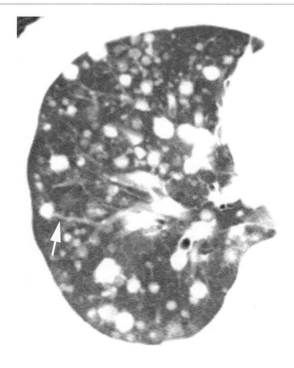

FIG. 6.28 **Pulmonary metastases with the feeding vessel sign.** Multiple well-defined nodules represent metastases from a renal cell carcinoma. Involvement of the peripheral lung is typical. A few of these nodules *(arrow)* appear to be related to a pulmonary vessel, the so-called *feeding vessel sign.*

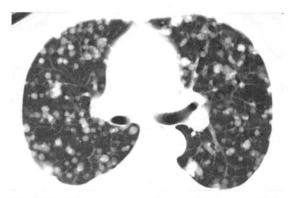

FIG. 6.27 **Pulmonary metastases.** CT shows multiple nodules with a diffuse distribution. Despite their small size, the nodules are sharply defined. They involve the pleural surfaces and have a diffuse and uniform distribution.

METASTASES

Hematogenous pulmonary metastases are typically diffuse or have a predilection for the peripheral and subpleural lung (Figs. 6.27 and 6.28); they may be small or large. Pulmonary metastases are typically round and well defined (Fig. 6.27). Some metastases with a surrounding hemorrhage can be ill defined or associated with the halo sign. Cavitation and calcification can be seen with some metastatic tumors. Pulmonary metastases may be seen to have a connection to a pulmonary artery branch, reflecting their embolic nature (i.e., the *feeding vessel sign*; Fig. 6.28). However, this finding can be present for other causes of pulmonary nodules, such as GPA and bland or septic emboli.

Small (<5 mm), scattered pulmonary nodules are commonly seen on CT in patients being followed up for a known neoplasm; most are benign, representing subpleural lymphoid aggregates and granulomas. Short-term follow-up CT (e.g., 3 months) is usually used to assess their significance. Metastases typically increase in size in untreated patients.

INVASIVE MUCINOUS ADENOCARCINOMA

In the classification of pulmonary adenocarcinoma reviewed earlier, what was formerly referred to as *diffuse* or *multifocal bronchioloalveolar carcinoma* is now termed *invasive mucinous adenocarcinoma* (IMA). This tumor presents with diffuse or patchy lung consolidation or GGO, or multiple lung nodules that may be centrilobular in location (Fig. 6.30). Although IMA is associated with lepidic growth, the tumor cells secrete mucin, which fills the alveoli and results in the consolidation on CT. The presence of visible opacified arteries within an area of consolidation on contrast-enhanced CT (termed the *CT angiogram sign*) has been reported to be suggestive of this tumor, but the same appearance can also be seen for other causes of consolidation, such as pneumonia. Bronchorrhea (excessive watery sputum production) can be associated with invasive mucinous adenocarcinoma. One lung or both lungs are often diffusely involved, and IMA has a poor prognosis.

LYMPHOMA AND LYMPHOPROLIFERATIVE DISEASE

Pulmonary parenchymal involvement is seen in 10% of patients with Hodgkin disease at the time of presentation. Direct extension from hilar nodes, focal discrete areas of consolidation, or mass-like lesions can be seen. Air bronchograms or areas of cavitation may be visible within the abnormal regions. In patients with untreated Hodgkin disease, lung involvement usually does not occur in the absence of radiographically demonstrable mediastinal (and usually ipsilateral hilar) adenopathy.

In patients with non-Hodgkin lymphoma, pulmonary disease can occur in the absence of lymph node enlargement (i.e., primary pulmonary lymphoma). This is common in patients with acquired immunodeficiency syndrome. Large, ill-defined nodules can be seen.

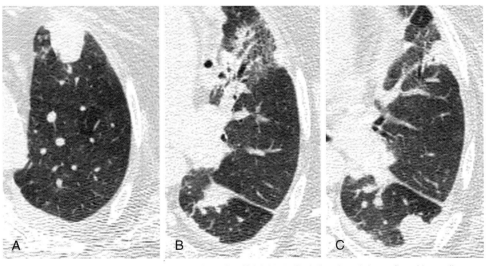

FIG. 6.29 **Nocardiosis with multiple nodules.** (A–C) Multiple ill-defined nodules reflect Nocardia pneumonia in an immunosuppressed patient.

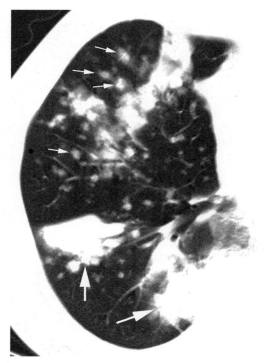

FIG. 6.30 Invasive mucinous adenocarcinoma with consolidation and multiple nodules. Focal areas of consolidation *(large arrows)* are visible in the right lung. Multiple nodules *(small arrows)* are also visible; these nodules are usually centrilobular in location and reflect endobronchial spread of tumor.

Other lymphoproliferative diseases, such as *focal lymphoid hyperplasia* and *posttransplant lymphoproliferative disorder*, can also result in multiple pulmonary nodules or masses.

INFECTIONS

In immunosuppressed patients, multiple nodules or masses suggest a fungal or, less likely, a nontuberculous mycobacterial or bacterial (e.g., *Nocardia*) infection (Fig. 6.29). The nodules may show the halo sign or cavitation. *Aspergillus* is most common among the fungal organisms resulting in lung infection in immunosuppressed patients.

Community-acquired fungal (e.g., histoplasmosis, coccidioidomycosis, blastomycosis, and cryptococcosis) and nontuberculous mycobacterial infections can be seen in immunocompetent patients. Focal consolidation or a solitary nodule or mass is more common than multiple nodules or masses, except when a massive inoculation of organisms has occurred (e.g., multinodular histoplasmosis in a cave explorer).

GRANULOMATOSIS WITH POLYANGIITIS

GPA is a multisystem disease of unknown cause associated with involvement of the upper respiratory tract (nasal, oral, or sinus inflammation), lower respiratory tract (airway or lung), and kidney. The presence of cytoplasmic antineutrophilic cytoplasmic antibody is characteristic and is seen in 90% of cases. Patients are usually aged between 30 and 60 years.

Multiple lung masses or cavities 2 to 4 cm in diameter are typical (Fig. 6.31). Usually fewer than a dozen nodules or masses are visible. A solitary nodule or mass may be seen, but this appearance is less common. With progression of the disease, nodules and masses tend to increase in size and number. With treatment, nodules usually resolve over a period of months. Typically, cavitary nodules and masses become thin walled and decrease in size with treatment. Complete resolution may occur. Pulmonary hemorrhage may also occur in GPA.

AMYLOIDOSIS

Patients with localized nodular amyloidosis are usually asymptomatic. Nodular amyloidosis may manifest itself as single or multiple lung nodules or masses that are usually well defined and round. Bilateral lung nodules are most typical, and they tend to be peripheral or subpleural in location. Nodules range from 0.5 to 5 cm in diameter in most cases but may be as large as 10 cm. Calcification is visible in 30% to 50% of cases, and may be stippled or dense. Cavitation may be seen in approximately 5% of cases. Nodules may grow slowly or remain stable over a number of years.

SUGGESTED READING

Camacho, J. C., Moreno, C. C., Harri, P. A., Aguirre, D. A., Torres, W. E., & Mittal, P. K. (2014). Posttransplantation lymphoproliferative disease: Proposed imaging classification. *Radiographics, 34,* 2025–2038.

Davis, S. D. (1991). CT evaluation for pulmonary metastases in patients with extrathoracic malignancy. *Radiology, 180,* 1–12.

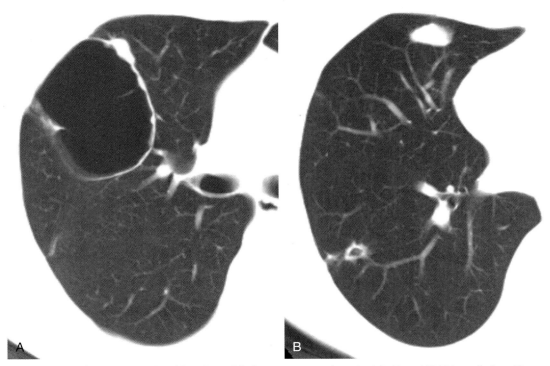

FIG. 6.31 Granulomatosis with polyangiitis (wegener granulomatosis). (A and B) Thin-walled cavities and nodules are present.

De Almeida, R. R., Zanetti, G., Pereira, E., et al. (2015). Respiratory tract amyloidosis. State-of-the-art review with a focus on pulmonary involvement. *Lung, 193,* 875–883.

Do, K. H., Lee, J. S., Seo, J. B., et al. (2005). Pulmonary parenchymal involvement of low-grade lymphoproliferative disorders. *J Comput Assist Tomogr, 29,* 825–830.

Hirakata, K., Nakata, H., & Haratake, J. (1993). Appearance of pulmonary metastases on high-resolution CT scans: Comparison with histopathologic findings from autopsy specimens. *AJR. Am J Roentgenol, 161,* 37–43.

Huang, R. M., Naidich, D. P., Lubat, E., et al. (1989). Septic pulmonary emboli: CT-radiographic correlation. *AJR. Am J Roentgenol, 153,* 41–45.

Georgiades, C. S., Neyman, E. G., Barish, M. A., et al. (2004). Amyloidosis: Review and CT manifestations. *Radiographics, 24,* 405–416.

Lee, K. S., Kim, T. S., Fujimoto, K., et al. (2003). Thoracic manifestation of Wegener's granulomatosis: CT findings in 30 patients. *Eur Radiol, 13,* 43–51.

Lee, K. S., Kim, Y., & Primack, S. L. (1997). Imaging of pulmonary lymphomas. *AJR. Am J Roentgenol, 168,* 339–345.

MacMahon, H., Naidich, D. P., Goo, J. M., et al. (2017). Guidelines for management of incidental pulmonary nodules detected on CT images: From the Fleischner Society 2017. *Radiology, 284,* 228–243.

Nachiappan, A. C., Rahbar, K., Shi, X., et al. (2017). Pulmonary tuberculosis: Role of radiology in diagnosis and management. *Radiographics, 37,* 52–72.

Sirajuddin, A., Raparia, K., Lewis, V. A., et al. (2016). Primary pulmonary lymphoid lesions: Radiologic and pathologic findings. *Radiographics, 36,* 53–70.

Travis, W. D., Brambilla, E., Noguchi, M., et al. (2011). International Association for the Study of Lung Cancer/American Thoracic Society/European Respiratory Society international multidisciplinary classification of lung adenocarcinoma. *J Thorac Oncol, 6,* 244–285.

E: AIRWAY ABNORMALITIES

THE TRACHEA

The trachea extends inferiorly from the thoracic inlet for a distance of 8 to 10 cm before bifurcating into the right and left main bronchi. It is usually round or oval and approximately 2 cm in diameter (see Chapter 2). Tracheal cartilage may be visible as a relatively dense horseshoe-shaped structure within the tracheal wall, with the open part of the horseshoe being posterior; calcification of tracheal cartilage is common in older patients, particularly women. The tracheal wall should be no more than 2 to 3 mm thick. The posterior tracheal membrane, which contains no cartilage, is very thin and may bow anteriorly with expiration.

Tracheal abnormalities are often associated with narrowing of the tracheal lumen. They can be considered as focal or diffuse. Tracheal abnormalities are uncommon and may be asymptomatic unless the tracheal lumen is reduced to a few millimeters in diameter.

Focal Tracheal Abnormalities
Tracheal Stenosis
Tracheal stenosis occurring because of previous intubation is a relatively common abnormality. It usually results in an hourglass-shaped narrowing of the trachea at the former site of the endotracheal tube balloon or tip. Narrowing of the tracheal lumen may result from intraluminal soft-tissue masses of reactive (granulation) tissue or collapse of the tracheal wall because of destruction of the tracheal rings and associated fibrosis.

Primary Tracheal Tumors
Primary tracheal tumors are rare. The most common primary malignancies are squamous cell carcinoma and cylindroma (adenoid cystic carcinoma). Squamous cell carcinoma is most common and typically arises in the distal part of the trachea. Adenoid cystic carcinoma is most common in the upper trachea and usually arises from the posterior tracheal wall (Fig. 6.32). CT can be helpful in choosing treatment in a patient with a malignant tracheal tumor. If there is no mediastinal invasion (as evidenced by a mediastinal mass), the lesion may be curable with a partial tracheal resection. Benign tumors such as hamartoma may arise in the trachea.

Tracheal Invasion or Metastases
Mediastinal tumor may compress, displace, or invade the trachea. Unless a mass is visible within the tracheal

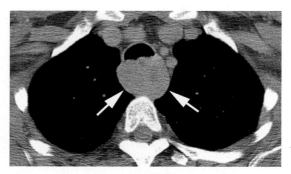

FIG. 6.32 Tracheal carcinoma (adenoid cystic carcinoma). The tumor is arising from the posterior tracheal wall and narrows the tracheal lumen. An extrinsic mass *(arrows)* is present.

lumen, tracheal invasion is difficult to diagnose with confidence. Neoplasms (e.g., thyroid carcinoma) may directly invade the trachea. The trachea can be involved by lung cancer as a result of direct extension from a tumor arising in a main bronchus. Hematogenous metastasis to the trachea from a distant tumor may occur.

Diffuse Tracheal Abnormalities
Saber-Sheath Trachea
Saber-sheath trachea is a common tracheal abnormality occurring in patients with chronic obstructive pulmonary disease (COPD). In this condition there is side-to-side narrowing of the intrathoracic trachea, with the anterior-to-posterior tracheal diameter being preserved or increased (Fig. 6.33); the extrathoracic trachea is normal. A focal segment of the trachea at the thoracic inlet may be involved first. The tracheal wall is of normal thickness. Saber-sheath trachea likely results from the trauma of chronic coughing with breakdown of tracheal rings.

Polychondritis
Polychondritis is an autoimmune disease involving cartilage, including the tracheal cartilage, nose, ears, and joints. It results in thickening of the anterior and lateral tracheal walls (i.e., where the cartilage is) because of inflammation, but the posterior tracheal membrane (containing no cartilage) appears normal (Fig. 6.34). Narrowing of the tracheal lumen typically occurs, and collapse occurs with expiration. The intrathoracic and extrathoracic trachea are both involved.

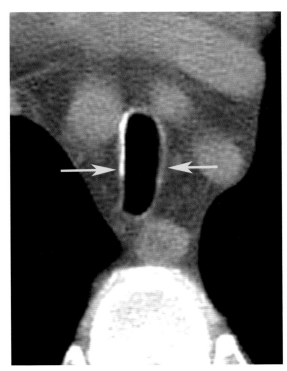

FIG. 6.33 **Saber-sheath trachea.** There is side-to-side narrowing of the trachea *(arrows)*. The tracheal wall is normal in thickness. Calcification of the tracheal cartilage is present.

Granulomatosis With Polyangiitis

GPA may involve the trachea and main bronchi, with thickening of the tracheal wall and narrowing of its lumen. It is most common in the subglottic trachea but may be diffuse.

Amyloidosis

Amyloidosis may involve the trachea and main bronchi, with diffuse or multifocal wall thickening and narrowing. Calcification is often present.

Other Diseases

Additional diseases that rarely result in multifocal or diffuse narrowing of the trachea and main bronchi include TB, scleroma, invasive tracheobronchial aspergillosis, sarcoidosis, and tracheobronchopathia osteochondroplastica.

BRONCHIAL ABNORMALITIES

Bronchiectasis

Bronchiectasis is defined as irreversible bronchial dilatation. It is commonly associated with chronic infection and chronic sputum production.

Spiral CT performed with thin slices should be used to diagnose bronchiectasis. In normal patients a bronchus and its adjacent pulmonary artery (bronchi and arteries travel together) are about the same size; on average, the lumen of a bronchus measures about 60% of the adjacent artery diameter.

In patients with bronchiectasis the dilated ring-shaped bronchus appears larger than the adjacent artery; together they mimic the appearance of a signet ring, a finding of bronchiectasis termed the *signet ring sign* (Fig. 6.35A).

By definition, the signet ring sign is present if the internal diameter of a bronchus exceeds the diameter of the adjacent artery. However, this appearance is occasionally seen in healthy individuals, particularly in those older than 60 years, or patients living at altitude. In patients with true bronchiectasis, because of infection or inflammation, bronchial wall thickening is also present in most cases, and the bronchus is considerably larger than the artery.

Mucus or pus may be seen filling abnormal bronchi in patients with bronchiectasis. Peripheral, small airway abnormalities may also be present. A finding termed *tree-in-bud* may be seen, corresponding to the presence mucus- or pus-filled, dilated bronchioles (Fig. 6.35).

Bronchiectasis is usually classified by its appearance as *cylindrical, varicose,* or *cystic,* but these designations are of little clinical significance. Cystic bronchiectasis may be associated with air-fluid levels in the dilated bronchi.

Bronchiectasis has many causes. Childhood infection, chronic airway infection, immunodeficiency, and cystic fibrosis are most common. Most patients with bronchiectasis have nonspecific findings, with patchy or lower lobe abnormalities. However, in some cases, and with some diseases, a particular distribution of abnormalities can help to limit the differential diagnosis. *Immune deficiency, childhood infections,* and *ciliary dysmotility* (e.g., *Kartagener syndrome*) are typically associated with lower lobe bronchiectasis (Fig. 6.35). *Cystic fibrosis* usually shows bilateral bronchiectasis involving the upper lobes and is most severe in the central (parahilar) lung regions. *Allergic bronchopulmonary aspergillosis* (ABPA) in patients with asthma also shows central bronchiectasis (Fig. 6.36A); mucous plugs in ABPA are common and are often high in attenuation because of calcium or metallic ions concentrated by the fungus (Fig. 6.36B). TB shows upper lobe bronchiectasis, which is often asymmetric. *Mycobacterium avium complex infection,* typical in older women (Fig. 6.37), is associated with bronchiectasis preferentially involving the middle lobe and lingula.

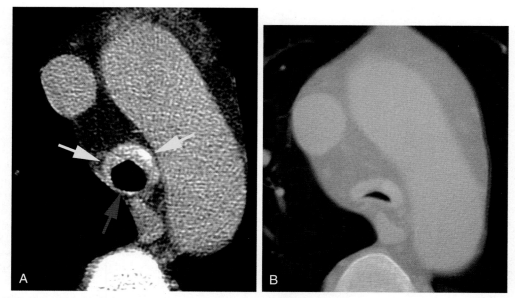

FIG. 6.34 **Tracheal narrowing caused by polychondritis.** (A) There is thickening of the anterior and lateral tracheal walls *(yellow arrows)*, but the posterior tracheal membrane is normal *(red arrow)*. The tracheal lumen is narrowed in a concentric fashion. This appearance is distinctly different from that of a saber-sheath trachea. (B) With expiration the tracheal walls collapse because of cartilage weakness, with marked reduction in the tracheal lumen.

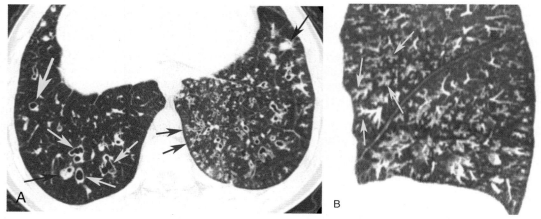

FIG. 6.35 **Bronchiectasis in a patient with ciliary dysmotility.** (A) High-resolution CT shows bronchiectasis at the lung bases. Thick-walled and irregularly dilated bronchi are visible in the right lower lobe *(yellow arrows)*. Their appearance would be classified as cylindrical or varicose. The dilated bronchi are considerably larger than the adjacent pulmonary artery and are examples of the signet ring sign *(large yellow arrow)*. Some bronchi *(red arrows)* are filled with mucus and are of soft-tissue attenuation. Numerous examples of the tree-in-bud pattern *(blue arrows)* are visible in the left lower lobe. (B) The tree-in-bud pattern *(arrows)* is shown on a sagittal reconstruction through the left lung base.

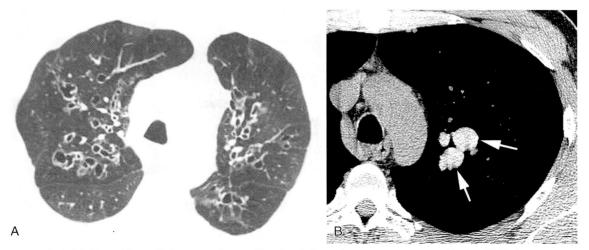

FIG. 6.36 **Bronchiectasis in two patients with allergic bronchopulmonary aspergillosis.** (A) High-resolution CT shows bronchiectasis in the central upper lobes. The lung parenchyma appears heterogeneous because of mosaic perfusion. (B) In another patient, mucous plugs *(arrows)* appear higher in attenuation than soft tissue when a mediastinal window is used. This finding strongly suggests allergic bronchopulmonary aspergillosis.

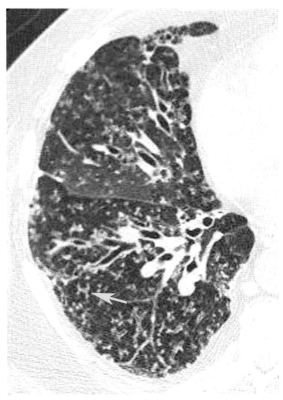

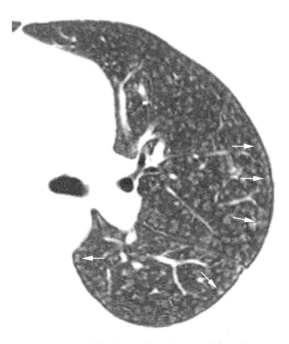

FIG. 6.38 **Centrilobular nodules in a patient with hypersensitivity pneumonitis.** Small, ill-defined nodules of ground-glass opacity are visible. The most peripheral nodules *(arrows)* are about 5 mm from the fissure or the pleural surfaces. The pleural surfaces are spared.

FIG. 6.37 *Mycobacterium avium* **complex infection.** In an elderly woman, bronchial wall thickening, bronchiectasis, and a tree-in-bud pattern *(arrow)* are visible. This combination is typical of *Mycobacterium avium* complex infection. Bronchiectasis is usually most severe in the middle lobe and lingula.

Bronchitis

Bronchial wall thickening without dilatation usually indicates inflammation (e.g., asthma, inflammatory bowel disease, and smoking-related chronic bronchitis) or airway infection and is termed *bronchitis*. When it is associated with infection, mucus or pus may be seen within the airway lumen, and tree-in-bud and/or nodules may be visible within the peripheral lung.

BRONCHIOLITIS (SMALL AIRWAYS DISEASE)

Bronchiole is a specific term used to describe airways that lack cartilage in their walls. The term *small airway* is often used to describe airways that are less than 3 mm in diameter; these often represent bronchioles. Three patterns of small airway (or bronchiolar) abnormalities are visible on HRCT; these have distinct appearances, but more than one may be seen in an individual patient. They relate to the presence of a cellular (inflammatory) bronchiolitis or bronchiolar obstruction.

Cellular Bronchiolitis With Tree-in-Bud

Tree-in-bud is a finding that looks like its name (Figs. 6.35 and 6.37). Branching opacities that are too big to represent normal vessels are visible in the lung periphery or in a centrilobular location, often with small nodules associated with the tips of branches. Tree-in-bud reflects the presence of mucus or pus filling dilated centrilobular bronchioles. Common causes include bacterial bronchopneumonia, chronic airway infection associated with bronchiectasis, endobronchial spread of TB or *Mycobacterium avium* complex infection (Fig. 6.22), and fungal and viral infections. When this finding is present, infection should be considered first; about 90% of patients showing tree-in-bud have infection. It uncommonly occurs in other conditions, including noninfectious inflammatory bronchiolitis (i.e., follicular bronchiolitis), mucoid impaction of bronchioles (as in ABPA), aspiration, and invasive mucinous adenocarcinoma. Tree-in-bud may be associated with either or both of the two patterns described next.

Cellular Bronchiolitis With Centrilobular Nodules

Centrilobular nodules can be seen in patients with infectious or inflammatory bronchiolitis. In patients with infection the nodules are often patchy in distribution and may be associated with tree-in-bud. In patients with noninfectious (inflammatory) cellular bronchiolitis, centrilobular nodules are often of GGO and diffuse (e.g., in hypersensitivity pneumonitis [Fig. 6.38] or respiratory bronchiolitis in a smoker). Centrilobular nodules are discussed later in the part on HRCT.

Obstructive Bronchiolitis With Mosaic Perfusion and Air Trapping

In patients with small airway obstruction because of cellular bronchiolitis or constrictive (obliterative) bronchiolitis, the lung parenchyma may appear heterogeneous in attenuation, with patchy and geographic areas of relative lucency. This finding or pattern is termed *mosaic perfusion* or *mosaic attenuation*. Mosaic perfusion reflects the presence of patchy (i.e., regional) differences in lung perfusion, with pulmonary vessels appearing smaller in the relatively lucent lung regions (Fig. 6.39).

Mosaic perfusion is most common with small airway obstruction; small airway obstruction results in vasoconstriction and reduced blood flow. It may also be seen with vascular occlusion, as in chronic pulmonary embolism. When it is as a result of airway obstruction, relatively lucent regions may correspond

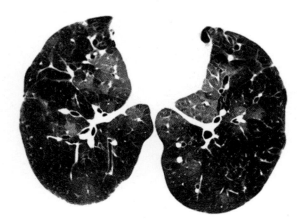

FIG. 6.39 **Constrictive bronchiolitis with mosaic perfusion.** In a patient with bronchiolitis obliterans resulting from a bone marrow transplantation and graft-versus-host reaction, the lung has a patchy appearance on high-resolution CT. Differences in lung density reflect differences in lung perfusion secondary to abnormal ventilation related to airway obstruction. The vessels look larger in the dense lung regions than in the lucent lung regions; this is an important clue to the presence of mosaic perfusion.

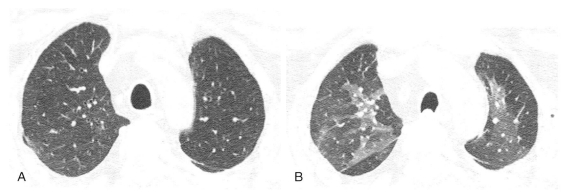

A   B

FIG. 6.40 Constrictive bronchiolitis with air trapping. High-resolution CT in a patient with constrictive bronchiolitis resulting from lung transplant rejection. (A) The inspiratory scan appears normal, without evidence of mosaic perfusion. (B) The expiratory scan shows patchy air trapping. The relatively dense lung is normal.

to secondary lobules, and air trapping is visible in lucent lung regions on expiratory scans. In some patients, expiratory scans show air trapping when inspiratory scans do not show mosaic perfusion (i.e., are normal; Fig. 6.40).

This pattern may accompany tree-in-bud and/or centrilobular nodules in patients with cellular bronchiolitis as a result of infection or inflammation. When findings of cellular bronchiolitis are absent, mosaic perfusion or air trapping is usually as a result of constrictive (obliterative) bronchiolitis, with fibrotic occlusion of small airways. *Constrictive bronchiolitis* has many causes, including some infections, inhalation of toxic fumes, collagen vascular disease, drugs, chronic lung transplant rejection, and graft-versus-host disease in bone marrow transplant patients.

SUGGESTED READING

Agarwal, R., Gupta, D., Aggarwal, A. N., et al. (2007). Clinical significance of hyperattenuating mucoid impaction in allergic bronchopulmonary aspergillosis: An analysis of 155 patients. *Chest, 132,* 1183–1190.

Aquino, S. L., Gamsu, G., Webb, W. R., & Kee, S. L. (1996). Tree-in-bud pattern: Frequency and significance on thin section CT. *J Comput Assist Tomogr, 20,* 594–599.

Arakawa, H., & Webb, W. R. (1998). Air trapping on expiratory high-resolution CT scans in the absence of inspiratory scan abnormalities: Correlation with pulmonary function tests and differential diagnosis. *AJR. Am J Roentgenol, 170,* 1349–1353.

Boiselle, P. M., O'Donnell, C. R., Bankier, A. A., et al. (2009). Tracheal collapsibility in healthy volunteers during forced expiration: Assessment with multidetector CT. *Radiology, 252,* 255–262.

Cartier, Y., Kavanagh, P. V., Johkoh, T., et al. (1999). Bronchiectasis: Accuracy of high-resolution CT in the differentiation of specific diseases. *AJR. Am J Roentgenol, 173,* 47–52.

Gruden, J. F., Webb, W. R., & Warnock, M. (1994). Centrilobular opacities in the lung on high-resolution CT: Diagnostic considerations and pathologic correlation. *AJR. Am J Roentgenol, 162,* 569–574.

Helbich, T. H., Heinz-Peer, G., Eichler, I., et al. (1999). Cystic fibrosis: CT assessment of lung involvement in children and adults. *Radiology, 213,* 537–544.

Jeong, Y. J., Lee, K. S., Koh, W. J., et al. (2004). Nontuberculous mycobacterial pulmonary infection in immunocompetent patients: Comparison of thin-section CT and histopathologic findings. *Radiology, 231,* 880–886.

Kligerman, S. J., Henry, T., Lin, C. T., et al. (2015). Mosaic attenuation: Etiology, methods of differentiation, and pitfalls. *Radiographics, 35,* 1360–1380.

Kwong, J. S., Müller, N. L., & Miller, R. R. (1992). Diseases of the trachea and main-stem bronchi: Correlation of CT with pathologic findings. *Radiographics, 12,* 647–657.

Lynch, D. A. (2008). Imaging of small airways disease and chronic obstructive pulmonary disease. *Clin Chest Med, 29,* 165–179.

Martinez, S., McAdams, H. P., & Batchu, C. S. (2007). The many faces of pulmonary nontuberculous mycobacterial infection. *AJR. Am J Roentgenol, 189,* 177–186.

Milliron, B., Henry, T. S., Veeraraghavan, S., & Little, B. P. (2015). Bronchiectasis: Mechanisms and imaging clues of associated common and uncommon diseases. *Radiographics, 35,* 1011–1030.

Müller, N. L., & Miller, R. R. (1995). Diseases of the bronchioles: CT and histopathologic findings. *Radiology, 196,* 3–12.

Okada, F., Ando, Y., Yoshitake, S., et al. (2007). Clinical/pathologic correlations in 553 patients with primary centrilobular findings on high-resolution CT scan of the thorax. *Chest, 132,* 1939–1948.

Park, C. M., Goo, J. M., Lee, H. J., et al. (2009). Tumors in the tracheobronchial tree: CT and FDG PET features. *Radiographics, 29*, 55–71.

Park, C. S., Müller, N. L., Worthy, S. A., et al. (1997). Airway obstruction in asthmatic and healthy individuals: Inspiratory and expiratory thin-section CT findings. *Radiology, 203*, 361–367.

Prince, J. S., Duhamel, D. R., Levin, D. L., et al. (2002). Nonneoplastic lesions of the tracheobronchial wall: Radiologic findings with bronchoscopic correlation. *Radiographics, 22*, S215–S230.

Rossi, S. E., Franquet, T., Volpacchio, M., et al. (2005). Tree-in-bud pattern at thin-section CT of the lungs: Radiologic-pathologic overview. *Radiographics, 25*, 789–801.

Shin, M. S., Jackson, R. M., & Ho, K. J. (1988). Tracheobronchomegaly (Mounier-Kuhn syndrome): CT diagnosis. *AJR. Am J Roentgenol, 150*, 777–779.

Ward, S., Heyneman, L., Lee, M. J., et al. (1999). Accuracy of CT in the diagnosis of allergic bronchopulmonary aspergillosis in asthmatic patients. *AJR. Am J Roentgenol, 173*, 937–942.

Webb, E. M., Elicker, B. M., & Webb, W. R. (2000). Using CT to diagnose nonneoplastic tracheal abnormalities: Appearance of the tracheal wall. *AJR. Am J Roentgenol, 174*, 1315–1321.

F: DIFFUSE LUNG DISEASE AND HIGH-RESOLUTION CT

HIGH-RESOLUTION CT TECHNIQUE

HRCT involves the use of thin slices and a high-resolution (sharp) algorithm (see Chapter 1); in patients with suspected diffuse infiltrative lung disease, images are usually obtained in both the supine position and the prone position, and expiratory imaging is often performed to detect air trapping (Fig. 6.40).

HRCT is sometimes used to evaluate patients with acute symptoms associated with a diffuse lung abnormality so as to characterize the abnormalities present and limit the differential diagnosis. Common causes of diffuse lung disease with an acute presentation include pneumonia, aspiration, various causes of pulmonary edema, and diffuse alveolar damage resulting in acute respiratory distress syndrome. In addition, because routine CT is often performed with thin slices, any chest CT can be regarded as HRCT, although routine CT is performed only with the patient supine.

HRCT is more commonly used to evaluate diffuse infiltrative lung diseases, particularly when they are chronic or progressive and the diagnosis is in question. The term *diffuse infiltrative lung disease* is used to describe a variety of conditions, both alveolar and interstitial, that manifest themselves as a generalized parenchymal abnormality.

In general, HRCT is used (1) to detect lung disease in patients with symptoms of respiratory distress or abnormal pulmonary function test results who have normal chest radiographs (approximately 10% to 15% of patients with infiltrative lung disease have normal chest radiographs), (2) to characterize lung disease in terms of its morphologic pattern (e.g., is there honeycombing?) and perhaps make a specific diagnosis, (3) to assess disease activity, and (4) to localize areas of abnormality in patients who are having a lung biopsy.

HRCT may be performed with (1) a spiral volumetric technique, (2) individual slices at 1- to 2-cm intervals, or (3) a combination of both techniques. In a patient with a diffuse lung disease, particularly when it is chronic or progressive, scans at 1- to 2-cm intervals provide a sampling of lung anatomy sufficient for diagnosis in many cases. A spiral technique results in a higher radiation dose but is more inclusive.

Scans are usually obtained during full inspiration in the supine position. Prone scans are commonly obtained in patients with a suspected interstitial lung disease to avoid misdiagnosis when posterior atelectasis develops with the patient lying supine. Some dependent lung collapse is often seen on CT and having scans in both positions allows one to differentiate this finding from subtle pathologic processes. Postexpiratory scans at three to five levels are often obtained to detect air trapping associated with small airways disease. They should be routine for the initial scan in most patients and for diagnosis of airway diseases.

HIGH-RESOLUTION FINDINGS IN HEALTHY INDIVIDUALS

The lung is a lobular organ made up of numerous *secondary pulmonary lobules*. Secondary pulmonary lobules (or simply pulmonary lobules) are polygonal in shape and are usually 1 to 3 cm in diameter. They are marginated to a varying degree by *interlobular septa* containing veins and lymphatic channels (Fig. 6.41). In the center of the lobule are pulmonary artery and bronchiolar branches.

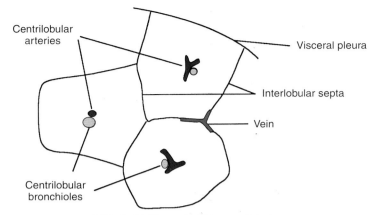

FIG. 6.41 **Normal pulmonary lobules.**

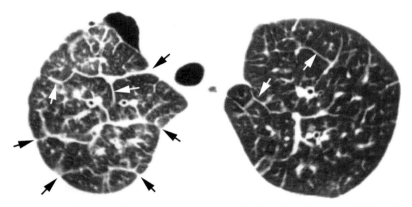

FIG. 6.42 **Thickening of interlobular septa.** In a patient with lymphangitic spread of breast carcinoma, high-resolution CT shows evidence of septal thickening *(arrows)* characteristic of this disease. Although the septal thickening is bilateral, it is most severe on the right side. A small right pneumothorax is also present.

On HRCT, normal interlobular septa are sometimes visible as very thin, straight lines of uniform thickness, 1 to 2 cm in length. Usually only a few well-defined septa, if any, are visible in a normal individual. A linear, branching, or dot-like opacity seen within the secondary lobule, or within 1 cm of the pleural surface, represents the *centrilobular artery* branch. The *centrilobular bronchiole* is not normally visible. In healthy individuals the pleural surfaces, fissures, and margins of central vessels and bronchi appear smooth and sharply defined.

ABNORMAL HIGH-RESOLUTION CT FINDINGS

Although the findings described next are typically associated with HRCT, they are applicable to routine CT diagnosis as well.

Reticular Patterns
Thickened Interlobular Septa

Thickening of interlobular septa can be seen in patients with a variety of interstitial lung diseases (Fig. 6.42). Within the central lung, thickened septa can outline lobules that appear hexagonal or polygonal and contain a visible central arterial branch. In the peripheral lung, thickened septa often extend to the pleural surface. Septal thickening can appear smooth, nodular, or irregular in different diseases.

Often, thickened septa in the peripheral lung reflect generalized interstitial thickening and are also associated with (1) thickening of fissures caused by subpleural interstitial thickening, (2) prominent centrilobular structures caused by thickening of the interstitial sheath of connective tissue that surrounds them, and (3) thickening of the interstitium surrounding central vessels and bronchi (i.e., peribronchial cuffing).

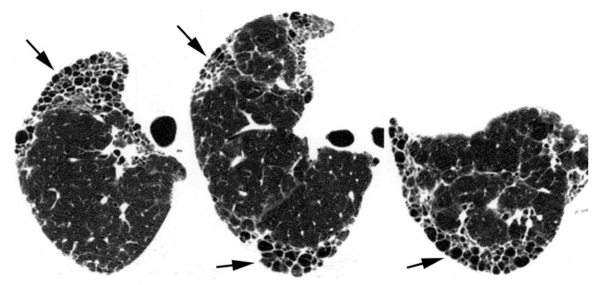

FIG. 6.43 Pulmonary fibrosis and honeycombing in rheumatoid arthritis. High-resolution CT of the right lung at three levels shows characteristic small, thick-walled cysts (honeycomb cysts) that are most evident peripherally *(arrows)*. This appearance is diagnostic of fibrosis and correlates with the presence of usual interstitial pneumonia.

Common causes of interlobular septal thickening as the predominant HRCT finding include:
- interstitial pulmonary edema (smooth thickening)
- lymphangitic spread of carcinoma (smooth or nodular septal thickening; Fig. 6.42)
- sarcoidosis (nodular when granulomas are present; irregular in fibrotic or end-stage disease)

Honeycombing

Honeycombing represents lung fibrosis associated with cystic areas of lung destruction. It results in a characteristic coarse reticular pattern or cystic appearance on HRCT that is typical (Figs. 6.43 and 6.44). Cystic spaces are usually several millimeters to 1 cm in diameter, are marginated by thick, clearly definable walls, and typically appear in rows and clusters in the peripheral and subpleural lung, with adjacent cysts sharing walls.

Unless a row or cluster of cysts is visible in the immediate subpleural lung, honeycombing cannot be diagnosed with certainty. The presence of honeycombing on HRCT means that fibrosis is present. Honeycombing usually indicates the presence of *usual interstitial pneumonia* (UIP), a histologic pattern. A confident diagnosis of UIP cannot be made on CT unless honeycombing is present. On the other hand, only about 70% of UIP cases show this finding.

Common causes of fibrosis with honeycombing as the predominant HRCT finding include:

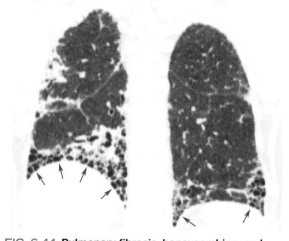

FIG. 6.44 Pulmonary fibrosis, honeycombing, and a usual interstitial pneumonia pattern in idiopathic pulmonary fibrosis. Coronal high-resolution CT reconstruction shows honeycombing *(arrows)* with a basal and subpleural predominance. This is typical of a usual interstitial pneumonia pattern.

- idiopathic pulmonary fibrosis (IPF; 60%–70% of UIP cases; Fig. 6.44)
- collagen vascular diseases with UIP, particularly rheumatoid arthritis and scleroderma (Fig. 6.43)

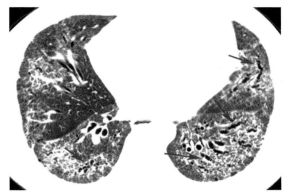

FIG. 6.45 Pulmonary fibrosis with reticulation and traction bronchiectasis in fibrotic nonspecific interstitial pneumonia. High-resolution CT in a patient with fibrotic nonspecific interstitial pneumonia associated with collagen vascular disease reveals abnormal lung reticulation associated with irregular dilatation of the bronchi (traction bronchiectasis; *arrows*). Note the relative sparing of the immediate subpleural lung. This is typical of nonspecific interstitial pneumonia.

- drug-related fibrosis with UIP
- asbestosis with UIP (in association with pleural thickening)
- end-stage hypersensitivity pneumonitis
- end-stage sarcoidosis (a small percentage of patients)

Irregular Reticulation and Traction Bronchiectasis

Irregular or nonspecific reticulation, appearing as a network of linear opacities, but not representing interlobular septal thickening or honeycombing, is commonly present in patients with lung fibrosis (Fig. 6.45) or lung infiltration.

When it results from fibrosis, it is typically associated with architectural distortion and traction bronchiectasis. *Traction bronchiectasis* represents dilatation of bronchi because of surrounding lung fibrosis; the dilated bronchi often have a very irregular, corkscrew appearance (Fig. 6.45). Traction bronchiectasis is a common finding in patients with fibrotic lung disease and may be associated with honeycombing. Any of the common causes of lung fibrosis and honeycombing listed above may be associated with this finding.

Conglomerate masses of fibrous tissue (i.e., *progressive massive fibrosis*) can be seen in the upper lobes of patients with sarcoidosis or silicosis. Traction bronchiectasis may be seen within the mass.

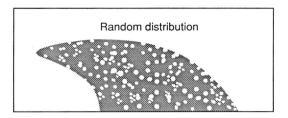

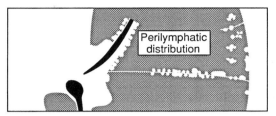

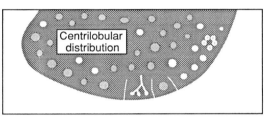

FIG. 6.46 Distributions of lung nodules. The tree-in-bud pattern is illustrated, along with centrilobular nodules and random distribution.

Nodular Patterns

Small nodules (a few millimeters in diameter), sometimes termed *micronodules*, can be detected on HRCT in patients with granulomatous diseases such as sarcoidosis and miliary TB, in patients with metastatic tumors, and in patients with small airways disease. Three distributions of lung nodules can be identified on HRCT (Fig. 6.46); recognition of one of these three patterns is invaluable in differential diagnosis.

Perilymphatic Nodules

Perilymphatic nodules occur in lung regions rich in lymphatic channels. They predominate:
- at the pleural surfaces (including the fissures)
- adjacent to large vessels and bronchi
- within interlobular septa
- in a centrilobular location

Not all patients show involvement of all four regions. Nodules are typically patchy in distribution. This pattern is most common in sarcoidosis (95% of cases; Figs. 6.46 and 6.47), silicosis, and lymphangitic carcinoma.

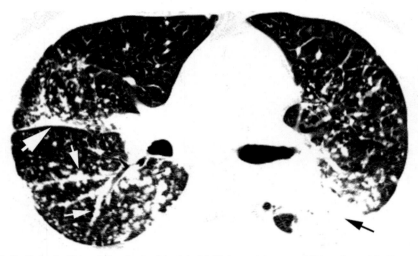

FIG. 6.47 Perilymphatic nodules (sarcoidosis). Multiple nodules are visible adjacent to the major fissure *(large white arrow)* and central bronchi and vessels *(small white arrows)*. This pattern is characteristic of sarcoidosis. Note the patchy distribution, whereby some lung regions are involved, whereas others appear normal. A conglomerate mass associated with satellite nodules is visible on the left *(black arrow)*.

Random Nodules

Random nodules also involve the pleural surfaces but involve the lung in a diffuse and uniform fashion, with a random distribution in relation to lung structures. They are most typical of hematogenous disease, such as miliary TB or fungal infection and hematogenous metastases (Figs. 6.27 and 6.46). Sarcoidosis uncommonly results in this pattern.

Centrilobular Nodules

Centrilobular nodules are centrilobular in location, and therefore spare the pleural surfaces (Figs. 6.22 and 6.38). They tend to be visible in relation to small vessels, with the most peripheral nodules being about 5 mm from the pleural surface. Because lobules are all about the same size, the nodules appear evenly spaced and can mimic a random pattern at first glance; however, pleural nodules are usually present with a random pattern.

Centrilobular nodules may be patchy or diffuse and may be of soft-tissue attenuation or GGO. Centrilobular nodules usually reflect diseases that occur in relation to centrilobular bronchioles and are common with endobronchial spread of infection (e.g., TB and bacterial bronchopneumonia; Fig 6.22), endobronchial spread of tumor tissue (e.g., invasive mucinous adenocarcinoma), and cellular bronchiolitis (e.g., hypersensitivity pneumonitis and respiratory bronchiolitis). Small vessel diseases (vasculitis) and abnormalities (edema or hemorrhage) can also result in centrilobular nodules,

but these are much less common. In patients with centrilobular nodules as a result of infection, a tree-in-bud pattern may also be visible.

Identifying the Nodular Pattern

When one is attempting to diagnose one of these three patterns of nodules, it is easiest to first decide if nodules are visible in relation to the pleural surfaces and fissures. If pleural nodules are absent, the distribution is likely centrilobular; if pleural or fissural nodules are present, then the overall distribution determines the pattern present. Nodules with a patchy distribution usually represent a perilymphatic distribution (look for involvement of the specific structures typically involved); a diffuse and uniform distribution indicates a random pattern. This method can be used to correctly categorize more than 90% of the cases seen.

Increased Lung Opacity (Attenuation)

Increased lung opacity may represent consolidation or GGO. The differential diagnoses of these two patterns overlap.

Consolidation

HRCT findings of air space consolidation have been described. Lung appears homogeneously opaque with obscuration of the pulmonary vessels. Air bronchograms are often present.

The differential diagnosis of consolidation is primarily based on the duration of the symptoms.

Consolidation associated with acute symptoms usually represents pneumonia (Fig. 6.3), severe pulmonary edema or hemorrhage, aspiration, or diffuse alveolar damage associated with acute respiratory distress syndrome. In patients with consolidation and chronic symptoms (i.e., longer than 4–6 weeks), common causes include organizing pneumonia, invasive mucinous adenocarcinoma (Fig. 6.30), chronic eosinophilic pneumonia, and lipoid pneumonia.

Ground-Glass Opacity

In some patients with minimal interstitial disease, alveolar wall thickening, or minimal air space consolidation, a hazy increase in lung density can be observed on HRCT; this is termed *ground-glass opacity* (GGO). GGO is differentiated from consolidation in that areas of increased opacity do not obscure underlying pulmonary vessels.

GGO is nonspecific and can be seen in a variety of diseases. As in patients with consolidation, the differential diagnosis of GGO is primarily based on the duration of symptoms. GGO associated with acute symptoms usually represents an atypical pneumonia (*Pneumocystis jiroveci* or viral pneumonia), edema (Fig. 6.48), hemorrhage, aspiration, or acute hypersensitivity pneumonitis. In patients with chronic symptoms (i.e., longer than 4–6 weeks), common causes include subacute hypersensitivity

pneumonitis, nonspecific interstitial pneumonia (NSIP), desquamative interstitial pneumonia (DIP), organizing pneumonia, invasive mucinous adenocarcinoma, lipoid pneumonia, and pulmonary alveolar proteinosis.

In all patients with acute symptoms, GGO indicates an active disease. In 60% to 80% of patients with chronic symptoms, this appearance correlates with some type of active lung disease. However, if GGO is seen only in lung regions that also show findings of fibrosis (e.g., honeycombing, reticulation, and traction bronchiectasis), it is likely that the GGO represents fibrosis rather than active disease. GGO in areas of fibrosis is common in patients with UIP and IPF.

Lung Cysts

Lung cysts are thin walled, air-filled spaces within the lung parenchyma. Multiple cysts are seen in honeycombing, bullous emphysema, and pneumonias resulting in pneumatocele formation (e.g., *Pneumocystis* pneumonia). Cystic bronchiectasis may mimic the appearance of a lung cyst.

Several rare lung diseases result in lung cysts as a primary manifestation of the disease. These include Langerhans cell histiocytosis, lymphangiomyomatosis (Fig. 6.49), lymphoid interstitial pneumonia or amyloidosis, particularly in association with Sjögren syndrome, and Birt-Hogg-Dubé syndrome.

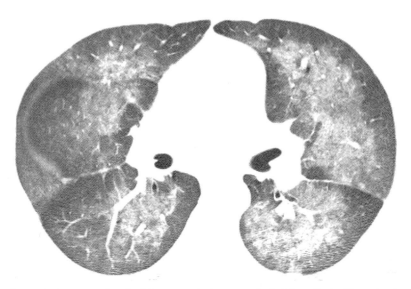

FIG. 6.48 **Ground-glass opacity.** Perihilar ground-glass opacity in this patient with acute dyspnea reflects pulmonary edema and hemorrhage related to an acute reaction to cocaine use.

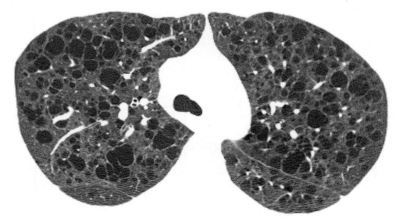

FIG. 6.49 **Lung cysts in lymphangiomyomatosis.** Diffuse, thin-walled, rounded lung cysts are visible in a young woman. This appearance is typical of lymphangiomyomatosis.

HIGH-RESOLUTION CT FINDINGS IN SPECIFIC DISEASES

Although more than 200 diseases can result in a diffuse pulmonary abnormality, knowledge of relatively few allows correct diagnosis of most cases observed. More than 90% of patients with diffuse lung disease have one of about a dozen diseases. Some of the entities described later are uncommon but have typical HRCT findings or are important to know about.

Metastatic Carcinoma

Although lymphangitic and hematogenous spread of carcinoma produce somewhat different patterns, overlap is common, and some patients show features of both.

Lymphangitic Spread of Carcinoma

In a patient with an appropriate history of malignancy and progressive dyspnea, the HRCT appearance of lymphangitic spread of neoplasm is diagnostic. It is characterized by:
- interlobular septal thickening that is smooth or nodular (Fig. 6.42)
- peribronchial interstitial thickening (peribronchial cuffing)
- thickening of fissures (smooth or nodular)
- a patchy or unilateral distribution (in some cases)
- lymph node enlargement (in some cases)

Hematogenous Spread

Hematogenous metastasis is more common than lymphangitic spread of tumor. It is characterized by:

- a random distribution of small nodules, sometimes with a peripheral predominance (Figs. 6.27 and 6.28)
- involvement of fissures and the pleural surfaces
- a bilateral distribution
- the presence of large nodules

Usual Interstitial Pneumonia and Idiopathic Pulmonary Fibrosis

Usual interstitial pneumonia (UIP) is a histologic pattern characterized by patchy lung fibrosis and honeycombing. When UIP is idiopathic, the disease is termed *idiopathic pulmonary fibrosis* (IPF); IPF accounts for two-thirds of cases of UIP. Other associations with UIP include collagen vascular diseases (particularly rheumatoid arthritis and scleroderma), drug-related fibrosis, asbestosis, end-stage hypersensitivity pneumonitis, and sometimes sarcoidosis.

UIP is one of the *idiopathic interstitial pneumonias*, a category that also includes NSIP, organizing pneumonia, and DIP, which are described later.

IPF may be diagnosed when a UIP pattern, seen on CT or pathology examination, is not associated with known diseases or exposures associated with this histologic pattern (i.e., it is idiopathic). Patients with IPF are usually older than 50 years, and most are men. Progressive dyspnea is typical. The prognosis is very poor without treatment. Recently two drugs have been approved for treatment of IPF; they inhibit fibrosis and slow progression of the disease.

A *UIP pattern* on HRCT is characterized by:
- subpleural and basal predominance (Fig. 6.44)
- reticulation (with traction bronchiectasis)

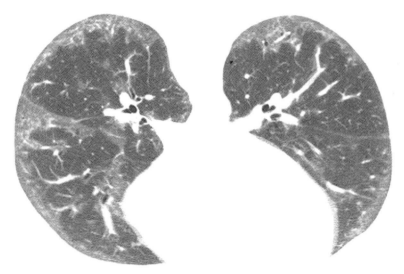

FIG. 6.50 **Cellular nonspecific interstitial pneumonia in a patient with scleroderma.** High-resolution CT of the patient in the prone position shows peripheral ground-glass opacity with subpleural sparing. This appearance is typical of nonspecific interstitial pneumonia.

- honeycombing (Figs. 6.43 and 6.44)
- absence of HRCT features considered inconsistent with UIP (i.e., findings typical of other lung diseases). These include:
    - upper, mid-lung, or peribronchial predominance
    - extensive GGO (greater than reticulation in extent)
    - profuse micronodules (bilateral, upper lobe)
    - discrete cysts not representing honeycombing
    - mosaic perfusion or air trapping (bilateral, multiple lobules)
    - segmental or lobar consolidation

If these four criteria are met, a *UIP pattern* should be diagnosed on HRCT. If the patient has no known disease (i.e., the UIP pattern is idiopathic), then the patient has IPF. Lung biopsy is not usually done if HRCT shows a UIP pattern; the CT appearance is highly specific, and biopsy can be risky.

If no honeycombing is present, but otherwise HRCT findings are typical, a diagnosis of *probable UIP* will be made. Specific criteria for making the diagnosis of a UIP pattern and IPF are listed in Raghu et al.

Nonspecific Interstitial Pneumonia

NSIP is a histologic pattern that, despite its name, is specific. It is commonly associated with collagen vascular disease or drug treatment but may be idiopathic as well. It is less common than UIP and IPF but is still relatively common in clinical practice. NSIP occurs in cellular (inflammatory) and fibrotic forms. It often responds to treatment in the cellular stage, and has a good prognosis.

NSIP is variable in appearance but often has the following characteristics:

- Predominance in the peripheral, posterior, and basal lung regions, with a concentric distribution (Figs. 6.45 and 6.50).
- Sparing of the immediate subpleural lung (seen in 50% of cases), a finding that is highly predictive of NSIP (Figs. 6.45 and 6.50).
- GGO in cellular NSIP (Fig. 6.50).
- Reticulation (Fig. 6.45).
- Traction bronchiectasis (usually but not always fibrotic NSIP; Fig. 6.45).
- Honeycombing is rare, and, if present, of limited extent.

Collagen Vascular Diseases

Rheumatoid lung disease, scleroderma, and other collagen diseases may result in findings of UIP, NSIP (Figs. 6.43, 6.45, and 6.50), organizing pneumonia, lymphoid interstitial pneumonia, or a combination of these in a given patient. Specific collagen diseases are also associated with disease-specific findings or common associations (e.g., esophageal dilatation in scleroderma).

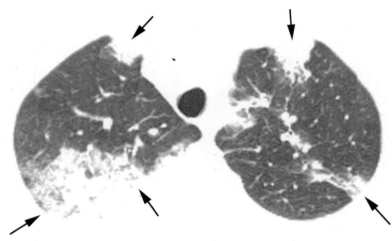

FIG. 6.51 Organizing pneumonia. Patchy areas of consolidation are noted in the peripheral lung *(arrows)*. This appearance in a patient with chronic symptoms is typical.

Organizing Pneumonia

Organizing pneumonia is a histologic pattern that can be idiopathic or result from infection, toxic exposure, drug reactions, or collagen diseases. It typically results in progressive dyspnea and low-grade fever, simulating pneumonia. The idiopathic form of this disease is termed *cryptogenic organizing pneumonia.* Steroids are used in treatment. It has a good prognosis.

HRCT features include the following:

- Patchy or nodular consolidation that is irregular in contour (Fig. 6.51).
- Patchy or nodular GGO.
- A peripheral and peribronchial distribution of nodular opacities (Fig. 6.51).
- The *atoll sign* or *reversed halo sign*, in which a ring of consolidation surrounds GGO. It is uncommonly seen in other diseases.

Chronic Eosinophilic Pneumonia

Chronic eosinophilic pneumonia is idiopathic and is characterized by filling of alveoli by a mixed inflammatory infiltrate consisting primarily of eosinophils. Blood eosinophilia is usually present. Typical symptoms include fever, cough, and shortness of breath. Treatment is with steroids, and resolution is often prompt.

HRCT features are very similar or identical to those of organizing pneumonia, including:

- patchy consolidation or GGO
- a peripheral or peribronchial distribution
- the atoll or reversed halo sign

Respiratory Bronchiolitis Associated–Interstitial Lung Disease and Desquamative Interstitial Pneumonia

These diseases are closely related and are caused by cigarette smoking in almost all cases. *Respiratory bronchiolitis* is a cellular bronchiolitis common seen on pathology in smokers; most are asymptomatic. When respiratory bronchiolitis is associated with symptoms, it is termed *respiratory bronchiolitis associated–interstitial lung disease* (RB-ILD). Both RB and RB-ILD are associated with the presence of pigment-laden macrophages in relation to bronchioles. In DIP, the macrophage infiltrate is more diffuse and lung involvement is extensive. Symptoms in RB-ILD and DIP include cough and dyspnea. Treatment includes smoking cessation or steroid administration. The prognosis is generally good.

HRCT features include:

- patchy or diffuse GGO (in DIP)
- centrilobular nodules of GGO (in RB-ILD)
- air-filled cysts within regions of GGO
- air trapping in some cases
- rare findings of fibrosis and honeycombing

Hypersensitivity Pneumonitis

Hypersensitivity pneumonitis is a common lung disease resulting from exposure to one of a number of organic dusts (e.g., bird-fancier's lung). In the acute and subacute stages, interstitial and alveolar infiltrates and ill-defined peribronchiolar granulomas are present. In the chronic stage, fibrosis and honeycombing occur. Hypersensitivity pneumonitis has a good prognosis if

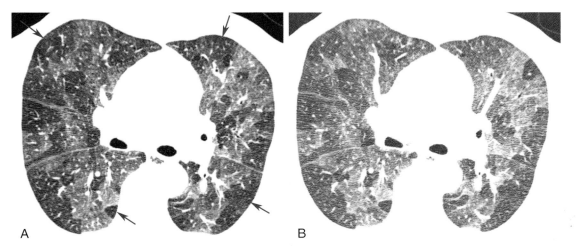

FIG. 6.52 **Ground-glass opacity and mosaic perfusion in hypersensitivity pneumonitis.** (A) Inspiratory HRCT. Multiple patchy areas of increased lung attenuation are typical of ground-glass opacity. Geographic areas of relative lucency reflect mosaic perfusion because of cellular bronchiolitis. This combination of ground-glass opacity and focal lucencies is typical of hypersensitivity pneumonitis and is termed the *headcheese sign.* (B) Expiratory scan shows air trapping (persistent lucency) in areas that appeared lucent in (A).

it is treated in the subacute stage with steroids or by removal the offending antigen from the environment. In 50% of cases the antigen cannot be identified.

In the subacute stage, HRCT typically shows:
- patchy or geographic GGO (80%; Fig. 6.52A);
- poorly defined centrilobular GGO nodules (50%; Fig. 6.38);
- upper or mid-lung predominance, with involvement of the entire cross section of the lung (i.e., there is no peripheral predominance);
- mosaic perfusion caused by bronchiolar obstruction (Fig. 6.52A);
- air trapping (commonly present on expiratory scans; Fig. 6.52B);
- a combination of patchy GGO and patchy mosaic perfusion (termed the *headcheese sign* because of its resemblance to a sausage of the same name; Fig. 6.52); the headcheese sign is typical of hypersensitivity pneumonitis.

In the chronic or fibrotic stage, hypersensitivity pneumonitis typically shows:
- patchy or geographic reticulation and traction bronchiectasis;
- honeycombing in some cases;
- upper or mid-lung predominance, with involvement of the entire cross-section of the lung;
- mosaic perfusion caused by bronchiolar obstruction;
- air trapping (commonly present on expiratory scans).

Sarcoidosis

Sarcoidosis can have a diagnostic appearance in many patients. Patients may be relatively asymptomatic despite extensive abnormalities. HRCT findings in patients with active and end-stage disease differ.

HRCT findings in patients with active sarcoidosis include the following:
- Perilymphatic nodules, 1 to 10 mm (particularly subpleural and peribronchial; Figs. 6.21 and 6.47); calcification can occur.
- Numerous peribronchial nodules can result in large parahilar masses with satellite nodules (i.e., the galaxy sign); air bronchograms may be present (Fig. 6.21).
- A patchy distribution, often asymmetric.
- Upper lobe predominance.
- Hilar and mediastinal node enlargement (helpful in diagnosis but not always present); calcification can be present.
- GGO (uncommon), reflecting the presence of small granulomas.

HRCT findings in patients with end-stage sarcoidosis and fibrosis include:
- irregular septal thickening
- architectural distortion
- parahilar conglomerate masses containing crowded, ectatic bronchi, often involving the upper lobes
- honeycombing (a small percentage)
- hilar and mediastinal node enlargement (not always present)

Silicosis and Coal Workers' Pneumoconiosis

Findings for silicosis and coal workers' pneumoconiosis can be similar to those for sarcoidosis, but significant differences are recognizable.

The findings include:
- perilymphatic nodules, 1 to 10 mm (particularly centrilobular and subpleural), with calcification in some cases;
- symmetric distribution;
- posterior lung predominance;
- upper lobe predominance;
- conglomerate masses of nodules or fibrosis in the upper lobes;
- hilar and mediastinal node enlargement; possible eggshell calcification.

Tuberculosis

TB has different appearances, depending on the form of the disease. In primary TB, CT may be normal or may show findings of pneumonia. In patients with disseminated TB, HRCT findings depend on the mode of spread.

Endobronchial Spread
- Centrilobular nodules (Fig. 6.22)
- Tree-in-bud (Fig. 6.22)
- Focal areas of consolidation
- Bronchial wall thickening or bronchiectasis
- Usually patchy or focal

Miliary Spread
- Random nodules of 1 to 5 mm (Fig. 6.46)
- Usually diffuse

Pulmonary Alveolar Proteinosis

Pulmonary alveolar proteinosis is characterized by filling of the alveolar spaces by a lipid-rich proteinaceous material. Most cases are idiopathic or autoimmune, but some are associated with exposure to dusts (particularly silica), hematologic or lymphatic malignancies, or chemotherapy, and a small percentage are as a result of gene mutations. Nocardial or mycobacterial superinfection may occur.

HRCT findings can be diagnostic and include (1) patchy or geographic GGO and (2) smooth, interlobular septal thickening in the regions of GGO. This combination is termed *crazy paving*. Although this finding is typical of pulmonary alveolar proteinosis, it is nonspecific.

Langerhans Cell Histiocytosis

Histiocytosis (Langerhans cell histiocytosis) is associated with centrilobular nodules early in the disease and cystic lesions late in the disease. Nodules and cysts can coexist. The disease is related to smoking and occurs in both men and women. It has the following features:
- centrilobular nodules, which may be cavitary
- thick- or thin-walled, very irregularly shaped lung cysts
- upper lobe predominance
- sparing of the costophrenic angles
- progression over time from nodules, to cavitary nodules, to thick-walled cysts, to thin-walled cysts

Lymphangiomyomatosis

Lymphangiomyomatosis may occur sporadically or in association with tuberous sclerosis, as a result of mutations in one or both tuberous sclerosis genes (*TSC1* or *TSC2*). Lymphangiomyomatosis typically occurs only in women of childbearing age. HRCT in lymphangiomyomatosis demonstrates thin-walled, rounded cysts involving the entire lung, with intervening lung appearing normal. When seen in a female patient with a characteristic history (i.e., dyspnea, spontaneous pneumothorax, and sometimes chylous pleural effusions), the findings are diagnostic.

HRCT features of lymphangiomyomatosis include:
- thin-walled, rounded lung cysts (Fig. 6.49)
- normal-appearing intervening lung
- a diffuse distribution, without sparing of the lung bases
- lymph node enlargement or pleural effusion in some patients
- renal angiomyolipoma in some patients

Emphysema

On HRCT or thin-slice spiral CT, emphysema is apparent in areas of low attenuation within surrounding normal lung parenchyma. Emphysema is usually distinguishable from honeycombing or cystic lung disease, because in most cases the lucent areas lack visible walls (Fig. 6.53). On CT, emphysema may be classified as centrilobular, panlobular, paraseptal, or bullous.

Centrilobular Emphysema

Centrilobular emphysema is most common, is usually associated with smoking, and is typically most severe in the upper lobes (Fig. 6.53). Sometimes it appears centrilobular on HRCT, but the presence of spotty upper lobe lucencies without visible walls is diagnostic.

Panlobular Emphysema

Panlobular emphysema is much less common and is often related to α_1-antitrypsin deficiency. It is diffuse or most severe at the lung bases and is manifest as an overall decrease in lung attenuation and in the size of pulmonary vessels (Fig. 6.54). Early panlobular emphysema can be quite difficult to detect. Focal lucencies may be absent.

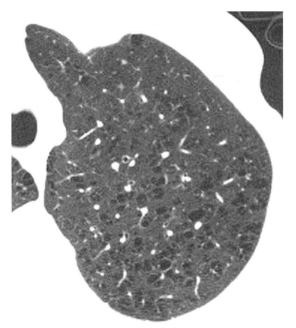

FIG. 6.53 **Centrilobular emphysema.** On high-resolution CT, multiple spotty areas of cystic lucency without visible walls are typical of centrilobular emphysema.

Paraseptal Emphysema

Paraseptal emphysema is common. It involves the subpleural lung adjacent to the chest wall and mediastinum. Emphysematous spaces several centimeters in diameter are typical, and their walls are seen easily (Fig. 6.55). It can occur as an isolated abnormality in young patients or may be associated with centrilobular emphysema. It has an upper lobe predominance.

Bullous Emphysema

Bullous emphysema is said to be present when bullae predominate. It is most often associated with paraseptal emphysema. Large bullae can be seen, particularly in young men. Bullae sometimes contain fluid as well as air, which may indicate infection.

Chronic Obstructive Pulmonary Disease

COPD is defined by pulmonary function test findings of airway obstruction that is not fully reversible. COPD is a nonspecific entity that can be associated with several disease processes, including emphysema, chronic bronchitis, and small airway obstruction. The airflow limitation in COPD, usually associated with cigarette smoking, is typically related to a combination of small airway obstruction and emphysema.

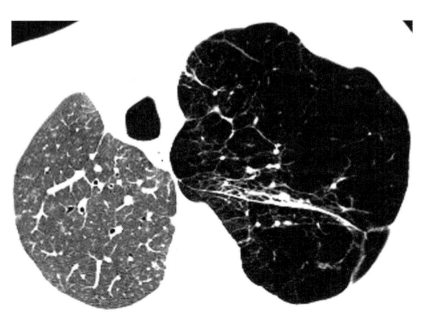

FIG. 6.54 **Panlobular emphysema.** Panlobular emphysema in a patient with a right lung transplant. The native left lung, involved by emphysema, is too lucent, and the vessels are abnormally small.

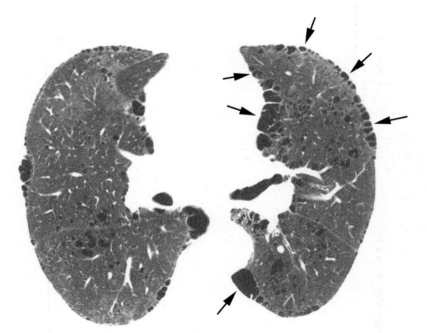

FIG. 6.55 Paraseptal emphysema. Subpleural lucency *(arrows)* is typical of paraseptal emphysema. Centrilobular emphysema is also present. Paraseptal emphysema is similar in appearance to honeycombing but typically occurs in a single layer, predominates in the upper lobes, and is not associated with findings of fibrosis.

Symptoms in patients with COPD usually include chronic cough, sputum production, and dyspnea. Although cough and sputum production are largely manifestations of chronic bronchitis in patients, respiratory disability often results from emphysema, small airway obstruction, or both.

In patients with COPD, HRCT may be used to determine the *COPD phenotype* present, on the basis of the preponderance of CT abnormalities visible, as either *emphysema predominant* or *airway predominant*, or in some patients a combination of both may be present.

Bronchial wall thickening (discussed in the previous section) is common in heavy cigarette smokers with chronic bronchitis, occurring because of bronchial inflammation and remodeling. However, the CT diagnosis of bronchial wall thickening is largely subjective and may be difficult to make.

Respiratory bronchiolitis is a cellular bronchiolitis, common in cigarette smokers and patients with COPD. Respiratory bronchiolitis is associated with large numbers of bronchiolar and peribronchiolar macrophages containing brown or black "smoker's" pigment. Respiratory bronchiolitis in patients with COPD may be visible on CT as poorly defined centrilobular nodules

of GGO, but abnormalities are often subtle or absent. Obstructive small airways disease is diagnosed on CT by identification of the presence of air trapping on expiratory scans.

SUGGESTED READING

Capobianco, J., Grimberg, A., Thompson, B. M., et al. (2012). Thoracic manifestations of collagen vascular diseases. *Radiographics, 32,* 33–50.

Chong, S., Lee, K. S., Chung, M. J., et al. (2006). Pneumoconiosis: Comparison of imaging and pathologic findings. *Radiographics, 26,* 59–77.

Criado, E., Sánchez, M., Ramírez, J., et al. (2010). Pulmonary sarcoidosis: Typical and atypical manifestations at high-resolution CT with pathologic correlation. *Radiographics, 30,* 1567–1586.

Foster, W. L., Gimenez, E. I., Roubidoux, M. A., et al. (1993). The emphysemas: Radiologic–pathologic correlations. *Radiographics, 13,* 311–328.

Frazier, A. A., Franks, T. J., Cooke, E. O., et al. (2008). From the archives of the AFIP. Pulmonary alveolar proteinosis. *Radiographics, 28,* 883–899.

Gruden, J. F., Webb, W. R., Naidich, D. P., & McGuinness, G. (1999). Multinodular disease: Anatomic localization at thin-section CT-multireader evaluation of a simple algorithm. *Radiology, 210,* 711–720.

Gruden, J. F., Webb, W. R., & Warnock, M. (1994). Centrilobular opacities in the lung on high-resolution CT: Diagnostic considerations and pathologic correlation. *AJR. Am J Roentgenol, 162*, 569–574.

Gupta, N., Vassallo, R., Wikenheiser-Brokamp, K. A., et al. (2015). Diffuse cystic lung disease. Part I. *Am J Respir Crit Care Med, 191*, 1354–1366.

Gupta, N., Vassallo, R., Wikenheiser-Brokamp, K. A., et al. (2015). Diffuse cystic lung disease. Part II. *Am J Respir Crit Care Med, 192*, 17–29.

Hansell, D. M., Bankier, A. A., MacMahon, H., McLoud, T. C., Muller, N. L., & Remy, J. (2008). Fleischner society: Glossary of terms for thoracic imaging. *Radiology, 246*, 697–722.

Hewitt, M. G., Miller, W. T., Jr., Reilly, T. J., & Simpson, S. (2014). The relative frequencies of causes of widespread ground-glass opacity: A retrospective cohort. *Eur J Radiol, 10*, 1970–1976.

Heyneman, L. E., Ward, S., Lynch, D. A., et al. (1999). Respiratory bronchiolitis, respiratory bronchiolitis-associated interstitial lung disease, and desquamative interstitial pneumonia: Different entities or part of the spectrum of the same disease process? *AJR. Am J Roengenol, 173*, 1617–1622.

Hirschmann, J. V., Pipavath, S. N. J., & Godwin, J. D. (2009). Hypersensitivity pneumonitis: A historical, clinical, and radiologic review. *Radiographics, 29*, 1921–1938.

Jeong, Y. J., Kim, K. I., Seo, I. J., et al. (2007). Eosinophilic lung diseases: A clinical, radiologic, and pathologic overview. *Radiographics, 27*, 617–639.

Johkoh, T., Müller, N. L., Cartier, Y., et al. (1999). Idiopathic interstitial pneumonias: Diagnostic accuracy of thin-section CT in 129 patients. *Radiology, 211*, 555–560.

Johkoh, T., Müller, N. L., Colby, T. V., et al. (2002). Nonspecific interstitial pneumonia: correlation between thin-section CT findings and pathologic subgroups in 55 patients. *Radiology, 225*, 199–204.

Kim, K. I., Kim, C. W., Lee, M. K., et al. (2001). Imaging of occupational lung disease. *Radiographics, 21*, 1371–1391.

Kim, S. J., Lee, K. S., Ryu, Y. H., et al. (2003). Reversed halo sign on high-resolution CT of cryptogenic organizing pneumonia: Diagnostic implications. *AJR. Am J Roentgenol, 180*, 1251–1254.

Lee, K. S., Kim, T. S., Han, J., et al. (1999). Diffuse micronodular lung disease: HRCT and pathologic findings. *J Comput Assist Tomogr, 23*, 99–106.

Lynch, D. A., Austin, J. H. M., Hogg, J. C., et al. (2015). CT-Definable subtypes of chronic obstructive pulmonary disease: A statement of the Fleischner Society. *Radiology, 277*, 192–205.

Lynch, D. A., Travis, W. D., Müller, N. L., et al. (2005). Idiopathic interstitial pneumonias: CT features. *Radiology, 236*, 10–21.

Miller, B. H., Rosado-de-Christenson, M. L., McAdams, H. P., & Fishback, N. F. (1995). Thoracic sarcoidosis: Radiologic-pathologic correlation. *Radiographics, 15*, 421–437.

Okada, F., Ando, Y., Yoshitake, S., et al. (2007). Clinical/pathologic correlations in 553 patients with primary centrilobular findings on high-resolution CT scan of the thorax. *Chest, 132*, 1939–1948.

Raghu, G., Remy-Jardin, M., Myers, J.L., et al. (2018). Diagnosis of idiopathic pulmonary fibrosis. An official ATS/ERS/JRS/ALAT clinical practice guideline. *Am J Respir Crit Care Med, 198*, e44–e68.

Rossi, S. E., Erasmus, J. J., McAdams, H. P., et al. (2000). Pulmonary drug toxicity: Radiologic and pathologic manifestations. *Radiographics, 20*, 1245–1259.

Silva, C. I. S., Müller, N. L., & Churg, A. (2007). Hypersensitivity pneumonitis: Spectrum of high-resolution CT and pathologic findings. *AJR. Am J Roentgenol, 188*, 334–344.

Travis, W. D., Costabel, U., Hansell, D. M., et al. (2013). An official American Thoracic Society/European Respiratory Society statement: Update of the international multidisciplinary classification of the idiopathic interstitial pneumonias. *Am J Respir Crit Care Med, 188*, 733–748.

Travis, W. D., Hunninghake, G., King, T. E., et al. (2008). Idiopathic nonspecific interstitial pneumonia: Report of an American Thoracic Society project. *Am J Respir Crit Care Med, 177*, 1338–1347.

Webb, W. R. (2006). Thin-section CT of the secondary pulmonary lobule: Anatomy and the image—the 2004 Fleischner lecture. *Radiology, 239*, 322–338.

CHAPTER 7

Pleura, Chest Wall, and Diaphragm

W. RICHARD WEBB

TECHNICAL CONSIDERATIONS

In general, the pleura and chest wall are adequately evaluated with routine thoracic CT techniques. Contrast medium infusion is helpful in showing pleural thickening and in allowing its differentiation from pleural fluid. Soft-tissue window settings and bone windows are most suitable for evaluating pleural abnormalities, the chest wall, and the diaphragm.

It should be kept in mind that the diaphragm and posterior pleural space extend well below the lung bases, and scans inferior to the diaphragmatic domes must be obtained for their complete evaluation. A good general rule is that if ribs are visible, then the pleural space is being imaged. Scanning with the patient in the prone position may be of assistance in evaluating pleural diseases; free pleural effusions shift to the dependent portion of the pleural space when the patient is moved from the supine position to the prone or decubitus position, whereas loculated effusions or fibrosis show little or no change. Prone scans in patients with pleural effusion are most commonly obtained when CT is being used for chest tube placement

PLEURA

Normal Anatomy

Because the lateral ribs are obliquely oriented, usually only a short segment of each rib is visible on a single CT slice. A more anterior rib represents one arising at a higher thoracic level than the rib posterior to it (Fig. 7.1). Thus, for example, at any given level, the fifth rib is anterior to the sixth, the fourth is anterior to the fifth, and so on. At the level of the lung apex, the first rib can be identified by its anterior position and by its articulation with the manubrium immediately below the level of the clavicle.

In many patients a bony spur projects inferiorly from the undersurface of the first rib at its junction with the manubrium. In cross section, with a lung window, this bony spur can appear to be surrounded by lung and can mimic a lung nodule. This appearance is usually bilateral and symmetric, providing a clue as to its true nature. As would be expected, it appears calcified at tissue windows.

Costal Pleura

On thin-slice CT in normal individuals, a 1- to 2-mm-thick opaque stripe is commonly seen in the intercostal spaces, between adjacent rib segments (Fig. 7.1). This stripe primarily represents the innermost intercostal muscle. In the paravertebral regions the innermost intercostal muscle is absent, and a much thinner line (or no line at all) is visible at the lung surface. The visceral and parietal pleura pass internal to the ribs and innermost intercostal muscles and are separated from them by a thin layer of extrapleural fat, but the pleural layers are not normally visible on CT.

Intrapulmonary Fissures

Intrapulmonary (interlobar) fissures are described and illustrated in Chapter 6 (Fig. 6.1). Normal collections of fat extending into the inferior aspects of the major fissures at the diaphragmatic surface can simulate fissural pleural thickening or effusion. They appear low in attenuation at mediastinal window settings.

Inferior Pulmonary Ligament

On each side below the inferior pulmonary vein, the parietal and visceral pleural layers join, forming a fold that extends inferiorly along the mediastinal surface of the lung and ends at the level of the diaphragm. This fold, the *inferior pulmonary ligament*, anchors the lower lobe. On CT images viewed at lung window settings, it appears as, or is related to, a small triangular opacity, 1 cm or less in size, with its apex pointing laterally into the lung and its base against the mediastinum. On each side, it usually lies adjacent to the esophagus (Fig. 7.2). Pleural effusion or pneumothoraces can be limited and marginated by the inferior pulmonary ligament.

A similar opacity can be seen on the right, lateral to the inferior vena cava (and thus anterior to the inferior pulmonary ligament), and on the left arising lateral to the left ventricle, extending inferiorly to the diaphragm, then extending laterally for several centimeters along the diaphragmatic surface (Fig. 7.2). These opacities represent the phrenic nerves and their pleural reflections. Their only significance is that they are commonly seen and just as commonly confusing.

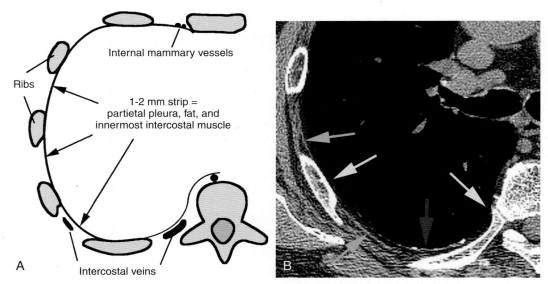

FIG. 7.1 Normal pleura. (A) A 1- to 2-mm line of opacity at the pleural surface primarily represents the innermost intercostal muscle, combined with the two pleural layers and the endothoracic fascia. In the paravertebral region, this stripe is much thinner or invisible. (B) In a patient with asbestos exposure, mild pleural thickening is visible posteriorly *(red arrow)*. The innermost intercostal muscle is visible as a 1- to 2-mm stripe *(green arrows)* between adjacent rib segments. Normal pleura *(yellow arrows)* in the paravertebral regions and internal to the ribs and intercostal muscles is invisible. The thickened pleura is partially calcified and is separated from the ribs and innermost intercostal muscle by a layer of fat.

Pleural Thickening and Look-alikes

Pleural thickening is visible on CT as a curvilinear soft-tissue stripe passing internal to the ribs and innermost intercostal muscles (Fig. 7.1B). A basic rule is that if the pleura is visible on CT, it is thickened. Thickened pleura enhances and is best seen after contrast medium infusion. Usually visible thickened pleura represents the parietal pleural layer.

In the presence of pleural thickening, the extrapleural fat layer is often thickened, and if this is the case, the visible pleural line is separated from the ribs and intercostal muscles by this fat layer (Fig. 7.1B). In the paravertebral regions or adjacent to the mediastinum, a distinct opaque stripe is visible in the presence of pleural thickening.

A small *pleural effusion* can mimic the appearance of pleural thickening; however, effusion is usually dependent on location and is crescentic. Thickened pleura can often be distinguished from small pleural fluid collections by contrast medium infusion; thickened pleura enhances, whereas fluid does not.

Normal *extrapleural fat pads* of a few millimeters in thickness can sometimes be seen internal to the ribs, particularly in the lower posterolateral thorax, and may not be easily distinguishable from pleural thickening or fluid with wide windows (1500 Hounsfield units [HU]). However, normal fat pads appear low in attenuation and are often symmetric, whereas pleural abnormalities generally are not.

The *subcostalis muscles* are sometimes visible posteriorly in the lower thorax as a 1- to 2-mm-thick stripe internal to one or more ribs. In contrast to pleural thickening, these muscles are smooth, uniform in thickness, and bilaterally symmetric.

Segments of *intercostal veins* are commonly visible in the paravertebral regions and can mimic focal pleural thickening. Continuity of these opacities with the azygos vein or hemiazygos vein can sometimes allow them to be identified correctly.

Pleural Effusion and Empyema
Diagnosis of Paradiaphragmatic Fluid Collections

The visceral pleura covers the surface of the lung, and its inferior extent is defined by the inferior extent of the lung parenchyma. The parietal pleura is contiguous with the chest wall and diaphragm and extends well below the level of the bases of the lungs, into the

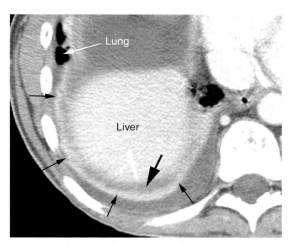

FIG. 7.3 **Subpulmonic effusion and a pseudodia-phragm mimicking ascites.** In a patient with a large right pleural effusion, the collapsed posterior lower lobe *(small black arrows)* simulates the diaphragm. Fluid *(large black arrow)* separating this opacity from the liver is in the region of the "bare area" of the liver. Ascites does not occur in this location. An aerated lower lobe *(white arrow)* is seen in association with the anterior aspect of the pseudodiaphragm.

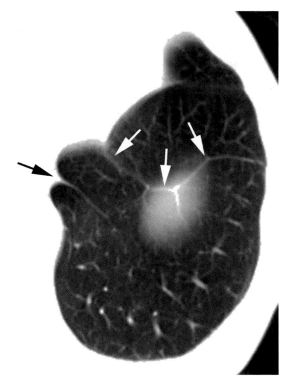

FIG. 7.2 **Inferior pulmonary ligament and phrenic Nerve.** A small triangular opacity *(black arrow)* arising adjacent to the esophagus represents the left inferior pulmonary ligament. Longer linear densities near the surface of the diaphragm *(white arrows)* represent pleural reflections adjacent to the phrenic nerve.

costophrenic angles. Thus pleural fluid collections in the costophrenic angles can be seen below the lung base and can mimic collections of fluid in the peritoneal cavity.

The parallel curvilinear configuration of the pleural and peritoneal cavities at the level of the perihepatic and perisplenic recesses allows fluid in either cavity to appear as an arcuate or semilunar opacity displacing the liver or spleen away from the adjacent chest wall. The relation of the fluid collection to the ipsilateral diaphragmatic crus (see later discussion) helps to determine its location. Pleural fluid collections in the posterior costophrenic angle lie posterior to the diaphragm and cause lateral displacement of the crus. Peritoneal fluid collections are anterior to the diaphragm and lateral to the crus, displacing it medially. Fluid seen posterior to the liver is within the pleural space; the peritoneal space does not extend into this region (this is the "bare area" of the liver).

A large pleural effusion allows the lower lobe to float anteriorly and lose volume. The posterior edge of the lower lobe when surrounded by fluid both anteriorly and posteriorly can appear to represent the diaphragm (a *pseudodiaphragm*), with pleural fluid posteriorly and ascites anteriorly (Fig. 7.3). Sequential scans at more cephalad levels, however, generally allow the correct interpretation to be made. Typically, the arcuate opacity of the atelectatic lower lobe becomes thicker superiorly, is contiguous with the remainder of the lower lobe, and may contain air bronchograms.

Fissural Fluid

Large effusions often extend into the major fissures, displacing the lower lobes medially and posteriorly. A localized collection of pleural fluid in a major or minor fissure can have a confusing appearance on CT scans and can be misinterpreted as representing a parenchymal mass. However, careful analysis of contiguous images will usually confirm the relation of the mass to the plane of the fissure. The edges of the fluid collection may be seen to taper, conforming to the fissure and forming a "beak" (Fig. 7.4).

Characterization of Pleural Effusion: Exudate or Transudate?

A pleural effusion is usually characterized by thoracentesis as being an *exudate* (a high-protein effusion

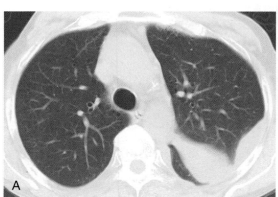 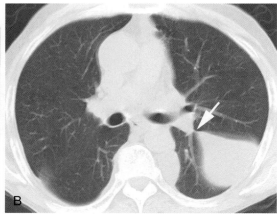

FIG. 7.4 **Fluid in a fissure.** (A and B) In this patient a free left pleural effusion extends into the major fissure. The fluid tapers medially in relation to the fissure (B, *arrow*), forming a "beak." Fissural fluid tends to be "localized" but not loculated.

TABLE 7.1
Common Causes of Exudates and Transudates

Exudates	Transudates
Parapneumonic effusion	Congestive heart failure
Empyema	Liver disease
Malignancy	Renal disease
Collagen vascular disease	Overhydration
Pulmonary embolism	Low serum protein level
Abdominal disease	
Hemothorax	
Chylothorax	

associated with pleural disease) or a *transudate* (a low-protein effusion associated with alteration in systemic factors governing the formation of pleural fluid) (Table 7.1). Exudates, being high in protein, tend to loculate, and tube drainage may be necessary. CT findings can help in diagnosing loculation and assessing the fluid collection.

On CT a crescentic and dependent fluid collection is likely, but not always, free (a definite diagnosis of free pleural effusion requires demonstration of a shift in effusion in association with a shift in patient position). A crescentic effusion may be a transudate or an exudate (Figs. 7.5 and 7.6). Lenticular (i.e., lens-shaped) fluid collections, and collections that are nondependent, are likely loculated, and thus very likely represent an exudate or an empyema (Figs. 7.6 and 7.10). When one is

describing an effusion on CT, its shape (crescentic or lenticular) and location (dependent or nondependent) should be indicated.

Most effusions appear to be near to water in attenuation, and measured CT numbers cannot be relied on to predict the specific gravity of the fluid or its nature (i.e., exudate or transudate). In patients with effusion the presence of pleural thickening on CT (Figs. 7.6 and 7.7) predicts that the effusion is an exudate rather than a transudate, with a specificity of nearly 100%. By definition, the pleura is considered thickened on CT if it is visible; contrast enhancement helps greatly in making this diagnosis. Transudates are not associated with pleural thickening (except in the unusual case of a patient with preexisting pleural disease who develops an unrelated transudate).

The absence of pleural thickening on contrast-enhanced CT in a patient with pleural effusion is less helpful; in this situation the effusion can be an exudate or a transudate (Fig. 7.7). Only about 50% to 60% of exudates are associated with visible pleural thickening on CT. However, the absence of pleural thickening on a contrast-enhanced scan makes empyema unlikely; empyema is almost always associated with parietal pleural thickening on contrast-enhanced CT.

Hemothorax

Hemothorax is defined as a pleural effusion having a hematocrit of at least 50% of the blood hematocrit. It may be traumatic or related to other causes of bleeding. Hemothorax may be dense (>50 HU) or may appear inhomogeneous, with some areas, particularly

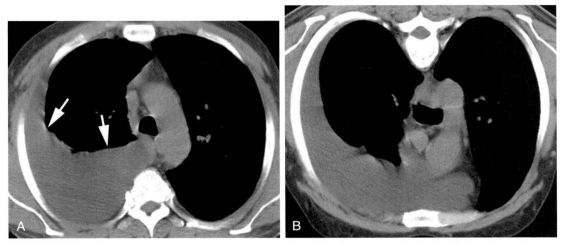

FIG. 7.5 **Free pleural effusion with a gravitational shift.** (A) A large crescentic fluid collection *(arrows)* is visible posteriorly on the right. (B) With the patient in the prone position, the fluid shifts to the anterior pleural space. This indicates it is free rather than loculated. No pleural thickening is seen.

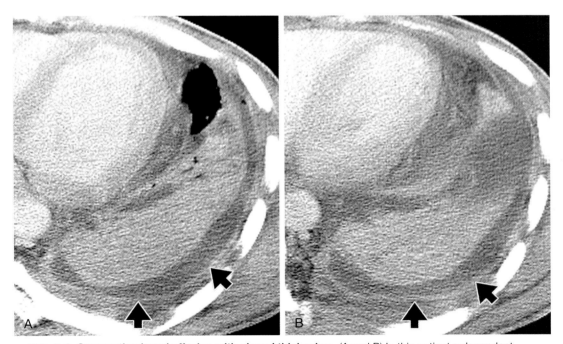

FIG. 7.6 **Crescentic pleural effusion with pleural thickening.** (A and B) In this patient a dependent and crescentic fluid collection is visible. Although this appearance suggests that the effusion is free, this is not always the case. Note that the parietal pleura is thickened (i.e., it is visible; *arrows*). Pleural thickening predicts the presence of an exudate; in this case it is an empyema. Extrapleural fat, between the thickened pleura and rib segments, is thick and edematous. The left lower lobe is collapsed.

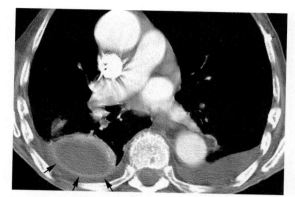

FIG. 7.7 Pleural effusions, with and without pleural thickening. Bilateral pleural effusions are present. The right pleural effusion is lenticular and is associated with pleural thickening *(arrows)* and the split pleura sign. It represents an empyema. The left pleural effusion is not associated with pleural thickening; this appearance is nonspecific. The left pleural effusion was transudative.

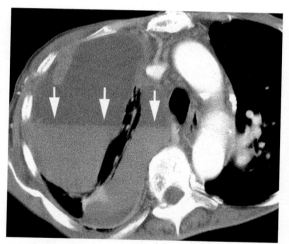

FIG. 7.8 Hemothorax. A large right pleural effusion shows a distinct fluid-fluid level or hematocrit effect, with dense blood or clot layered posteriorly *(arrows)*.

dependent regions, having an attenuation greater than that of the surrounding fluid. A fluid-fluid level (a hematocrit effect) or dependent clot may be seen with hemothorax (Fig. 7.8).

Parapneumonic Effusion

Pleural fluid can accumulate in patients with pneumonia, even when the pleural space is uninfected. This is termed a *simple parapneumonic effusion*, and it results from increased permeability of the visceral pleura

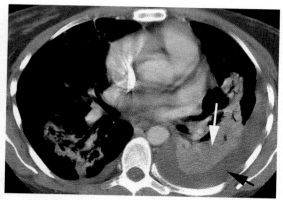

FIG. 7.9 Parapneumonic pleural effusion. A patient with left lower lobe pneumonia *(white arrow)* has a left pleural effusion *(black arrow)*. The effusion is dependent and crescentic in appearance; it is not associated with pleural thickening.

associated with the inflammation. The effusion is usually an exudate.

Parietal pleural thickening is present in about half of patients with parapneumonic effusion, whereas visceral pleural thickening is seen in one-fourth of patients. Because loculation is not usually present, the effusion is typically crescentic and dependent (Fig. 7.9).

Empyema

Empyemas are often associated with pneumonia but may occur in the absence of lung infection. Empyema is diagnosed if pleural fluid contains infectious organisms on smear or culture.

Classically, an empyema is associated with the *split pleura sign*. This sign is said to be present when the thickened visceral and parietal pleural layers are split apart by and surround the infected fluid collection (Figs. 7.7 and 7.10); the two pleural layers are generally similar in thickness. However, the split pleura sign is not always present in patients with empyema. Although empyema is nearly always associated with parietal pleural thickening on contrast-enhanced CT, visceral pleural thickening (and thus the split pleura sign) is present in only half of cases (Fig. 7.6).

Empyemas can be free or loculated, and crescentic (Fig. 7.6), rounded, elliptic, or lenticular (Figs. 7.6, 7.7, and 7.10). Loculated effusions are typically, but not always, elliptic. Multiple loculations may be present (Fig. 7.10B).

In patients with a dependent and crescentic effusion associated with pleural thickening, simple parapneumonic effusion and empyema cannot be distinguished.

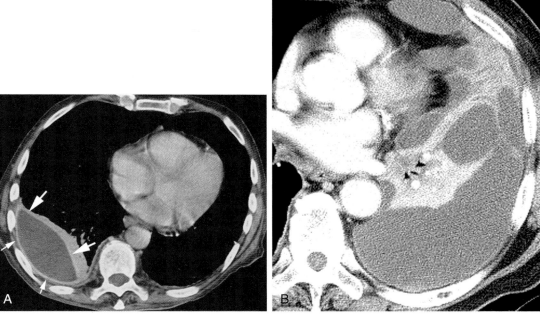

FIG. 7.10 **Empyema in two patients.** (A) A classic empyema is lenticular and well defined. After contrast medium injection, the thickened visceral *(large white arrows)* and parietal pleura *(small white arrows)* and the split pleura sign are visible. (B) An empyema is associated with a large left pleural effusion, pleural thickening, and multiple loculations. The left lower lobe is collapsed.

However, loculation is not usually present in simple parapneumonic effusion and predicts empyema.

The presence of air within an empyema is almost always due to recent thoracentesis, but may also indicate bronchopleural fistula (Fig. 7.11) or the presence of a gas-forming organism. In the absence of thoracentesis, this finding is usually an indication for tube drainage.

Extension of an empyema to involve the chest wall is termed *empyema necessitatis*. Two-thirds of cases result from tuberculosis, but other responsible organisms include *Actinomyces* and *Nocardia*. CT findings include low-attenuation fluid collections within the chest wall.

Differentiation of Empyema From Lung Abscess

Distinguishing empyema from lung abscess is sometimes important in patients who are clinically infected; empyema is often treated by tube drainage, whereas lung abscess generally is not. CT can be helpful in making this distinction, particularly when contrast medium is infused.

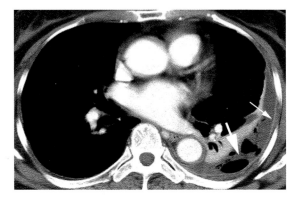

FIG. 7.11 **Empyema and bronchopleural fistula.** A crescentic left pleural effusion associated with pleural thickening *(small arrow)*. Multiple collections of air *(large arrow)* in the left effusion result from a bronchopleural fistula. The presence of multiple discrete air bubbles indicates the presence of a multiseptated pleural effusion.

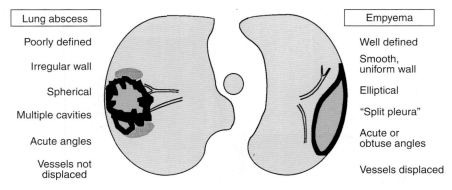

FIG. 7.12 **Empyema versus lung abscess.**

The outer edge of an empyema is sharply demarcated from adjacent lung, and on contrast-enhanced scans the empyema wall appears smooth and uniform in thickness. When a bronchopleural fistula is present and air is contained within the empyema cavity, or when air is introduced into the empyema during thoracentesis, its inner margin also appears smooth.

In contrast, lung abscesses are irregularly shaped and may contain multiple areas of low-attenuation necrosis or collections of air and fluid (Fig 6.26). On contrast-enhanced scans the abscess wall is generally opacified relative to fluid in the abscess cavity (Fig 6.26). The inner surfaces of an abscess may appear irregular and ragged, and their outer edges may be poorly defined or irregular because of adjacent pulmonary parenchymal consolidation.

At their point of contact with the chest wall, empyemas can show acute or obtuse angles (Fig. 7.12), whereas abscesses typically have acute angles. Empyemas also tend to compress and displace the lung and vessels, acting as a space-occupying mass, whereas lung abscesses usually destroy the lung without displacing it.

Organizing Empyema (Pleural Peel)

In patients with chronic empyema, especially if it is tuberculous in origin, ingrowth of fibroblasts can result in pleural fibrosis and the development of chronic pleural thickening. CT may show a thickened pleural peel (Fig. 7.13). The presence of a decreased volume of the affected hemithorax is an important finding (Fig. 7.13). Calcification, which typically is focal in its early stages, may become extensive (Fig. 7.14). Frequently, a thickened layer of extrapleural fat is also visible, separating the parietal pleura and the ribs (this layer is considerably thicker than the fat pads, which can be seen normally) (Fig. 7.14). Treatment usually requires pleural stripping.

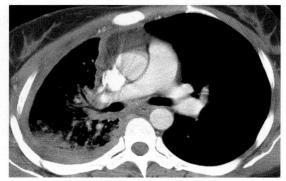

FIG. 7.13 **Pleural peel.** A patient with prior empyema shows extensive smooth thickening of the right pleura. Note that the hemithorax is reduced in volume. This is typical of pleural fibrosis.

Dense pleural thickening, even with calcification, does not indicate that the pleural disease is inactive. Loculated fluid collections resulting from active infection (Fig. 7.14) may be seen on CT within the thickened pleura.

Thoracostomy Tubes

Infected pleural fluid collections often become loculated and can be difficult to drain. CT is sometimes indicated to evaluate thoracostomy tube position when the tube is functioning poorly. Malpositioned chest tubes can lie within a fissure, within a loculated fluid collection (whereas other collections remain undrained), or outside the empyema.

Pleural Calcification and Talc Pleurodesis

Pleural thickening with calcification may be seen with chronic empyema, particularly if it is tuberculous in nature (Fig. 7.14), and with resolved hemothorax, asbestos exposure (Figs. 7-1B, 7.15, and 7.19), and

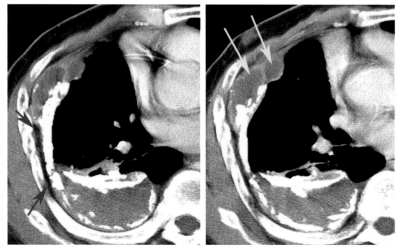

FIG. 7.14 **Calcified pleural thickening associated with tuberculosis.** The parietal and visceral pleura are densely calcified. Thickened extrapleural fat *(red arrows)* is visible external to the calcified parietal pleura. Residual fluid is evident in the pleural space, and loculated collections anteriorly *(yellow arrows)* reflect active infection.

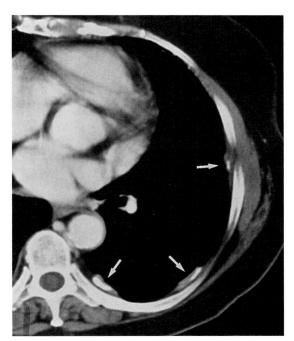

FIG. 7.15 **Asbestos-related pleural plaques.** Typical calcified pleural plaques *(arrows)* are visible. They are often internal to the ribs.

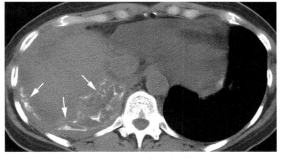

FIG. 7.16 **Talc pleurodesis.** Streaky high-attenuation opacities in the posterior right hemithorax represent talc injected for pleurodesis *(arrows)*. This appearance mimics pleural thickening with calcification.

Asbestos-Related Pleural Disease

Asbestos-related pleural thickening has a typical appearance on CT. Early pleural thickening is discontinuous, with the intervening pleura appearing normal; focal areas of pleural thickening are termed *pleural plaques* (Figs. 7.1B, 7.15, and 7.19). The pleural disease is typically bilateral. Calcification is common. Diffuse pleural thickening, which is probably the result of prior asbestos-related benign pleural effusion, can also be seen. In patients with asbestos-related pleural disease, the pleural thickening, plaques, or calcification typically involves the parietal pleura, but this is difficult to recognize on CT unless the presence of pleural fluid separates the visceral and parietal pleural layers.

rarely in pleural sarcomas. Pleurodesis using talc can mimic pleural calcification. The talc is dense and typically accumulates in the posterior and inferior hemithorax (Fig. 7.16).

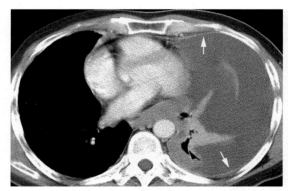

FIG. 7.17 **Malignant effusion caused by metastatic carcinoma.** A large left pleural effusion is associated with left lung atelectasis, mediastinal displacement to the right, and pleural thickening *(arrows)*.

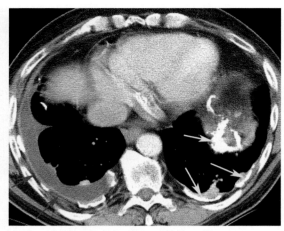

FIG. 7.19 **DMM in a patient with asbestos exposure.** Bilateral calcified pleural plaques *(yellow arrows)* reflect asbestos exposure; note the presence of a calcified plaque on the surface of the left hemidiaphragm. A new right pleural effusion associated with parietal pleural thickening *(red arrows)* is nonspecific, but in this patient indicates the presence of mesothelioma.

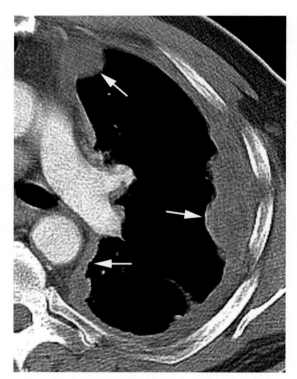

FIG. 7.18 **CT findings of malignancy in DMM.** There is circumferential and nodular left pleural thickening *(arrows)*. The mediastinal pleura is thickened, and the pleural thickening exceeds 1 cm. These four findings predict a malignancy.

The diaphragmatic pleura is commonly involved in patients with asbestos-related pleural disease (Fig. 7.19). However, the diaphragm lies roughly in the scan plane, and detection of uncalcified pleural plaques on the diaphragmatic surface can be difficult. In some patients, diaphragmatic pleural plaques are visible deep in the posterior costophrenic angle, below the lung base. Pleural plaques along the mediastinum have been considered unusual in patients with asbestos-related pleural disease, but they are visible on CT scans in about 40% of these patients. Paravertebral pleural thickening is also common.

Although it is unusual, pleural thickening can involve a fissure and result in a localized fissural pleural plaque; this may simulate a lung nodule on CT unless the plane of the fissure is identified.

Pleural Neoplasm: CT Findings

Neoplasm, primary or metastatic, is a common cause of pleural effusion, pleural thickening, and/or pleural mass.

Pleural Effusion

In patients with malignancy, pleural effusion can result from primary or metastatic tumor involvement of the pleura or lymphatic obstruction in the hila or mediastinum. In both instances an exudate is typically present, and effusions may be large. The term *malignant effusion* means that malignant cells are present in the pleural fluid. In patients with malignant effusion, pleural thickening or mass may or may not be visible on contrast-enhanced CT (Fig. 7.17).

CT Findings of Malignancy

CT findings that strongly suggest the diagnosis of malignant involvement of the pleura, either primary or metastatic, (Fig. 7.18) include:

- nodular pleural thickening
- a pleural thickness of more than 1 cm
- thickening that concentrically involves the pleura, encasing the lung
- thickening of the mediastinal pleura

Primary Pleural Neoplasms

Primary pleural neoplasms have recently been reclassified by the World Health Organization as mesothelial, mesenchymal, or lymphoproliferative. Mesothelioma and solitary fibrous tumor (SFT) are most common. Primary effusion lymphoma and various sarcomas are less frequently seen.

Diffuse Malignant Mesothelioma

Diffuse malignant mesothelioma (DMM) is a highly aggressive mesothelial neoplasm with an extremely poor prognosis. Morphologically, it is characterized by nodular pleural thickening. However, hemorrhagic pleural effusion is often present and may obscure the underlying pleural thickening, which can be minimal in early cases. In most patients, this tumor is related to asbestos exposure; although it is rare in the general population, the incidence in workers heavily exposed to asbestos is about 5%.

In patients with DMM, CT can expedite the initial diagnosis and define the extent of tumor. Usually, irregular or nodular pleural thickening is visible (Fig. 7.18), although a new pleural effusion or diffuse pleural thickening may be the only recognizable finding (Fig. 7.19). Pleural thickening is usually most pronounced in the inferior thorax. Contrast medium infusion can allow tumor to be distinguished from associated fluid collections. Scans with the patient in the prone or decubitus position can also help in distinguishing underlying mesothelioma from pleural fluid.

Although DMM is visible most frequently along the lateral chest wall, mediastinal pleural thickening or concentric pleural thickening is seen with extensive disease (Fig. 7.18). The abnormal hemithorax can appear contracted and fixed, with little change in size on inspiration. Thickening of the fissures, particularly the lower part of the major fissures, can reflect tumor infiltration. DMM typically spreads by local invasion, involving the mediastinum and sometimes the chest wall. Although hematogenous pulmonary metastases or distant metastases occur in about 30% of cases, these are usually clinically insignificant; local invasion usually determines prognosis.

Mesothelioma is staged with a TNM system similar to that used with lung cancer. The T classification is most important in determining treatment. Patients most commonly present locally advanced disease (stage III, 40%) or advanced disease (stage IV, 35%). Local disease stages (stage I or stage II) account for only 25% of patients.

Localized Malignant Mesothelioma

Localized malignant mesothelioma is rare. It appears as a localized pleural lesion and has a better prognosis than DMM.

Solitary Fibrous Tumor

Solitary fibrous tumor (SFT), formerly termed *localized fibrous tumor of the pleura*, is an uncommon fibroblastic mesenchymal tumor. SFT accounts for less than of 5% of primary pleural tumors. Approximately 10% of SFTs are malignant, although they have a good prognosis. SFT is unassociated with asbestos exposure. It is usually detected incidentally, but can be associated with chest pain, hypoglycemia because of production of insulin-like growth factor type 2, and hypertrophic pulmonary osteoarthropathy.

SFT usually arises from the visceral pleura and most commonly involves the costal pleural surface (Figs 7.20 and Fig. 7.21); occasionally, it can be seen within a fissure. On CT, these tumors are solitary, smooth, sharply defined, and often large, and contact a pleural surface (Figs. 7.16 and 7.21).

SFT usually appears homogeneous on CT. However, large tumors can appear heterogeneous with or without contrast medium infusion, and calcification may be present (Fig. 7.21). Although it is generally stated that pleural abnormalities result in obtuse angles at the point of contact between the lesion and the chest wall, SFT may show acute angles and pleural thickening adjacent to the mass (Fig. 7.20). This thickening may reflect a small amount of fluid accumulation in the pleural space at the point at which the visceral and parietal pleural surfaces are separated by the mass. A similar "beak" or "thorn" sign is often visible on plain radiographs in patients with a SFT in a fissure.

Pleural Metastases

Metastatic malignant pleural effusion may or may not be associated with visible pleural thickening or other pleural abnormality.

In some cases, pleural metastases result in large pleural nodules visible on CT. In most such cases, pleural effusion is also present. Nodular pleural metastases

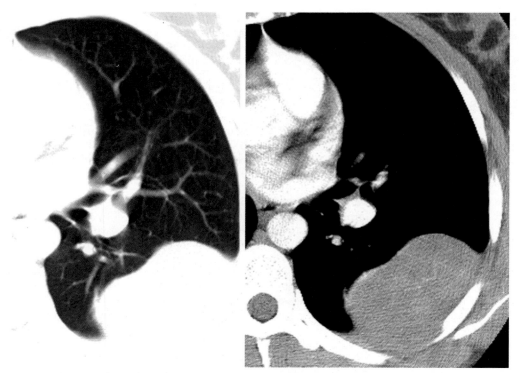

FIG. 7.20 **Localized Fibrous Tumor of the Pleura.** The large homogeneous mass is smooth and sharply defined. Slight beak-shaped pleural thickening is seen adjacent to the mass, probably related to a small amount of pleural fluid.

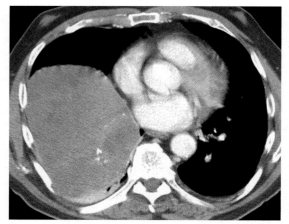

FIG. 7.21 **Localized fibrous tumor of the pleura.** A large heterogeneous and calcified mass appears smooth and sharply defined.

are more easily seen on contrast-enhanced scans, being higher in attenuation than associated fluid (Figs. 7.22 and 7.23). Invasive thymoma and some other tumors can result in pleural nodules unassociated with pleural effusion (Fig 4.18).

Pleural metastatic tumor can diffusely infiltrate the pleura, resulting in an appearance indistinguishable from that of DMM (Fig. 7.24). Metastatic tumor may extend into the fissures; thickening of the fissure or fissural nodules may be present (Fig. 7.25).

Lymphoma

Pleural effusions occur in 15% of patients with Hodgkin disease and usually reflect lymphatic or venous obstruction by a mediastinal or hilar tumor rather than by pleural involvement; effusions in Hodgkin disease tend to resolve after local mediastinal or hilar radiation. Pericardial effusions, however, present in 5% of patients, usually indicate direct involvement of the pericardium. Masses involving the pleura or extrapleural chest wall can sometimes be seen in Hodgkin lymphoma or non-Hodgkin lymphoma (Fig. 7.26); these may or may not be associated with effusion.

Primary effusion lymphoma is a rare and aggressive B-cell non-Hodgkin lymphoma, usually presenting with malignant pleural, pericardial, or peritoneal effusions, without visible tumor masses. Primary effusion lymphoma is associated with human herpesvirus 8 (also known as Kaposi sarcoma–associated herpesvirus).

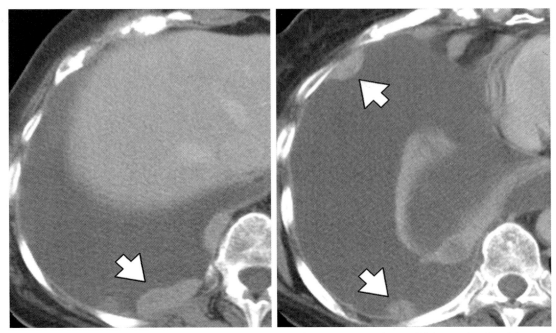

FIG. 7.22 **Pleural metastases from colon carcinoma.** On a contrast-enhanced CT scan, focal nodular pleural masses *(arrows)* are visible arising from the parietal pleura. A large pleural effusion is also present.

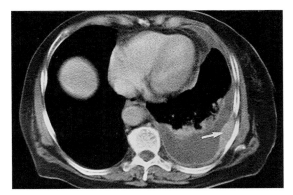

FIG. 7.23 **Pleural metastasis.** Pleural thickening is evident after contrast medium infusion. An enhanced pleural mass *(arrow)* and pleural effusion are visible.

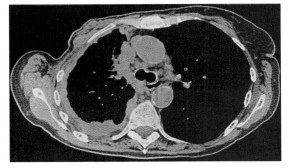

FIG. 7.24 **Pleural metastasis.** Diffuse nodular pleural thickening in a patient with breast cancer simulates mesothelioma.

Patients are immunosuppressed (HIV infection, after organ transplantation), and 70% of cases occur with concurrent Epstein-Barr virus infection. The prognosis of primary effusion lymphoma is poor.

CHEST WALL
Lung Cancer With Chest Wall Invasion

Direct invasion of the chest wall by a peripheral lung carcinoma is common. In the lung cancer staging system (Table 4.3), tumors invading the parietal pleura, chest wall (including the superior sulcus), phrenic nerve, or parietal pericardium are classified as *T3* and are usually considered resectable. Tumors invading the vertebral body, diaphragm, recurrent laryngeal nerve, or great vessels at the lung apex are considered *T4*; these may be resectable if lymph node metastases are limited to the hila, often following chemotherapy and/or radiation therapy.

Hodgkin disease can involve structures of the chest wall by direct invasion from the mediastinum or lung in a small percentage of cases. Diffuse (malignant) mesothelioma commonly invades the chest wall.

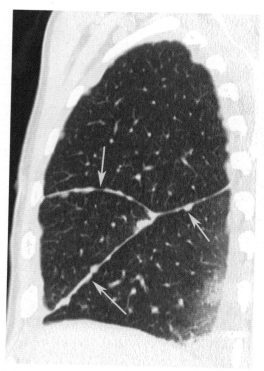

FIG. 7.25 Pleural metastases with nodules involving the fissures. Nodular thickening of the major and minor fissures *(arrows)* on this sagittal reconstruction is as a result of pleural metastases from colon carcinoma. A small pleural effusion is visible in the posterior costophrenic angle.

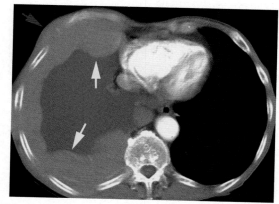

FIG. 7.26 Mantle cell non-hodgkin lymphoma with pleural and chest wall involvement. Gross nodular pleural thickening *(yellow arrows)* is present on the right in association with a large pleural effusion. Tumor also involves the adjacent chest wall *(red arrow)*. A mediastinal mass was visible at higher levels.

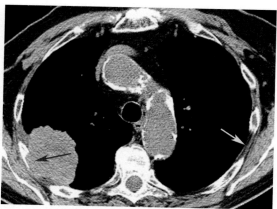

FIG. 7.27 Lung carcinoma with chest wall invasion. This patient shows a number of findings that predict or are diagnostic of chest wall invasion, including more than 3 cm of contact between the tumor and chest wall, obtuse angles with the pleural surface, and a contact length between the tumor and the chest wall of more than 70% of the maximum tumor diameter. Also note the obliteration *(red arrow)* of normal extrapleural fat, rib destruction, and chest wall mass adjacent to the tumor. Normal fat planes *(yellow arrow)* are shown on the left.

The CT diagnosis of chest wall invasion can be difficult, but a variety of CT findings can help in prediction. The most accurate CT findings of chest wall invasion in order of increasing specificity (Figs. 7.27 and 7.28) are:

- obtuse angles at the point of contact between tumor and pleura
- extensive contact between the tumor and chest wall (>3 cm or 70% of the tumor diameter)
- obliteration of extrapleural fat planes
- infiltration of soft tissues
- a chest wall mass
- bone destruction

Diagnosing chest wall invasion when a tumor simply abuts the pleura should be avoided. Tumors adjacent to the pleura, even when associated with focal pleural thickening and pleural effusion, may not be invasive. In a patient with lung cancer, pleural effusion can occur for a variety of reasons, including obstructive pneumonia and lymphatic or pulmonary venous obstruction by tumor. Only patients with demonstration of tumor cells in the pleural fluid (malignant effusion) or pleural nodules are considered to have unresectable disease (M1a in the staging system; Table 4.3).

Superior Sulcus (Pancoast) Tumors

Invasive tumors arising in the superior pulmonary sulcus produce the characteristic clinical findings of Horner

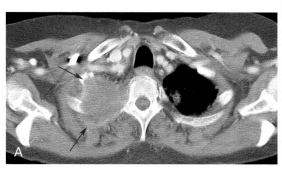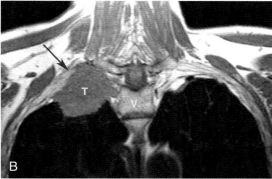

FIG. 7.28 **Pancoast tumor with chest wall invasion.** (A) On CT a right apical mass is associated with invasion of the chest wall and rib destruction *(arrows)*. Although the tumor appears to contact the vertebral body, it appears intact. (B) Coronal magnetic resonance imaging shows the relationship of the tumor *(T)* to the vertebral body *(V)* and the brachial plexus *(arrow)*, which appears to be involved.

syndrome and shoulder and arm pain; this presentation is termed *Pancoast syndrome*. Previously, tumors of the superior sulcus were considered to have a poor prognosis, but combined therapy with radiation, followed by resection of the upper lobe, chest wall, and adjacent structures, has resulted in 5-year survival rates of up to 30%. In patients being considered for this combined therapy, CT scans can provide information on the anatomic extent of tumor spread that is useful in planning both the radiation therapy and the surgical approach to the tumor. However, magnetic resonance imaging has been shown to be more accurate than CT in showing the apical extent of tumors.

Extension of a tumor posteriorly or laterally at the lung apex primarily involves the chest wall (Fig. 7.28). Although such chest wall invasion does not prevent resection, extensive chest wall and bone involvement makes surgical treatment difficult, and the prognosis for patients with extensive chest wall disease is relatively poor. Invasion of tumor tissue posteromedially involves the ribs or vertebral bodies. This occurs in one-third to half of cases and is usually visible on CT. Anterior and medial extension of a tumor can involve the esophagus, trachea, and brachiocephalic vessels. Invasion of these structures or the vertebral body precludes resection in most cases.

Axillary Space

As usually defined, the axilla is bordered by the fascial coverings of the following muscles: the pectoralis major and pectoralis minor anteriorly; the latissimus dorsi, teres major, and subscapularis posteriorly; the chest wall and serratus anterior medially; and the coracobrachialis and biceps laterally. However, when patients are scanned with their arms above their heads, the axilla is open laterally.

The axilla contains the axillary artery and vein, branches of the brachial plexus, some branches of the intercostal nerves, and a large number of lymph nodes, all surrounded by fat. The axillary vessels and the brachial plexus extend laterally, near the apex of the axilla, close to the pectoralis minor muscle. In general, the axillary vein lies below and anterior to the axillary artery, whereas the brachial plexus is largely above and posterior to the artery. Although these vessels can usually be seen on CT scans, in many healthy individuals it is impossible to distinguish artery and vein within the axilla unless the vein is opacified by contrast medium.

Lymphadenopathy

Axillary lymph nodes, which are usually up to 1 cm but occasionally are 1.5 cm in diameter, can be seen in normal individuals. Lymph nodes larger than 1 cm (short-axis or least diameter) should be considered suspicious when an abnormality is suspected on clinical grounds; lymph nodes of 2 cm or greater in diameter are considered pathologic regardless of the history. Axillary lymphadenopathy is seen most frequently in patients with lymphoma or metastatic carcinoma. Lymph node masses are detected most easily by observation of both axillae for symmetry. Enlarged lymph nodes high within the axilla lie beneath the pectoral muscles (subpectoral nodes) and may not be palpable, but these nodes can be detected by CT. Axillary masses in relation to nerves of the brachial plexus can also be demonstrated with CT.

Breast

Soft tissues of the breasts are seen on CT scans of female patients in the supine position. Localized breast masses are occasionally visible, but their CT appearance is usually nonspecific. Enhancing masses are suggested of carcinoma. Breast masses detected incidentally on CT images generally should be evaluated by physical examination and mammography.

Breast Carcinoma

Other than for staging, CT is not used in the routine evaluation of patients with breast cancer. However, CT can aid the planning of radiation therapy by providing an accurate measurement of chest wall thickness and by detecting internal mammary lymph node metastases.

Mastectomy

In women who have had a mastectomy, uncommon in current practice, characteristic alterations in chest wall anatomy are seen, depending on the surgical procedure performed. CT is sometimes used to evaluate suspected local tumor recurrence and to guide needle biopsy.

Surgery for breast cancer is often limited to lumpectomy, and little is visible on CT except for a local scar. Some residual breast tissue remains when segmental or partial mastectomy is performed. Simple mastectomy consists of removal of the breast. Axillary lymph node dissection may be performed with any of these approaches. Typically, surgical clips are present within the axilla, and focal scarring remains visible on CT. Postoperative scarring is visible as irregular soft tissue within the axillary fat. Localized postoperative fluid collections may be seen in the breast or axilla.

A radical mastectomy consists of complete removal of the breast tissue and pectoralis major and pectoralis minor muscles and extensive axillary lymph node dissection. On CT, although most of the pectoralis muscles are absent, residual pectoralis major muscle is sometimes seen at its sternal or costal attachment. This should not be misinterpreted as a recurrent tumor.

Modified radical mastectomy consists of removal of the breast and the pectoralis minor muscle and axillary lymph node dissection. In patients who have undergone a modified radical mastectomy, the amount of pectoralis minor muscle remaining is variable. Without careful clinical correlation, it is sometimes difficult to distinguish postsurgical changes from tumor recurrence.

Keep in mind that if a patient has difficulty in elevating both arms symmetrically for the CT scan because of surgery, asymmetry of the breasts, axillae, and underlying musculature may be present (e.g., the pectoralis muscle may look thicker on one side). This asymmetry should not be misinterpreted as abnormal.

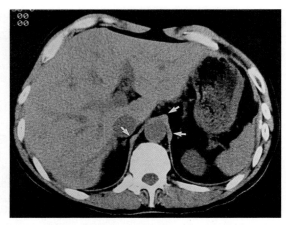

FIG. 7.29 **Normal diaphragm.** The diaphragm is outlined by retroperitoneal fat. Where it contacts the liver and spleen, it is not usually visible as a discrete structure. The diaphragmatic crura can appear quite lumpy *(arrows)*. Here they pass anterior to the aorta to form the aortic hiatus.

DIAPHRAGM
Anatomy

Because of the transaxial plane of CT, the central portion of the diaphragm does not appear as a distinct structure, and its position can be inferred only by the position of the lung base above and the upper abdominal organs below. However, as the more peripheral portions of the diaphragm extend caudad toward their sternal and costal attachments, the anterior, posterior, and lateral portions of the diaphragm become visible adjacent to retroperitoneal fat (Fig. 7.29). Where the diaphragm is contiguous with the liver or spleen, it is sometimes outlined as a distinct structure because of a subdiaphragmatic fat layer.

Diaphragmatic Crura

The right and left diaphragmatic crura are tendinous structures arising inferiorly from the anterior surfaces of the upper lumbar vertebral bodies and intervening disks and are continuous with the anterior longitudinal ligament of the spine. The crura ascend anterior to the spine on each side of the aorta, and then pass medially and anteriorly, joining the muscular diaphragm anterior to the aorta to form the aortic hiatus (Fig. 7.29). The right crus, which is larger and longer than the left crus, arises from the first three lumbar vertebral levels; the left crus arises from the first two lumbar segments.

The diaphragmatic crura can be mistaken for enlarged lymph nodes or masses because of their rounded appearance; para-aortic lymph nodes can indeed be seen in a similar position. However, on contiguous CT scans, the crura merge gradually with the diaphragm at more

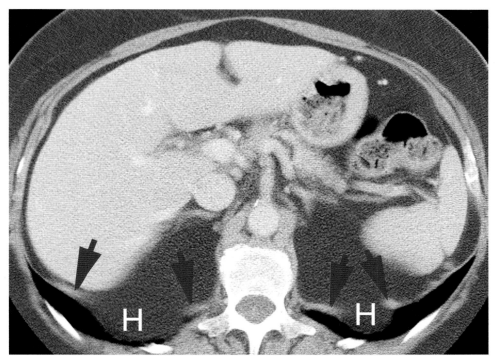

FIG. 7.30 Bochdalek hernias. In this patient, bilateral Bochdalek hernias *(H)* consist of retroperitoneal fat. The edges of the diaphragm *(arrows)* outline the defects leading to herniation.

cephalad levels. The diameter of the crura also varies with lung volume, increasing at full inspiration compared with expiration.

Openings in the Diaphragm

The diaphragm is perforated by several openings that allow structures to pass from the thorax to the abdomen. The aortic hiatus is posterior; it is bounded posteriorly by the vertebral body and anteriorly by the crura. Through it pass the aorta, the azygos and hemiazygos veins, the thoracic duct, the intercostal arteries, and the splanchnic nerves. The esophageal hiatus is situated more anteriorly, in the muscular portion of the diaphragm. Through it pass the esophagus, the vagus nerves, and small blood vessels. The foramen of the inferior vena cava pierces the fibrous central tendon of the diaphragm anterior and to the right of the esophageal hiatus.

Of these three structures, the aortic hiatus is defined most easily. On CT scans the esophageal foramen is visible as an opening at the junction of the esophagus and stomach. The foramen of the inferior vena cava must be inferred from the position of the inferior vena cava. The foramina of Morgagni and of Bochdalek are not visible on CT scans in normal individuals.

Diaphragmatic Abnormalities
Hernias

Abdominal or retroperitoneal contents can herniate into the chest through congenital or acquired areas of weakness in the diaphragm or through traumatic diaphragmatic ruptures. Hernias of the stomach through the esophageal hiatus are the most common.

Hernias through the foramen of Bochdalek occur in as many as 5% of healthy adults. Most are left-sided, and although they are often located in the posterolateral diaphragm, they can occur anywhere along the posterior costodiaphragmatic margin (Fig. 7.30). Bochdalek hernias in adults usually contain retroperitoneal fat or, much less commonly, kidney.

Parasternal hernias through the foramen of Morgagni are relatively rare. Most Morgagni hernias occur on the right and, in contrast to Bochdalek hernias, usually contain an extension of the peritoneal sac. Their contents can include omentum, liver, or bowel.

An understanding of the anatomy of the anterior portion of the diaphragm is essential in correctly diagnosing a Morgagni hernia. The presence of bowel anterior to the heart can suggest the presence of a hernia, but this is not usually the case.

Diaphragmatic rupture can result from penetrating or nonpenetrating trauma to the abdomen or thorax. In nearly all cases the left hemidiaphragm is affected, with ruptures of the central or posterior diaphragm being the most frequent. The diaphragmatic defect may appear as a localized absence of visible diaphragm, associated with thickening of the adjacent visible portion of the diaphragm or ipsilateral crus. Omentum, stomach, small or large intestine, spleen, and kidney may all herniate through a diaphragmatic rent. CT reconstructions in the sagittal or coronal plane may help in diagnosis; the hernia may show a "neck" at the site of herniation.

If diaphragmatic rupture is associated with splenic rupture, small bits of splenic tissue may seed the left pleural space. This is termed *thoracic splenosis*. CT can show small, left-sided pleural nodules, usually associated with findings of splenectomy and diaphragmatic injury.

Tumors

Tumors involving the diaphragm usually represent pleural tumors (e.g., mesothelioma), pleural metastases, or upper abdominal tumors with local invasion. Primary diaphragmatic tumors are rare. Pleural lipoma is occasionally seen as an incidental finding.

Diaphragmatic Eventration and Paralysis

Local eventration of the right hemidiaphragm with superior displacement of the liver can be confused radiographically with a peripheral pulmonary or pleural mass. CT scans after infusion of contrast medium can demonstrate opacification of normal intrahepatic vessels in the apparent mass, allowing its identification.

Hemidiaphragm elevation is seen in patients with diaphragmatic paralysis. The ipsilateral diaphragm may appear thinner than the opposite hemidiaphragm if the paralysis is chronic.

SUGGESTED READING

Aquino, S. L., Chen, M. Y., Kuo, W. T., & Chiles, C. (1999). The CT appearance of pleural and extrapleural disease in lymphoma. *Clinical Radiology, 54*, 647–650.

Aquino, S. L., Webb, W. R., & Gushiken, B. J. (1994). Pleural exudates and transudates: Diagnosis with contrast-enhanced CT. *Radiology, 192*, 803–808.

Bligh, M. P., Borgaonkar, J. N., Burrell, S. C., et al. (2017). Spectrum of CT findings in thoracic extranodal non-Hodgkin lymphoma. *Radiographics, 37*, 439–461.

Choi, J. A., Hong, K. T., Oh, Y. W., et al. (2001). CT manifestations of late sequelae in patients with tuberculous pleuritis. *AJR. American Journal of Roentgenology, 176*, 441–445.

Desir, A., & Ghaye, B. (2012). CT of Blunt diaphragmatic rupture. *Radiographics, 32*, 477–498.

Dynes, M. C., White, E. M., Fry, W. A., & Ghahremani, G. G. (1992). Imaging manifestations of pleural tumors. *Radiographics, 12*, 1191–1201.

Federle, M. P., Mark, A. S., & Guillaumin, E. S. (1986). CT of subpulmonic pleural effusions and atelectasis: Criteria for differentiation from subphrenic fluid. *AJR. American Journal of Roentgenology, 146*, 685–689.

Ferretti, G. R., Chiles, C., Choplin, R. H., & Coulomb, M. (1997). Localized benign fibrous tumors of the pleura. *AJR. American Journal of Roentgenology, 169*, 683–686.

Halvorsen, R. A., Fedyshin, P. J., Korobkin, M., et al. (1986). Ascites or pleural effusion? CT differentiation: Four useful criteria. *Radiographics, 6*, 135–149.

Harish, M. G., Konda, S. D., MacMahon, H., & Newstead, G. M. (2007). Breast lesions incidentally detected with CT: What the general radiologist needs to know. *Radiographics, 27*, S37–S51.

Im, J.-G., Webb, W. R., Rosen, A., & Gamsu, G. (1989). Costal pleura: Appearances at high-resolution CT. *Radiology, 171*, 125–131.

Leung, A. N., Müller, N. L., & Miller, R. R. (1990). CT in differential diagnosis of diffuse pleural disease. *AJR. American Journal of Roentgenology, 154*, 487–492.

Nandalur, K. R., Hardie, A. H., Bollampally, S. R., et al. (2005). Accuracy of computed tomography attenuation values in the characterization of pleural fluid: An ROC study. *Academic Radiology, 12*, 987–991.

Nason, L. K., Walker, C. M., McNeeley, M. F., et al. (2012). Imaging of the diaphragm: Anatomy and function. *Radiographics, 32*, E51–E70.

Nickell, L. T., Lichtenberger, J. P., III, Khorashadi, L., et al. (2014). Multimodality imaging for characterization, classification, and staging of malignant pleural mesothelioma. *Radiographics, 34*, 1692–1706.

Santamarina, M. G., Beddings, I., Holmgren, G. V. L., et al. (2017). Multidetector CT for evaluation of the extrapleural space. *Radiographics, 37*, 1352–1370.

Stark, D. D., Federle, M. P., Goodman, P. C., et al. (1983). Differentiating lung abscess and empyema: Radiography and computed tomography. *AJR. American Journal of Roentgenology, 141*, 163–167.

Takasugi, J. E., Godwin, J. D., & Teefey, S. A. (1991). The extrapleural fat in empyema: CT appearance. *The British Journal of Radiology, 64*, 580–583.

Travis, W. D., Brambilla, E., Burke, A. P., Marx, A., & Nicholson, A. G. (Eds.). (2015). *WHO Classification of Tumours of the Lung, Pleura, Thymus and Heart* (4th ed). Lyon: International Agency for Research on Cancer.

Tyszko, S. M., Marano, G. D., Tallaksen, R. J., & Gyure, K. A. (2007). Malignant mesothelioma. *Radiographics, 27*, 259–264.

Walker, C. M., Takasugi, J. E., Chung, J. H., et al. (2012). Tumorlike conditions of the pleura. *Radiographics, 32*, 971–985.

CHAPTER 8

Introduction to CT of the Abdomen and Pelvis

WILLIAM E. BRANT

Despite marked advances in limiting image times for magnetic resonance imaging, CT remains the primary modality for most indications for imaging the abdomen and pelvis. The technology of multidetector CT (MDCT) scanners continues to advance, with progressive increases in the number of detectors, now exceeding 128 detector rows, and progressive decrease in acquisition times. Concern is now focused on CT radiation dose and overuse as thin-slice rapid scanning during multiple phases of contrast enhancement has rapidly expanded the indications for body CT. Isotropic voxel scanning allows CT data obtained in the axial plane to be reconstructed with the same resolution in any plane. (An isotropic voxel is of the same size in all directions.) Coronal, sagittal, and oblique plane reconstructions have become routine. CT angiography, enterography, and colonography are commonly used.

Evaluation of the abdomen and pelvis by CT requires greater attention to patient preparation, technique, and individualization than CT evaluation of any other area of the body. The best quality studies are produced when the radiologist evaluates the patient clinically, assesses the nature of the imaging problem, and tailors the study to optimize the information that the examination provides.

TECHNICAL CONSIDERATIONS

When a request is presented for an abdomen-pelvis CT scan, the radiologist should assess the clinical problem to be evaluated by reviewing the available patient history and all pertinent available previous imaging studies. Medical history of importance to CT examination includes the current indication for the study, the risk of administering contrast agents, including history of allergic reactions or impaired renal function, the presence of cardiac or other diseases, past abdominal surgical procedures, history of malignancies and radiation therapy, and the findings and availability of previous imaging studies performed elsewhere. Previous imaging studies are reviewed to ensure that all previously identified abnormalities and questionable findings are appropriately reevaluated.

Decisions to be made to individualize the examination include:

- Area scanned: anatomic landmarks and scan extent.
- Radiation dose (tube current, peak tube potential), pitch, scan speed, rotation time specific to the size of the patient. Specific pediatric protocols should be used.
- Beam collimation (detector width and number of detector rows).
- Type and concentration of contrast agent to be administered: intravenous, oral, rectal, or intracavitary.
- Intravenous contrast agent concentration, administration rates, method of administration, and scan timing for arteriography and venography, or for arterial phase, venous phase, and delayed phase enhancement of solid organs and tissues.
- Slice thickness, reconstruction intervals, reconstruction planes, and three-dimensional image reconstructions.

Most institutions have developed standard protocols for a variety of indications, which depend in part on the scanner manufacturer and the number of detector rows. These may be modified as needed to appropriately address the patient problem.

GASTROINTESTINAL CONTRAST AGENTS

Nearly all CT scans of the abdomen require the administration of intraluminal contrast agents to demonstrate the lumen of and to distend the gastrointestinal tract. Radiopaque agents may be dilute concentrations of barium or iodinated contrast agents. Iodinated agent concentrations of 1% to 3% are optimal for intraluminal opacification for CT, as compared with the 30% to 60% solutions used for fluoroscopy. Barium mixtures and water-soluble iodinated agents are equally effective as opaque oral contrast agents.

Air and water are excellent as low-attenuation contrast agents. Carbon dioxide is preferred for instillation into the rectum to insufflate the colon for CT colonography. Effervescent crystals with a small volume of water may be given orally to distend the stomach with gas. Water serves as an excellent low-density contrast agent for the upper gastrointestinal tract. Urine in the distended bladder provides excellent contrast for bladder lesions. Patient preparation may include having the patient avoid urination or clamping an indwelling Foley catheter. Low-attenuation barium-based contrast agents are used for CT enterography.

INTRAVENOUS CONTRAST AGENTS

Intravenous contrast agents improve the quality of abdominal CT by opacifying blood vessels, increasing the CT attenuation of abdominal organs, confirming perfusion, and increasing image contrast between lesions and normal structures. MDCT allows multiphase imaging to demonstrate the passage of contrast agent through the arterial system, organs and tumors, and the venous system. Delayed images show contrast agent excretion by the kidneys, late enhancement, or prolonged retention of intravenous contrast agent in organs and lesions. For most applications, intravenous contrast agents are administered by power injectors that provide accurate control of the rate and volume of administration.

Low-osmolarity "nonionic" iodine-based agents are the intravenous contrast agents of choice for most abdominal scanning because of their lower rate of adverse reactions. Sterile iodinated contrast agents approved for intravenous injection can be injected into indwelling catheters, drainage tubes, sinus tracts, and fistulas to evaluate the extent of disease. For intravenous administration, iodine concentrations of 60% and 75% are most commonly used. Older ionic contrast agents of higher osmolality are no longer used for intravascular injection because of significantly higher rates of adverse reactions. However, these cheaper ionic agents may be used for intracavitary injection, where adverse reactions are rare. For injection into the bladder for CT cystography, or through indwelling catheters for demonstration of fistulas, sinus tracts, or abscess cavities, the contrast agent is usually diluted to an iodine concentration of 2% to 3%.

Although detailed review of adverse reactions and safe use of intravenous contrast agent is beyond the scope of this text, patient safety is always the first priority. Adverse reactions associated with intravenous contrast agent administration include anaphylaxis, cardiac and respiratory arrest, nephrotoxicity, and hives. The reader is referred to the Suggested Reading section for several excellent reviews on safe use of iodinated intravenous contrast agents.

HOW TO INTERPRET CT SCANS OF THE ABDOMEN AND PELVIS

When one is just beginning to learn to interpret body CT scans, it is very useful to develop a checklist to ensure that all structures are inspected and that all key observations are noted to make accurate and comprehensive diagnoses. A system of structured reporting or dictation templates aids in ensuring complete review of all elements of the study.

Because of the dramatic increase in the number of images obtained by MDCT, image viewing is best performed on a computer workstation using the reconstructed digital images obtained directly from the CT scanner. Image display workstations allow rapid scrolling through serial images, the ability to conveniently change window level and window width settings, and the ability to perform rapid image reformatting in multiple anatomic planes and with three-dimensional techniques.

Each CT image of the abdomen contains much more information than can be displayed by any one window width and level setting. Routine "soft-tissue" windows (window width ~400 Hounsfield units [HU]; window level 30–50 HU) define most abdominal anatomy. However, the liver may also be inspected using narrower "liver windows" (window width ~100–150 HU; window level 70–80 HU) to increase image contrast within the liver and improve visibility of subtle lesions. The lung bases are included on scans through the upper abdomen and should be inspected using "lung windows" (window width 1000–2000 HU; window level 600–700 HU). Lung windows are also used to detect free intraperitoneal air and gas collections. Lastly, inspection of the bones using "bone windows" (window width ~2000 HU; window level ~600 HU) may yield important clues to pathologic findings within the abdomen and pelvis (Fig. 8.1).

Each organ and structure should be systematically examined on serial images obtained through all phases of the CT examination. No interpretation will be accurate without consideration of the "phase" of contrast enhancement (arterial, venous, cortical, nephrogram, delayed, etc.).
- Lung bases: nodules, infiltrates, scars, pleural effusions, atelectasis
- Liver: size, homogeneous parenchymal attenuation, uniform enhancement, portal veins, hepatic veins, hepatic arteries, lesions cystic or solid, enhancement of lesions

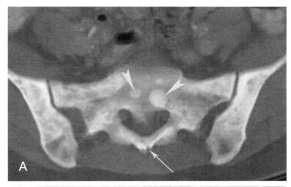

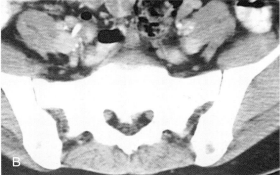

FIG. 8.1 **Bone windows.** Metastatic lesions *(arrowheads)* from prostate carcinoma to the sacrum and iliac bones are obvious on "bone window" (A) but cannot be seen on routine "soft-tissue window" (B). An occult spina bifida defect *(arrow)* is also evident.

- Biliary tree and gallbladder: visible bile ducts, wall thickness, presence and distention of the gallbladder, low density stones, high density stones
- Spleen: size (normal up to 14 cm), inhomogeneous enhancement early, homogeneous enhancement late, splenules, splenic vein, splenic artery
- Adrenals: Y or V shape, limb thickness less than 1 cm, no convex margins
- Pancreas: size and position, head, neck, body, tail, size of the pancreatic duct, patent splenic vein, lucent peri-pancreatic fat
- Kidneys: normal length 9-13 cm in adults, symmetric enhancement, calyces and pelvis and ureter, position and orientation
- Lymph nodes: retroperitoneum, mesentery, omentum, porta hepatis, pelvis
- Blood vessels: aorta, inferior vena cava, celiac axis and branches, superior and inferior mesenteric arteries, renal arteries, renal veins, splenic vein, superior mesenteric vein, portal vein

- Stomach: position, distention, contents, wall thickness, fold thickness
- Duodenum and small bowel: position, distention, wall thickness, surrounding fat, mesentery
- Colon and rectum: position, distention, wall thickness, luminal contents, diverticula
- Uterus and ovaries: size, position, endometrium, follicles, assess appropriateness for the patient's age and phase of the menstrual cycle, uterine and adnexal masses
- Prostate and seminal vesicles: size, contour, definition, calcifications
- Bladder: distension, wall thickness, luminal contents
- Bones: degenerative changes, metastatic disease, mineralization

After diligent use of a checklist, detailed inspection of the images becomes automatic and familiar. Remember that you "see" what you look for and that it is hardest to "see" what is not there: absent gallbladder, ectopic kidney, etc.

ARTIFACTS IN BODY CT
Patient Motion

Patient motion during CT scanning causes anatomic structures to be displaced, distorted, and blurred. Anomalous white bands and dark spots may be displayed on the image as a result of motion during scan acquisition. The rapid scan times of modern MDCT scanners diminishes but does not totally eliminate the effect of cardiac motion, vessel pulsation, and bowel peristalsis. Most patients can hold their breath for the 20 seconds or less required to scan the abdomen. Uncooperative patients may breathe or move during scanning, causing severe artifacts and limiting diagnostic information (Fig. 8.2).

Volume Averaging

By design a CT scanner irradiates a three-dimensional slab of tissue to create a two-dimensional image. All CT images are "volume averaged" in that a finite thickness of patient tissue is summated to create the two-dimensional image (Fig. 8.3). The effect of this technique is to display the summed average of densities within the slice thickness instead of separate individual densities. For example, *volume averaging* of opaque oral contrast agent within the duodenum may create the appearance of a high-density stone in the gallbladder when no stone is present. Volume averaging is diminished, and spatial resolution is increased by use of thin slices. MDCT has the capability to obtain a large number of thin slices over a short period to minimize volume averaging artifacts.

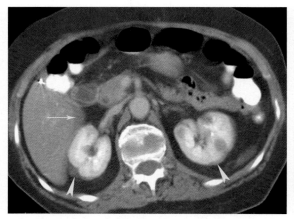

FIG. 8.2 Motion artifact. Patient breathing motion has caused blurring of the margins of both kidneys *(arrowheads)* and the edge of the liver *(arrow)*, simulating subcapsular fluid. The pancreas, bowel, and cysts in the left kidney are also indistinct.

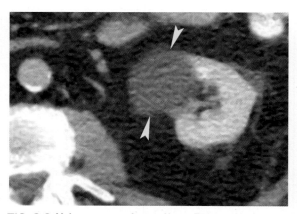

FIG. 8.3 Volume averaging artifact. The margin *(arrowheads)* of the cyst extending from the left kidney is blurred because its contour is rounded, and attenuation of the cyst is averaged with attenuation of the adjacent fat within this 5-mm CT slice.

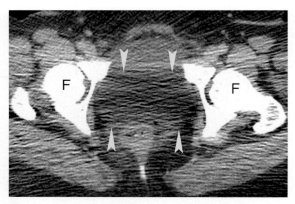

FIG. 8.4 Beam hardening artifact. The alternating light and dark streaks of beam hardening artifact (between *arrowheads*) are prominent on this CT image of the pelvis in an obese patient. The dense bone of the femoral heads *(F)* and acetabuli selectively absorb lower energy X-ray photons, resulting in higher average energy of the transmitted X-ray beam. The artifact is accentuated by the increased absorption of radiation in the "thicker" patient.

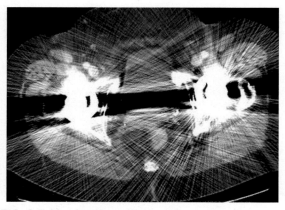

FIG. 8.5 Metal artifact. (A) Bilateral metallic hip prostheses ruin the CT image of the pelvis with dense dark and light bands and streaks.

Beam Hardening

Beam hardening refers to an increase in the mean energy of an X-ray beam when it passes through an object. Low-energy X-ray photons are preferentially absorbed, whereas higher-energy X-ray photons are more likely to pass through the structure. Radiographically dense structures that strongly absorb X-ray photons "harden the beam" and may produce streak artifacts on the CT image. This artifact is most commonly seen in body CT between the dense bones of the hips (Fig. 8.4) and

those of the shoulders. Dense metallic objects such as surgical clips, bullets, and orthopedic hardware produce dramatic beam hardening and prominent streak artifact (Fig. 8.5), which is further accentuated by motion.

Noise: Quantum Mottle

Image reconstruction in CT requires a large amount of data to produce an adequate image. The data are generated by X-ray photons coursing through and being absorbed by the patient, with transmitted photons

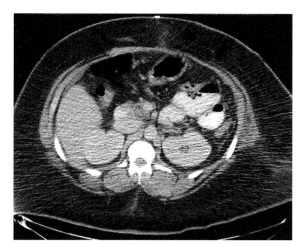

FIG. 8.6 **Quantum mottle artifact.** CT image of the abdomen in an obese patient showing a generalized prominent salt-and-pepper (light and dark dots) appearance of the image. This is called *quantum mottle* or *noise artifact* and is created by a deficiency in the number of photons used to create the image. Low CT technique (low milliamperes), reduced slice thickness, and large size of the patient are factors that increase image noise.

striking CT detectors; the more transmitted photons, the better the data. The smaller the number of X-ray photons that strike the detectors, the more limited are the data. The more absorbed photons, the higher the radiation dose to the patient. The use of MDCT has resulted in valuable multiphase imaging to assess organ and tumor perfusion in arterial, venous, and delayed phases of contrast enhancement. This valuable additional diagnostic information comes at the cost of increased radiation exposure to the patient as the patient is scanned multiple times. Current CT scanners and MDCT scanning protocols are designed to emphasize use of the lowest radiation dose needed to produce an acceptable diagnostic image. This drive to lower radiation dose protocols leads to noisier images. *Quantum mottle* resulting from a low-dose technique with limited numbers of photons producing the image results in a salt-and-pepper grainy appearance of the CT image (Fig. 8.6). With MDCT, choices must be made to find the balance between radiation dose to the patient and acceptable noise in the image. The size of the patient significantly affects the requirement for the radiation exposure needed to produce diagnostic CT images. An obese patient with large axial dimensions requires a far higher radiation dose than a small child. It is essential that CT dose parameters be adjusted to correlate with the size of the patient. Reducing slice thickness to

increase resolution and decrease the volume averaging effect will reduce the number of photons used to create the image and cause increased noise (quantum mottle artifact) in the image. Thinner slices require higher radiation exposure to produce a diagnostic image.

RADIATION DOSE IN CT

The continuing expansion of the indications for CT for diagnostic imaging combined with the popularity and widespread use of MDCT has caused a dramatic increase in radiation exposure to patients. CT now accounts for more than 40% of all radiation exposure to patients from diagnostic imaging. As many as 65 million CT examinations may be performed each year in the United States. Approximately 11% of these examinations are performed on infants and children, who are more susceptible to the adverse effects of radiation. The radiation dose profile for MDCT is 27% higher than for single-detector helical CT. The individual doses to the kidneys, uterus, ovaries, and pelvic bone marrow may be 92% to 180% higher with MDCT than with single-detector helical CT. The dose "penalty" with MDCT increases with decreasing slice thickness and repeated scanning during the different phases of contrast enhancement. These considerations mandate a responsibility for the radiologist and the ordering physician to limit CT to definitive indications, provide dose-efficient CT imaging protocols, offer alternative imaging techniques for young children, who are at the greatest risk from radiation, work with manufacturers to limit the radiation dose, and educate patients and health care providers on the potential risk of low-dose radiation. Guidelines for imaging of the pregnant patient are provided in Suggested Reading.

SUGGESTED READING

American College of Radiology Committee on Drugs and Contrast Media. (2016). *Manual on Contrast Media. Version 10.2.* Reston: American College of Radiology.

Barrett, J. F., & Keat, N. (2004). Artifacts in CT: Recognition and avoidance. *Radiographics, 24,* 1679–1691.

Chintipalli, K. N., Montgomery, R. S., Hatab, M., et al. (2012). Radiation dose management: Part 1, minimizing radiation dose in CT-guided procedures. *AJR. American Journal of Roentgenology, 198,* W352–W356.

Dalrymple, N. C., Prasad, S. R., El-Merhi, F. M., & Chintapalli, K. N. (2007). Price of isotropy in multidetector CT. *Radiographics, 27,* 49–62.

Fält, T., Söderberg, M., Hörberg, L., et al. (2013). Seesaw balancing radiations dose and IV contrast dose: Evaluation of a new abdominal CT protocol for reducing age-specific risk. *AJR. American Journal of Roentgenology, 200,* 383–388.

Goldberg-Stein, S. A., Liu, B., Hahn, P. F., & Lee, S. I. (2012). Radiation dose management: Part 2, estimating fetal radiation risk from CT during pregnancy. *AJR. American Journal of Roentgenology, 198*, W347–W351.

Hendee, W. R., & O'Connor, M. K. O. (2012). Radiation risks of medical imaging: Separating fact from fantasy. *Radiology, 264*, 312–321.

Maldijian, P. D., & Goldman, A. R. (2013). Reducing radiation dose in body CT: A primer on dose metrics and key CT technical parameters. *AJR. American Journal of Roentgenology, 200*, 741–747.

Raman, S. P., Mahesh, M., Blasko, R. V., & Fishman, E. K. (2013). CT scan parameters and radiation dose: Practical advice for radiologists. *Journal of the American College of Radiology, 10*, 840–846.

Tirada, N., Dreizin, D., Khati, N. J., et al. (2015). Imaging pregnant and lactating patients. *Radiographics, 35*, 1751–1765.

CHAPTER 9

Peritoneal Cavity, Vessels, Nodes, and Abdominal Wall

WILLIAM E. BRANT

PERITONEAL CAVITY

Anatomy

The various recesses and spaces of the peritoneal cavity are easiest to recognize on CT when ascites is present. Identifying the precise compartment that an abnormality is in goes a long way toward identifying the nature of the abnormality and deciding on a plan for intervention. The peritoneum is a thin membrane that produces serous fluid, which lubricates the abdominal and pelvic cavity. Parietal peritoneum lines the abdominal wall and covers the retroperitoneum. Visceral peritoneum covers organs and bowel. Whereas all the spaces of the peritoneal cavity potentially communicate with one another, diseases, such as abscesses, tend to loculate within one or more specific locations. The right subphrenic space communicates around the liver with the anterior subhepatic and posterior subhepatic space (Morison pouch). The left subphrenic space communicates freely with the left subhepatic space. The right and left subphrenic spaces are separated by the falciform ligament and do not communicate directly. The lesser sac is the isolated peritoneal compartment between the stomach and the pancreas. It communicates with the rest of the peritoneal cavity (greater sac) through the small opening of the foramen of Winslow.

The right subphrenic and subhepatic spaces communicate freely with the pelvic peritoneal cavity by means of the right paracolic gutter. The phrenicocolic ligament prevents free communication between the left subphrenic/subhepatic spaces and the left paracolic gutter. Free fluid, blood, infection, and peritoneal metastases commonly settle in the pelvis because the pelvis is the most dependent portion of the peritoneal cavity, and the pelvic recesses communicate freely with both sides of the abdomen.

The small bowel mesentery is a double layer of peritoneum that suspends the jejunum and ileum and contains branches of the superior mesenteric artery and vein, as well as mesenteric lymph nodes. The mesentery extends like a fan obliquely across the abdomen from the ligament of Treitz in the left upper quadrant to the region of the right sacroiliac joint. Disease originating from above the ligament is directed toward the right lower quadrant. Disease originating from below the ligament has open access to the pelvis.

The greater omentum is a double layer of peritoneum that hangs from the greater curvature of the stomach and descends in front of the abdominal viscera. The greater omentum encloses fat and a few blood vessels. It serves as fertile ground for implantation of peritoneal metastases.

Fluid in the Peritoneal Cavity

Fluid in the peritoneal cavity originates from many different sources and differs greatly in composition. *Ascites* refers to accumulation of serous fluid within the peritoneal cavity and results from cirrhosis, hypoproteinemia, congestive heart failure, or venous obstruction. Exudative ascites is associated with inflammatory processes such as pancreatitis, peritonitis, and bowel perforation. Neoplastic ascites is caused by intraperitoneal tumor. Chylous ascites is due to obstruction of or traumatic injury to the thoracic duct or cisterna chyli. Urine and bile may spread through the peritoneal cavity owing to obstruction of or injury to the urinary or biliary tracts. *Hemoperitoneum* is an important sign of abdominal injury in blunt trauma. When the anatomy of the peritoneal cavity is known, recognition of fluid density within its recesses on CT is easy. Paracentesis is required for precise differentiation of the exact type of fluid present in the peritoneal cavity. However, CT can offer some clues:

- Free intraperitoneal fluid occupies and distends the recesses of the peritoneal cavity. Bowel loops tend to float to the central abdomen. The diaphragm may be elevated by a large volume of ascites.
- Serous ascites has an attenuation value near that of water (-10 to 15 Hounsfield units [HU]) and tends to accumulate in the greater peritoneal space, sparing the lesser sac.

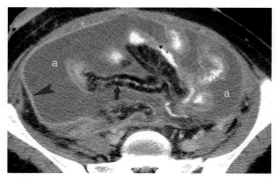

FIG. 9.1 **Peritonitis and ascites.** Ascites *(a)* resulting from pancreatitis occupies and distends peritoneal recesses. Small bowel loops float within the fluid suspended on fat-filled mesentery *(arrow)*. The parietal peritoneum *(arrowhead)* is thickened and is enhanced following intravenous contrast medium administration, indicating peritoneal inflammation.

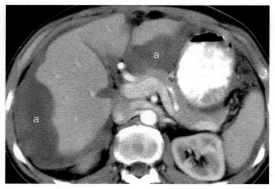

FIG. 9.2 **Pseudomyxoma peritonei.** High-attenuation gelatinous ascites *(a)* is loculated in peritoneal recesses and causes scalloping and mass effect on adjacent organs. The cause was mucinous adenocarcinoma of the stomach metastatic to the peritoneum.

- Hemoperitoneum has a higher attenuation value, averaging 45 HU, and is usually above 30 HU. Blood tends to accumulate in greatest amount about the site of hemorrhage. The presence of higher-attenuation clots in the fluid is a clue to the fluid being blood.
- Exudative ascites due to pancreatitis tends to preferentially accumulate within the lesser sac. Exudative and neoplastic ascites have intermediate attenuation values that overlap those of serous ascites and blood. With peritonitis (Fig. 9.1) the peritoneum appears thickened and enhances following intravenous contrast medium administration.
- Loculations of peritoneal fluid due to benign or malignant adhesions may simulate cystic abdominal masses. Tense loculated ascites may accumulate in confined spaces such as the lesser sac and compress and displace bowel loops. Loculated ascites, however, tends to conform to the general shape of the recesses it occupies. Cystic masses make their own space, cause greater displacement of adjacent structures, and have more varied internal consistency.
- *Pseudomyxoma peritonei* is an unusual complication of mucocele of the appendix or of mucinous cystadenocarcinoma manifested by filling of the peritoneal cavity with gelatinous mucin. The mucinous fluid is typically loculated and causes scalloping and mass effect on the liver and involved bowel (Fig. 9.2). Septations, mottled densities, and calcification within the fluid may be seen on CT. Soft-tissue peritoneal implants are sometimes apparent.

Free Air in the Peritoneal Cavity

Free air within the peritoneal cavity is an important sign of a perforated intestinal tract but may be surprisingly difficult to recognize on CT when the volume of pneumoperitoneum is small:

- The diagnosis is based on recognizing that the air is outside the bowel lumen (Fig. 9.3). Images should be routinely examined at "lung windows" (window level -400 to -600 HU; window width 1000–2000 HU) for free intraperitoneal air. Free intraperitoneal air is easiest to recognize anterior to the liver and in nondependent recesses that do not contain bowel. The very thin wall of distended bowel may be difficult to appreciate. A clue is that the air within bowel appears confined, whereas free intraperitoneal air is not confined. Rolling the patient into a decubitus position and rescanning will assist in interpretation of difficult cases.
- Before pneumoperitoneum is ascribed to bowel perforation, a thoracic source, such as pneumothorax or mechanical ventilation, or an iatrogenic source such as a recent paracentesis or a recent surgical procedure should also be considered.

Peritoneal Carcinomatosis

Diffuse metastatic seeding of the peritoneal cavity occurs commonly with abdominopelvic tumors. The most common tumors to spread by this method are ovarian carcinoma in females and stomach, pancreas, and colon carcinoma in both sexes. The preferential sites for tumor implantation are the pouch of Douglas, the right paracolic gutter, and the greater omentum. CT findings with peritoneal tumor seeding include:

- Ascites is usually present and is commonly loculated.
- Tumor nodules appear as soft-tissue masses on, or thickening of, the parietal peritoneum (Fig. 9.4). Implants and involved peritoneum may show contrast enhancement.

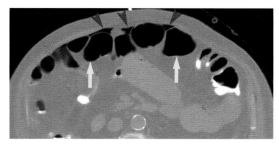

FIG. 9.3 **Pneumoperitoneum.** Small pockets of free intraperitoneal air are recognized on an abdominal CT image viewed on lung windows by the characteristic triangular and linear appearance *(red arrowheads)* between bowel loops in the nondependent areas of the abdomen. Note the more rounded appearance of air within bowel confined by the thin bowel wall *(yellow arrows)*.

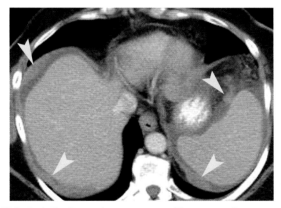

FIG. 9.4 **Peritoneal metastases.** Metastases *(arrowheads)* from ovarian carcinoma to the peritoneum appear as focal areas of peritoneal thickening and nodules.

- The term *omental cake* describes the thickened nodular appearance of tumor involving the greater omentum. The tumor cake displaces bowel away from the anterior abdominal wall (Fig. 9.5).
- Tumor nodules and enlarged lymph nodes may be seen in the mesentery (Fig. 9.6).
- Thickening and nodularity of the bowel wall is due to tumor implantations on the bowel serosa.
- Minute implants, which may be painfully obvious and diffuse at surgery, are commonly missed by CT owing to their small size. The presence of ascites in patients with known abdominopelvic tumor, especially ovarian carcinoma, should be regarded as suspicious for peritoneal seeding, even if distinct tumor nodules are not evident. Calcification of tumor implants may aid in their CT identification. Calcified peritoneal carcinomatosis is most commonly associated with serous adenocarcinoma of the ovary, colon, or stomach.

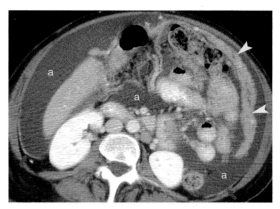

FIG. 9.5 **Omental cake.** Ascites *(a)* is present throughout the peritoneal cavity. The parietal peritoneum *(red arrows)* is thickened and is enhanced following intravenous contrast medium administration, indicating that the ascites is neoplastic or inflammatory. Omental cake *(yellow arrowheads)* manifests itself as a layer of irregular soft tissue that displaces bowel away from the anterior abdominal wall.

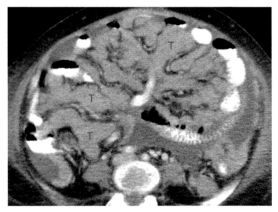

FIG. 9.6 **Mesenteric carcinomatosis.** Tumor nodules *(T)* from intraperitoneal spread of ovarian cancer cause diffuse thickening of the folds of the small bowel mesentery.

- Tuberculous peritonitis mimics peritoneal carcinomatosis and may cause calcification of the peritoneum. Thickening of the peritoneum caused by tuberculous peritonitis is diffusely smooth, whereas that of peritoneal carcinomatosis is irregular and nodular.

Primary Neoplastic Diseases of the Peritoneum and Mesentery

Primary neoplastic diseases of the peritoneum are rare and diverse, with nonspecific imaging characteristics that mimic other lesions, particularly carcinomatosis:

- Although most malignant mesotheliomas originate in the pleura, 20% to 40% of mesotheliomas arise

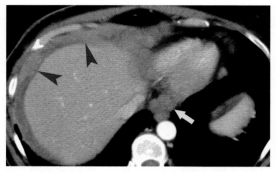

FIG. 9.7 Peritoneal mesothelioma. Tumor nodules *(red arrowheads)* on peritoneal surfaces are apparent. The appearance is indistinguishable from peritoneal carcinomatosis, but biopsy confirmed peritoneal mesothelioma. Adenopathy *(yellow arrow)* is seen adjacent to the esophagus.

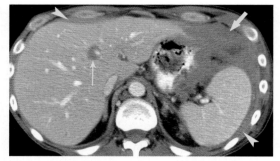

FIG. 9.8 Peritoneal lymphoma. Postcontrast CT revels homogeneous soft-tissue thickening of peritoneal surfaces *(arrowheads)* and soft-tissue mass infiltrating the perigastric and perisplenic areas *(fat arrow)*. A focus of lymphoma is also present in the liver *(skinny arrow)*.

within the abdomen. Mesothelioma is a rare tumor with a rapidly fatal course. Asbestos exposure is a significant risk factor. CT shows an enhanced solid tumor in the mesentery, in omentum, or on peritoneal surfaces (Fig. 9.7). It may cause diffuse irregular thickening of the peritoneum, multiple small nodules, or a focal peritoneal mass. Ascites is present in most cases.

- Multilocular mesothelioma appears as a large (>10 cm) multicystic mass with enhancing septa. The lesion mimics metastatic cystadenoma of the ovary. The clinical course is benign or indolent.
- Desmoplastic small round cell tumor is an aggressive malignancy that mimics Wilms tumor. It occurs most commonly in patients aged 15 to 25 years. CT shows diffuse intra-abdominal soft-tissue masses with peritoneal thickening.
- Primary serous carcinoma of the peritoneum is an extraovarian malignancy that occurs in postmenopausal women. CT shows diffuse peritoneal tumor and marked ascites with absence of an ovarian mass. Calcification of the tumor nodules is common (30%).
- Lymphoma may be primary to the peritoneum or secondary to widespread disease. Primary peritoneal lymphoma occurs nearly always in immune compromised patients. CT (Fig. 9.8) reveals diffuse thickening of the peritoneum, multiple peritoneal nodules, ascites, and often extensive adenopathy.

Abscess

CT is commonly performed to search for and plan percutaneous or surgical drainage of suspected abdominal and pelvic abscesses. Once an abdominal or pelvic abscess has been found, percutaneous aspiration confirms the diagnosis and provides material for culture. Image-directed catheter placement is commonly used for drainage ("pus busting"). Most abscesses occur as complications of abdominal trauma, surgery, pancreatitis, or bowel perforation (ruptured appendicitis, diverticulitis). Intraperitoneal abscesses are commonly located in the pelvic cavity and the subphrenic and subhepatic spaces. CT features of abscess include:

- Most abscesses appear as loculated fluid collections displacing bowel and adjacent organs. Internal debris, fluid-fluid levels, septations, sometimes air-fluid levels, or bubbles of air (Fig. 9.9) are often present within the collection.
- Definable walls with irregular thickening are usually identifiable.
- Nearby fascia is thickened, and fat planes are infiltrated or obliterated because of inflammation.
- Ascites, pleural effusions, and lower lobe pulmonary infiltrates commonly accompany abdominal abscesses.
- Any fluid collection within the abdomen is suspect in patients in whom infection or abscess is suggested clinically. Fine-needle aspiration is a safe and definitive way to exclude or confirm the diagnosis.

Cystic Abdominal and Pelvic Masses

Cystic masses in the abdomen and pelvis commonly present challenges in diagnosis. Differential considerations include:

- Abscess—evidence of loculation, air bubbles, air-fluid levels.
- Loculated ascites—displaces organs and tissues.
- Pancreatic pseudocyst (see Chapter 13).

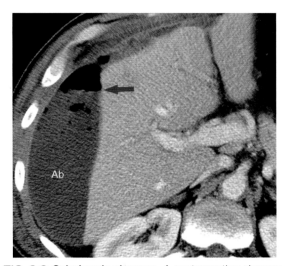

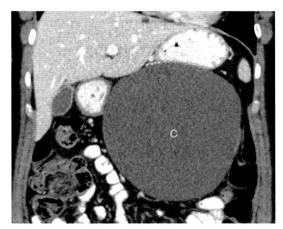

FIG. 9.9 **Subphrenic abscess.** A postoperation abscess *(Ab)* is seen as a fluid collection between the diaphragm and the liver. Mass impression on the liver is evidence of fluid loculation. An air-fluid level *(arrow)* is evidently caused by gas-producing *Escherichia coli*. This abscess was successfully treated by CT-guided percutaneous catheter drainage.

FIG. 9.10 **Cystic lymphangioma.** Coronal CT image showing a well-defined cystic mass *(C)* that is centered in the mesentery and displaces loops of small bowel without causing bowel obstruction. Pathology following surgical removal revealed a mesenteric cystic lymphangioma. Note the uniform low attenuation and imperceptibly thin wall.

- Ovarian/paraovarian cyst/cystic tumor (see Chapter 18).
- Lymphocele—a cystic mass containing lymphatic fluid that occurs as a complication of surgery or trauma that disrupts lymphatic channels. It may be of any size and appears days to years after surgery.
- Cystic lymphangioma—a congenital counterpart of lymphocele believed to arise from congenital obstruction of lymphatic channels (Fig. 9.10). Most are thin walled and may be unilocular or multilocular. Attenuation ranges from water to fat density. *Mesenteric cysts* are cystic lymphangiomas of the mesentery. *Omental cysts* are less common cystic lymphangiomas of the greater omentum.
- Enteric duplication cysts are a congenital focal cystic malformation of the gastrointestinal tract lined with gastrointestinal mucosa. They are usually attached to normal bowel and occur along the mesenteric border. On CT they appear as round or oval fluid-filled masses with a mildly enhanced wall. Often asymptomatic, reported complications include bowel obstruction, volvulus, perforation, and intussusception.
- Cystic teratoma may arise in the retroperitoneum, mesentery, or omentum. CT shows a complex cystic and solid mass with areas of water and fat attenuation and calcifications.

- Peritoneal inclusion cyst (see Chapter 18).
- Spinal meningeal cyst (see Chapter 18).

VESSELS
Anatomy

The abdominal aorta descends anterior to the left side of the spine to its bifurcation at the level of the iliac crest. The normal aorta does not exceed 3 cm in diameter and tapers progressively as it proceeds to its bifurcation. The inferior vena cava (IVC) lies to the right of the aorta. On axial imaging its shape ranges from round to oval to slit-like depending on the breath-holding technique and intravascular fluid balance. The common iliac arteries and veins appear oval in cross section as they diverge from the midline. The common iliac vessels bifurcate at the pelvic brim, which one identifies by noting the shape of the sacrum change from convex anteriorly (the sacral promontory) to concave. The external iliac vessels course anteriorly to the inguinal triangle, whereas the internal iliac (hypogastric) vessels have many small branches in the posterior pelvis. The iliac arteries normally do not exceed 1.5 cm in diameter.

The celiac axis originates from the anterior aspect of the aorta at the level of the aortic hiatus in the diaphragm. The superior mesenteric artery originates anteriorly from the aorta 1 cm below the celiac axis. The renal arteries arise from the lateral aspect of the aorta within 1 cm of the superior mesenteric artery. The inferior mesenteric artery is a tiny anterior branch off the aorta just above the bifurcation.

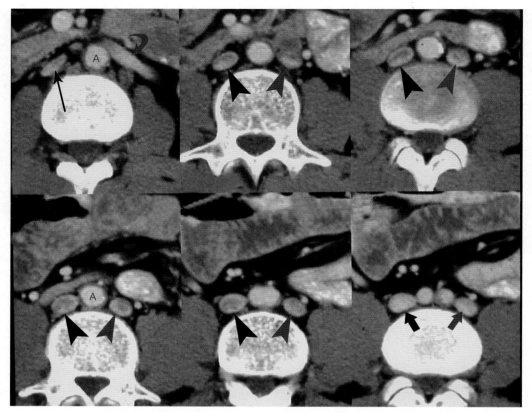

FIG. 9.11 Duplication of the inferior vena cava. Sequential CT images show the persistent left inferior vena cava (IVC) *(red arrowheads)* extends as the continuation of the left common iliac vein *(fat red arrow)* along the left side of the aorta *(A)* to end in the left renal vein *(curved arrow)*, which drains into the normal right suprarenal IVC *(skinny black arrow)*. The normal right IVC *(black arrowheads)* extends from the right common iliac vein *(fat black arrow)* to follow its normal course through the liver. Blood flow from the left IVC flows into the right IVC via the left renal vein.

Anatomic Variations

A number of vascular anomalies must be recognized to avoid misinterpretation as abnormalities:

- *Duplication of the IVC* (Fig. 9.11) may be identified as a persistent left IVC extending between the left common iliac vein and the left renal vein on the left side of the aorta. The enlarged left renal vein drains into the normal suprarenal IVC on the right. The right common iliac vein continues as the right IVC until it is joined by the left renal vein carrying blood from the left leg.
- The *left IVC* results from persistence of the left supracardinal vein with regression of the right supracardinal vein. The left IVC is formed by confluence of the common iliac veins, ascends to the left of the aorta, and joins the left renal vein, which drains into the normal suprarenal IVC on the right.

- Left renal veins may course posterior instead of anterior to the aorta (*retroaortic left renal vein*) (Fig. 9.12), or duplicated left renal veins may course both anterior and posterior to the aorta (circumaortic left renal veins).
- The intrahepatic segment of the IVC may be absent, with drainage continuing to the superior vena cava by means of the azygos system (*azygous continuation of the IVC*).

Technical Considerations

Thin-section multidetector CT combined with three-dimensional reconstruction techniques has made CT angiography (CTA) a useful diagnostic and surgical planning tool. Compared with conventional catheter angiography, CTA is less invasive, less costly, can be performed more quickly, and is capable of demonstrating

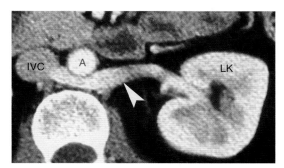

FIG. 9.12 **Retroaortic left renal vein.** The left renal vein *(arrowhead)* courses posterior instead of anterior to the aorta *(A)* to join the inferior vena cava *(IVC)*. *LK,* Left kidney.

important nonvascular abnormalities that would be missed by conventional angiography.

CT venography of the lower limbs may be combined with CTA of the pulmonary arteries to allow complete evaluation of the patient for venopulmonary thromboembolism. CT venography has reported sensitivity of 89% to 100%, with specificity of 94% to 100% for venous thrombosis. Optimal venous enhancement of the lower limbs is obtained at 3.5 minutes following onset of intravenous contrast medium injection into the upper extremity. Images are viewed at 1.75 to 2.5-mm slice thickness. Three-dimensional reconstructions provide the big picture.

Abdominal Aortic Aneurysm

Aneurysms are defined as circumscribed dilatations of an artery. A true aneurysm involves all three layers of the arterial wall (intima, media, and adventitia). Most are due to atherosclerotic disease that weakens the vessel wall and allows the lumen to dilate as a result of high intra-aortic blood pressure. Risk factors for abdominal aortic aneurysms (AAAs) include age more than 60 years, smoking, hypertension, and Caucasian ethnicity.

- Fusiform, saccular, or spherical dilatation of the aorta is the key finding (Fig. 9.13) of AAA. Care must be taken to avoid overestimation of aortic size because the vessel is tortuous and imaged obliquely.
- Outer-to-outer diameter of the abdominal aorta greater than 3 cm is evidence of AAA. Risk of rupture depends largely on the size of the aneurysm. The risk is about 3% to 15% per year for a 5- to 6-cm AAA, 10% to 20% per year for a 6- to 7-cm AAA, 20% to 40% per year for a 7- to 8-cm AAA, and 30% to 50% per year for AAAs with diameter larger than 8 cm. Risk of rupture is also affected by the rate of aneurysm expansion, continued smoking, and persisting hypertension.
- Failure of the aorta to taper distally as it gives off branches is another sign of aneurysm (Fig. 9.14).

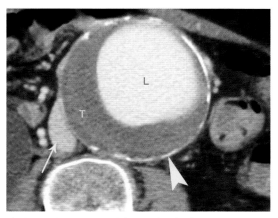

FIG. 9.13 **Aneurysm of the abdominal aorta.** A large aortic aneurysm is evident. The aorta exceeds 5 cm in diameter. A large amount of thrombus *(T)* partially surrounds the patent, contrast-enhanced lumen *(L)*. Note the atherosclerotic calcification *(arrowhead)* in the wall of the aneurysm. The inferior vena cava *(arrow)* is compressed by the large aneurysm.

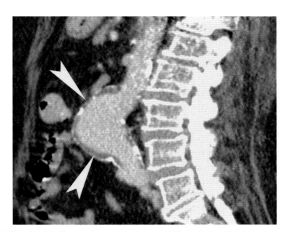

FIG. 9.14 **Saccular aneurysm of the abdominal aorta.** Sagittal reconstructed image showing focal saccular dilatation *(arrowheads)* of the abdominal aorta. Note the atherosclerotic calcifications throughout the aorta of this 81-year-old woman.

Distal dilatation is evidence of aneurysm even if the diameter is less than 3 cm.
- Iliac artery aneurysms are defined by vessel diameter greater than 1.5 cm (Fig. 9.15).
- The patent lumen enhances with intravenous contrast medium. Thrombus within the aneurysm remains low attenuation. Atherosclerotic plaques may be of low attenuation or may be calcified.

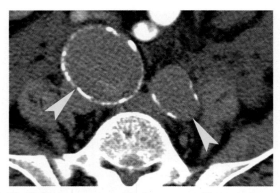

FIG. 9.15 Aneurysms of both common iliac arteries. CT without intravenous contrast medium reveals bilateral aneurysms of the iliac arteries *(arrowheads)* measuring 4 cm on the right and 2.5 cm on the left.

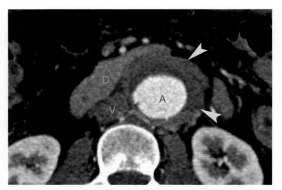

FIG. 9.16 Inflammatory abdominal aortic aneurysm. Axial image from a CT angiogram showing an enhanced dilated lumen of the infrarenal abdominal aorta *(A)* surrounded by a thick cuff of soft tissue *(arrowheads)*. The transverse duodenum *(D)* and inferior vena cava *(V)* are closely applied to the inflammatory tissue.

- Calcification is commonly present in the wall of the aneurysm as well as in atherosclerotic plaques lining the aorta. Occasionally long-standing intraluminal thrombus may also calcify.
- The proximal extent of the AAA must be defined for treatment planning. Most (90%) are begin below the origin of the renal arteries (infrarenal AAA). An origin above the renal arteries (suprarenal AAA) must be identified because more complicated surgical repair is required.
- *Inflammatory AAA* accounts for 5% to 10% of AAAs and differs from atherosclerotic AAA in several important ways. Both types primarily affect the infrarenal abdominal aorta; however, patients with inflammatory AAA are typically younger males and are usually symptomatic with back pain or abdominal pain. CT shows a characteristic rind of soft-tissue inflammation surrounding the aneurysm (Fig. 9.16). The inflammatory tissue may be enhanced. The wall of the aneurysm is thickened with fibrosis extending to and binding adjacent tissues to the aneurysm. The inflammatory tissue may envelop and obstruct the ureters, causing renal failure. The cause is unknown but is believed to be related to immune reaction in the vessel wall. Erythrocyte sedimentation rate is elevated. Typically only the abdominal aorta is involved, without inflammation of other arteries. The risk of rupture is less than for atherosclerotic AAA.

Rupture of an Abdominal Aortic Aneurysm

Acute rupture of an AAA is highly lethal (mortality reported as 77%–94%). The classic presentation is acute severe abdominal pain, hypotension, and pulsatile abdominal mass. Because ruptured AAAs are commonly confused clinically with other diseases,

CT is used to confirm the diagnosis. Unenhanced CT is adequate to demonstrate characteristic findings of a ruptured AAA. Rapid intervention is needed.
- An AAA, usually large, is evident.
- Adjacent periaortic hemorrhage dissects tissue planes of the pararenal and perirenal retroperitoneum (Fig. 9.17) resulting in a retroperitoneal hematoma adjacent to the AAA.
- The draped aorta sign refers to absence of visualization of the posterior wall of an AAA. The wall is indistinct and follows the contour of the adjacent vertebral bodies.
- Active arterial bleeding may be demonstrated with intravenous contrast medium administration. Streaks and puddles of contrast medium are seen outside the aorta within the retroperitoneal hematoma.
- Iliac artery aneurysms, especially those larger than 3.5 cm, may also be the site of rupture producing similar findings.

Signs of Impending Rupture of an Abdominal Aortic Aneurysm

Early diagnosis of the signs that indicate impending rupture of an AAA can be lifesaving. The following is evidence of impending rupture; however, no imaging findings may be present in an AAA about to rupture:
- Acute abdominal pain may indicate impending rupture of an AAA.
- A rapid rate of enlargement correlates with increasing risk of rupture. The risk of rupture doubles with every 5-mm increase in diameter. An aneurysm growth rate exceeding 1 cm per year justifies elective repair.

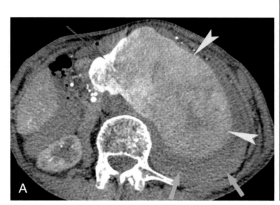 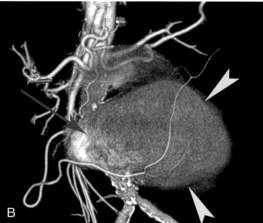

FIG. 9.17 **Rupture of aortic aneurysm.** (A) Axial postcontrast CT demonstrates prominent high-attenuation active retroperitoneal hemorrhage *(yellow arrowheads)* extending into a lower-attenuation thrombus *(green arrows)*. Note the disruption *(red arrow)* of the wall of the aortic aneurysm. (B) Three-dimensional maximum intensity projection reconstruction showing the active hemorrhage *(yellow arrowheads)* extending into a retroperitoneal thrombus from the rent *(red arrow)* in the aneurysm.

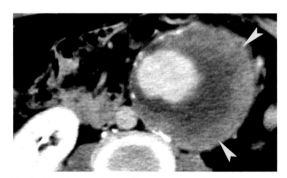

FIG. 9.18 **Hyperattenuating crescent sign.** Routine follow-up CT of an abdominal aortic aneurysm documented a rapid increase in size. The crescent of increased density *(arrowheads)* in the periphery of the aneurysm is highly indicative of impending rupture.

- The *hyperattenuating crescent sign* refers to a crescent-shaped area of high attenuation within the wall or within the intraluminal thrombus of an AAA (Fig. 9.18). The sign is indicative of impending rupture of an AAA. It is caused by acute blood dissecting into the intraluminal thrombus and dissecting to the weak outer wall of the aneurysm. Progressive damage of the wall leads to rupture. This sign is 77% sensitive and 93% specific for impending rupture.
- Focal discontinuity of intimal calcifications can indicate an impending rupture site.
- Focal bulging of the wall of an aneurysm (an aortic *bleb*) may indicate impending rupture.

- Enhanced infiltrating blood within the intraluminal thrombus indicates fissuring of the thrombus and weakening of the wall of the aneurysm.

Infected Aneurysms

Infected aneurysms are rare, difficult to suspect clinically, and highly prone to rupture (53%–75% incidence). Infected aneurysms are also called *mycotic aneurysms*; however, this term applies to all infected aneurysms, not just fungal infections. Most infected aneurysms occur as a result of bacterial infection of the intima in a normal arterial wall or in a preexisting aneurysm, commonly in association with bacterial endocarditis. *Salmonella* is the most common causative organism. Urgent surgical repair is needed.

- The aneurysm is saccular in shape with a lobulated contour in nearly all cases (Fig. 9.19). It may be found anywhere in the aorta or branch arteries. Gas is occasionally present in the soft tissues. The aneurysm may enlarge rapidly over a short period.
- Periarterial soft-tissue stranding and fluid is commonly present.
- Findings of osteomyelitis may be seen in the vertebral body adjacent to an infected AAA.

Aortic Dissection

Dissection of blood into the media through a tear in the intima results in a dilated segment of artery with two lumina. Branch vessels may be occluded by the process or may be fed by the new (false) lumen or the original (true) lumen. Most dissections begin in the thoracic aorta but commonly extend into the abdominal aorta.

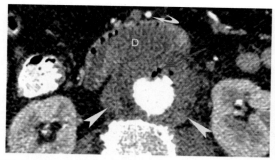

FIG. 9.19 **Mycotic aneurysm.** This mycotic aneurysm *(arrowheads)* contains bubbles of gas *(red arrow)* and threatens rupture into the third portion of the duodenum *(D)*. The *curved arrow* indicates the contrast-enhanced superior mesenteric artery anterior to the retroperitoneal duodenum.

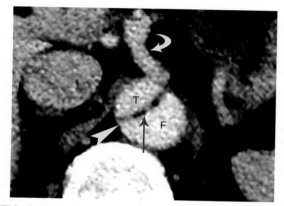

FIG. 9.20 **Aortic dissection.** A dissection of the thoracic aorta extends into the abdominal aorta. The intimal flap *(red arrow)* is readily apparent within the enhancing aorta. The true lumen *(T)* supplies the celiac axis *(curved arrow)*. The false lumen *(F)* is identified by the "beak sign" *(arrowhead)*.

- The key finding is an intimal flap separating the true and false lumens (Fig. 9.20).
- Thrombosis of the false lumen may preclude visualization of the intimal flap.
- Differentiation of the true and false lumens is important in treatment planning. The false lumen is usually larger and commonly contains a thrombus. Thrombus is generally not seen in the true lumen. The junction of the flap with the outer wall of the false lumen produces an acute angle, called the *beak sign*. Intimal calcifications may be seen on the intimal flap and in the wall of the true lumen.
- Intimal plaque calcification is internally displaced.
- The true lumen may be compressed by expanding hematoma in the false lumen.

- Branch vessels may be compressed or occluded, resulting in ischemia or infarction of supplied organs.
- *Intramural hematoma* refers to aortic dissection without rupture of the intima. The hematoma results from hemorrhage of the vasa vasorum into the aortic wall, weakening the media but without tearing of the intima. Noncontrast CT shows high-attenuation blood within the wall of the aorta (Fig. 9.21). Intimal calcifications are displaced toward the aortic lumen. The luminal surface is smooth compared with the irregular surface of the more common intraluminal thrombus. Intramural hematomas may resolve or progress to aortic dissection.
- *Penetrating atherosclerotic ulcer* is an atherosclerotic lesion with ulceration that is a precursor to intramural hemorrhage. CT shows a focal ulcer extending into a subintimal hematoma (Fig. 9.22). Treatment is controversial but may involve resection and replacement of the aortic wall with a surgical graft or endoluminal stenting of the affected section of the aorta.
- *Acute aortic syndrome* refers to a clinical presentation of acute intense chest or abdominal pain typically described as ripping, pulsating, or tearing. Pathologic causes include acute aortic dissection, aortic intramural hematoma, and penetrating atherosclerotic ulcer. Each condition is life-threatening with high mortality when it presents as acute aortic syndrome.

Retroperitoneal Fibrosis

Retroperitoneal fibrosis describes a range of diseases characterized by proliferation of collagen-rich inflammatory tissue that surrounds the infrarenal abdominal aorta, IVC, and iliac vessels frequently encasing and obstructing the ureters. Two-thirds of cases are idiopathic. Known causes include drugs (ergot alkaloids), neoplasms (lymphoma, metastases, sarcoma), retroperitoneal hemorrhages (leaking AAA), and infections (tuberculosis, fungus).

- CT shows a well-defined but irregularly shaped soft-tissue periaortic mass extending from the renal arteries to the iliac vessels. The mass partially surrounds the anterior and lateral aspect of the aorta, characteristically sparing the posterior aspect of the aorta (Fig. 9.23). The aorta is not displaced.
- Encasement of the ureters causes obstruction and hydronephrosis, often presenting with renal failure.
- Noncontrast attenuation of the mass is similar to that of muscle. Avid enhancement characterizes early-stage disease, whereas little or no enhancement is present in late, inactive disease.
- Additional findings may include deep vein thrombosis, focal lymphadenopathy, and involvement of the renal vessels.

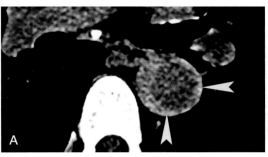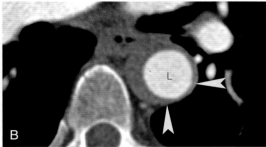

FIG. 9.21 Intramural hematoma. (A) Noncontrast CT demonstrates high-attenuation hemorrhage *(arrowheads)* in the wall of the descending thoracic aorta indicative of intramural hematoma. The unopacified patent lumen *(L)* of the aorta is low in attenuation compared with the hematoma. (B) Postcontrast CT with the patent lumen *(L)* now very high in attenuation, obscuring the high attenuation of acute intramural hematoma *(arrowheads)*, which appears as a bland thrombus.

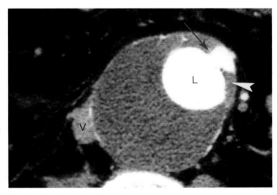

FIG. 9.22 Penetrating atherosclerotic ulcer. Contrast-enhanced CT reveals a focal contrast-defined ulceration *(red arrow)* within a high-attenuation intramural thrombus *(yellow arrowhead)* within a large aortic aneurysm. The ulcer communicates with the contrast-enhanced lumen *(L)* of the aortic aneurysm. A large volume of intraluminal thrombus *(T)* is also present. The inferior vena cava *(V)* is displaced by the large aneurysm.

Deep Vein Thrombosis

Venous thrombi may be bland, septic, or associated with tumor invasion.

- Thrombus appears as a low-attenuation mass within the vein causing complete or partial obstruction (Fig. 9.24). Dilatation of the vein at the site of thrombosis is evidence that the process is acute.
- Upstream veins may be dilated compared with veins of the contralateral side, and soft tissues may show streaks and strands of edema (thrombophlebitis).
- The wall of the affected vein may show contrast enhancement provided by the vasa vasorum.
- Chronic thrombosis appears as an irregular intraluminal clot that may calcify. The wall of the affected

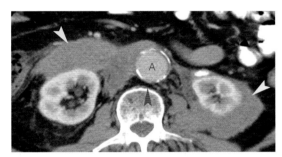

FIG. 9.23 Retroperitoneal fibrosis. On this contrast-enhanced CT image a band *(yellow arrowheads)* of soft-tissue attenuation surrounds the left kidney and partially envelops the aorta *(A)* and the right kidney. The inferior vena cava is compressed and not visible. Note the characteristic sparing of the posterior aspect of the aorta *(red arrowhead)* by the process of retroperitoneal fibrosis.

vein is commonly thickened. The diameter of the lumen may be normal or reduced.

- Flow artifacts and layering of contrast medium may mimic thrombosis. Confirmation with venous compression and Doppler ultrasound imaging may be needed in questionable cases.
- Extrinsic displacement and compression may also be difficult to differentiate from thrombosis. The tumors most likely to extend into the IVC as tumor thrombus are renal, hepatic, and adrenal carcinomas.

NODES
Anatomy

Normal lymph nodes are oblong and homogeneous in CT attenuation. Most are oriented parallel to their accompanying vessels. Abdominoaortic nodal groups surround the aorta and IVC and are commonly involved in abdominal and pelvic malignancy.

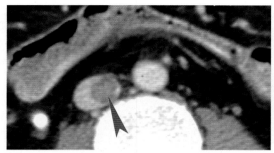

FIG. 9.24 Thrombosis in the inferior vena cava.
Thrombus appears as a low-attenuation filling defect
(arrowhead) in the contrast-enhanced inferior vena cava.
Care must be taken to inspect serial images to ensure this
is really thrombus as flow of opacified blood from the lower
extremities may cause lucencies in the opacified inferior
vena cava.

Visceral nodes drain adjacent organs and include mesenteric, hepatic, splenic, and pancreaticoduodenal
nodal groups.

Nodal Metastases

Lymph node metastases are associated with poor
prognosis of many abdominal malignancies. Size
is the major CT criterion for diagnosis of abnormal
lymph nodes. Nodes are considered to be pathologically enlarged when they exceed 10 mm in short axis
in the abdomen or pelvis or 6 mm in the retrocrural
and porta hepatis region. Multiple 8- to 10-mm nodes
in the abdomen or pelvis are considered suspicious.
Benign lymph nodes are usually oval, whereas malignant lymph nodes tend to be spherical. Interpretation
must always be made in clinical context. Even minimally enlarged nodes should be viewed with suspicion
when they are present in an area where a known malignancy is highly likely to metastasize.

Unfortunately, involvement of nodes with metastatic tumor does not usually change the CT attenuation of the node and, in some cases, will not enlarge
the node sufficiently to be interpreted as pathologic by
size criteria. Nodes may be enlarged because of benign
disease (false-positive interpretation) or be of normal
size and yet be involved (false-negative interpretation).

- Fat density within a lymph node is usually a sign of
  benignity.
- Calcification of a lymph node usually represents
  granulomatous disease; however, treated lymphoma
  and germ cell tumors as well as some calcifying tumors may also show nodal calcification
- Large nodes that are internally heterogeneous represent necrosis that is usually associated with malignancy.

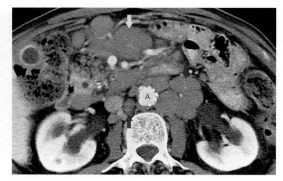

FIG. 9.25 Lymphoma. Enlarged lymph nodes *(red arrows)* surround the aorta *(A)* and inferior vena cava *(V)* and
are seen in the small bowel mesentery *(yellow arrow)*.

- Cystic change within a lymph node usually represents malignancy, especially with nonseminomatous germ cell tumors.
- Heterogeneous contrast enhancement of a lymph
  node is a sign of malignant involvement.

Lymphoma

Lymphomas account for 5% to 6% of all malignancies. More than 50 types of lymphomas are recognized
by the World Health Organization in a classification
system that is periodically revised. Lymphomas typically enlarge involved lymph nodes and may spread
to involve any organ. CT features of lymphoma in the
abdomen and pelvis include:

- Enlargement of isolated lymph nodes, a regional
  group of lymph nodes, multiple isolated groups of
  lymph nodes, or nearly all lymph nodes.
- Multiple enlarged individual nodes (>10 mm in
  short axis), typically of homogeneous attenuation.
- Increased number of small lymph nodes.
- Coalescence of enlarged nodes to form rounded
  multilobular nodal masses that may encase vessels,
  displace organs, and obstruct ureters (Fig. 9.25).
- Conglomerate nodal masses that are typical of lymphoma and are rarely seen with metastatic disease
  or other conditions.
- Calcifications of lymphomatous nodes that usually
  occurs only after treatment.

Signs of extranodal spread of lymphoma to solid organs of the abdomen include diffuse increased organ
size, multiple hypodense nodules, multiple enhancing
masses, solitary intraparenchymal mass, organ invasion
from external nodal mass, circumferential encasement
of organs, and diffuse nodular wall thickening in the
gastrointestinal tract. Positron emission tomography
CT provides improved lymphoma staging accuracy
compared with CT alone.

Acquired Immunodeficiency Syndrome

Medications have dramatically slowed the progression of acquired immunodeficiency syndrome (AIDS). However, manifestations of AIDS on CT remain dominated by signs of intra-abdominal opportunistic infections, AIDS-related lymphoma, and Kaposi sarcoma. Most CT findings are a manifestation of a complicating disease rather than human immunodeficiency virus (HIV) infection alone. The most common findings on CT include the following.

- Lymphadenopathy involving the retroperitoneal, pelvic, and mesenteric nodes is caused by disseminated *Mycobacterium avium-intracellulare* infection (30%), AIDS-related lymphoma (30%), Kaposi sarcoma, or other infection. Lymph node enlargement is unlikely to be due to HIV infection alone. Unexplained adenopathy warrants biopsy.
- Hepatosplenomegaly without focal lesions may result from *M. avium-intracellulare* infection, histoplasmosis, and hepatocellular disease.
- Focal small (<1 cm) low-attenuation lesions in the liver are usually due to *Mycobacterium tuberculosis*, AIDS-related lymphoma, Kaposi sarcoma, or histoplasmosis.
- Focal small (<1 cm) low-attenuation lesions in the spleen are caused by *M. tuberculosis*, *M. avium-intracellulare*, coccidiomycosis, candidiasis, bacillary peliosis, Kaposi sarcoma, AIDS-related lymphoma, and *Pneumocystis carinii* infection.
- Focal bowel wall thickening or focal bowel mass is nearly always caused by AIDS-related lymphoma.
- Calcifications in spleen, lymph nodes, and liver usually result from *P. carinii* infection.
- Nephromegaly with striated nephrogram after contrast medium administration is a sign of HIV nephropathy.
- *Mycobacterial infections* cause lymph node enlargement, small low-density lesions in solid organs, hepatosplenomegaly, and bowel wall thickening.
- *P. carinii* infections cause punctate or nodular calcifications in solid organs and lymph nodes and low-attenuation lesions in the spleen.
- *Kaposi sarcoma* causes adenopathy and hepatosplenomegaly. Less common findings include focal bowel wall thickening, low-density nodules in the liver, and intrahepatic low-density bands in the periportal region.
- *AIDS-related lymphoma* must be suspected for any solid mass anywhere in the abdomen. Additional findings include multiple sites of adenopathy, bowel involvement with wall thickening and focal masses, and focal masses in the spleen, liver, and kidney.

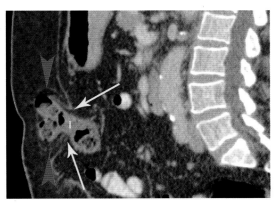

FIG. 9.26 **Incisional hernia.** Sagittal plane reconstruction shows a loop of small intestine (*l*) herniating through a defect (*yellow arrows*) in the anterior abdominal wall at the site of a previous surgical incision. The hernia sac is seen as a thin membrane (*red arrowheads*).

ABDOMINAL WALL

Anatomy

CT is an excellent imaging technique for evaluation of abnormalities of the abdominal wall. The muscles of the abdominal wall are outlined by subcutaneous and extraperitoneal fat. The rectus abdominis muscles are anterior within the rectus sheath. The flanks are defined by three muscle layers formed by the external and internal oblique and transversus abdominis muscles. The posterior muscles are the latissimus dorsi, the quadratus lumborum, and the paraspinal muscles.

Abdominal Wall Hernia

Obesity makes hernias of the abdominal wall difficult to diagnose clinically. Hernias may cause intermittent pain or bowel obstruction. Hernia sacs contain fat, which is usually omentum, and may contain bowel and occasionally ascites. Complications include bowel obstruction, incarceration, strangulation, traumatic injury, and hernia recurrence after surgical repair.

- *Incisional hernias* are common ventral hernias with protrusion of abdominal contents through the abdominal wall weakened by a surgical incision (Fig. 9.26). They commonly occur near a stoma.
- *Inguinal hernias* are classified as indirect or direct. Indirect hernias are congenital lesions seen to protrude anterior to the spermatic cord (males) or round ligament (females) and lateral to the inferior epigastric vessels (Fig. 9.27). Direct inguinal hernias are always acquired and are seen to arise medial to the inferior epigastric vessels. Hernia contents may protrude into the scrotum or labia majora.

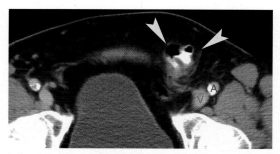

FIG. 9.27 **Inguinal hernia.** Bowel *(arrowheads)* protrudes through the left internal inguinal ring and into the inguinal canal. The left femoral vein *(V)* and left femoral artery *(A)* serve as anatomic landmarks. Both femoral arteries have calcified atherosclerotic plaques.

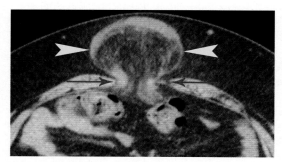

FIG. 9.28 **Paraumbilical hernia.** CT of a very obese woman reveals a large paraumbilical hernia *(yellow arrowheads)* containing fat density greater omentum. The defect *(red arrows)* in the anterior abdominal wall near the umbilicus is apparent.

- *Umbilical hernias* are the most common ventral hernia. The hernia protrudes through the umbilicus.
- *Paraumbilical hernias* protrude through the linea alba above or below the umbilicus (Fig. 9.28).
- *Spigelian hernias* are uncommon but carry a high risk of bowel incarceration and strangulation. They protrude through a defect in the spigelian aponeurosis between the linea semilunaris and the lateral edge of the rectus abdominis (Fig. 9.29). They are difficult to recognize clinically, often requiring imaging diagnosis by CT or other modalities.
- *Lumbar hernias* occur through defects in the posterior fascia or lumbar muscles below the 12th rib and above the iliac crest. The hernia sac may contain retroperitoneal fat, bowel loops, a kidney, or another organ.
- *Richter hernias* involve only a portion of the antimesenteric wall of the bowel in the hernia sac. The entire circumference of the bowel wall is not

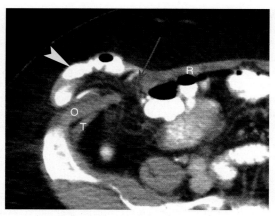

FIG. 9.29 **Spigelian hernia.** Magnified view of the right lower quadrant from an axial CT slice of an obese patient showing a defect *(red arrow)* in the anterior abdominal wall at the lateral edge of the rectus muscle *(R)*. Small bowel *(yellow arrowhead)* extends through the defect into the subcutaneous tissues. The internal and external oblique muscles *(O)* are fused and retracted. The transversus abdominis muscle *(T)* is evident.

compromised. However, if the involved portion of the bowel wall becomes strangulated and infarcts, bowel perforation occurs, making this a dangerous type of hernia. Laparoscopic port sites are common locations for Richter hernias to occur.

Abdominal Wall Hematomas

Bleeding into the abdominal musculature may complicate bleeding disorders or anticoagulant therapy or may result from trauma. Hematomas enlarge the involved muscle, on CT are hyperdense acutely, and progressively decrease in attenuation with time (Fig. 9.30). Hematomas or seromas are commonly visualized in surgical wounds during the postoperative period. Infection results in abscess formation with increased stranding densities in subcutaneous fat, gas formation, and fluid levels. Confirmation of infection requires percutaneous aspiration.

Abdominal Wall Tumors and Subcutaneous Nodules

Fatty tissue provides an optimal background for CT demonstration of nodules and masses in the subcutaneous tissues. Diagnostic considerations include the following:

- Hematogenous metastases to the skin are characteristic of malignant melanoma (Fig. 9.31). Other primary tumors to consider include breast, stomach, ovary, renal, and lung carcinomas. Nodules are often well defined and enlarge over time.

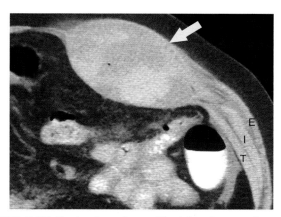

FIG. 9.30 **Rectus hematoma.** The left rectus muscle *(arrow)* is markedly enlarged and shows irregular high attenuation indicative of intramuscular hematoma. Bleeding occurred as a complication of dialysis. The flank muscles are well shown. *E,* External oblique; *I,* internal oblique; *T,* transversus abdominis.

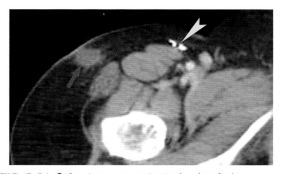

FIG. 9.31 **Subcutaneous metastasis.** A soft-tissue nodule *(red arrow)* with spiculated margins is seen in the subcutaneous fat. Biopsy confirmed metastatic melanoma. Surgical clips *(yellow arrowhead)* are present in the right inguinal region from previous lymph node dissection. The primary lesion had been removed from the right thigh 2 years previously.

- Desmoid tumors are locally invasive dysplastic tumors of connective tissue that involve the muscles and fascia of the anterior abdominal wall. Local recurrence is common after surgical removal. Familial desmoid tumors occur with Gardner syndrome.
- Benign fibromas, hemangiomas, and lipomas arising in the anterior abdominal wall are relatively common.
- Injection hematomas and granulomas are usually seen in the lower anterior abdominal wall.
- Sebaceous cysts range in size and are attached to the skin surface.

- Enlarged subcutaneous vessels are round, oval, or tubular. They may be related to portal hypertension or venous thrombosis. Contrast medium administration shows enhancement.
- Endometriomas result from implants of endometrium in surgical scars. They characteristically bleed and become painful during menstruation.

SUGGESTED READING

Peritoneal Cavity
McLaughlin, P. D., Filippone, A., & Maher, M. M. (2013). Neoplastic diseases of the peritoneum and mesentery. *AJR. American Journal of Roentgenology, 200,* W420–W430.

Pickhardt, P. J., & Bhalla, S. (2005). Unusual nonneoplastic peritoneal and subperitoneal conditions: CT findings. *Radiographics, 25,* 719–730.

Tirkes, T., Sandrasegaran, K., Patel, A. A., et al. (2012). Peritoneal and retroperitoneal anatomy and its relevance for cross-sectional imaging. *Radiographics, 32,* 437–451.

Tomar, B. S. (2016). Pediatric ascites revisited. *International Journal of Gastroenterology & Hepatology Transplant Nutrition, 1,* 55–73.

Vessels
Caiafa, R. O., Vinuesa, A. S., Izquierdo, R. S., et al. (2013). Retroperitoneal fibrosis: Role of imaging in diagnosis and follow-up. *Radiographics, 33,* 535–552.

Hellmann, D. B., Grand, D. J., & Freischlag, J. A. (2007). Inflammatory abdominal aortic aneurysm. *JAMA, 297,* 395–400.

Smillie, R. P., Shetty, M., Boyer, A. C., et al. (2015). Imaging evaluation of the inferior vena cava. *Radiographics, 35,* 578–592.

Vu, K.-M., Kaitoukov, Y., Morin-Roy, F., et al. (2014). Rupture signs on computed tomography, treatment and outcome of abdominal aortic aneurysms. *Insights Imaging, 5,* 281–293.

Wadgaonkar, A. D., Black, J. H., III, Weihe, E. K., et al. (2015). Abdominal aortic aneurysms revisited: MDCT with multiplanar reconstructions for identifying indicators of instability in the pre- and postoperative patient. *Radiographics, 35,* 254–268.

Nodes
Ganeshalingam, S., & Koh, D.-M. (2009). Nodal staging. *Cancer Imaging, 9,* 104–111.

Johnson, S. A., Kumar, A., Matasar, M. J., et al. (2015). Imaging for staging and response assessment in lymphoma. *Radiology, 276,* 323–338.

Swerdlow, S. H., Campo, E., Pileri, S. A., et al. (2016). The 2016 revision of the World Health Organization classification of lymphoid neoplasms. *Blood, 127,* 2375–2390.

Abdominal Wall
Cabarrus, M. C., Yeh, B. M., Phelps, A. S., et al. (2017). From inguinal hernias to spermatic cord lipomas: Pearls, pitfalls, and mimics of abdominal and pelvic hernias. *Radiographics, 37,* 2063–2082.

CHAPTER 10

Abdominal Trauma

WILLIAM E. BRANT

Multidetector CT (MDCT) is the imaging method of choice for the diagnosis of intra-abdominal injury following blunt abdominal trauma. Treatment is directed by characterization of the precise nature of the injury, or by the reliable demonstration of the absence of significant injury. CT is particularly valuable when physical examination of the abdomen is equivocal or unreliable, such as with head trauma or impairment of consciousness caused by drugs or alcohol. CT has the advantage of evaluating the entire abdomen and pelvis in a single comprehensive study. The sensitivity of CT for detecting intra-abdominal injury exceeds 90%.

Patients who have had significant blunt abdominal trauma and who are hemodynamically stable are candidates for trauma CT of the abdomen. Patients who are hemodynamically unstable, who have signs of peritonitis, or who have had penetrating abdominal trauma are candidates for immediate exploratory surgery, which should not be delayed by CT. On the other hand, patients with a history of blunt abdominal trauma who do not have physical examination evidence of traumatic injury to the abdomen receive little benefit from trauma CT.

At many institutions limited ultrasound examination is used to perform a rapid screening of the abdomen and pelvis to detect the presence of free intraperitoneal fluid (focused abdominal sonography for trauma [FAST] scan). If fluid is present, trauma CT of the abdomen and pelvis is performed. If fluid is absent and clinical assessment is low risk, trauma CT may be deferred, although not all significant intra-abdominal injuries are associated with hemoperitoneum. The sensitivity of ultrasound imaging for free intraperitoneal fluid is 63%. It is limited primarily by lack of bladder filling impairing visualization of fluid in the cul-de-sac. Routine filling of the bladder with 200 to 300 mL of sterile saline increases sensitivity to 84%. In females of reproductive age and in children, free fluid limited to the cul-de-sac is most likely physiologic.

SCAN TECHNIQUE

Intravenous contrast agent administration is the most critical component in the performance of trauma CT of the abdomen. Solid organ enhancement confirms the presence of blood flow and provides the optimal detection of lacerations and hematomas, which may be isodense in unenhanced organs. All trauma CT scans must include both the abdomen and the pelvis. Extensive hemorrhage may settle dependently in the pelvis and be barely detectable on scans confined to the abdomen. All CT images should be viewed with lung windows to detect pneumothorax and pneumoperitoneum, with bone windows to detect bone injuries, and with routine soft-tissue windows to reveal organ injury.

The use of oral contrast agent before trauma CT scans remains controversial, with most institutions now scanning without oral contrast agent in the setting of trauma. Extended patient preparation with oral contrast agent may inappropriately delay CT scanning. Patients may vomit or aspirate oral contrast agent. Oral contrast agent may interfere with the performance of angiography, if needed in the treatment of active hemorrhage. Oral contrast agent is often poorly distributed through the bowel because of ileus induced by trauma. At our institution we routinely scan acute trauma patients without oral contrast agent. A number of studies, including our own, have documented no significant change in the accuracy of trauma CT without the use of oral contrast agent. Water may serve as an effective agent to distend the stomach and proximal part of the bowel without the disadvantages of positive contrast agents. When possible and without causing delay in obtaining the CT scan, 400 to 700 mL of water may be given orally or via a nasogastric tube.

For trauma CT scans, helical MDCT is performed with a 70-second delay (portal venous phase scan) following intravenous injection of 150 mL of iodinated contrast agent by a power injector at 3.5 mL per second. Images are viewed at 2.5- to 5.0-mm slice thickness. Delayed scans through the kidneys at 5 to 10 minutes are performed to evaluate patients for rupture of the collecting system if the initial scan shows perirenal fluid or other signs of renal injury. The entire abdomen and pelvis are scanned from the dome of the diaphragm through the ischial tuberosities. If the chest is also being evaluated by panscan CT, imaging is continued throughout the abdomen and pelvis without overlap. In select cases an arterial phase scan at 25 to 30 seconds after intravenous contrast agent injection may be added to assess patients for active hemorrhage. Indications for the arterial phase scan include severe mechanism of injury, clinical suspicion of active bleeding, and known displaced fractures of the pelvis.

CT cystography should be performed if bladder injury is suspected because of gross hematuria, significant trauma to the pelvis, the presence of pelvic fractures, or stranding or fluid around the bladder. The bladder must be actively distended to a minimum of 250 mL to demonstrate or to exclude bladder rupture. Passive filling of the bladder by intravenous contrast agent is not sufficient to exclude bladder injury. CT cystography is performed by instillation of 250 to 300 mL of 3% to 5% iodinated contrast agent into the bladder via a Foley catheter. Scans are obtained through the pelvis before and after contrast agent instillation with images reconstructed at 3- to 5-mm thickness. Post–bladder drainage scans are not necessary.

TRAUMA CT AND THE PREGNANT PATIENT

In the pregnant patient radiation exposure is an appropriate concern. However, trauma is a leading cause of nonobstetric maternal death and fetal loss. Pregnancy itself increases the risk of intra-abdominal traumatic injury. Maternal death nearly always results in fetal death. Although each case should be evaluated individually, in the setting of major abdominal trauma to the pregnant patient the risk of a missed or delayed diagnosis of major traumatic injury far outweighs the low risk of radiation exposure. Care should be taken to ensure that the lowest possible radiation dose be used to obtain a diagnostic trauma CT scan. Ultrasonography is used to determine the well-being of the fetus.

CT FINDINGS OF TRAUMATIC INJURY

CT findings of traumatic injury within the abdomen or pelvis include the following:
- *Hemoperitoneum.* Blood within the peritoneal cavity is a highly reliable sign of intra-abdominal injury (Fig. 10.1). Fresh unclotted blood measures 30 to

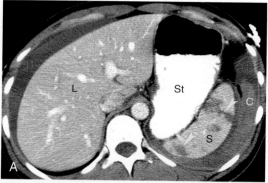

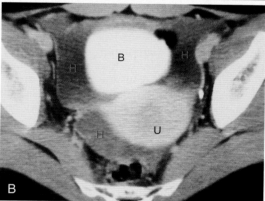

FIG. 10.1 **Hemoperitoneum.** (A) Contrast-enhanced CT through the upper abdomen shows hemoperitoneum *(H)* enveloping the liver *(L)* and spleen *(S)*. Multiple lacerations of the spleen are evident as low-attenuation clefts *(yellow arrowheads)* through the enhanced splenic parenchyma. A higher-attenuation blood clot *(C)* is seen adjacent to the spleen. Note the difference in attenuation between clot and liquid blood *(red arrow)*. This patient received an oral contrast agent, which distends the stomach *(St)*. (B) CT image of the pelvis showing blood *(H)* settling in the peritoneal recesses of the pelvis surrounding the bladder *(B)* and uterus *(U)*.

45 Hounsfield units (HU) compared with 0 to 15 HU of ascites or serum. Separation of clotted blood and serum may result in visible fluid layers *(hematocrit effect)*. Fresh blood flows from the area of injury to dependent peritoneal recesses in the abdomen and pelvis. Small volumes of low-attenuation fluid (10–15 HU) may be considered a normal finding in children, adult males, and females during their menstrual cycle. Rarely attenuation of liquid blood may be less than 20 HU if the patient has anemia or preexisting ascites.

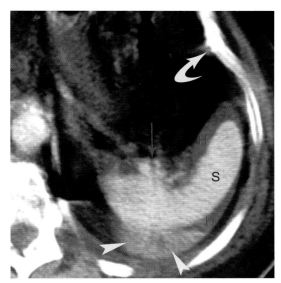

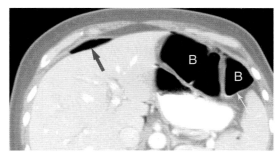

FIG. 10.4 **Pneumoperitoneum.** CT image of the abdomen shown with lung windows demonstrating an extraluminal collection of air *(red arrow)* anterior to the liver. This patient had a traumatic laceration of the jejunum. Serial images are inspected to ensure that no bowel containing gas in the lumen is in this area. Compare this with gas within the bowel *(B)* limited by a thin bowel wall *(yellow arrow)*.

FIG. 10.2 **Sentinel clot.** A high-attenuation blood clot *(yellow arrowheads)* serves as a marker of a poorly visible laceration *(red arrow)* in the spleen *(S)*. Lower-attenuation blood *(H)* is seen in the recesses of the peritoneal cavity around the spleen. A rib fracture *(curved arrow)* is also present.

- *Sentinel clot.* A focal collection of clotted blood (45–70 HU) is an accurate marker of injury to the adjacent organ (Figs. 10.1A and 10.2). Occasionally the sentinel clot is the only positive finding of specific organ injury. The higher-density clot stands out in relief compared with lower-density unclotted blood or serum.
- *Active bleeding.* Active hemorrhage may be detected by scanning during the arterial phase of dynamic intravenous contrast agent administration. Active extravasation is seen as hyperdense foci within areas of lower-density liquid blood (Fig. 10.3). The attenuation of active hemorrhage ranges from 85 to 370 HU and is usually within 20 HU of the attenuation of nearby arteries such as the aorta. On delayed images the focal contrast agent collection fades into the surrounding hematoma. This finding is a sign of life-threatening hemorrhage and often necessitates immediate angiographic or surgical therapy.
- *Free air* in the peritoneal cavity is a sign of transmural bowel laceration (Fig. 10.4). Unfortunately this sign is neither sensitive nor specific. Extraluminal air is found in only 32% to 55% of cases of bowel laceration. Free air may also result from diagnostic peritoneal lavage, barotrauma, or mechanical ventilation. Additional findings of bowel injury must be present before this finding is definitively ascribed to bowel perforation. Pneumoperitoneum appears as very low attenuation extraluminal collections of gas in the anterior abdomen in the supine patient. Free air is best detected on lung windows.

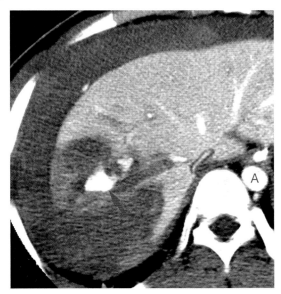

FIG. 10.3 **Active hemorrhage.** Contrast-enhanced trauma CT of the liver during the arterial phase shows a focus of active hemorrhage *(arrow)* seen as an amorphous extravascular collection of contrast agent within a low-attenuation hepatic hematoma. Compare the attenuation of the contrast agent collection with that of the enhanced aorta *(A)*. Extensive hemoperitoneum *(H)* is evident.

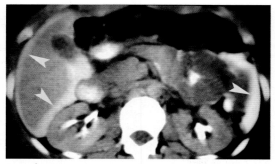

FIG. 10.5 **Free intraperitoneal contrast agent.** Image through the upper abdomen revealing high-density contrast agent in the peritoneal recesses *(arrowheads)*. This patient had an intraperitoneal rupture of the bladder. Contrast agent excreted in the urine was extravasated through the hole in the bladder into the peritoneal cavity.

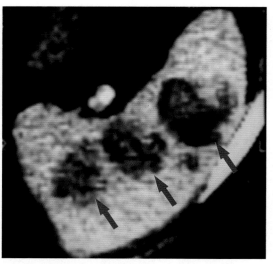

FIG. 10.7 **Intraparenchymal hematomas.** Multiple intraparenchymal hematomas *(arrows)* are seen as low-attenuation defects within the contrast-enhanced splenic parenchyma.

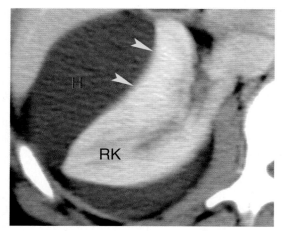

FIG. 10.6 **Subcapsular hematoma.** The contour *(arrowheads)* of the right kidney *(RK)* is compressed and distorted by a hematoma *(H)* confined within the restricted space bounded by the renal capsule. This finding is indicative of subcapsular location of the hematoma.

- *Free contrast agent* in the peritoneal cavity may occur with extravasation of oral contrast agent through a bowel perforation or from leakage of contrast-opacified urine from the urinary tract (Fig. 10.5). Extraluminal oral contrast agent is found in only 14% of bowel transections. Additional findings such as bowel wall thickening and blood in the mesentery confirm bowel injury as the source of extraluminal contrast agent. Extravasated contrast agent–containing urine should be seen on delayed images after the re-

nal collecting systems, ureter, and bladder fill with contrast agent.

- *Subcapsular hematomas* appear as crescent-shaped collections that flatten and indent the organ parenchyma (Fig. 10.6). Attenuation is lower than that of contrast-enhanced organ parenchyma. The outer border of the collection is sharply defined by the capsule of the involved organ. The inner margin compresses adjacent parenchyma.

- *Intraparenchymal hematomas* are seen as irregularly shaped rounded low-attenuation collections within contrast-enhanced parenchyma (Fig. 10.7). Small intraparenchymal hematomas are commonly called *contusions.* Flow defects during contrast enhancement of the normal spleen should not be mistaken for intrasplenic hematomas (see Fig. 14.3).

- *Lacerations* are jagged linear, often branching, defects in organ tissue that are defined by lower-density blood within the laceration (Fig. 10.8). Most lacerations extend through the organ capsule and are associated with hemoperitoneum.

- *Shattered organs* are disrupted by multiple lacerations (Fig. 10.9). Shattered organs are frequently associated with multiple infarcted segments of parenchyma. Portions of enhanced and nonenhanced organ parenchyma may be widely dispersed by hemorrhage.

- *Absence of parenchymal enhancement* is an indication of loss of vascular supply (Fig. 10.10). The supplying

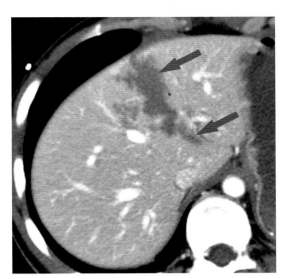

FIG. 10.8 Liver laceration. Traumatic laceration *(arrows)* of the liver is seen as a jagged low-attenuation defect with the enhanced liver parenchyma. Blood and bile within the laceration are responsible for the low attenuation of the laceration. Contrast enhancement of the liver accentuates the lesion.

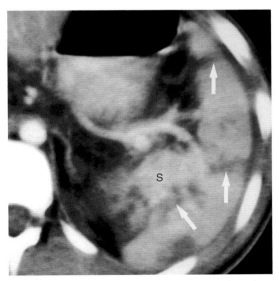

FIG. 10.9 Shattered spleen. Multiple lacerations *(arrows)* are seen as jagged defects in the parenchyma of the spleen *(S)*.

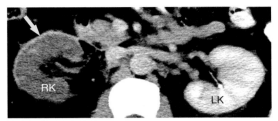

FIG. 10.10 Renal pedicle injury. The right kidney *(RK)* shows a diffuse lack of enhancement compared with the left kidney *(LK)*. Failure of an organ to be enhanced with intravenous contrast agent is evidence of injury to its vascular supply. In this case the main right renal artery thrombosed because of a traumatic tear of the intima. Faint enhancement of the periphery of the kidney is seen, demonstrating the *cortical rim sign (arrow)*. Arteries supplying the renal capsule do not arise from the main renal artery and thus remain patent when the main renal artery is occluded. These capsular branches provide blood supply to a thin rim of peripheral cortex. The cortical rim sign becomes apparent approximately 8 hours after the vascular insult.

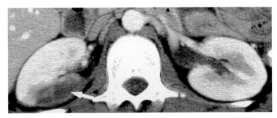

FIG. 10.11 Renal infarction. A wedge-shaped portion *(arrow)* of the right kidney fails to be enhanced. This is evidence of renal infarction resulting from occlusion or tear of a branch renal artery. The left kidney is enhanced normally.

artery may be lacerated or thrombosed. The entire organ, or only a portion of the organ, may be affected.

- *Infarctions* are seen as sharply demarcated, often wedge-shaped, areas of decreased contrast enhancement that extend to the organ capsule (Fig. 10.11). Infarctions are caused by thrombosis or lacerations of segmental arteries.

SPLEEN TRAUMA

The spleen is the most frequently injured intraabdominal organ. Current management strives to avoid splenectomy. Patients who undergo splenectomy have a significantly increased risk of infection and overwhelming sepsis. Patients who are hemodynamically stable may be treated conservatively with

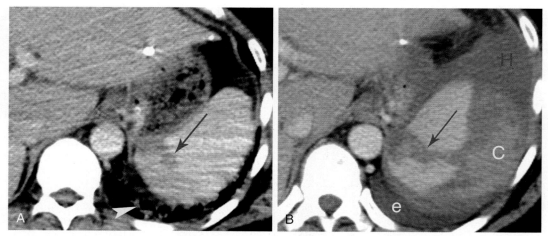

FIG. 10.12 Delayed rupture of the spleen. (A) The initial posttrauma CT scan shows a small in-trasplenic hematoma *(red arrow)* and atelectasis *(yellow arrowhead)* in the left lower lobe of the lung. No hemoperitoneum is present. (B) On the third day after trauma the patient experienced increasing left upper quadrant pain and generalized abdominal pain. A subsequent CT scan revealed completed rupture of the spleen *(red arrow)* with generalized hemoperitoneum *(H)*, a sentinel clot *(C)* adjacent to the spleen, and a left pleural effusion (e).

close observation. *Delayed rupture of the spleen* may occur up to 10 days following trauma (Fig. 10.12). Delayed rupture is associated with low-grade splenic injuries, including intraparenchymal and subcapsular hematomas. Surgery or angiographic intervention is reserved for patients who have active bleeding, large nonperfused portions of the spleen, or who have formed pseudoaneurysms. Up to 40% of patients with splenic injury have associated left lower rib fractures. Extraperitoneal hemorrhage may be present in association with splenic injury and intraperitoneal hemorrhage. Blood tracks into the anterior pararenal space along the splenic vessels and pancreas. Both arterial and portal venous phase imaging are currently recommended to evaluate patients for blunt splenic injury. With rapid bolus administration of intravenous contrast agent and the rapid scanning of MDCT, early irregular enhancement of the spleen (Fig. 10.13) is a common normal finding. Contrast agent diffuses relatively slowly through the pulp of the spleen. These defects in enhancement must not be mistaken for splenic injury or other abnormalities. Delayed images will demonstrate uniform splenic enhancement.

LIVER TRAUMA

The liver is the second most commonly injured abdominal organ. However, liver laceration is associated with

important complications and twice the morbidity of spleen laceration. Up to 45% of patients with liver injury also have spleen injury. When the liver capsule is intact, the liver will usually heal within 1 to 6 months. Nonsurgical management is preferred whenever possible.

- Lacerations are the most common liver injury. They tend to be linear and branching, paralleling the course of the hepatic arteries.
- Diffuse fatty infiltration makes identification of lacerations and hematoma more difficult. Hematomas may appear with high density rather than low density relative to enhanced liver parenchyma.
- *Periportal low attenuation* (Fig. 10.14) may be found with blood tracking adjacent to portal vessels, or with dilated periportal lymphatics associated with elevated central venous pressure caused by vigorous fluid resuscitation. Injuries to the biliary tree or intrahepatic lymphatic system are additional causes of periportal low attenuation. This nonspecific finding does not preclude nonsurgical management of liver trauma.
- Delayed complications affect up to 20% of liver injuries. Bile in liver hematomas delays healing and may result in bilomas (Fig. 10.15). Vascular injury may result in pseudoaneurysms or arterioportal fistulas. The mass effect of bilomas or hematomas may cause obstructive jaundice. Other complications include persistent bile leak, liver

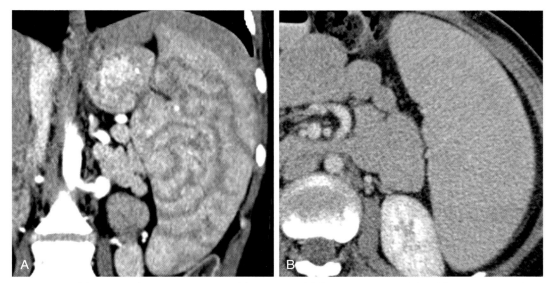

FIG. 10.13 **Early mottled enhancement of the spleen.** (A) Coronal plane multislice CT image obtained during arterial enhancement showing irregular enhancement of the splenic parenchyma with multiple linear defects caused by normal slow diffusion of contrast agent through the splenic pulp. (B) Delayed image of the normal spleen in the same patient shown in axial projection showing uniform splenic enhancement.

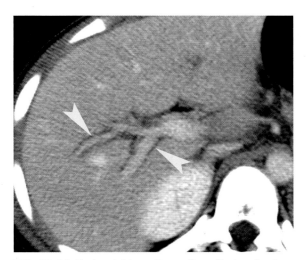

FIG. 10.14 **Periportal low attenuation.** Postcontrast trauma CT image of a 10-year-old child showing linear low attenuation *(arrowheads)* adjacent to the enhanced portal veins. A careful search must be made for additional evidence of liver laceration. In this case the periportal low attenuation was caused by aggressive intravenous hydration.

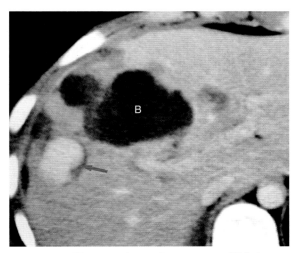

FIG. 10.15 **Biloma and pseudoaneurysm.** CT 3 days following injury reveals a biloma *(B)* appearing as a well-defined low-attenuation fluid collection. Nearby is an avidly enhanced rounded structure *(arrow)* representing a pseudoaneurysm.

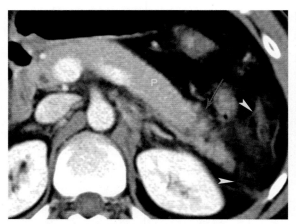

FIG. 10.16 Pancreas laceration. Trauma CT shows a laceration *(red arrow)* extending through the tail of the pancreas *(P)*. Hemorrhage and edema *(yellow arrowheads)* in the peripancreatic fatty tissue is minimal.

abscess, biliary strictures, and delayed hemorrhage. Hepatobiliary scintigraphy accurately detects biliary leaks.

- Liver injuries in the superomedial bare area of the liver may be associated with retroperitoneal hematomas rather than hemoperitoneum.

PANCREAS TRAUMA

Injury to the pancreas is uncommon but carries high morbidity and is frequently clinically occult. Penetrating trauma, knife and gunshot wounds, causes most pancreatic injuries (75%). Blunt abdominal trauma, often associated with child abuse, is the most common cause of pancreatitis in children. The body of the pancreas is compressed against the spine and is prone to contusion, laceration (Fig. 10.16), transection, pancreatitis, and focal hemorrhagic necrosis.

- Tissue displacement may be minimal, making pancreatic lacerations difficult to identify. Fluid tracking adjacent to the splenic vein, unexplained thickening of the anterior renal fascia, and fluid in the lesser sac or anterior pararenal space are CT clues to possible pancreatic injury. The sensitivity of CT for pancreatic injury is reported as 67% to 90%.
- Complications of traumatic injury to the pancreas are common, with mortality as high as 20%. Complications include pseudocyst formation, necrotizing pancreatitis, abscess, and fistula.

- The pancreas and duodenum are commonly injured simultaneously.

BOWEL AND MESENTERY TRAUMA

Injuries to the bowel and mesentery occur in about 5% of patients following blunt abdominal trauma. CT findings associated with these injuries are often subtle and are easily overlooked. Delays in diagnosis increase the risk of sepsis and peritonitis. The accuracy of CT in diagnosis of bowel and mesentery injuries is reported as 77% to 93%.

- The bowel segments most commonly injured are the proximal part of the jejunum near the ligament of Treitz, and the distal part of ileum near the ileocecal valve. The duodenum may be injured by a blow to the midabdomen from a steering wheel or the handlebars of a bicycle.
- Bowel injury is common (34% incidence) when three or more abdominal organs are injured.
- As mentioned, free intraperitoneal air or oral contrast agent is highly suggestive but is not a specific sign of bowel injury. Many cases of bowel injury lack these findings.
- Hemoperitoneum in the absence of detected solid organ injury should promote a diligent search for subtle abnormalities of the bowel and mesentery. Fluid between bowel loops is highly suggestive of bowel injury.
- Focal mesenteric hematoma in association with focal thickening of the bowel wall indicates a high likelihood of significant bowel injury requiring surgery.
- Focal mesenteric hematoma without focal thickening of the bowel wall is a nonspecific finding found in association with lesions that require surgery and those that do not. Isolated mesenteric hematoma does not require surgery (Fig. 10.17).
- Discontinuity of the bowel wall is the most specific CT sign of bowel injury.
- Thickening of the bowel wall may be circumferential or eccentric (Fig. 10.18). High-density hematoma within the bowel wall is highly indicative of bowel injury. Wall thickening greater than 3 mm with the lumen well distended is considered to be abnormal.
- Intense enhancement of the bowel wall associated with bowel wall thickening and free intraperitoneal fluid is strongly indicative of bowel perforation and peritonitis.
- Retroperitoneal air or oral contrast agent is highly indicative of laceration of the duodenum.

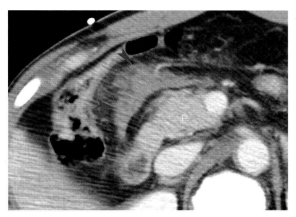

FIG. 10.17 **Mesenteric haematoma.** Hemorrhage *(arrowheads)* into the mesentery is seen as an amorphous density enveloping mesenteric blood vessels. The head of the pancreas *(P)* is adjacent to the hematoma. In this case the mesenteric hematoma was an isolated injury.

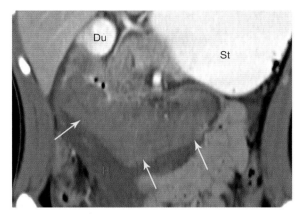

FIG. 10.19 **Duodenal hematoma.** Coronal postcontrast CT image showing marked distention of the oral contrast agent–filled stomach *(St)* and duodenal bulb *(Du)* by a large intramural hematoma *(arrows)* thickening the wall and obstructing the lumen of the descending and transverse duodenum. Hemorrhage *(H)* extends into the retroperitoneum.

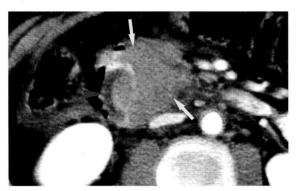

FIG. 10.18 **Torn duodenum.** The descending duodenum is filleted open by an extended longitudinal tear. A large hematoma *(yellow arrows)* occupies its lumen and envelops retroperitoneal vessels. The duodenal wall *(red arrowhead)* is thickened. This is a retroperitoneal injury without hemoperitoneum.

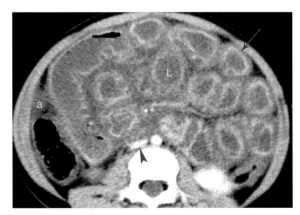

FIG. 10.20 **Shock bowel.** Postcontrast CT image of the midabdomen of a 7-year-old girl injured in a motor vehicle collision showing diffuse distension of the small bowel with striking enhancement *(arrow)* of the bowel wall. The small bowel lumen *(L)* is distended with fluid, and ascites *(a)* is present in peritoneal recesses and between bowel loops. The inferior vena cava *(arrowhead)* is flattened.

- Wall thickening of the transverse duodenum is indicative of intramural duodenal hematoma (Fig. 10.19). The stomach and proximal part of the duodenum may be obstructed.
- Laceration or transection of the jejunum or ileum results in peritonitis and dilated small bowel within about 12 hours. Free air is seen in only about 50% of cases. Subtle findings include focal wall thickening and sentinel clot. Look for discontinuity of bowel loops.
- Colonic injury may result in intraperitoneal or extraperitoneal findings.

- *Shock bowel* results from severe hypotension and hypoperfusion in trauma patients. CT findings include diffuse dilatation of the small bowel with wall thickening and increased contrast enhancement of the bowel wall (Fig. 10.20). The colon remains normal. The inferior vena cava is flattened, and the kidneys show intense contrast enhancement of the parenchyma.

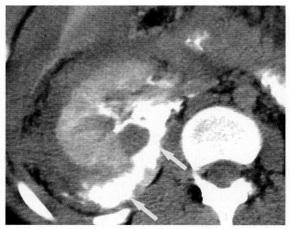

FIG. 10.21 Tear of the renal collecting system.
Delayed image through the right kidney showing extravasation of contrast agent *(arrows)* from the renal pelvis into the perirenal space already distended with blood *(H)* and urine. Early postcontrast images showed no early contrast agent extravasation, excluding active bleeding.

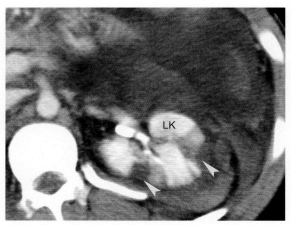

FIG. 10.22 Shattered kidney. The left kidney *(LK)* has multiple lacerations and foci of parenchyma that are not enhanced *(arrowheads)*, indicating devascularization. A large perirenal hematoma *(H)* is present. Hemoperitoneum *(HP)* caused by a spleen laceration is also evident. This severely damaged kidney was surgically removed.

- Fluid overload resulting from aggressive fluid resuscitation may cause diffuse edema of the small bowel wall associated with dilatation of the inferior vena cava, periportal edema, and normal enhancement of the bowel wall and renal parenchyma.

RENAL TRAUMA

The kidneys are injured in 8% to 10% of patients with blunt trauma abdominal injuries. Minor injuries are most common (75%–85%) and are managed without surgery, and include contusions, subcapsular hematomas, and minor lacerations with limited perinephric hematomas, and small cortical infarcts. Gross hematuria, although not always present, is a reliable sign of injury to the urinary tract.

- Injury to the renal collecting system is diagnosed on delayed images by extravasation of contrast-opacified urine into the renal sinus and medial perirenal space (Fig. 10.21). Deep renal lacerations may be associated with urine leakage into the lateral perirenal space. Urinary extravasation will heal spontaneously as long as there is no obstruction to normal antegrade urine flow. Obstruction requires stent placement or surgical repair.
- Catastrophic injuries require surgical intervention. These include shattered kidneys and injuries to the renal vascular pedicle. Shattered kidneys (Fig. 10.22) have multiple lacerations, severe impairment of contrast agent excretion, extensive hemorrhage, lacerations of the renal collecting system with urine leakage, and often active arterial bleeding. Devitalized segments of kidney may be present.
- Thrombosis of the main renal artery is caused by stretching of the renal pedicle with tearing of the intima, which is less elastic than the media and adventitia. The intimal flap initiates thrombosis, which propagates distally. The entire kidney, or a segmental portion of the kidney, fails to be enhanced (see Fig. 10.10). Abrupt termination of enhancement of the renal artery may be visualized with high-quality helical CT. Most occlusions occur in the proximal 2 cm of the renal artery. This injury usually occurs in the absence of perirenal hematoma. The *cortical rim sign* is a delayed finding of renal arterial occlusion, appearing several days after the acute renal artery thrombosis (see Fig. 10.10). Only the periphery of the kidney, supplied by collaterals to the renal capsule, is enhanced. The bulk of the kidney supplied by the main renal artery, which lacks collateral pathways, is not enhanced.
- Avulsion of the renal artery is rare and usually life ending. Patients with avulsion who survive to be examined have absent renal enhancement, have large perinephric hematomas, and may show arterial extravasation.
- Ureteropelvic junction (UPJ) injuries are caused by sudden deceleration, which tears the UPJ. Urinomas are seen medially or occasionally surrounding the kidney, but no perinephric hematoma is usually

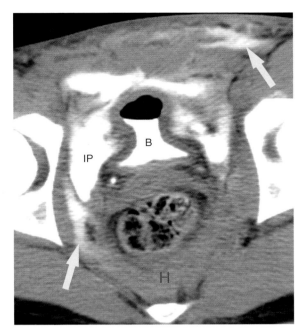

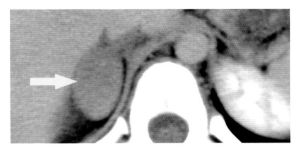

FIG. 10.24 **Adrenal hemorrhage.** A solid mass *(arrow)* replaces the right adrenal gland in a patient with multiple injuries from a motor vehicle accident. Follow-up CT confirmed the return of the right adrenal gland to a normal appearance, confirming posttraumatic right adrenal hemorrhage. Unilateral adrenal hemorrhage requires no treatment.

FIG. 10.23 **Combined intraperitoneal and extraperitoneal bladder rupture.** CT cystogram demonstrates free spill of contrast agent from the bladder *(B)* into the peritoneal cavity *(IP)* and extraperitoneal spaces *(arrows)*. The bladder is compressed by surrounding hemorrhage and urine. Hemorrhage *(H)* extends into the extraperitoneal presacral space.

present. Complete transections at the UPJ show contrast agent in the renal pelvis but not in the distal part of the ureter. UPJ lacerations are characterized by visualization of contrast agent in both the renal pelvis and the distal part of the ureter. Absence of CT visualization of contrast agent in the ureter is an indication for retrograde pyelography.

BLADDER TRAUMA

Rupture of the bladder occurs in up to 10% of patients with pelvic fractures. In most cases (80%) the bladder is lacerated by a spicule of fractured bone, and urine (with contrast agent) leaks into extraperitoneal spaces. Rupture of the bladder into the peritoneal cavity (20%) occurs as a result of a blow to the lower abdomen when the bladder is distended. The sudden increase in intracystic pressure ruptures the bladder at its dome, resulting in leakage of urine into the peritoneal cavity. Both types of bladder rupture are effectively demonstrated by CT following contrast agent administration either intravenously or by a bladder catheter. However, the

bladder must be distended to at least 250 mL to reliably demonstrate small ruptures.

- The presence of free fluid or hematoma in the pelvis, or fractures of the pubic rami, sacrum, or ileum, suggest possible bladder injury. CT cystography should be considered.
- *Extraperitoneal bladder rupture* is characterized by contrast agent leakage into the retropubic space with extension along fascial planes into the abdominal wall, scrotum, thigh, and retroperitoneum. The contrast agent collections tend to be linear and poorly defined. Extraperitoneal bladder ruptures usually heal without surgery.
- *Intraperitoneal bladder rupture* is characterized by contrast agent leakage into the peritoneal cavity surrounding loops of the bowel and extending along the paracolic gutters. The contrast agent collections are sharply defined by visceral and parietal peritoneum. Intraperitoneal bladder rupture usually requires surgical repair.
- Combined extraperitoneal and intraperitoneal ruptures occur in about 5% of patients (Fig. 10.23).
- *Bladder contusions* appear as focal areas of thickening of the bladder wall. Hemorrhage in the bladder wall may produce focal high attenuation.
- *Urethral injuries* should be suspected in patients with pelvic fractures, bladder injuries, and pelvic hematomas. Clinical findings include blood at the urethral meatus and inability to void. Urethral injuries are diagnosed by retrograde urethrogram.

ADRENAL TRAUMA

Hemorrhage into the adrenal gland is seen in about 2% of adults with severe trauma. Posttraumatic hemorrhage has a striking propensity to involve the right adrenal gland (90% of cases). The predilection for the right adrenal gland has been attributed to compression of the gland between the liver and spine. Hemorrhage is bilateral in 25% of cases. Bilateral hemorrhage places the patient at risk of development of adrenal insufficiency.

- Acute hemorrhage produces a hyperdense (50–75 HU) round to oval mass replacing the affected adrenal gland (Fig. 10.24).
- Fat adjacent to the adrenal gland is infiltrated with streaks of soft-tissue density representing bleeding into the periadrenal fat.
- The hemorrhage decreases in density and shrinks over time. Calcifications may develop in the gland within a few months.

HYPOPERFUSION COMPLEX

Persistent hypovolemic shock may be caused by severe blood loss from traumatic injury. The heart is unable to pump enough blood, resulting in generalized inadequate circulation impairing organ function. CT signs of hypovolemic shock include:

- flattening of the infrahepatic inferior vena cava and renal veins;
- decreased size of the abdominal aorta;
- shock bowel seen as diffuse thickening and hyperenhancement of the wall of the small bowel;
- decreased enhancement of the renal medulla on delayed postcontrast images;
- decreased enhancement of the spleen in early-phase imaging.

The latter two findings are associated with poor clinical prognosis for patients with hypovolemic shock.

SUGGESTED READING

Bates, D. D. B., Wasserman, M., Malek, A., et al. (2017). Multidetector CT of surgically proven blunt bowel and mesenteric injury. *Radiographics, 37*, 613–625.

Bonatti, M., Lombardo, F., Vezzali, N., et al. (2015). MDCT of blunt renal trauma: Imaging findings and therapeutic implications. *Insights Imaging, 6*, 261–271.

Boscak, A. R., Shanmuganathan, K., Mirvis, S. E., et al. (2013). Optimizing trauma multidetector CT protocol for blunt splenic injury: Need for arterial and portal venous phase scans. *Radiology, 268*, 79–88.

Hamilton, J. D., Kumaravel, M., Censullo, M. L., et al. (2008). Multidetector CT evaluation of active extravasation in blunt abdominal and pelvic trauma patients. *Radiographics, 28*, 1603–1616.

Joshi, G., Kim, E. Y., Hanna, T. N., et al. (2018). CT cystography for suspicion of traumatic urinary bladder injury: Indications, technique, findings, and pitfalls in diagnosis. *Radiographics, 38*, 9293.

Patlas, M. N., Dreizin, D., Manias, C. O., et al. (2017). Abdominal and pelvic trauma: Misses and misinterpretations at multidetector CT. *Radiographics, 37*, 703–704.

Ramchandani, P., & Buckler, P. M. (2009). Imaging of genitourinary trauma. *AJR. American Journal of Roentgenology, 192*, 1514–1523.

Raptis, C. A., Mellnick, V. M., Raptis, D. A., et al. (2014). Imaging of trauma in the pregnant patient. *Radiographics, 34*, 748–763.

Soto, J. A., & Anderson, S. W. (2012). Multidetector CT of blunt abdominal trauma. *Radiology, 265*, 678–693.

CHAPTER 11

Liver

WILLIAM E. BRANT

ANATOMY

In 2000 the Terminology Committee of the International Hepato-Pancreato-Biliary Association refined the accepted terminology of hepatic anatomy and liver resections. The international classification system divides the liver into eight independent segments (Couinaud [pronounced "kwee-NO"] segments) (Fig. 11.1, Tables 11.1 and 11.2). Each segment is a self-contained unit that can be surgically resected without damaging the remainder of the liver. Each segment has its own dual vascular inflow (hepatic artery and portal vein), its own biliary drainage, and a shared vascular outflow (hepatic veins). The portal triads (bile ducts, hepatic arteries, portal veins) course through the center of each segment, whereas the hepatic veins define the periphery of the segment and the plane of surgical dissection. This segmental anatomy provides a useful and widely accepted method for identification of the location of lesions seen on CT and other imaging studies.

The right, middle, and left hepatic veins enter the intrahepatic inferior vena cava (IVC) just before it pierces the diaphragm about 2 cm below the right atrium. Whereas the right hepatic vein usually enters the IVC separately, the middle and left hepatic veins often (65%–85%) form a common trunk before joining the IVC. In most patients these three major hepatic veins drain the entirety of the liver except for the caudate lobe. Short hepatic veins drain the caudate lobe separately directly into the IVC. As an anatomic variant, accessory hepatic veins drain segment 5 or segment 6 independently into the IVC.

The portal vein is formed by the junction of the splenic vein with the superior mesenteric vein just anterior to the IVC and just posterior to the neck of the pancreas. It ascends behind the duodenum in company with the hepatic artery and common bile duct to the porta hepatis, where it divides into a short fatter right portal vein and a longer thinner left portal vein.

The hepatic artery has variable anatomy. In its "classic" form (55%) the right and left hepatic arteries branch from a proper hepatic artery that is a continuation of the common hepatic artery arising from the celiac axis. In 10% of individuals the left hepatic artery arises as a branch of the left gastric artery. In 11% of individuals the right hepatic artery arises from the superior mesenteric artery. In this case the "replaced" right hepatic artery passes through the portocaval space from the superior mesenteric artery to the right hepatic lobe.

Division of the liver into eight segments is based on a concept of three vertical planes and one transverse plane. A vertical plane through the middle hepatic vein, IVC, and gallbladder fossa divides the liver into right and left lobes. A vertical plane through the right hepatic vein divides the right lobe into anterior (7 and 5) and posterior (7 and 6) segments. A vertical plane through the left hepatic vein divides the left lobe into medial (4a and 4b) and lateral (2 and 3) segments. A transverse plane through the left portal vein divides the left lobe into superior (4a and 2) and inferior (4b and 3) segments. An oblique transverse plane through the right portal vein divides the right lobe into superior (8 and 7) and inferior (5 and 6) segments (Table 11.1).

Segment 1 is the caudate lobe, which is separated from the rest of the liver by the fissure of the ligamentum venosum anteriorly and the IVC posterolaterally. It is supplied by branches of the right and left hepatic arteries and portal veins and drains venous blood directly into the IVC by numerous small hepatic veins. The papillary process of the caudate lobe extends toward the lesser sac and may appear separate from the rest of the caudate lobe, simulating a mass or an enlarged lymph node.

Segment 2 and *segment 3* make up the lateral division of the left lobe. The plane of the left portal vein divides segments 2 and 3. Segment 2 makes up the left superior and lateral contour of the liver. Segment 3 makes up the left inferior and lateral contour of the liver. *Segment 4* makes up the medial division of the left lobe. The plane of the left portal vein divides the medial segment of the left lobe into segments 4a (superior) and 4b (inferior). In older literature, segment 4 was called the *quadrate lobe*.

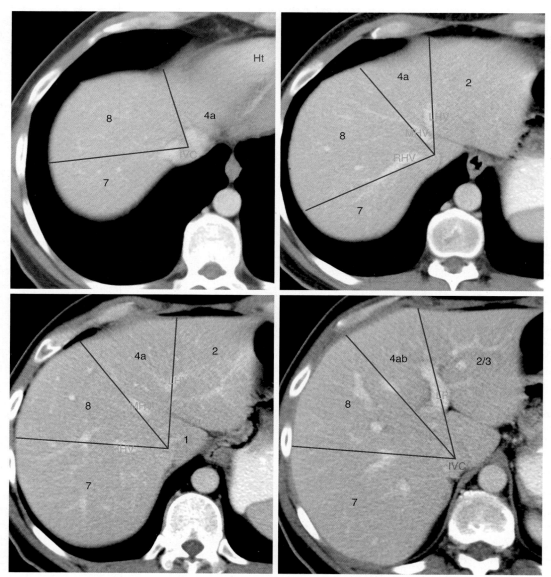

FIG. 11.1 Anatomic segments of the liver. A series of axial postcontrast CT images demonstrating the anatomic landmarks and segmental anatomy of the liver. Segments are labeled 1 to 8. The vertical planes defined by the right hepatic vein *(RHV)*, middle hepatic vein *(MHV)*, and left hepatic vein *(LHV)* are shown as straight lines. Other key landmarks are identified. Note the difficulty of applying straight geometric planes to curving vessels. This patient has had a cholecystectomy. *ARPV,* Anterior branch of the RPV; *FLT,* fissure of the ligamentum teres; *FLV,* fissure of the ligamentum venosum; *GBF,* gallbladder fossa; *Ht,* heart; *IVC,* inferior vena cava; *LPV,* left portal vein; *MPV,* main portal vein; *PRPV,* posterior branch of the right portal vein; *RPV,* right portal vein.

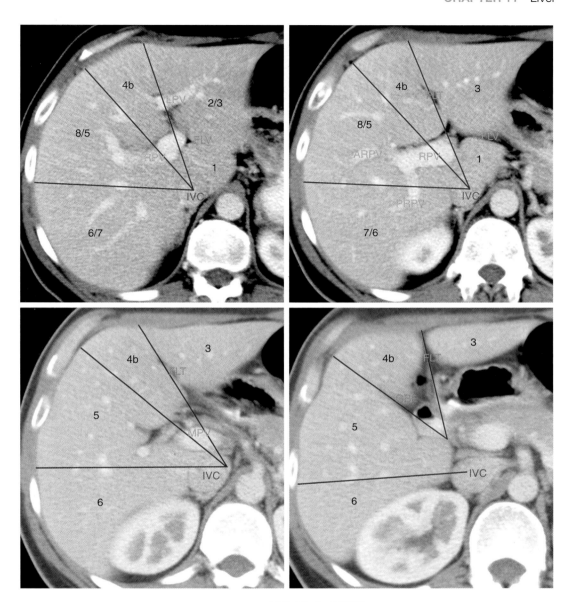

FIG. 11.1, cont'd

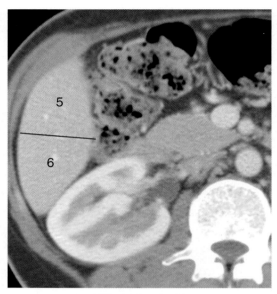

FIG. 11.1, cont'd

TABLE 11.1
Nomenclature for Anatomic Segments of the Liver

Couinaud Segment	Anatomic Description	Traditional Nomenclature
1	Caudate lobe	Caudate lobe
		Left lobe
2	Left lateral superior subsegment	Lateral segment
3	Left lateral inferior subsegment	Lateral segment
4a	Left medial superior subsegment	Medial segment
4b	Left medial inferior subsegment	Medial segment
		Right lobe
5	Right anterior inferior subsegment	Anterior segment
8	Right anterior superior subsegment	Anterior segment
6	Right posterior inferior subsegment	Posterior segment
7	Right posterior superior subsegment	Posterior segment

The anterior segments (5 and 8) of the right lobe are separated from the posterior segments (6 and 7) by the plane of the right hepatic vein. The lateral contour of the anterior right lobe is formed by *segment 8* superiorly and *segment 5* inferiorly. *Segment 7* lies posterior to segment 8, and *segment 6* lies posterior to segment 5. The plane of the right portal vein separates anterior segment 8 from anterior segment 5 and separates posterior segment 7 from posterior segment 6.

Unfortunately, natural anatomic variation in blood supply does not adhere perfectly to the concept of flat geometric planes dividing the segments. In reality the vascular territorial boundaries between segments have more variable and curving undulations to their borders than the concept of flat planes indicates. In addition, many three-dimensional drawings in the literature are misleading as to the location of the lobes. Segment 7 is posterior to and hidden by segment 8 in a frontal projection rather than lateral to segment 8 as shown in some drawings. Likewise, segment 6 is posterior, not lateral, to segment 5. The axial images in Fig. 11.1 are an attempt to localize the segments as demonstrated by CT. Correlate the anatomic description of the lobes in Table 11.1 with their location as shown in Fig. 11.1 to

TABLE 11.2
Nomenclature for Surgical Resection of Liver Segments

Term for Surgical Resection[a]	Segments Removed	Anatomic Term
Right hepatectomy	5, 6, 7, 8	Right hemiliver
Left hepatectomy	2, 3, 4	Left hemiliver
Right anterior segmentectomy	5, 8	Right anterior section
Right posterior segmentectomy	6, 7	Right posterior section
Left medial segmentectomy	4	Left medial section
Left lateral segmentectomy	2, 3	Left lateral section
Right trisegmentectomy	4, 5, 6, 7, 8	Right hemiliver plus left medial section
Left trisegmentectomy	2, 3, 4, 5, 8	Left hemiliver plus right anterior section
Segmentectomy	Any one of segments 1–9	Segments 1–9 (e.g., segmentectomy 6)
Bisegmentectomy	Any two of segments 1–9	Two contiguous segments (e.g., bisegmentectomy 5,6)

[a]Some surgeons use the term *sectionectomy* in lieu of *segmentectomy*.
Modified from Terminology Committee of the International Hepato-Pancreato-Biliary Association (2000). The Brisbane 2000 terminology of liver anatomy and resections. *HPB, 2*, 333–339.

learn the segments. Recognize that anatomic variation in blood supply makes localization of lesions to specific segments quite inaccurate. Also, many liver lesions will involve two or more segments.

Several fissures and ligaments deserve special mention either because they are particularly prominent or because they define important perihepatic spaces. The *falciform ligament* consists of two closely applied layers of peritoneum extending from the umbilicus to the diaphragm in a parasagittal plane. The caudal free end of the falciform ligament contains the ligamentum teres, which is the remnant of the obliterated umbilical vein. The reflections of the falciform ligament separate over the posterior dome of the liver to form the coronary ligaments that define the *"bare area"* of the liver not covered by peritoneum. The coronary ligaments reflect between the liver and the diaphragm and prevent access of intraperitoneal fluid from covering the bare area of the liver. The absence of fluid over the bare area is an important sign in the differentiation of ascites from pleural effusion on CT. The remainder of the falciform ligament and ligamentum teres continues into the liver to form a prominent fat-filled fissure that defines the left intersegmental fissure dividing the medial and lateral segments of the left lobe.

The *fissure of the ligamentum venosum* contains the remnant of the ductus venosus, which in fetal life carried oxygenated blood from the umbilical vein to the

IVC. This fissure is commonly fat filled and prominent on CT, separating the caudate lobe and the left lobe.

The *lesser omentum* suspends the lesser curve of the stomach and the duodenal bulb from the inferior surface of the liver, attaching within the fissure of the ligamentum venosum. The lesser omentum is subdivided into the gastrohepatic ligament and the hepatoduodenal ligament. The gastrohepatic ligament contains coronary veins that serve as an important sign of portal hypertension when they become dilated. The right free edge of the hepatoduodenal ligament carries the portal vein, hepatic artery, and common bile duct between the porta hepatis and the duodenum. The hepatoduodenal ligament provides the anterior border of the foramen of Winslow, which opens into the lesser sac.

The normal liver is homogeneous in CT attenuation, measuring 55 to 65 Hounsfield units (HU) on unenhanced CT. The unenhanced liver parenchymal attenuation is normally greater than that of blood vessels and 7 to 8 HU greater than that of splenic parenchyma. Anemia lowers the CT attenuation of blood vessels and may make the liver parenchyma appear falsely increased in density. The contour of the liver is smooth and convex adjacent to the diaphragm, with a sharp inferior border and a concave undersurface. Fissures may be fat filled and prominent. The right lobe is usually larger than the left lobe and may extend far caudad as a *Riedel lobe*, a normal variant. The left lobe

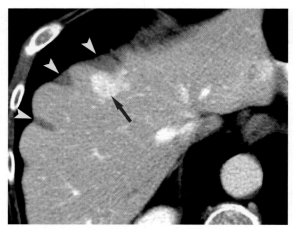

FIG. 11.2 Diaphragmatic slips. Folds in the diaphragm *(yellow arrowheads)* in this 78-year-old woman create defects in the liver. These diaphragmatic slips are more common in older patients. They are recognized by their peripheral location and characteristic linear infolded appearance. An enhancing hemangioma *(red arrow)* is partially visualized.

is more variable in size, and its lateral segment may extend far to the left and wrap partially around the spleen. Congenital absence of the left lobe is a rare anomaly. *Diaphragmatic slips* are infoldings of the diaphragm that indent the normal smooth contour of the liver (Fig. 11.2). These invaginations of diaphragmatic muscle occur with increasing frequency with age greater than 60 years and should not be mistaken for masses in the liver or on the diaphragm.

TECHNICAL CONSIDERATIONS

Multidetector CT (MDCT) allows scanning of the entire liver with thin collimation during a single 10- to 25-second breath hold. Acquisition is routinely repeated several times during various phases of contrast medium enhancement.

Dynamic contrast-enhanced liver CT offers the opportunity to accurately characterize lesion enhancement patterns and significantly increase the specificity of diagnosis. Various lesions are detected best, or sometimes only, in specific phases of postcontrast scanning. Intravenous contrast medium is administered by a power injector using a contrast medium iodine concentration of 300 mg/mL at a rate of 4 to 5 mL per second for a volume of 100 to 150 mL. Routine scan delays for MDCT are 25 seconds following initiation of contrast medium injection for the arterial phase and 65 seconds following initiation of contrast medium

injection for the portal venous phase. With MDCT, images are routinely acquired at 1.25- to 2.50-mm collimation but are viewed at 5-mm slice thickness. Thin collimation acquisitions allow highly detailed multiplanar reconstructions. Enhancement of the normal liver is homogeneous throughout the parenchyma on all enhancement phases.

- *Noncontrast scans* are commonly obtained to provide a baseline for the degree of lesion enhancement. Many liver lesions are detected, but small lesions are often mistaken for unopacified vessels. Noncontrast scans are superior to postcontrast scans for diagnosis of fatty infiltration and other alterations of parenchymal attenuation.
- *Arterial phase* acquisition is optimal for visualization of hypervascular lesions supplied by the hepatic artery such as hepatoma, carcinoid metastases, and focal nodular hyperplasia (FNH). Lesions are conspicuous because they are enhanced more than the surrounding parenchyma. A variety of perfusion anomalies and abnormalities are seen only on arterial phase images.
- *Portal venous phase* imaging shows overall the best lesion detection because parenchymal enhancement is maximum during this phase. Lesions are conspicuous because they are of low attenuation within a background of maximally enhanced liver parenchyma.
- The *equilibrium phase* occurs at 2 to 3 minutes after initiation of contrast medium injection. During the equilibrium phase the concentration of contrast medium is approximately equal in the intravascular and extravascular spaces, rendering most liver lesions invisible.
- *Delayed phase* images, acquired at 10 to 20 minutes after contrast medium injection, are obtained to demonstrate delayed contrast medium fill-in of hemangiomas and to detect fibrotic tumors such as cholangiocarcinoma.

LIVER HEMODYNAMICS AND PERFUSION ABNORMALITIES

The liver has a distinctive dual blood supply, with approximately 25% of its blood volume normally coming from the hepatic artery and approximately 75% arriving from the portal vein. Although this distribution pattern holds for the liver as a whole, it is not uniform throughout the liver. Alterations in arterial and venous supply to portions of the liver result in transient perfusion abnormalities that are demonstrated on postcontrast CT. Some perfusion abnormalities result from transient conditions, whereas others are congenital or chronic conditions that cause metabolic alterations in the liver resulting in abnormalities such as focal steatosis or focal sparing in diffuse fatty liver. Temporary conditions that may cause transient perfusion abnormalities include compression of the liver capsule by ribs or by infoldings of the diaphragm (slips) during breath hold for CT. Variations in vascular supply, termed *third inflow*, are chronic conditions that may result in focal metabolic changes in the liver parenchyma. Third inflow is a normal variant that involves small volumes of the liver that are supplied by aberrant systemic veins, in addition to the usual hepatic artery and portal venous supply.

Perfusion abnormalities usually represent an increase of arterial blood flow to a portion of the liver in response to a focal decrease in portal venous flow. In most cases the perfusion abnormality manifests itself as increased enhancement of a segment or subsegment of the liver during the arterial phase, with normal parenchymal enhancement returning during the portal venous phase. When the blood flow anomaly is persistent, resulting metabolic abnormalities manifest themselves as focal steatosis or focal fatty sparing. Most perfusion disorders are asymptomatic but must be recognized to avoid mistaking them for significant lesions.

Third inflow by systemic veins causes perfusion abnormalities in predictable areas of the liver and is thus relatively easy to recognize. Systemic veins communicate with portal venous branches to focally decrease portal venous flow, resulting in an increase in hepatic arterial flow in the same area. The following are prime areas for focal fatty infiltration or focal fatty sparing:

- The liver parenchyma adjacent to the gallbladder in segments 4 and 5 is sometimes supplied by the cholecystic vein draining the gallbladder. This pathway allows direct spread of gallbladder carcinoma into the liver.
- An aberrant right gastric vein may drain directly into the liver instead of into the portal or splenic vein. This results in an area of hyperenhancement at the posterior edge of segment 4.
- An aberrant left gastric vein drains directly into the liver instead of into the left portal vein, creating an area of hyperenhancement in the posterior aspect of segments 2 and 3.
- Aberrant gastric veins allow direct spread of gastric carcinoma into the liver.
- The dorsal aspect of segment 4 adjacent to the porta hepatis may be supplied by the parabiliary veins draining the distal part of the stomach and the head of the pancreas.

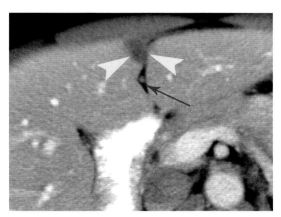

FIG. 11.3 Pseudolesion caused by third inflow. Early portal venous phase image showing a low-attenuation nodular focus *(yellow arrowheads)* adjacent to the fissure of the ligamentum teres. This should be recognized as a common pseudolesion related to third inflow. The remnant of the falciform ligament *(red arrow)* is seen as a soft-tissue density within the fissure.

- The anterior aspect of segments 3 and 4 adjacent to the fissure of the ligamentum teres is often supplied by the epigastric-paraumbilical veins draining blood from the anterior abdominal wall directly into the liver (Fig. 11.3). This venous plexus may be enlarged and prominently visualized on CT in the presence of obstruction of either the superior vena cava or the IVC. In portal hypertension these collaterals are enlarged and blood flow may reverse to drain out of the liver instead of into the liver.

Extrinsic compression of the liver capsule causes low-attenuation defects with the following features:

- A poorly marginated low-attenuation defect is seen during the portal venous phase beneath a concave indentation of the liver capsule caused by diaphragmatic slips or ribs.
- No abnormalities are seen in the same area on unenhanced, arterial phase, equilibrium phase, or delayed images.
- The offending ribs or diaphragmatic slips are evident. Metastatic disease on the peritoneal surface of the liver and subcapsular fluid collections may cause similar perfusion findings.

Tumors may affect perfusion in adjacent liver parenchyma in several ways:

- Hypervascular tumors may have intratumoral arterioportal shunts. These produce transient, peripheral wedge-shaped enhancement zones during the arterial phase in the parenchyma peripheral to the tumor

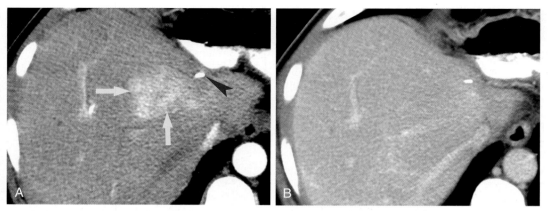

FIG. 11.4 **Transient arterial perfusion abnormality.** (A) Arterial phase image of the liver in a patient who has had a left hepatectomy showing a poorly marginated area of bright arterial enhancement *(yellow arrows)*. Serial images showed no evidence of a mass in this region. A metallic staple *(red arrowhead)* placed during surgery is noted. (B) Portal venous phase image through same region showing normal parenchymal enhancement. This perfusion defect was believed to be caused by postsurgical occlusion of portal venous branches to this area, resulting in a compensatory increase in hepatic arterial flow.

and early enhancement of peripheral portal vein branches before the main portal vein is enhanced. The peripheral enhancement may be mistaken for additional tumor, resulting in overestimation of tumor size.

- Tumor invasion, induced thrombosis, or vein compression may obstruct the portal vein or its branches. This results in decreased attenuation of affected parenchyma on noncontrast scans as a result of edema and transient increased enhancement during the arterial phase because of increased arterial flow (Fig. 11.4). Thrombi may be seen in portal veins.

- Hypervascular tumors, such as large hepatocellular carcinomas (HCCs), may parasitize and enlarge regional hepatic arteries. The tumor may either "steal" blood from adjacent parenchyma or cause increased arterial blood flow to adjacent parenchyma (Fig. 11.5). Thus on arterial phase images, parenchyma adjacent to large hypervascular tumors may show either increased or decreased enhancement.

DIFFUSE LIVER DISEASE
Fatty Liver

Fatty infiltration of the liver (hepatic steatosis) is one of the most common abnormalities diagnosed by liver CT. Fatty infiltration is a nonspecific response of hepatocytes to a variety of insults, including alcoholism, obesity, diabetes, hyperlipidemia, viral hepatitis,

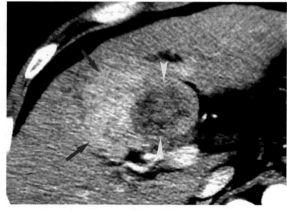

FIG. 11.5 **Parenchymal hyperenhancement caused by tumor.** Postcontrast CT reveals a large area of liver parenchymal hyperenhancement *(red arrows)* peripheral to hepatocellular carcinoma. The size of the tumor is shown by the yellow arrowheads.

chemotherapy, corticosteroid therapy, hyperalimentation, and malnutrition. The varied appearances of fatty infiltration include the following:

- Fatty infiltration lowers the CT attenuation of the involved liver parenchyma. The findings are most accurately assessed on noncontrast CT. The normal liver parenchymal attenuation is at least 10 HU greater than that of the spleen parenchyma. With fatty infiltration, attenuation of involved liver is at

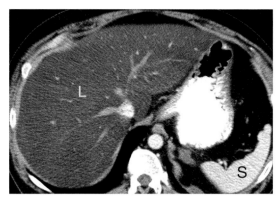

FIG. 11.6 **Diffuse fatty infiltration.** On this postcontrast CT image the liver parenchyma *(L)* is diffusely and markedly lower in attenuation than the spleen parenchyma *(S)*, indicating diffuse hepatocellular fatty infiltration. The blood vessels in the liver show normal distribution and tapering without evidence of a mass effect.

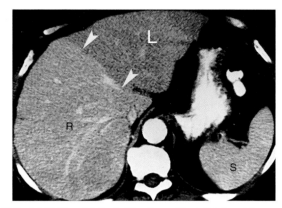

FIG. 11.7 **Focal fatty infiltration.** The left lobe of the liver *(L)* is lower in attenuation than the right lobe of the liver *(R)* and the spleen *(S)*. A strikingly sharp boundary *(arrowheads)* separates the left and right lobes. This appearance is characteristic of focal fatty infiltration.

least 10 HU lower than that of the spleen. Hepatic vessels course through areas of fatty infiltration unchanged. Fatty change is more difficult to judge on postcontrast CT because of the variability of the timing of the scan and the fact that maximum liver enhancement is delayed compared with maximum spleen enhancement. CT attenuation below –40 HU on postcontrast CT is strong evidence of hepatic steatosis but is insensitive to mild cases.

- *Diffuse fatty infiltration.* In most cases the entire liver is uniformly reduced in density (Fig. 11.6). Vessels stand out in prominent relief but run their normal course through the liver without displacement or narrowing by mass effect. The liver is usually enlarged, and the parenchyma is enhanced minimally. This pattern is the most common and is easiest to recognize. In some cases the fatty infiltration is diffuse throughout the liver but is nonuniform and patchy in severity.
- *Focal fatty infiltration.* A geographic or fan-shaped portion of the liver shows fat infiltration, whereas the remainder of the liver is of normal density (Fig. 11.7). The low-attenuation area may extend to the liver surface, but no bulge in contour is seen. Vessels run their normal course through the area of involvement. Margins between fat-infiltrated and normal liver are frequently straight and well-defined, reflecting blood flow territories as the fat infiltration is confined to segments and subsegments. Areas of the liver supplied by third inflow systemic veins are commonly affected: adjacent to

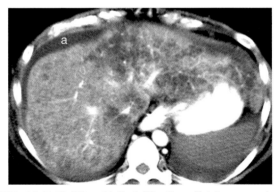

FIG. 11.8 **Multifocal fatty infiltration.** Patchy areas of low-attenuation fatty infiltration permeate the liver parenchyma. The enhanced intrahepatic blood vessels follow a normal course without a mass effect. Ascites *(a)* is present.

the gallbladder, the fissure of the ligamentum teres, and the porta hepatis.

- *Multifocal fatty infiltration.* Patchy areas of decreased attenuation are scattered throughout the liver (Fig. 11.8). Tumors may be simulated by the islands of fatty infiltration surrounded by normal parenchyma or by islands of normal parenchyma surrounded by fatty infiltration. The pattern tends to be geographic with straight margins rather than rounded masses. Areas of involvement may interdigitate with normal parenchyma.
- *Focal sparing.* Islands of normal parenchyma are surrounded by large areas of diffuse fatty infiltration

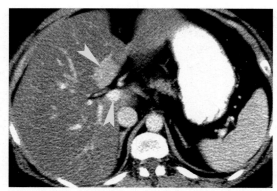

FIG. 11.9 **Focal sparing.** Islands of normal parenchyma (*arrowheads*) in segment 4b and the caudate lobe (segment 1) simulate mass lesions in a liver with extensive fatty infiltration. Most of the liver parenchyma is fatty infiltrated, making these islands of normal parenchyma appear of high attenuation by comparison.

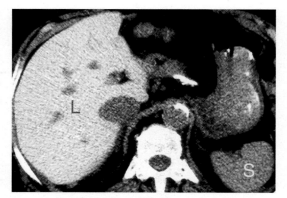

FIG. 11.10 **High-attenuation liver.** Noncontrast CT demonstrates markedly high attenuation of the liver (L) compared with the spleen (S) in this patient receiving chronic amiodarone therapy for cardiac arrhythmias.

and may simulate neoplasms (Fig. 11.9). As previously mentioned, the patterns of focal steatosis and focal sparing are related to chronic perfusion abnormalities such as systemic venous drainage into the liver. Focal sparing is most common in the same areas of the liver most often affected by focal steatosis.

- *Nonalcoholic fatty liver disease (NAFLD)* refers to hepatic steatosis with causes other than alcohol abuse. It is one of the most common liver diseases, with a global prevalence estimated at 24%. Although the exact cause is uncertain, causative factors include obesity; metabolic syndrome; insulin resistance and diabetes mellitus type 2; hyperlipidemia; drugs, including corticosteroids, tamoxifen, and methotrexate; and genetic predisposition in Native Americans, South Americans, and other groups. *Nonalcoholic steatohepatitis (NASH)* is a severe form of NAFLD with fatty infiltration complicated by inflammation and fibrosis, progression to cirrhosis, and risk of HCC. NASH progresses to cirrhosis in 20% of patients.

The following findings are most useful in making a confident diagnosis of fatty infiltration:

- Angulated geometric margins (nonspherical) between normal and fatty tissue.
- Interdigitating margins with slender fingers of normal or fatty tissue.
- Absence of mass effect, vessel displacement, or narrowing by encasement.
- Rapid change over time. Fatty changes can be seen within 3 weeks after the insult and can resolve within 6 days after removal of the insult.

- Further confirmation of fatty replacement can be provided by other imaging tests. Ultrasonography will show the areas of fatty infiltration as corresponding areas of increased parenchymal echogenicity. This gives rise to a "flip-flop" sign: fat is dark on CT and is bright on ultrasonography. Chemical shift magnetic resonance imaging with in-phase and out-of-phase images is highly sensitive to the presence of fat. Percutaneous biopsy is an option in difficult cases.
- Ultrasonography is the screening method of choice for fatty liver disease, with low cost and high sensitivity. Magnetic resonance spectroscopy and imaging are most accurate for quantifying fat in the liver. Ultrasound and magnetic resonance elastography detect and quantitate liver fibrosis to distinguish NASH from NAFLD.

Increased Liver Attenuation

Normal liver attenuation on unenhanced CT is 55 to 65 HU and is at least 10 HU higher than the attenuation of the spleen. Increased liver attenuation is usually in the range of 75 to 140 HU. On noncontrast CT, portal and hepatic veins stand out as dark tubular structures in a background of bright liver parenchyma. Causes include:

- *Iodine.* Amiodarone is toxic to the liver and raises its attenuation by deposition of iodine-containing metabolites (Fig. 11.10). Amiodarone is used to treat cardiac arrhythmias.
- *Gold.* Rheumatoid arthritis therapy with gold salts may lead to deposition of gold in the liver parenchyma.

- *Iron.* Hemochromatosis raises liver attenuation by deposition of iron. Primary hemochromatosis is characterized by increased intestinal absorption of iron, with deposition of hemosiderin in hepatocytes, and in the parenchyma of the pancreas and other organs, eventually causing cellular injury and loss of function. In secondary hemochromatosis (also called *hemosiderosis*) iron overload from multiple blood transfusions is taken up by reticuloendothelial cells in the liver, spleen, and bone marrow. Hemochromatosis commonly progresses to cirrhosis. Magnetic resonance imaging is the most sensitive for confirming the presence of iron excess in the liver.
- *Copper.* Wilson disease is associated with increased liver attenuation by deposition of copper.
- *Glycogen.* Glycogen storage diseases mildly raise liver attenuation.
- *Thorium.* Thorotrast, containing thorium dioxide, was used as a radiographic contrast agent from 1928 to the 1950s. Thorium is weakly radioactive and was found to be associated with development of hepatic angiosarcoma, cholangiocarcinoma, and HCC. High-attenuation thorium deposition in the reticuloendothelial system of the liver, spleen, and lymph nodes may be apparent even on conventional radiographs.

Cirrhosis

Cirrhosis is a chronic diffuse liver disease characterized by progressive destruction of liver parenchyma with distortion of hepatic architecture by extensive fibrosis and nodular regeneration of liver tissue. Common causes of cirrhosis include chronic alcoholism, chronic viral hepatitis, NASH, chronic biliary stasis associated with primary sclerosing cholangitis and primary biliary cirrhosis, and genetic diseases such as autoimmune hepatitis, Wilson disease, and hemochromatosis. Patients with cirrhosis show the following CT findings:

- In the earliest stages of cirrhosis the liver may appear normal on CT.
- Fatty infiltration with hepatomegaly is evidence of active hepatocyte injury.
- Heterogeneous parenchymal attenuation on non-contrast CT is as a result of patchy fatty infiltration and irregular fibrosis (Fig. 11.11). Contrast enhancement is heterogeneous as well and accentuates the diverse appearance of the liver tissue.
- The surface contour of the liver is finely nodular or irregular lobulated caused by areas of parenchymal atrophy and regenerative nodules (Fig. 11.12).

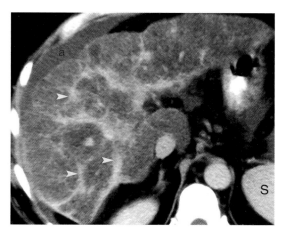

FIG. 11.11 Advanced cirrhosis with fatty infiltration. Delayed portal venous phase CT image showing the liver to be misshapen and nodular in contour. Overall parenchymal attenuation significantly lower than that of the spleen *(S)* is indicative of fatty infiltration and continuing liver injury. Prominent scars and bands of fibrosis *(arrowheads)* are seen throughout the liver. Ascites *(a)* is present.

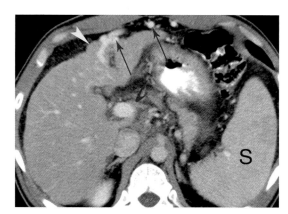

FIG. 11.12 Cirrhosis with portal hypertension. Post-contrast CT reveals the liver to be nodular in contour *(yellow arrowhead)* with patent enlarged paraumbilical veins *(straight red arrows)* and splenomegaly *(S)*, findings indicative of portal hypertension. Mildly enlarged portosystemic collateral vessels *(curved red arrow)* are also evident in the gastrohepatic ligament.

- Atrophy of the right lobe with hypertrophy of the left and caudate lobes is common and characteristic of alcoholic (Laënnec) micronodular cirrhosis. This finding is related to absorption of alcohol directly from the stomach with preferential flow of blood from the stomach to the right hepatic lobe in the portal venous system.

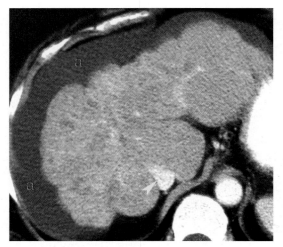

FIG. 11.13 **Advanced cirrhosis.** The liver is shrunken, with markedly nodular contour and heterogeneous parenchyma. Hepatic vessels are distorted and poorly visualized. Ascites *(a)* is present. The inferior vena cava *(arrowhead)* is compressed and distorted by liver atrophy and progressive fibrosis.

- With progressive cirrhosis, total liver volume decreases and the liver appears shrunken and deformed (Fig. 11.13).
- The size and prominence of the porta hepatis and intrahepatic fissures increase because of atrophy of adjacent liver tissue.
- Ascites, splenomegaly, and other signs of portal hypertension are commonly present.
- Serous cysts may develop adjacent to intrahepatic and extrahepatic bile ducts. These peribiliary cysts may mimic biliary dilatation when present in a linear configuration. More typically they appear as a row of cysts with thin but visible cyst walls.
- Enlarged lymph nodes (>1 cm) are commonly seen in the porta hepatis and portocaval space in patients with advanced cirrhosis. These are usually benign, associated with the development of cirrhosis, and not indicative of a malignant process.
- Ultrasound and magnetic resonance elastography are used to quantitate liver fibrosis in patients with suspected cirrhosis.
- Percutaneous liver biopsy, often guided by ultrasound, remains the gold standard for evaluation of cirrhosis.
- Mimics of cirrhosis include treated breast cancer metastases causing retraction of the liver capsule, irregular liver contour, and heterogeneous parenchymal nodularity; sarcoidosis with noncaseating granulomas causing fine nodularity of the liver surface and parenchymal granularity; miliary metastases causing surface nodularity; Budd-Chiari syndrome; and fulminant hepatic failure causing loss of parenchyma with distortion of liver contour.

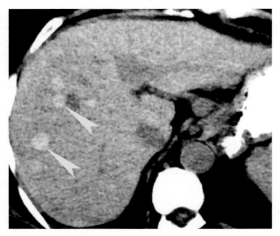

FIG. 11.14 **Siderotic regenerative nodules.** Noncontrast CT demonstrates several high-attenuation nodules *(arrowheads)* within a cirrhotic liver. These are siderotic regenerative nodules with high iron content.

Nodules in Cirrhosis

Nodular lesions in cirrhosis may be regenerative nodules, dysplastic nodules, or small HCCs. Regenerative nodules are present in all cirrhotic livers but are visualized on CT in only 25% of cases. They represent a local reparative response to injury with focal proliferation of hepatocytes and supporting stroma. Dysplastic nodules are premalignant; a nodular collection of hepatocytes that have cellular atypia and dysplastic features but no frank malignancy. HCC may develop spontaneously or as a result of progression of focal dysplasia.

- Regenerative nodules, although nearly always present pathologically, are usually not demonstrated on noncontrast CT because they are too small or are isodense with surrounding tissue. However, they may accumulate iron and show high attenuation on noncontrast CT (Fig. 11.14). These are termed *siderotic nodules.* Siderotic nodules usually disappear on postcontrast CT. When seen, regenerative nodules typically are not enhanced on arterial phase postcontrast CT. On portal venous phase, regenerative nodules are either not seen because they are enhanced homogeneously with surrounding tissue or appear hypodense because they are enhanced less than surrounding tissue (Fig. 11.15). Visualized regenerative nodules are typically smaller than 10 mm.

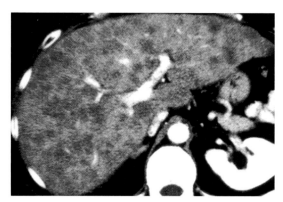

FIG. 11.15 **Regenerative nodules.** Portal venous phase postcontrast CT reveals numerous small (<10 mm) low-attenuation nodules in a cirrhotic liver. This shows unusually prominent visualization of regenerative nodules.

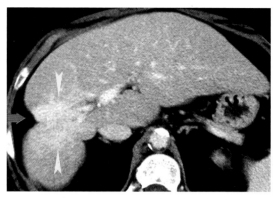

FIG. 11.16 **Confluent fibrosis.** Postcontrast axial CT image showing an ill-defined enhancing fibrotic mass *(yellow arrowheads)* extending from the liver periphery toward the porta hepatis associated with marked retraction *(red arrow)* of the liver capsule. This is the characteristic appearance of focal confluent fibrosis.

- A unique but very helpful finding is that often regenerative nodules appear larger on portal venous and delayed phase images than they do on precontrast or in arterial phase. This finding is not found with malignant nodules.
- Dysplastic nodules are not often demonstrated on CT. When seen, dysplastic nodules are slightly hypoattenuating or hyperattenuating on noncontrast CT. On postcontrast CT, most dysplastic nodules are enhanced homogeneously with surrounding liver tissue on both arterial and portal venous phase and are not detectable and show no enhancement on arterial, portal, and equilibrium postcontrast images. Siderotic nodules larger than 10 mm are considered dysplastic. A small number of dysplastic nodules demonstrate homogeneous enhancement on arterial phase images, and are isodense with parenchyma on portal venous, equilibrium, and delayed phase images. These are distinguishable from HCC only by biopsy.
- Small HCC nodules are hypointense or isointense to surrounding tissue on noncontrast CT. Hyperintense homogeneous enhancement in arterial phase images is the key finding that suggests HCC. The hallmark findings of HCC, considered to be diagnostic without biopsy, are near isointensity on noncontrast CT with hyperenhancement in arterial phase images and rapid contrast agent washout in portal venous phase images. Up to 50% of pathologically proven small HCC nodules are not detectable because they are isodense to parenchyma on all pre- and post contrast phase images.

- Diffuse metastatic disease, especially associated with breast cancer, may mimic cirrhosis with nodules. Medical history usually provides the differentiation. Innumerable small metastases may also be seen with small cell lung carcinoma, melanoma, carcinoid, and occasionally pancreatic carcinoma.
- Hemangiomas are rarely seen in cirrhotic livers. The process of parenchymal injury and scarring results in complete fibrosis of most hemangiomas, so they are not detected.
- Hepatic cysts are present at the same frequency as in noncirrhotic livers but are usually easily diagnosed by uniform low attenuation, sharp margination with imperceptible wall, and lack of contrast enhancement.

Focal Confluent Fibrosis

Focal confluent fibrosis describes a process of progressive hepatic parenchymal tissue loss with replacement by a fibrotic mass that occurs commonly in cirrhotic livers, especially those related to alcohol abuse.

- The lesion appears as a focal, commonly wedge-shaped, fibrotic mass extending from the porta hepatis to the liver periphery associated with retraction or flattening of the liver capsule caused by tissue loss (Fig. 11.16). The lesion is of low attenuation on noncontrast CT and shows delayed but persistent enhancement extending into the equilibrium phase.
- Serial imaging over time shows moderate progression of tissue loss and capsular retraction.

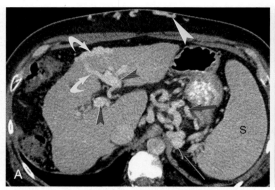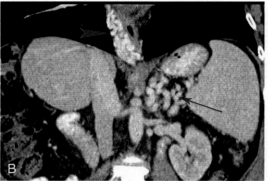

FIG. 11.17 Portal hypertension. (A) Axial postcontrast CT shows signs of advanced portal hypertension in a patient with cirrhosis. The liver is shrunken and nodular in contour. The right and left portal veins *(red arrowheads)* are enlarged, each measuring 15 mm. Dilated and tortuous cardinal veins *(fat red arrow)* are seen in the gastrohepatic ligament and retroperitoneum *(skinny red arrow)*. Paraumbilical collateral veins are patent and dilated, extending through the fissure of the ligamentum teres and falciform ligament *(yellow curved arrows)* and as subcutaneous collaterals *(yellow arrowhead)*. Visualization of patent paraumbilical collateral veins is the most specific CT sign of portal hypertension. The spleen *(S)* is enlarged. (B) Coronal CT image of the same patient showing dramatic paraesophageal varices *(arrowhead)* and the tangle of the retroperitoneal and perigastric collaterals *(arrow)*.

Portal Hypertension

Portal hypertension, defined as pathologic increase in portal venous pressure, results from progressive fibrosis of the hepatic vascular bed with development of portosystemic collateral vessels and eventually hepatofugal flow (i.e., flow away from, instead of into, the liver). Portal hypertension causes major morbidity in the patient with cirrhosis because of hepatic encephalopathy and variceal hemorrhage. Portal hypertension can be diagnosed on CT by the presence of the following anatomic signs:

- Portosystemic collateral vessels enlarge as they shunt blood between the portal and systemic veins (Fig. 11.17). Findings include esophageal, paraesophageal, and gastric varices; enlarged paraumbilical veins that connect with enlarged subcutaneous veins around the umbilicus (caput medusae); splenorenal shunts; and perisplenic collaterals. Varices appear as well-defined, round, serpentine structures that are enhanced homogenously with contrast agent during portal venous and delayed phases (Fig. 11.17B).
- The portal vein and branches are enlarged (>13 mm) (Fig. 11.17A).
- The splenic and superior mesenteric veins are enlarged (>10 mm). With engorgement of the mesenteric veins the bowel often appears edematous and thick walled.

- When a splenorenal shunt is present, the left renal vein is enlarged.
- Splenomegaly is usually evident because of splenic congestion.
- Ascites is often present.
- The enlarged collateral vessels characteristic of portal hypertension may be subtle and easily missed or may be mistaken for other structures. You see what you look for!

Portal Vein Thrombosis

Thrombosis of the portal vein is found in association with cirrhosis, hepatoma, hypercoagulability, pancreatitis, pancreatic cancer, trauma, or mesenteric inflammation. Portal vein thrombosis can cause or exacerbate portal hypertension. Thrombosis may be partial or complete, acute or chronic. Thrombosis may be classified as bland or as neoplastic if tumor extends into the portal veins. HCC is the most common cause of tumor extending into the portal vein. In patients with large HCC, bland portal vein thrombus is reported as present in as many as 20% of patients and tumor thrombus is present in as many as 33%. Thrombus may extend into the splenic and superior mesenteric veins. The signs of portal vein thrombosis include the following:

- *Bland thrombus* is of low attenuation and nonenhancing filling or partially filling the lumen of the portal vein or branches the portal (Fig. 11.18).

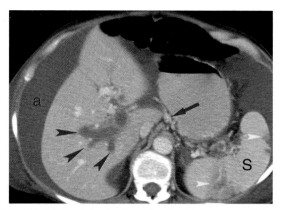

FIG. 11.18 **Portal vein thrombosis.** Postcontrast CT shows low-attenuation thrombus *(red arrowheads)* filling and distending the right portal vein and branches. Collaterals have formed in the gastrohepatic ligament *(red arrow)*. The spleen *(S)* shows multiple infarctions *(yellow arrowheads)*. The splenic vein (not shown) was also thrombosed. Ascites *(a)* is present.

- The diameter of the portal vein is often increased (>15mm).
- If thrombosis is complete, the portal vein is not enhanced on postcontrast scans. Failure to visualize the portal vein suggests complete thrombosis. When partial thrombosis is present, contrast-opacified blood outlines the low-attenuation clot.
- Nonmalignant partial portal vein thrombosis will spontaneously resolve in about half of cases.
- *Tumor thrombus* within the portal vein is of low attenuation on noncontrast CT. Contrast agent administration shows enhancement of tumor within the vein most prominent on arterial phase images. Intraluminal tumor enhancement parallels the timing and degree of enhancement of the primary tumor. The presence of tumor thrombus in patients with HCC usually excludes them as candidates for liver transplantation.
- *Cavernous transformation* refers to the development of numerous periportal collateral veins in response to chronic portal vein thrombosis, usually in patients with cirrhosis. CT demonstrates a nest of collateral vessels in the porta hepatis.
- Calcification may be seen within the portal vein when thrombus is chronic.
- Altered blood flow results in arterial perfusion changes within the liver parenchyma. Where venous blood flow is decreased, hepatic arterial blood flow is increased, showing hyperenhancement during the arterial phase. Parenchyma with chronic decreased

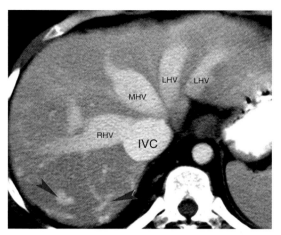

FIG. 11.19 **Passive hepatic congestion.** The inferior vena cava *(IVC)*, right hepatic vein *(RHV)*, middle hepatic vein *(MHV)*, and left hepatic vein *(LHV)* are massively dilated in this patient with chronic right-sided heart failure. Similar in physiology to Budd-Chiari syndrome, intrahepatic collateral vessels *(arrowheads)* have enlarged and are visualized as enhanced tubular and comma-shaped structures.

blood flow may atrophy, whereas lesser affected or unaffected parenchyma may show compensatory hypertrophy.

Passive Hepatic Congestion

In the presence of right-sided heart failure, constrictive pericarditis, or pericardial effusion the volume of returning venous blood exceeds the capacity of the right side of the heart, causing a rise in central venous pressure with dilatation of the IVC and hepatic veins. Chronic congestion and stasis in the hepatic sinusoids causes ischemic injury to hepatocytes, resulting in fatty infiltration and eventually cirrhosis.

- The hepatic veins and IVC are distended because the failing heart cannot accommodate venous return (Fig. 11.19). Perivascular edema may be present, seen as low-attenuation zones encircling the portal veins and intrahepatic IVC.
- Contrast medium injection into the upper extremities characteristically shows prominent retrograde flow of contrast medium deep into the hepatic veins. This pathologic finding must be differentiated from bland reflux of contrast medium into the upper IVC and distal hepatic veins sometimes seen with high-volume power injection.
- Hepatic parenchyma may be enhanced in a mottled mosaic pattern (termed *nutmeg liver*) similar to that seen with Budd-Chiari syndrome.

- Cardiomegaly, pleural and pericardial effusions, ascites, and hepatomegaly are frequently present.
- Decreased blood flow, hypoxia, and increased venous pressure lead to diffuse hepatocellular necrosis progressing to cirrhosis. Cardiac cirrhosis may be irreversible even if cardiac function improves.
- Magnetic resonance and ultrasound elastography are used to assess liver stiffness and the development of fibrosis in chronic cases.

Budd-Chiari Syndrome

Budd-Chiari syndrome refers to the manifestations of hepatic venous outflow obstruction, which causes elevated pressure in the sinusoids and decrease in portal venous flow, resulting in severe centrilobular congestion, hepatocellular necrosis, and parenchyma atrophy. Acute thrombosis of the main hepatic veins or IVC is associated with pregnancy, oral contraceptive use, chemotherapy, radiation therapy, and polycythemia vera. Neoplastic obstruction of the hepatic veins or IVC occurs with HCC, renal cell carcinoma, and adrenal carcinoma. Chronic fibrosis is idiopathic and affects small sublobular and central hepatic veins. Congenital causes include webs or diaphragms that obstruct the IVC. CT findings are variable depending on the chronicity of the disease.

- In acute Budd-Chiari syndrome (1–3 months), the liver is enlarged and hypoattenuating but with normal morphology on noncontrast CT. The IVC and hepatic veins are narrowed. Thrombus within the veins may be hyperattenuating. After contrast medium administration, the caudate lobe and liver surrounding the IVC show early arterial enhancement, with decreased enhancement of the liver periphery reflecting sinusoidal congestion. In the portal venous phase the liver periphery is enhanced while the contrast medium is washed out of the central liver, resulting in decreased attenuation. This has been termed the *flip-flop appearance* of liver enhancement. The hepatic veins and IVC show low attenuation with enhancement of the vein walls.
- In chronic Budd-Chiari syndrome the caudate lobe is enlarged, whereas the remainder of the liver is dysmorphic, with atrophy and multiple regenerative nodules. The caudate lobe is spared from injury because of its separate hepatic vein drainage directly into the IVC. The IVC and hepatic veins are collapsed and usually not visualized. Parenchymal enhancement is inhomogeneous, appearing as a mosaic pattern (Fig. 11.20). Parenchymal nodules, 1 to 4 cm in size, show hyperenhancement in the arterial phase persisting into the portal venous phase. Portal

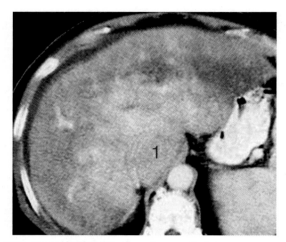

FIG. 11.20 Budd-Chiari syndrome. Portal venous phase postcontrast image showing a markedly abnormal mottled pattern of liver parenchymal enhancement with the central liver well enhanced and the peripheral liver poorly enhanced. Venography (not shown) demonstrated occlusion of the intrahepatic inferior vena cava and hepatic veins. The caudate lobe *(1)* is characteristically enlarged.

hypertension is present, resulting in splenomegaly and the presence of intrahepatic and extrahepatic portosystemic collateral vessels. Characteristic intrahepatic collateral vessels are seen as comma-shaped enhancing vessels, as is seen with passive hepatic congestion (Fig. 11.19). The azygos vein is enlarged, providing an alternative pathway for return of blood to the heart.

- Regenerative nodules are prominent and resemble multifocal HCC. The key finding is that regenerative nodules in Budd–Chiari syndrome remain relatively hyperdense in the portal venous phase, whereas early washout of contrast medium in the portal venous phase is characteristic of HCC.

Hereditary Hemorrhagic Telangiectasia

Also called *Osler-Weber-Rendu syndrome*, hereditary hemorrhagic telangiectasia (HHT) demonstrates prominent perfusion abnormalities on CT of the liver. HHT is an autosomal dominant disorder with variable penetrance characterized by multiorgan telangiectasias and arteriovenous malformations. The liver is involved in most cases (60%–75%), although liver involvement is often asymptomatic. The skin, mucous membranes, lungs, and brain are prominently affected. Patients present in adulthood with hemoptysis, epistaxis, and mucocutaneous telangiectasias. Many patients are asymptomatic when the disease is recognized by its

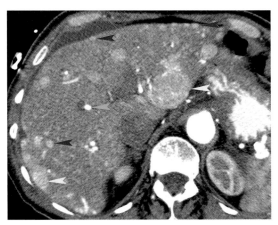

FIG. 11.21 **Hereditary hemorrhagic telangiectasia.**
Arterial phase postcontrast CT shows markedly heterogeneous enhancement of liver parenchyma with distinct
telangiectasias *(red arrowheads)*, confluent vascular channels *(yellow arrowheads)*, and early filling of portal veins
(blue arrowhead). Additional images (not shown) showed a
dilated and tortuous common hepatic artery.

imaging findings. CT findings are striking on arterial
phase images (Fig. 11.21).
- *Telangiectasias* are the most common findings in the
  liver. They are dilated small vessels that may be capillaries, venules, or arterioles. On CT they appear as
  hypervascular rounded masses from 1 to 10 mm in
  size. They appear hyperdense on early and late arterial
  phase images and become isodense with liver parenchyma on venous phase images. The overall appearance of diffuse telangiectasis is marked early phase
  heterogeneous enhancement of the liver parenchyma.
- Large *confluent vascular channels* (>1cm) form from
  coalescence of telangiectasias. Typically they are
  enhanced in the arterial phase, showing persisting
  enhancement as contrast medium pools within the
  vascular channels on venous phase.
- Vascular malformations are characterized by early
  contrast opacification and dilation of portal and hepatic veins. Arterial phase filling of the portal vein is
  indicative of arterioportal (hepatic artery to portal
  vein) shunts. Arterial phase filling of the hepatic vein
  is indicative of arteriovenous (hepatic artery to hepatic vein) shunts. Visualization of a vessel connecting
  portal veins to hepatic veins or the IVC is indicative
  of portovenous (portal vein to hepatic vein) shunts.
- As a result of extensive vascular shunting the common hepatic artery is dilated and tortuous, often
  exceeding 10 mm in diameter. A dilated common
  hepatic artery associated with diffuse heterogeneous

parenchymal enhancement is considered diagnostic
of HHT.
- Involvement of the liver by HHT may remain asymptomatic or result in portal hypertension caused by
  numerous shunts, hepatic encephalopathy, biliary
  disease, or high-output heart failure.
- Biliary disease in HHT is characterized by bile duct
  cysts, biliary strictures, and biliary dilatation. The
  findings are believed to result from biliary ischemia
  caused by extensive arteriovenous shunting. The ischemic biliary system is at risk of infection.
- Pancreatic lesions, including telangiectasias, arteriovenous fistulas, and arterial and venous aneurysms,
  are seen in 10% to 30% of patients.
- Thorax CT may show cardiomegaly, enlarged pulmonary arteries, and arteriovenous malformations
  in the lungs. Arteriovenous malformations may also
  be evident in the pancreas, gastrointestinal tract,
  and other organs.

Hepatic Sarcoidosis
Sarcoidosis is characterized by the presence of noncaseating granulomas scattered diffusely through multiple
organs and lymph nodes. The diagnosis is usually made
by the presence of characteristic findings in the chest.
The liver is affected pathologically in 94% of cases,
although most patients are asymptomatic with respect
to their liver disease. About 70% of patients with liver
involvement also have spleen involvement.
- The most common CT finding is hepatomegaly.
- Noncontrast CT may show innumerable small (sub-
  millimeter to 2 cm) hypoattenuating lesions in the
  liver and spleen. The appearance overlaps that of
  lymphoma.
- The lesions are hypovascular, showing little enhancement during the arterial phase, but may become isoattenuating with liver parenchyma in the
  portal venous phase.
- Diffuse lymphadenopathy is often present (30%)
  and sometimes massive (>2 cm nodes) (10%).
- A key to differentiating liver sarcoid from lymphoma, metastatic disease, or microabscesses is to note
  that the patient is young and generally not clinically
  ill or symptomatic.

Viral Hepatitis
The various forms of viral hepatitis are the most common
cause of liver disease worldwide. Acute viral hepatitis is
most commonly caused by hepatitis A virus, hepatitis B
virus, hepatitis C virus, or hepatitis E virus. Other viral
causes include hepatitis D virus, human immunodeficiency virus (HIV), Coxsackie virus, and herpes simplex

virus. Diagnosis is usually made clinically and by laboratory testing. Imaging may be obtained to exclude other conditions.

- On CT acute viral hepatitis may show heterogenous enhancement, periportal edema, focal low-attenuation areas, and gallbladder wall thickening.
- Acute fulminant viral hepatitis with liver failure appears on CT as an enlarged and edematous liver, heterogeneously low in attenuation on noncontrast CT. With contrast agent administration the liver parenchyma is enhanced irregularly and remains heterogeneous. Findings of confluent fibrosis and scarring are often evident on follow-up.
- Chronic viral hepatitis often appears normal on CT but may progress to hepatic fibrosis, cirrhosis, portal hypertension, ascites, and splenomegaly.

FOCAL LIVER MASSES

CT of the abdomen performed for any reason may reveal liver lesions that require accurate characterization. Clinically significant liver lesions require immediate treatment or follow-up and include malignancies, infections, and lesions that may hemorrhage or become malignant. Examples include metastases, HCC, choriocarcinoma, lymphoma, hepatic angiosarcoma, abscesses, and hepatic adenomas. Incidental liver lesions must be confidently diagnosed so that the patient can be reassured. Examples include benign liver cysts, hemangiomas, FNH, and focal fatty infiltration or sparing.

Predominantly Solid Liver Masses

Predominantly solid liver masses displace or replace hepatic parenchyma, have internal blood vessels, and are firm and stable in shape. Most predominantly solid masses may undergo cystic degeneration or necrosis.

Metastases

Metastases are the most common malignant tumors in the liver, outnumbering primary malignant tumors by a ratio of 18:1. Metastatic liver disease is a common cause of death in cancer patients. Liver metastases can originate from almost any primary malignant tumor, but most arise from the gastrointestinal tract, especially the colon. Usually, metastases are multiple, but the greatest problems in differentiation occur when they are solitary. A wide spectrum of CT appearance is possible:

- A well-defined low-attenuation solid mass with vague peripheral enhancement producing a target appearance is most common.

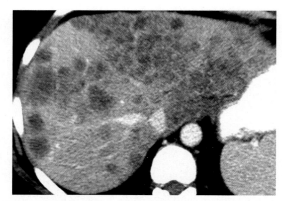

FIG. 11.22 **Metastases.** Postcontrast CT in the delayed phase shows innumerable ill-defined low-attenuation nodules throughout the enhanced liver. Many nodules show confluent growth. Hepatic vessels are distorted by the mass effect of these metastases from colon carcinoma.

- Hypovascular metastases are best seen during the portal venous phase, appearing with low density in a background of enhanced liver parenchyma. Metastases from colon cancer are characteristically hypovascular (Fig. 11.22).
- Hypervascular metastases show diffuse enhancement during the arterial phase, appearing bright on a background of darker liver parenchyma. Most hypervascular metastases show washout of contrast medium in the delayed phase. The most common hypervascular metastases are carcinoid, choriocarcinoma, melanoma, pancreatic neuroendocrine tumor, pheochromocytoma, renal cell carcinoma, and thyroid carcinoma. About 15% of breast cancer metastases to the liver are hypervascular. If the primary lesion is known to be hypervascular, arterial phase imaging is required for detection. Hypervascular metastases may not be detectable on portal venous phase imaging alone.
- Tiny liver nodules that cause perfusion changes in liver parenchyma are likely to be metastases.
- Metastases may appear with high attenuation on noncontrast scans, especially when the liver is fatty infiltrated.
- Cystic/necrotic tumors are nonenhancing and low in attenuation centrally. Common primary tumors include mucinous colon carcinoma, lung carcinoma, melanoma, and carcinoid.
- Metastases may be calcified when the primary neoplasm is mucinous adenocarcinoma, osteosarcoma, or chondrosarcoma.
- Diffusely infiltrating metastases mimic cirrhosis and may not appear as distinct masses.
- Metastases are uncommon in cirrhotic livers.

TABLE 11.3
LI-RADS Categories and Management

LI-RADS Category	Examples	Management
LR-1: definitely benign	Benign cyst, hemangioma, focal fat deposition or sparing, perfusion alteration such as arterioportal shunt, vascular anomalies, definite confluent fibrosis or focal scar, hypertrophic pseudomass	Continued routine surveillance, as appropriate
LR-2: probably benign	Examples as listed for LR-1 but with less confident findings	Continued routine surveillance, as appropriate
LR-3: intermediate probability of HCC	Includes nodules with features of focal nodular hyperplasia or hepatic adenoma	Variable follow-up (depends on clinical considerations)
LR-4: probably HCC		Additional imaging, biopsy, treatment, or close follow-up
LR-5: definitely HCC	100% certainty of HCC	Treat without biopsy Radiologic TMN staging
LR-TIV: definitely tumor invading vein		Treat without biopsy Radiologic TMN staging
LR-TR: treated, posttreatment observation categories		Close follow-up to assess treatment response. Retreat if needed
LR-M: probably or definitely malignant but not HCC	Cholangiocarcinoma, lymphoma, metastases	Biopsy, additional imaging, treatment, or close follow-up
LR-NC: not categorizable	Because of omission or degradation of key images or phases of contrast enhancement	

HCC, Hepatocellular carcinoma. *TMN staging*, American Joint Committee on Cancer tumor-node-metastases staging.
Modified from American College of Radiology. CT/MRI LI-RADS v2017. https://www.acr.org/Clinical-Resources/Reporting-and-Data-Systems/LI-RADS/CT-MRI-LI-RADS-v2017.

In summary, metastases can look like almost every other lesion in the liver and must always be considered a possibility.

Hepatocellular Carcinoma
Hepatoma is the most common primary hepatic malignancy. In Western countries, 80% of HCCs arise in cirrhotic livers. Most patients are older than 50 years. Elevated serum alpha-fetoprotein level is a common clinical clue to the diagnosis. Chronic hepatitis B and hepatitis C are major risk factors for development of HCC. About 12% of patients with chronic hepatitis develop HCC. HCC occurs in 3% to 6% of patients with other causes of cirrhosis. Detection of HCC on CT is limited by the extensive abnormalities seen with cirrhosis. Historically as many as 40% of all HCCs in cirrhotic livers are missed by CT.

To improve image detection, especially of small HCCs, the American College of Radiology created the Liver Imaging Reporting and Data System (LI-RADS) as a system for standardized acquisition, interpretation, reporting, and data collection specifically and solely for patients with cirrhosis, chronic hepatitis B viral infection, or current or prior HCC. LI-RADS does not apply to patients younger than 18 years or patients with cirrhosis caused by vascular disorders or congenital hepatic fibrosis. The system, periodically updated, applies to CT, magnetic resonance imaging, and contrast-enhanced ultrasound imaging findings. Liver lesions are characterized as to the relative risk of HCC using a defined lexicon and scoring algorithm (Table 11.3). See Suggested Reading for the American College of Radiology weblink for complete details and the most recent updates of LI-RADS.

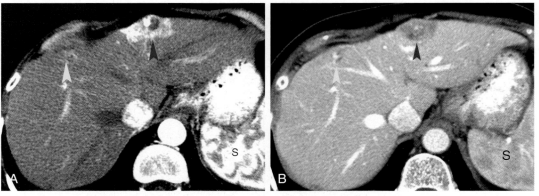

FIG. 11.23 **Small hepatocellular carcinomas.** Early arterial phase (A) and portal venous phase (B) CT images showing avid enhancement of a small lesion *(red arrowhead)* in the arterial phase with rapid wash-out in the portal venous phase, characteristic of hepatocellular carcinoma. A second smaller lesion *(yellow arrowhead)* with similar characteristics is partially seen. Note the exaggerated enhancement pattern of the spleen *(S)* in this patient with cirrhosis caused by chronic hepatitis C.

Small HCC, defined as less than 2 cm in diameter, overlap the appearance of high-grade dysplastic nodules. Detection leading to treatment of small HCC is a major goal of hepatic imaging in cirrhosis and LI-RADS (Fig. 11.23).

Major criteria used by LI-RADS for diagnosis of HCC include:

- Hyperenhancement of the lesion in the arterial phase definitely greater than that of liver parenchyma.
- Lesion "washout" defined as visual hypointensity of the lesion compared with liver parenchyma on portal venous and delayed phases.
- Peripheral rim of hyperenhancement of the capsule or pseudocapsule of the lesion on portal venous and delayed phase images.
- Threshold growth defined as an increase in diameter of the mass by at least 5 mm and 50% or greater increase in lesion diameter compared with the findings of imaging examinations performed less than 6 months previously, or 100% or greater increase in lesion diameter compared with the findings of examination performed more than 6 months previously, or a new 10-mm lesion regardless of the time interval. The size of the lesion is measured in the same phase and the same plane in serial CT or magnetic resonance imaging examinations.

Tumor in vein by LI-RADS criteria include:

- unequivocal enhanced soft tissue in hepatic or portal veins (definitive) (Fig. 11.24);
- occluded vein with ill-defined walls (not definitive);

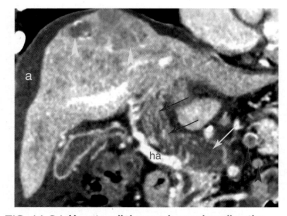

FIG. 11.24 **Hepatocellular carcinoma invading the portal vein.** Early arterial phase CT shown as a coronal plane image shows enhancing tumor vessels *(red arrows)* in a greatly dilated main portal vein. The tumor thrombus caused bland thrombosis of the splenic vein *(yellow arrow)* and mesenteric veins *(red arrowheads)*. The primary tumor shows as multiple nodules *(yellow arrowheads)* throughout the cirrhotic liver. Ascites *(a)* is present. The hepatic artery *(ha)* is dilated and tortuous.

- occluded or obscured vein in contiguity with malignant mass (not definitive);
- heterogeneous vein enhancement not attributable to artifact (nondefinitive).

Ancillary signs specifically favoring HCC by LI-RADS criteria include:

- nonenhancing capsule (smooth, uniform, sharp border around nodule);

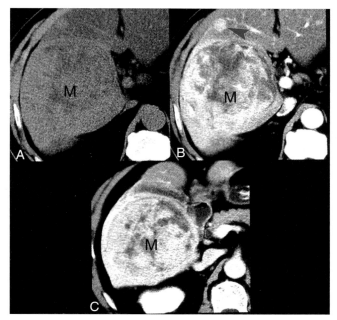

FIG. 11.25 **Hepatocellular carcinoma.** Noncontrast (A), arterial phase (B), and portal venous phase (C) images demonstrating early heterogenous enhancement of this hepatocellular carcinoma *(M)*. The tumor contains areas of hemorrhage and necrosis. A satellite tumor nodule *(red arrowhead)* is seen on the arterial phase image.

- "nodule-in-nodule" appearance (small nodule within a larger nodule and with imaging features different from those of the larger, outer nodule);
- mosaic architecture (randomly distributed small internal nodules with different imaging features);
- fat in mass, more than in adjacent liver;
- hemorrhage within or adjacent to the lesion without a history of biopsy or intervention.

Ancillary signs favoring malignancy (not specifically HCC) by LI-RADS criteria include:
- discrete nodule visible on ultrasonography as well as on CT or magnetic resonance imaging;
- increase in size of nodule but less than threshold criteria;
- relative paucity of fat in solid nodule relative to diffuse fatty liver.

Ancillary signs favoring benignity by LI-RADS criteria include:
- stable size for more than 2 years;
- unequivocal reduction in size;
- enhancement pattern that parallels blood pool enhancement;
- vessels traverse mass without displacement or distortion;
- presence of iron in mass.

Additional imaging features of HCC, especially tumors larger than 2 cm, include the following:
- HCCs show three major patterns of tumor growth: solitary tumor (50%), diffuse infiltrative tumor (30%), and multinodular tumor (20%) (see Fig. 11.26). Particularly characteristic is a dominant mass with nearby satellite lesions (Fig. 11.25).
- The infiltrative form of HCC consists of minute nodules spread throughout large regions of the liver, usually over multiple segments, an entire lobe, or even the entire liver. Prognosis is poor.
- The degree of hyperenhancement in the arterial phase varies with the grade of malignancy and the size of the tumor. HCCs larger than 2 cm typically show avid contrast enhancement in the arterial phase with washout in the portal venous or equilibrium phase.
- Well-differentiated HCC may be visualized best on portal venous phase CT images.
- Areas of tumor necrosis in larger tumors are common, and calcification is present in 25%.
- Tumor invasion of hepatic (12%–54%) and portal (29%–65%) veins is frequent (Fig. 11.24). Tumor extension into the IVC and right atrium may occur. A liver tumor seen in association with portal vein

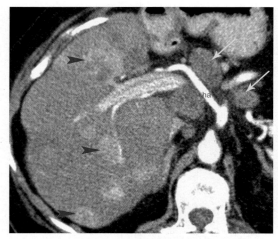

FIG. 11.26 **Multinodular hepatocellular carcinoma with lymph node metastases.** Late arterial phase CT image showing multiple enhancing nodules *(red arrowheads)* in the liver. These nodules showed washout on late portal venous phase images (not shown). This patient previously had the left hepatic lobe resected for a solitary hepatocellular carcinoma. Multiple lymph nodes *(yellow arrows)* involved with metastatic disease surround the common hepatic artery *(ha)*.

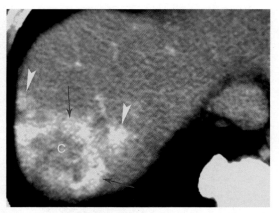

FIG. 11.27 **Peripheral mass-forming cholangiocarcinoma.** Arterial phase CT shows a poorly defined hyperenhancing mass in the right dome of the liver. Note the avid enhancement *(red arrows)* in the periphery of the tumor, while centrally *(C)* the tumor remains hypodense. Enhanced satellite nodules *(yellow arrowheads)* are present. Pathology confirmed cholangiocarcinoma.

thrombosis is very likely HCC, although peripheral cholangiocarcinomas may also invade the portal vein.
- Fat deposition may occur within HCC. Small well-differentiated HCC may show diffuse fatty change, lowering the attenuation of the nodule on noncontrast CT. Larger tumors tend to show patchy focal fatty metamorphosis.
- In patients with HIV and hepatitis C virus coinfection, HCC is more likely to be of diffuse infiltrative type, to invade the portal vein, and to have a dramatically worse prognosis.
- Extrahepatic spread of HCC to the lungs and pleura, lymph nodes in the abdomen (Fig. 11.26), bones, and adrenal glands is most common. Direct invasion by tumor may involve the diaphragm.

Intrahepatic Cholangiocarcinoma

Peripheral mass-forming intrahepatic cholangiocarcinoma (ICC) is the second most common primary malignant liver tumor, after HCC. As such it should be considered along with HCC in the differential diagnosis of focal solid liver tumors. It is an adenocarcinoma arising from the epithelium of the peripheral bile ducts. ICC accounts for 5% to 10% of all cholangiocarcinomas and 10% to 20% of all primary malignant liver tumors.

- Tumors appear as solid mass lesions with sharp-rounded, lobulated, or ill-defined margins. Most tumors are large at diagnosis, up to 15 cm in diameter. Retraction of the liver capsule, satellite nodules, and bile duct dilatation peripheral to the tumor are additional typical features. Invasion of adjacent peripheral branches of the portal vein is common and characteristic.
- On noncontrast CT most tumors are of low attenuation. Some are isodense with unenhanced liver parenchyma
- Following contrast medium administration, tumors typically show peripheral enhancement in arterial phase (Fig. 11.27). In portal venous phase most tumors wash out and become hypodense or isodense with liver parenchyma. This is followed by gradual central enhancement on delayed images. This marked homogeneous enhancement on delayed images is most characteristic of ICC. Most active tumor cells are peripheral and are enhanced early, whereas dense slowly enhancing fibrous stroma typically occupies the center of the tumor. A few tumors, especially those smaller than 3 cm, show diffuse hyperenhancement in arterial phase.
- Imaging features that differentiate ICC from HCC include the following: the presence of fat in HCC, not found in ICC; persistent central enhancement in ICC on delayed phase images, whereas HCC is

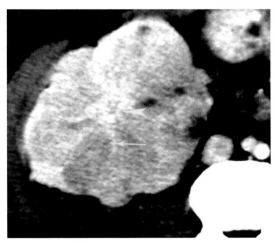

FIG. 11.28 **Fibrolamellar carcinoma.** Portal venous phase image showing a fibrolamellar carcinoma in a 37-year-old man replacing most of the right lobe of the liver. An enhanced central scar *(arrowhead)* with enhancing radiating fibrous bands *(arrow)* is faintly visualized.

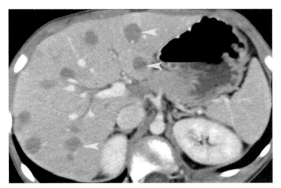

FIG. 11.29 **Secondary hepatic lymphoma.** Portal venous phase CT image revealing multiple low-attenuation nodules *(arrowheads)* in the liver in this patient with non-Hodgkin lymphoma. The spleen does not appear to be involved.

usually of homogeneous or heterogenous low attenuation on delayed phase images; peripheral bile duct dilatation favors ICC over HCC; both tumors commonly invade the portal vein.

- Periductal infiltrating and intraductal growing cholangiocarcinomas are reviewed in Chapter 12.

Fibrolamellar Carcinoma

Fibrolamellar HCC is a rare (<1% of all HCCs) entity distinct from HCC. It is a slow-growing tumor that usually arises in normal liver. Patients are younger (usually <40 years) than most HCC patients, and elevated serum alpha-fetoprotein level is not present. Prognosis is good if the tumor is completely resected.

- A large hepatic mass (often >12 cm in diameter) within a normal liver in a young adult or adolescent is characteristic.
- Noncontrast CT demonstrates a large low-attenuation lobulated mass with well-defined margins.
- On postcontrast scans the lesion is enhanced prominently and heterogeneously during both the arterial phase and the portal venous phase. Enhancement becomes more homogeneous and remains evident on delayed scans.
- Fibrous tissue extends through the mass separating the tumor into islands and commonly coalescing into a central scar (Fig. 11.28). The scar is visible on CT in up to 60% of cases. The scar is best seen on delayed scans and may calcify (33%–55%). Typically, enhancement

of the scar is not present on arterial and portal venous images but may be evident on delayed scans.

- Cirrhosis, vascular invasion, and multifocal disease common with HCC are rare with fibrolamellar carcinoma.
- Fibrolamellar carcinoma may be difficult to differentiate from FNH. Heterogeneous enhancement of the tumor with delayed enhancement of the central scar is a features that differentiates fibrolamellar carcinoma from FNH.
- Enlarged lymph nodes are present near the porta hepatis in 50% of cases.

Lymphoma

Secondary involvement by systemic lymphoma involves the liver in more than half of all patients with lymphoma; however, detection of liver involvement by CT is uncommon. Secondary lymphoma is diffuse or multiple, whereas very rare primary liver lymphoma is usually solitary.

- Diffuse infiltration may cause only hepatomegaly without altering parenchymal density.
- Multiple well-defined, large, homogeneous low-attenuation nodules are most characteristic of secondary lymphoma, especially Hodgkin lymphoma (Fig. 11.29). Lesions may show a target appearance with enhancement.
- The spleen is usually also involved, and abdominal adenopathy is usually present with secondary lymphoma.
- Primary liver lymphoma presents as a solitary large multilobulated mass (Fig. 11.30). Enhancement is usually weak.

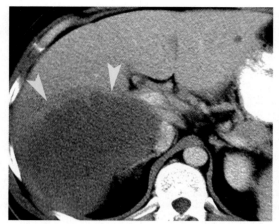

FIG. 11.30 Primary hepatic lymphoma. Portal venous phase CT reveals a large homogeneous poorly enhanced mass *(arrowheads)* largely replacing the right lobe. Chest-abdomen-pelvis CT showed no additional evidence of lymphoma. Biopsy confirmed primary hepatic lymphoma.

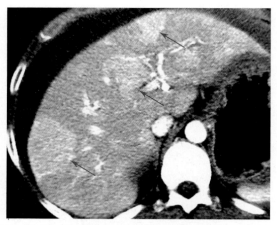

FIG. 11.31 Multiple hepatic adenomas. Arterial phase image showing homogeneous enhancement of multiple hepatic adenomas *(arrows)* in this woman with hepatic adenomatosis. Ascites is present because of associated impaired liver function.

Hepatic Adenoma

Hepatocellular adenoma is a rare benign tumor seen most often in young women (90%) who use oral contraceptives, in men who take anabolic steroids, and in patients with glycogen storage disease type 1. It is a significant lesion because of the risk of major hemorrhage associated with its presence. Hepatic adenomas are composed of neoplastic well-differentiated hepatocytes and lack bile ducts and portal triads. Kupffer cells are occasionally present but are nonfunctional. Most patients are asymptomatic and have normal liver function study findings. Surgical removal is often recommended because of the risk of rupture and malignant transformation. The imaging findings include the following:

- On unenhanced CT many adenomas, consisting of well-differentiated hepatocytes, are isoattenuating to normal liver parenchyma.
- In some tumors the hepatocytes become filled with fat and the lesion approaches fat density. Lipid content in adenomas tends to be more diffuse, whereas that in larger HCC tends to be focal and patchy. Patients typically do not have cirrhosis or viral hepatitis, and alpha-fetoprotein levels are not elevated.
- Hemorrhage may be most apparent on noncontrast scans. Fresh hemorrhage is of high attenuation, whereas old hemorrhage appears as heterogeneous low attenuation. Intratumoral hemorrhage is common, seen in 25% to 40% of adenomas.

- Calcifications are seen in 10% of tumors.
- Arterial phase postcontrast scans show early homogeneous enhancement (Fig. 11.31). Contrast medium washes out relatively rapidly, and the tumors become near isodense with liver parenchyma on portal venous phase and delayed postcontrast scans.
- Because Kupffer cells are few in number and dysfunctional, uptake of technetium-99m sulfur colloid is absent within the tumor on radionuclide scans.
- Tumors are solitary in 70% to 80% of cases. Lesions range in size from 1 to 15 cm.
- Multiple tumors are seen in patients with glycogen storage disease type 1 and hepatic adenomatosis (Fig. 11.31). Hepatic adenomatosis is defined as having 10 or more adenomas in the liver. Adenomatosis occurs with equal frequency in men and women.
- Tumors lack the central scar that is often present in FNH.

Focal Nodular Hyperplasia

In contrast to hepatic adenoma, FNH contains all the histologic elements of normal liver, including Kupffer cells. It is the second most common benign liver tumor, after cavernous hemangioma. Fibrous bands and central stellate fibrous scars are characteristic. Hemorrhage and necrosis are rare. Most patients are asymptomatic, and the tumor is discovered incidentally. Because the tumor is benign and without

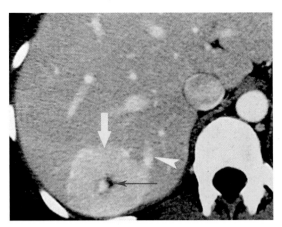

FIG. 11.32 **Focal nodular hyperplasia.** A brightly enhanced mass *(yellow arrow)* in the posterior segment of the right hepatic lobe has a characteristic central low-attenuation scar *(red arrow)*. A large draining vein *(yellow arrowhead)* is evidence of the hypervascular nature of the mass.

malignant potential or risk of rupture, no treatment is indicated. FNH is now considered a response of liver parenchyma to a preexisting vascular malformation such as an arteriovenous malformation or telangiectasia.

- Typically FNH is discovered incidentally as an asymptomatic solitary solid mass lesion in a young woman.
- Lesions are solitary (80%–95%) and usually smaller than 5 cm.
- On unenhanced CT, lesions are isodense or very slightly hypodense to normal liver parenchyma. The central scar may be hypodense (20%) or invisible (80%).
- The hallmark finding of immediate intense homogeneous enhancement is seen on arterial phase postcontrast CT. A central scar, if present, may remain hypodense (Fig. 11.32). Large feeding arteries may be evident.
- In portal venous phase, the lesion becomes nearly isodense with enhanced parenchyma. Large draining veins result in rapid washout of contrast agent.
- On delayed phase postcontrast images the lesion is usually isodense to parenchyma but the central scar may show enhancement.
- Normal (40%) or increased (10%) radionuclide uptake within the tumor on technetium-99m sulfur colloid–labeled liver scan is the most specific finding. However, 50% of the lesions show as a nonspecific cold defect.

Cavernous Hemangioma

Cavernous hemangiomas are the second most common focal mass lesion in the liver, exceeded in frequency only by metastases. They are the most common benign liver lesion, found in up to 7% of individuals. They are often discovered incidentally during hepatic imaging. They may be found at any age and are more common in women. Although most are solitary, 10% of affected patients have multiple lesions that may be mistaken for metastases. The lesions consist of large, thin-walled, blood-filled vascular spaces lined by epithelium and separated by fibrous septa. Blood flow through the complex of vascular spaces is very slow, resulting in characteristic prolonged retention of contrast agents on CT. Most lesions are less than 5 cm in diameter, are asymptomatic, and pose no threat to the patient. The lesions carry no risk of malignant transformation. Larger giant cavernous hemangiomas (20 cm or larger) may cause symptoms by pressure effect, hemorrhage, or arteriovenous shunting. About 90% of lesions show classic features on CT.

- On unenhanced CT hemangiomas appear as a well-defined hypodense mass of the same attenuation as other blood-filled spaces, such as the IVC or portal vein. Isoattenuation with blood vessels is an important diagnostic finding.
- Postcontrast arterial phase images show early, peripheral, discontinuous nodules of contrast enhancement equal in density to the enhancement of the aorta (Fig. 11.33).
- Portal venous phase images show progressive fill-in enhancement from the periphery, with the lesion eventually becoming uniformly enhanced.
- Delayed images show prolonged enhancement as a result of the characteristic slow washout of contrast agent. Contrast enhancement usually persists within the lesion for 20 to 30 minutes after contrast agent injection.
- Because blood flow is slow through the lesion, thrombosis may occur, leading to irregular areas of fibrosis, which remain unenhanced throughout the postcontrast phases of CT. Occasionally these fibrotic portions of the lesion may show particulate or dense calcification.
- Small hemangiomas, especially those smaller than 1 cm, may show immediate homogeneous enhancement during the arterial phase, mimicking HCC and hypervascular metastases. Differentiation is made by observing the slow washout and persistent enhancement during the portal venous phase and on delayed images that is characteristic of hemangiomas but not the hypervascular tumors.

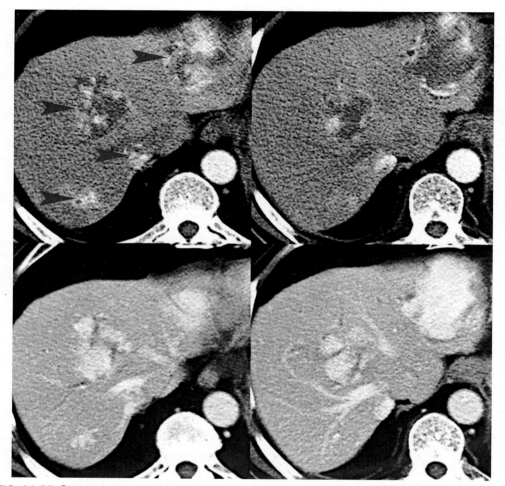

FIG. 11.33 **Cavernous hemangiomas.** Arterial phase (top row) and portal venous phase (bottom row) images demonstrating the characteristic enhancement pattern of multiple cavernous hemangiomas *(arrowheads)*. Early contrast medium enhancement appears nodular and at the periphery. Enhancement proceeds centrally to complete opacification, except for areas of fibrous scarring in large lesions.

- Most hemangiomas remain stable in size over time.
- When classic findings are observed, the CT examination can be considered diagnostic of cavernous hemangioma with a high degree of confidence. In questionable cases, tagged red blood cell scintigraphy is usually diagnostic.
- Hemangiomas are rarely seen in cirrhotic livers. This soft lesion is obliterated by progressive fibrosis.

Predominantly Cystic Liver Masses

Predominantly cystic liver masses contain fluid that may differ widely in composition. Cystic masses may contain simple fluid, protein-rich fluid, pus, bile, blood, and combinations of fluid types. Identification of solid components in cystic lesions is a key imaging finding.

Hepatic Cysts

Simple benign hepatic cysts are developmental unilocular cysts lined by a single thin layer of cuboidal bile duct epithelium. They are found in up to 20% of the population, most commonly in patients aged 40 to 70 years. They cause no symptoms and are usually discovered incidentally. They have no malignant potential but must be differentiated from significant lesions. Multiple very tiny cysts may mimic early metastases.

- On unenhanced CT cysts are well defined and of low density with internal attenuation of water (<20 HU). The cyst wall is not perceptible (Fig. 11.34). They are a few millimeters to several centimeters in size. They may be solitary or multiple.

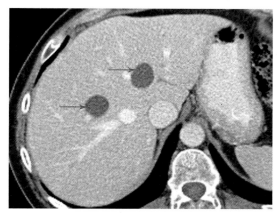

FIG. 11.34 **Simple hepatic cysts.** Postcontrast CT shows the classic appearance of simple hepatic cysts *(arrows)*. Simple hepatic cysts have uniform low internal density and sharp margins with the surrounding hepatic parenchyma. No cyst walls are evident. The lesions do not enhance with intravenous contrast medium administration.

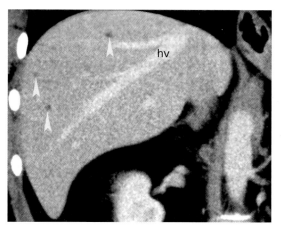

FIG. 11.35 **Biliary hamartomas.** Coronal plane post-contrast CT shows the typical appearance of tiny biliary hamartomas *(arrowheads)*. The diagnosis was confirmed by magnetic resonance imaging, which showed many more lesions. *hv,* Middle hepatic vein.

- No enhancement is seen in any phase of postcontrast scans.
- Very tiny cysts may not measure the low attenuation of water because of volume averaging. A confident diagnosis of a benign cyst can be made by noting uniform low attenuation, sharply defined borders, and stability over time.

Biliary Cystadenomas

Biliary cystadenomas are uncommon cystic neoplasms that arise from mucin-secreting columnar epithelium of the bile ducts similar to cystadenomas of the pancreas and ovary. They occur predominantly in middle-aged women and have the potential to develop into cystadenocarcinomas. The risk of malignant transformation is about 20%.

- Lesions appear as a complex cystic mass ranging in size from 3 to 40 cm. They have a well-defined, thick fibrous capsule, and most have internal septations. Attenuation of internal fluid is usually of water density but may be higher if internal hemorrhage has occurred. Calcifications may occur in the cyst wall and septa. The tumor may cause peripheral dilation of the bile ducts.
- Septa and the cyst wall demonstrate contrast enhancement.
- Enhanced tumor nodules and papillary projections may be seen with both cystadenomas and cystadenocarcinomas, which cannot be differentiated by imaging. Because of the risk of malignancy, surgical removal is often recommended.

Biliary Hamartomas

Biliary hamartomas (von Meyenburg complexes) are multiple small predominantly cystic lesions that occur throughout the liver and result from failure of involution of embryologic bile ducts. They are considered benign, are asymptomatic, and do not require treatment. However, a few isolated case reports indicate possible degeneration into cholangiocarcinoma.

- Biliary hamartomas are small (<15 mm), usually innumerable, hypoattenuating lesions scattered throughout the liver (Fig. 11.35). Lesions typically appear as simple cysts with predilection for the subcapsular region. Larger lesions may show rim enhancement. Absence of communication with the biliary tree differentiates them from Caroli disease. Lesions may appear more prominent and numerous on magnetic resonance imaging than on CT.

Polycystic Liver Disease

Polycystic liver disease occurs in association with autosomal dominant polycystic kidney disease (70% of cases), or as a genetically distinct autosomal dominant polycystic liver disease without renal involvement. Most patients are asymptomatic. Despite often massive replacement of liver parenchyma by cysts, most patients maintain normal liver function. Complications are uncommon but include massive hepatomegaly, abdominal pain, intracystic hemorrhage and infection, and portal hypertension. Two types of cysts may be identified:

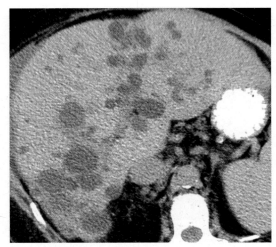

FIG. 11.36 Polycystic liver disease. Noncontrast CT of the liver in a patient with autosomal dominant polycystic kidney disease shows innumerable hepatic cysts of variable sizes.

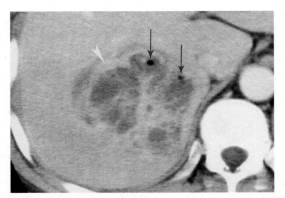

FIG. 11.37 Pyogenic liver abscess. A liver abscess containing *Escherichia coli* has a thick enhanced wall *(yellow arrowhead)*, has irregular septations, and contains a few bubbles of air *(red arrows)*. Because of the multiple loculations, this abscess did not respond to percutaneously placed catheter drainage but required surgical débridement.

- Most cysts are peripheral and resemble simple cysts in appearance with thin walls and internal fluid contents of water attenuation (Fig. 11.36). These cysts are numerous, replacing and displacing hepatic parenchyma. They may be large, exceeding 8 cm in diameter.
- Peribiliary cysts are smaller (<1 cm) and multiple, appearing as a string of multiple cysts paralleling the course of the portal triads.

Infected or hemorrhagic cysts show increased attenuation of the internal fluid, fluid-fluid levels, thickened walls with enhancement, and rarely intracystic gas bubbles. Old infected or hemorrhagic cysts may have calcifications in the cyst wall.

Pyogenic Abscess

Bacterial hepatic abscess is a localized collection of pus and debris within an area of destroyed liver parenchyma. Bacterial seeding occurs by way of the portal vein, hepatic artery, or biliary tree, by direct extension from bowel infection (appendicitis, diverticulitis), or as a result of trauma. Approximately 85% of liver abscesses in the United States are pyogenic, most caused by *Escherichia coli*. Patients are usually clinically septic and are often jaundiced.

- Bacterial abscess is usually solitary but often multiloculated with thickened enhancing walls. Internal fluid measures 0 to 45 HU. When multiple, lesions are often grouped and consist of many microabscesses. Masses are hypodense with a peripheral rim that is usually enhanced with contrast medium.

- Gas bubbles are present within the lesion in 20% of cases (Fig. 11.37). Gas may also be seen in bile ducts.
- Fine-needle aspiration is indicated for bacterial culture. Catheter or surgical aspiration and drainage and intravenous antibiotics are needed.
- Biliary obstruction and thrombophlebitis are the most common associated findings.

Amebic Abscess

Amebic abscess occurs in 3% to 7% of patients with amebiasis (*Entamoeba histolytica*). Amebic abscesses account for 6% of liver abscesses in the United States. Amebic serology findings are positive in 95% of cases. Patients present acutely ill with high temperature and right upper quadrant pain. Amebic abscesses are most common in Africa, Southeast Asia, India, South America, Central America, and Mexico. Patients with the disease in the United States often have a history of recent travel to these areas.

- The abscess (Fig. 11.38) is usually solitary (85%) and in the right lobe (72%).
- The CT appearance overlaps that of pyogenic abscess. The wall is well-defined, thickened (3–15 mm), sometimes nodular, and enhances with contrast agent administration. The liver parenchyma adjacent to the wall of the abscess is also commonly enhanced, producing a double-rim target appearance. The cavity may show fluid-debris levels, hemorrhage, gas bubbles, and multiple septa.
- Right pleural effusion and right lower lobe infiltration are often present. The abscess may rupture through the diaphragm, resulting in empyema.

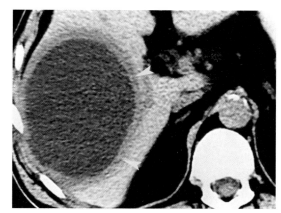

FIG. 11.38 **Amebic abscess.** An American living in Thailand returned to the United States with this mass in his liver. Although the internal density is homogeneously low, a distinct thick wall *(arrowheads)* is present and was observed to be enhanced with intravenous contrast medium administration. Serologic titers were positive for amebiasis.

Hydatid Cyst

Hydatid disease is produced by the larval stage of the tapeworm *Echinococcus granulosus*. The liver is the most common site of disease. The disease is not endemic in the United States, so cases are seen mainly in immigrants and travelers to endemic areas, primarily sheep-grazing areas in South America, Australia, New Zealand, Africa, the Middle East, and the Mediterranean. The disease is acquired from contaminated food. Most patients have eosinophilia. Serology findings are positive in only 25% of patients.

- The appearance of the hydatid cyst (Fig. 11.39) depends on its stage of growth. The cyst may be unilocular, contain daughter cysts, or completely calcified (dead).
- The cyst wall is usually of high attenuation and is commonly calcified (50%). The internal fluid is usually of near water attenuation. Layering debris (hydatid sand) is commonly present within the cysts. Detached floating membranes are sometimes evident.
- Daughter cysts present a cyst-within-a-cyst appearance. The daughter cysts may be separated by a hydatid matrix that produces a spoke wheel appearance.

Fungal Infection: Microabscesses

Fungal infection usually occurs only in immune-compromised patients. Fungal infection in the liver typically manifests itself as numerous disseminated tiny microabscesses. *Candida albicans* is the most common causative organism. Infection is spread hematogenously via the portal venous system from the intestinal tract. Complications include cholangitis and rupture of the microabscesses.

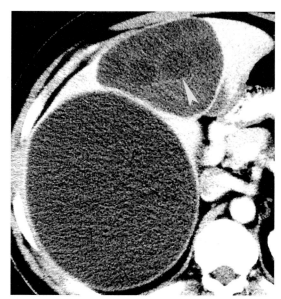

FIG. 11.39 **Hydatid cysts.** Two hydatid cysts are seen in the right lobe of the liver. Several daughter cysts *(arrowhead)* are faintly visualized in the anterior lesion. Ultrasonography confirmed the presence of the daughter cysts and revealed thin internal membranes and hydatid sand.

- CT shows innumerable hypoattenuating hypovascular lesions (2–20 mm in size) throughout the liver, usually best seen on arterial phase images. Peripheral ring enhancement may occur, but the lesions are not enhanced centrally.
- Similar lesions are commonly present in the spleen and kidneys.
- With healing, the lesions may calcify.

SUGGESTED READING

American College of Radiology. CT/MRI LI-RADS v2017. https://www.acr.org/Clinical-Resources/Reporting-and-Data-Systems/LI-RADS/CT-MRI-LI-RADS-v2017.

Bächler, P., Baladron, M. J., Menias, C., et al. (2016). Multimodality imaging of liver infections: Differential diagnosis and potential pitfalls. *Radiographics, 36*, 1001–1023.

Bandali, M. F., Mirakhur, A., Lee, E. W., et al. (2017). Portal hypertensions: Imaging of portosystemic collateral pathways and associated image-guided therapy. *World Journal of Gastroenterology, 23*, 1735–1746.

Borhani, A. A., Wiant, A., & Heller, M. T. (2014). Cystic hepatic lesions: A review and an algorithmic approach. *AJR. American Journal of Roentgenology, 203*, 1192–1204.

Elsayes, K. M., Shaaban, A. M., Rothan, S. M., et al. (2017). A comprehensive approach to hepatic vascular disease. *Radiographics, 27*, 813–836.

Ferral, H., Behrens, G., & Lopera, J. (2012). Budd-Chiari syndrome. *AJR. American Journal of Roentgenology, 199*, 737–745.

Ganeshan, D., Szklaruk, J., Kundra, V., et al. (2014). Imaging features of fibrolamellar hepatocellular carcinoma. *AJR. American Journal of Roentgenology, 202*, 544–552.

Huber, A., Ebner, L., Heverhagen, J. T., & Christe, A. (2015). State-of-the-art imaging of liver fibrosis and cirrhosis: A comprehensive review of current applications and future perspectives. *Eur J Radiol Open, 2*, 90–100.

Jha, P., Poder, L., Wang, Z. J., et al. (2010). Radiologic mimics of cirrhosis. *AJR. American Journal of Roentgenology, 194*, 993–999.

Kim, H. J., Kim, A. Y., Kim, T. K., et al. (2005). Transient hepatic attenuation difference in focal hepatic lesions: Dynamic CT features. *AJR. American Journal of Roentgenology, 184*, 83–90.

Kouri, B. E., Abrams, R. A., Al-Refaie, W., et al. (2016). ACR appropriateness criteria radiologic management of hepatic malignancy. *Journal of The American College of Radiology, 13*, 265–273.

Lawrence, D. A., Oliva, I. B., & Isreal, G. M. (2012). Detection of hepatic steatosis on contrast-enhanced CT images: Diagnostic accuracy of identification of areas of presumed focal fatty sparing. *AJR. American Journal of Roentgenology, 199*, 44–47.

Lee, S. S., & Park, S. H. (2014). Radiologic evaluation of non-alcoholic fatty liver disease. *World Journal of Gastroenterology, 20*, 7392–7402.

Pal, P., & Ray, S. (2016). Alcoholic liver disease: A comprehensive review. *European Medical Journal, 1*, 85–92.

Pickhardt, P. J., Hahn, L., Muñoz del Rio, A., et al. (2014). Natural history of hepatic steatosis: Observed outcomes for subsequent liver and cardiovascular complications. *AJR. American Journal of Roentgenology, 202*, 752–758.

Seo, N., Kim, D. Y., & Choi, J.-Y. (2017). Cross-sectional imaging of intrahepatic cholangiocarcinoma: Development, growth, spread, and prognosis. *AJR. American Journal of Roentgenology, 209*, W64–W75.

Sneag, D. B., Krajewski, K., Giardino, A., et al. (2011). Extrahepatic spread of hepatocellular carcinoma: Spectrum of imaging findings. *AJR. American Journal of Roentgenology, 197*, W658–W664.

Strasberg, S. M., & Phillips, C. (2013). Use and dissemination of the Brisbane 2000 nomenclature of liver anatomy and resections. *Annals of Surgery, 257*, 377–382.

Terminology Committee of the International Hepato-Pancreato-Biliary Association. (2000). The Brisbane 2000 terminology of liver anatomy and resections. *HPB, 2*, 333–339.

Tomasian, A., Sandrasegaran, K., Elsayes, K. M., et al. (2015). Hematologic malignancies of the liver: Spectrum of disease. *Radiographics, 35*, 71–86.

Venkatesh, S. K., Chandan, V., & Roberts, L. R. (2014). Liver masses: A clinical, radiologic, and pathologic perspective. *Clinical Gastroenterology and Hepatology, 12*, 1414–1429.

Vilgrain, V., Lagadec, M., & Ronot, M. (2016). Pitfalls in liver imaging. *Radiology, 278*, 34–51.

Wells, M. L., Fenstad, E. R., Poterucha, J. T., et al. (2016). Imaging findings of congestive hepatopathy. *Radiographics, 36*, 1024–1037.

Wu, J. S., Saluja, S., Garcia-Tsao, G., et al. (2006). Liver involvement in hereditary hemorrhagic telangiectasia: CT and clinical findings do not correlate in symptomatic patients. *AJR. American Journal of Roentgenology, 187*, W399–W405.

Younossi, Z., Anstee, Q. M., Marietti, M., et al. (2018). Global burden of NAFLD and NASH: Trends, predictions, risk factors, and prevention. *Nature Reviews of Gastroenterology and Hepatology, 15*, 11–20.

CHAPTER 12

Biliary Tree and Gallbladder

WILLIAM E. BRANT

BILIARY TREE

Primary imaging of the biliary tree depends increasingly on CT, ultrasonography, magnetic resonance imaging, and magnetic resonance cholangiopancreatography, and with diminishing reliance on invasive endoscopic retrograde cholangiopancreatography. Multidetector CT (MDCT) with thin sections and multiplanar reformats can clearly demonstrate the normal anatomy, anatomic variants, stones, tumors, and inflammatory disease of the biliary system.

Anatomy

The bile ducts arise as biliary capillaries between hepatocytes. Bile capillaries coalesce to form intrahepatic bile ducts. Intrahepatic bile ducts branch in a predictable manner corresponding to the segments of the liver. Interlobular bile ducts combine to form two main trunks from the right and left lobes of the liver. The 3- to 4-cm-long common hepatic duct is formed in the porta hepatis by the junction of the main right and left bile ducts. The cystic duct runs posteriorly and inferiorly from the gallbladder neck to join the common hepatic duct and form the common bile duct (CBD). The 6- to 7-cm-long CBD courses ventral to the portal vein and to the right of the hepatic artery, descending from the porta hepatis along the free right border of the hepatoduodenal ligament to behind the duodenal bulb. Its distal third turns directly caudad, descending in the groove between the descending duodenum and the head of the pancreas just ventral to the inferior vena cava. The CBD tapers distally as it ends in the sphincter of Oddi, which protrudes into the duodenum as the ampulla of Vater. The CBD and the pancreatic duct share a common orifice in 60% of cases and have separate orifices in the remainder. In any case, they are in such close proximity that tumors of the ampullary region will generally obstruct both ducts.

Thin collimation (1–2.5-mm) MDCT with dynamic bolus intravenous contrast enhancement reveals normal intrahepatic ducts in about 40% of patients. Normal intrahepatic ducts are 2 mm in diameter in the central liver and taper progressively toward the periphery. The common hepatic duct is usually seen in the porta hepatis, and the CBD is routinely visualized descending adjacent to the descending duodenum. It is fair to use the generic term *common duct* to refer to both the common hepatic duct and the CBD because the cystic duct junction marking their anatomic partition is not routinely visualized on CT. The normal common duct does not exceed 6 mm in diameter in most adult patients. In elderly patients the normal common duct diameter increases by about 1 mm per decade (i.e., 7 mm is normal for patients in their 70s, and 8 mm is normal for those in their 80s). Contrast medium enhancement improves identification of both normal and dilated bile ducts by enhancing blood vessels and the surrounding parenchyma. Bile ducts are seen as lucent branching tubular structures. The bile ducts may be difficult to differentiate from blood vessels without contrast agent administration.

Technique

Evaluation for biliary obstruction is the most common reason to perform CT of the bile ducts. Water is preferred as an oral contrast agent in this clinical setting because high-density contrast in the duodenum may cause streaks and obscure stones in the adjacent CBD.

- The patient drinks 300 mL of water in 15 to 20 minutes just before CT examination.
- Thin sections (0.625–2.5 mm) with MDCT provide high-resolution images of the bile ducts.
- Multiphase imaging is commonly used. Stones may be seen best on noncontrast images. Scanning during the arterial phase demonstrates pancreatic lesions best. Delayed imaging at 15 to 20 minutes after intravenous contrast medium administration shows the delayed enhancement characteristic of cholangiocarcinomas.
- Isotropic voxel imaging allows high-resolution image reconstruction in multiple anatomic planes and in three dimensions.

Biliary Obstruction

CT is about 96% accurate in determining the presence of biliary obstruction, 90% accurate in determining its level, and 70% accurate in determining its cause.

TABLE 12.1
Causes of Obstructive Jaundice in Adults

Gallstone impacted in bile duct
Bile duct stricture
    Trauma/surgery/instrumentation
    Chronic pancreatitis
    Primary sclerosing cholangitis
    Recurrent pyogenic cholangitis
    AIDS-associated cholangitis
    Benign tumors of the biliary tract
Malignancy
    Pancreas head carcinoma
    Duodenal/ampullary carcinoma
    Cholangiocarcinoma
    Gallbladder carcinoma
    Metastases
Parasites (*Ascaris, Clonorchis, Fasciola*)
AIDS-related cholangiopathy
Choledochal cyst

AIDS, Acquired immunodeficiency syndrome.

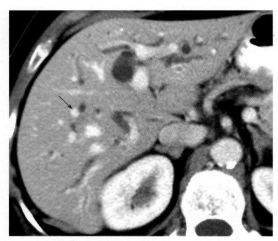

FIG. 12.1 **Dilated bile ducts.** Postcontrast image showing dilated bile ducts *(green arrowheads)* in the liver as low-attenuation round and oval structures or as tortuous tubes. Note that in cross section the dilated bile duct *(green arrow)* is slightly larger in diameter than the adjacent portal vein *(blue arrow)*. The diameter of normal intrahepatic bile ducts should not be larger than 40% of the diameter of the adjacent portal vein.

The major causes of biliary obstruction are gallstones, tumor, stricture, and pancreatitis (Table 12.1). A rare but interesting cause of biliary obstruction is *Mirizzi syndrome*. A gallbladder stone impacted in the cystic duct induces cholangitis or erodes into the common duct to cause obstructive jaundice. Tumors include cholangiocarcinoma, pancreatic head carcinoma, ampullary carcinoma, gallbladder carcinoma, and benign tumors of the bile duct such as biliary cystadenomas and granular cell tumors.

CT diagnosis of biliary obstruction depends on the demonstration of dilated bile ducts. The biliary tree dilates proximal to the point of obstruction, whereas bile ducts distal to the obstruction remain normal or are reduced in size. When cirrhosis, cholangitis, or periductal fibrosis prohibits dilation of the bile ducts in obstructive jaundice, the CT findings will be falsely negative. The CT findings of biliary obstruction include:

- multiple branching, round or oval, low-density tubular structures, representing dilated intrahepatic biliary ducts, coursing toward the porta hepatis. (Figs. 12.1–12.3);
- dilatation of the common duct in the porta hepatis seen as a tubular or oval, fluid density tube greater than 7 mm in diameter;
- dilatation of the CBD in the pancreatic head seen as a round fluid density tube larger than 7 mm;
- enlargement of the gallbladder to more than 5 cm in diameter, when the obstruction is distal to the cystic duct.

Clues to the cause of biliary obstruction are illustrated in Fig. 12.4.

- Abrupt termination of a dilated CBD is characteristic of a malignant process (Fig. 12.5) even in the absence of a visible mass. Common tumors causing biliary obstruction include pancreatic head carcinoma, ampullary carcinoma, and cholangiocarcinoma. A small mass may be recognized at the point of biliary obstruction by careful inspection of noncontrast, arterial phase, portal venous phase, and delayed postcontrast CT images. Occasional benign biliary tumors may cause similar findings.
- Gradual tapering of a dilated duct is seen most commonly with benign disease such as inflammatory stricture or pancreatitis (Fig. 12.6). Calcifications in the pancreas are a clue to the presence of chronic pancreatitis.
- The presence of choledocholithiasis (Fig. 12.7) may be difficult to recognize because of the wide variation in the CT appearance of gallstones. Stones differ in CT attenuation from fat density to calcific.

Choledocholithiasis

Stones in the biliary tree are a common cause of pancreatitis, jaundice, biliary colic, and cholangitis. However, stones in the bile ducts may also be asymptomatic.

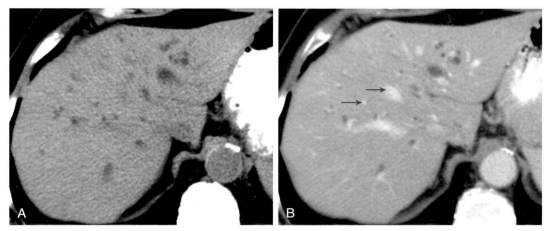

FIG. 12.2 Dilated bile ducts. (A) On noncontrast CT dilated bile ducts are difficult to recognize, appearing as ill-defined foci of low attenuation difficult to differentiate from unopacified blood vessels. (B) Following intravenous contrast agent administration the dilated low-attenuation bile ducts *(green arrowheads)* are much better defined and the enhanced now high-attenuation blood vessels *(blue arrows)* are now well seen.

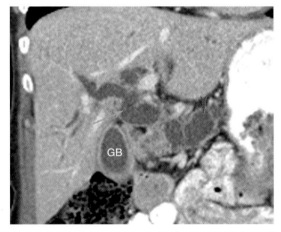

FIG. 12.3 Dilated common duct. Postcontrast coronal plane CT in a patient with pancreatic head carcinoma (not shown) reveals tortuous dilatation of the common bile duct *(green arrow)* in the porta hepatitis, as well as dilatation of the main pancreatic duct *(red arrowhead)*. The gallbladder *(GB)*, incompletely shown on this CT slice, was also dilated.

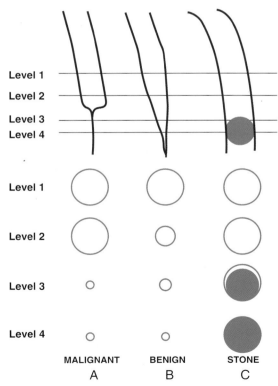

FIG. 12.4 Clues to the cause of biliary obstruction. (A) Malignant tumors cause abrupt termination of the distal part of the common bile duct. (B) Inflammatory strictures and pancreatitis cause progressive tapering of the distal part of the common bile duct. (C) Impacted gallstones may be seen as rounded structures in the distal part of the common bile duct. The CT density of gallstones ranges from calcific density to fat density.

Most stones (95%) in the bile ducts form in the gallbladder although stones may also develop primarily within the bile ducts, especially when the gallbladder has been removed or is chronically obstructed. CT demonstrates approximately 75% of stones in the CBD.

- Gallstones in the bile ducts are seen as calcific (calcium bilirubinate stones), soft-tissue (mixed stones), or fat (cholesterol stones) density structures. Stones

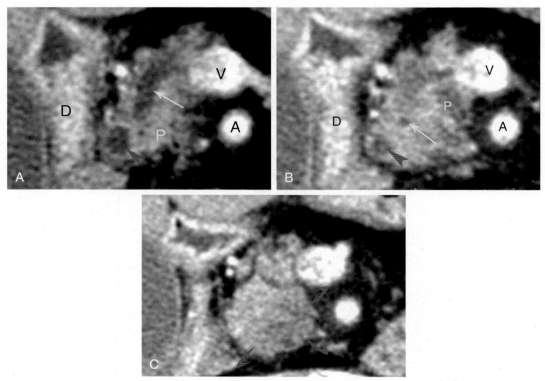

FIG. 12.5 Malignant tumor obstructing the common bile duct. Magnified images from sequential slices of contrast-enhanced CT, proceeding from superior to inferior. (A) The common bile duct *(red arrowhead)*, in the head of the pancreas *(P)*, is mildly dilated to 10 mm. The nearby pancreatic duct *(yellow arrow)* is also dilated. (B) The common bile duct *(red arrowhead)* and the pancreatic duct *(yellow arrow)* become narrowed as they encounter the tumor in the head of the pancreas. (C) Both ducts disappear within the subtly defined tumor *(curved red arrows)*. Pathology confirmed pancreatic adenocarcinoma. *A,* Superior mesenteric artery; *D,* duodenum; *V,* superior mesenteric vein.

may be isodense with bile and not visualized by CT (15%–25% of gallstones). Stones may also contain nitrogen gas and show foci of air attenuation.

- The stone may appear as a central density surrounded by a rim or crescent of lower-density bile—the target or crescent sign (Fig. 12.7).
- Low-attenuation stones may be defined by a higher-attenuation outer rim, called the *rim sign.*
- Abrupt termination of the CBD proximal to the ampulla is suggestive of a stone in the CBD.

Cholangiocarcinoma

Cholangiocarcinoma is a slow-growing adenocarcinoma arising from the epithelium of the bile ducts. It may occur as a complication of choledochal cyst, primary sclerosing cholangitis (PSC), Caroli disease, intrahepatic stone disease, or clonorchiasis.

Prognosis is poor, with recurrence rates of 60% to 90% after surgical resection. The growth patterns of cholangiocarcinoma are mass-forming intrahepatic (see Fig. 11.27), periductal infiltrating, and intraductal growing. Tumors occur in the periphery of the liver (10%), in the hilum (25%), or in the extrahepatic bile ducts (65%). The tumors are hypovascular and markedly fibrotic, resulting in poor contrast enhancement and limited CT detection especially on early postcontrast scans. Delayed scans at 10 to 20 minutes after contrast medium injection are recommended for optimal tumor detection.

- Intrahepatic mass-forming cholangiocarcinoma appears as a homogeneous tumor with irregular borders and remarkably low attenuation. The mass is highly fibrotic and often shows only weak peripheral enhancement on early postcontrast images (see

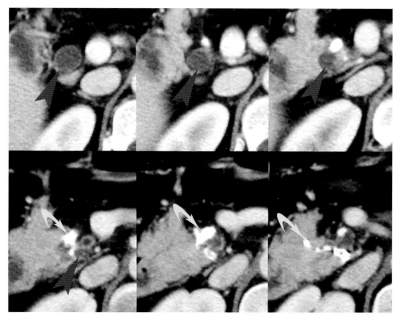

FIG. 12.6 **Benign stricture of the common bile duct as a result of chronic pancreatitis.** Magnified sequential postcontrast CT images demonstrating progressive tapering of the distal common bile duct *(red arrowheads)* as it passes through the head of the pancreas. The pancreatic head is deformed, and multiple calcifications *(curved yellow arrows)* and cystic changes indicate chronic pancreatitis.

Fig. 11.27). Delayed images (up to several hours) may show central or diffuse enhancement. Bile ducts peripheral to the tumor are often obstructed and dilated.

- Periductal-infiltrating lesions grow along the bile ducts in an elongated, branching pattern. Irregular narrowing of the duct produces obstruction. Tumor-involved ducts are narrowed with thick walls, whereas peripheral ducts are dilated with thin walls. Visible tumor mass is minimal. Cholangiocarcinomas occurring at the confluence of the right and left hepatic bile ducts are frequently small and infiltrating, causing early biliary obstruction (Fig. 12.8). These have been termed *Klatskin tumor.*
- Intraductal tumors are polypoid or sessile papillary lesions that extend superficially along the bile duct mucosa. Some of these tumors produce large amounts of mucin, which disproportionately dilates the biliary system.
- Extrahepatic cholangiocarcinomas may appear as a duct-obstructing polypoid tumor nodule 1 to 2 cm in diameter (Fig. 12.9), as an abrupt stricture with wall thickening up to 1 cm, or as single or multiple intraductal frond-like masses.

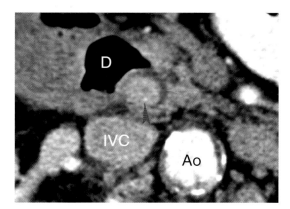

FIG. 12.7 **Stone in the common bile duct.** Magnified image of the distal common bile duct near the ampulla in a patient with biliary obstruction showing a gallstone *(red arrowhead)* as a slightly high-attenuation focus with the common bile duct. A thin rim of bile *(green arrow)* partially surrounds the obstructing stone. *Ao,* aorta; *D,* duodenum; *IVC,* inferior vena cava.

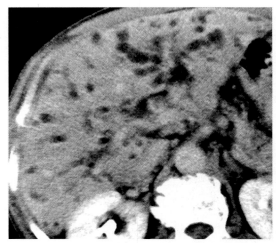

FIG. 12.8 Infiltrating hilar cholangiocarcinoma. An infiltrating cholangiocarcinoma at the junction of the right and left bile ducts (a Klatskin tumor) causes generalized dilatation of the intrahepatic biliary tree. The primary tumor is not visualized with CT, but its location is indicated by diffuse dilatation of intrahepatic bile ducts without dilatation of extrahepatic bile ducts.

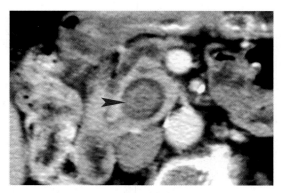

FIG. 12.9 Intraductal polypoid cholangiocarcinoma. Magnified axial CT image of the distal part of the common bile duct showing polypoid cholangiocarcinoma *(arrowhead)* that caused obstructive jaundice with marked dilatation of the common bile duct. Note the similarity in appearance to the low-attenuation stone shown in Fig. 12.7.

Cholangitis

Cholangitis refers to inflammation of the bile ducts.

- *Primary sclerosing cholangitis* (PSC) is an idiopathic inflammatory condition characterized by progressive fibrosis of the bile ducts leading to obstruction, cholestasis, and biliary cirrhosis. PSC is strongly associated (70% of cases) with ulcerative colitis and

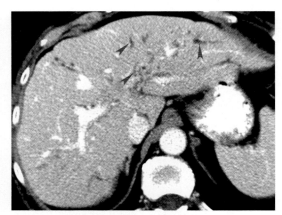

FIG. 12.10 Primary sclerosing cholangitis. Postcontrast CT shows patchy irregular dilatation of the intrahepatic bile ducts *(arrowheads)*. Only the focally dilated portions of the bile ducts are evident. The strictured portions are not seen but can be inferred from this pattern of dilated ducts.

other inflammatory bowel diseases. CT in PSC demonstrates multiple segmental strictures with thickening (2–5 mm) of the bile duct walls alternating with normal-caliber or slightly dilated duct segments that produce a beaded appearance (Fig. 12.10). Stones are seen in the ducts in 30% of patients.

- *Acute pyogenic cholangitis* occurs when bacteria contaminate an obstructed biliary system. Liver abscesses and sepsis may occur. Patients present with acute abdominal pain, fever, and intermittent jaundice. Acute bacterial cholangitis may complicate biliary drainage procedures. CT findings include periductal low-attenuation edema (Fig 12.11), bile duct dilatation, and inhomogeneous enhancement of the liver parenchyma. Infecting bacteria may produce gas in the biliary tree (Fig. 12.12).

- *Recurrent pyogenic cholangitis* (sometimes termed *Oriental cholangitis*) refers to recurrent episodes of acute pyogenic cholangitis associated with pigmented stones and multifocal biliary strictures and dilatations. Infestations with *Clonorchis sinensis* and *Ascaris lumbricoides*, malnutrition, and portal vein bacteremia all play a role in its cause. Persistent inflammation leads to bile duct fibrosis, strictures, stasis, and stone formation. The condition is endemic in Southeast Asian and Chinese populations and is seen predominantly in immigrants in Western countries. Dilated bile ducts with enhanced thickened walls are filled with stones and pus (Fig. 12.13). Marked dilatation of the CBD is characteristic. Complications include liver abscesses, portal vein thrombosis, and cholan-

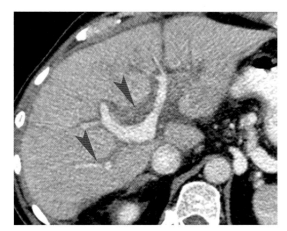

FIG. 12.11 **Acute pyogenic cholangitis.** Postcontrast CT in a patient with a liver transplant presenting with acute abdominal pain and fever shows marked periductal and periportal edema *(arrowheads)*. Further evaluation showed stricture at the biliary anastomosis. Bile culture yielded *Escherichia coli*.

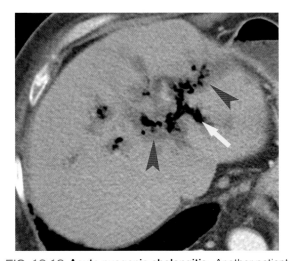

FIG. 12.12 **Acute pyogenic cholangitis.** Another patient with an obstructing pancreatic tumor after endoscopic retrograde cholangiography developed acute pain and fever. Noncontrast CT revealed gas *(yellow arrow)* within the biliary tree and marked periductal/periportal edema *(red arrowheads)*. Urgent biliary drainage was needed. Bile culture yielded gas-producing *Escherichia coli*.

giocarcinoma. Pneumobilia is commonly caused by infection with gas-forming organisms.

- *AIDS-cholangiopathy* is associated with opportunistic infection with *Cryptosporidium* or cytomegalovirus.

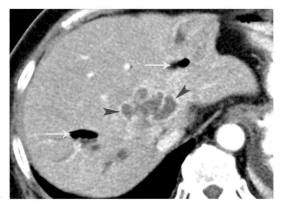

FIG. 12.13 **Recurrent pyogenic cholangitis.** Axial postcontrast CT image showing cystic structures *(red arrowheads)* with thick enhancing walls representing dilated bile ducts. Other bile ducts are dilated with gas *(yellow arrows)*. This Asian immigrant had recurrent pyogenic cholangitis.

Intrahepatic bile ducts show focal narrowing and dilatation similar to that in PSC. Striking thickening and enhancement of the walls of the bile ducts and gallbladder is often evident. The distal part of the CBD is commonly strictured.

- *Autoimmune pancreatitis-associated cholangitis.* Autoimmune pancreatitis includes a subset of patients with involvement of the biliary tree. IgG4-positive lymphocytes infiltrate the wall of intrahepatic and extrahepatic bile ducts. Thickening and enhancement of the wall of the bile ducts occurs in association with multiple strictures. The distal part of the CBD is most commonly affected. The gallbladder wall may also show diffuse thickening. Imaging features of autoimmune pancreatitis are present (see Chapter 13).

Choledochal Cyst

Choledochal cysts are congenital dilatations of any portion of the biliary tree. Most are discovered in childhood. Adult patients with undetected biliary cysts may present with pancreatitis, cholangitis, jaundice, or unexplained abdominal pain, nausea, or vomiting. Complications include gallstones, cholangitis, pancreatitis, and cholangiocarcinoma. CT demonstrates cystic structures in the course of the intrahepatic bile ducts or CBD and separate from the gallbladder. Todani classified choledochal cysts into five types:

- Type I (50%–80%), classic choledochal cyst, is localized cystic dilatation of the CBD (Fig. 12.14). This may appear large and saccular, or small and fusiform.

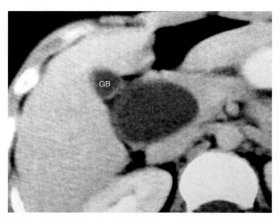

FIG. 12.14 Choledochal cyst, type i. The common bile duct *(C)* is massively dilated, characteristic of a type I choledochal cyst. The neck of the gallbladder *(GB)* is seen adjacent to the dilated common bile duct.

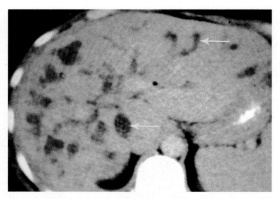

FIG. 12.15 Caroli disease. Abnormally dilated intrahepatic bile ducts *(arrows)* are seen as tubular and rounded cystic lucencies in the liver.

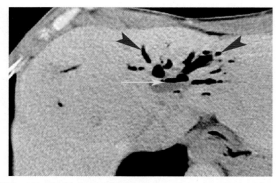

FIG. 12.16 Air in the biliary tree. Air is seen in the bile ducts *(red arrowheads)* of the left lobe of the liver in this patient with a choledochojejunostomy performed as part of a Whipple procedure. Air fills the left hepatic bile ducts in a supine patient and the right hepatic bile ducts in a prone patient. Note the air-bile level *(yellow arrow)*.

- Type II (2%) is a diverticulum arising from the CBD or common hepatic duct. The remainder of the biliary system is normal.
- Type III (1.4%–4.5%), choledochocele, is rare bulbous dilatation of the intramural portion of the distal part of the CBD that protrudes into the lumen of the duodenum. Choledochoceles are most commonly detected in adults. Stones are commonly present in the biliary tree.
- Type IV (15%–35%) is divided into type IV-A, which is cystic dilatation of the intrahepatic bile ducts associated with saccular dilatation of the CBD, and type IV-B (extremely rare), which is multiple cystic dilatations of the extrahepatic bile ducts with normal intrahepatic bile ducts.
- Type V is Caroli disease.

Caroli Disease

Caroli disease is a rare congenital anomaly of the biliary tract characterized by saccular dilatation of the intrahepatic biliary tree, cholangitis, and gallstone formation in the absence of cirrhosis or portal hypertension. Patients are at greatly increased risk of bile duct carcinoma (7% of patients). *Caroli syndrome* is the combination of Caroli disease with congenital hepatic fibrosis.

- CT demonstrates cystic dilatation of the intrahepatic biliary tree with focal areas of tubular and saccular enlargement (Fig. 12.15). The extrahepatic biliary tree remains normal.

Gas or Contrast Material in Biliary Tree

Gas or contrast material in the biliary tree (Fig. 12.16) is an abnormal finding that must be explained. Most often the cause is iatrogenic. The differential diagnosis is listed in Table 12.2.

GALLBLADDER
Anatomy

The gallbladder lies in the fossa formed by the junction of the right and left lobes of the liver. Although the position of the fundus differs, the neck and body of the gallbladder are invariably positioned in the porta hepatis and major interlobar fissure. The

TABLE 12.2
Reflux of Gas or Bowel Contrast Medium into the Biliary Tree

Recent instrumentation of the biliary system
    Endoscopic retrograde cholangiopancreatography
    Percutaneous cholangiography
Iatrogenic
    Sphincterotomy
    Choledochojejunostomy
    Whipple procedure
Gallstone fistula
    Cholecystoduodenal fistula
Perforated ulcer
    Choledochoduodenal fistula
Carcinoma
    Choledochoenteric fistula

gallbladder is close to the duodenal bulb and hepatic flexure of the colon. The normal gallbladder is 3 to 5 cm in diameter and 10 cm in length and has a capacity of roughly 50 mL. Normal gallbladder wall thickness is 3 mm or less. *Agenesis* of the gallbladder is extremely rare (<0.02%), and duplication of the gallbladder occurs in about 1 in 4000 individuals. Folds in the gallbladder, producing a Phrygian cap deformity, are common (1%–6% incidence) and not clinically significant.

Ultrasonography, not CT, is the primary modality for imaging the gallbladder. However, significant gallbladder disease may be diagnosed by CT, especially when the acutely ill patient is screened. Normal bile is of fluid density (0–20 Hounsfield units [HU]) on CT. Higher-density bile suggests bile stasis (sludge), hemorrhage, or infection (pus). The gallbladder wall enhances avidly with bolus contrast agent administration.

Gallstones

Although gallstones may be detected by CT, the sensitivity of CT is only about 85%, much less than that of ultrasonography or magnetic resonance imaging. Dual-energy CT may improve gallstone detection over conventional CT. Gallstones differ in CT density from negative values on the HU scale, indicating the fat attenuation of cholesterol stones, to high positive values on the HU scale of calcified stones (Fig. 12.17). Fissured stones may contain linear streaks of gas, known to be nitrogen. Some gallstones may not be seen on CT because they are isodense with bile or because they are too small. Contrast agents in adjacent bowel loops may obscure, or mimic, gallstones.

Acute Cholecystitis

Acute cholecystitis is usually diagnosed clinically, by ultrasonography, or by radionuclide hepatobiliary scan. Cases are studied with CT usually because the patient has unexplained right upper quadrant pain, has atypical symptoms, or is suspected to have complicated cholecystitis. *Gangrenous cholecystitis* may lead to perforation, abscess, fistula, or peritonitis. *Acalculous cholecystitis* (without gallstones present) (~5%–10% of cases) occurs most commonly in critically ill patients, especially after surgery, trauma, or burns, or in patients receiving hyperalimentation. Acalculous cholecystitis is induced by biliary stasis, ischemia, and bacteremia. *Emphysematous cholecystitis* is a severe form of cholecystitis that tends to occur in elderly people and in people with diabetes. It may produce deceptively mild symptoms but carries high morbidity and mortality. The CT findings in acute cholecystitis are as follows:

- Gallstones are shown by CT to be present in the gallbladder in 75% of cases of acute cholecystitis (Fig. 12.18).
- The gallbladder is usually distended to 4 to 5 cm in diameter, reflecting cystic duct obstruction.
- The gallbladder wall is thickened (>3 mm) and appears indistinct because of inflammation and edema. The wall is commonly enhanced brightly, reflecting inflammatory hyperemia.
- Transient early-phase hyperenhancement of the liver adjacent to the gallbladder is strong evidence of hyperemia and inflammation.
- A halo of subserosal edema in the gallbladder wall and stranding in the pericholecystic tissues reflects inflammation of the wall.
- Pericholecystic fluid collection is associated with perforation and abscess.
- Increase in bile density (>20 HU) is caused by biliary stasis, intraluminal pus, hemorrhage, or cellular debris.
- The CT findings of *acalculous cholecystitis* are identical to those of calculous cholecystitis except that gallstones are absent. This condition occurs only in patients with the predisposing conditions listed.
- Air in the gallbladder wall or lumen is seen with *emphysematous cholecystitis*, a severe form of acute cholecystitis caused by gas-forming organisms and associated with high mortality (Fig. 12.19).

Porcelain Gallbladder

Calcification of the gallbladder wall (Fig. 12.20), in association with chronic cholecystitis, is termed *porcelain gallbladder*. The calcification may be broad and continuous or punctate and discontinuous. Gallstones

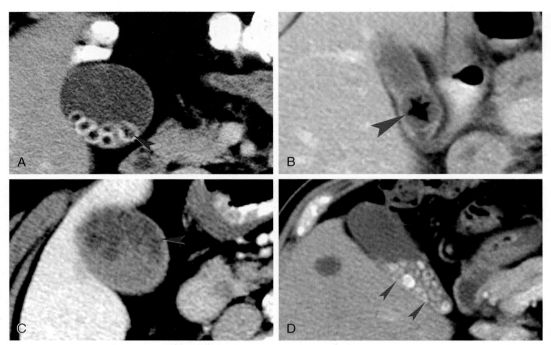

FIG. 12.17 **Gallstones.** (A) Gallstones *(arrowhead)* settle dependently in the gallbladder. These stones consist of low-attenuation centers of high cholesterol content and calcified outer margins. (B) A gallstone with a very faintly calcified rim contains nitrogen gas *(arrowhead)*. (C) Very low attenuation gallstone *(arrowhead)* suspended within the gallbladder is faintly visible because of its cholesterol content. Gallstones may be entirely of the same attenuation as bile and may be undetectable on CT. (D) Numerous gallstones *(arrowheads)* of differing size and shape layer dependently within the gallbladder. A benign hepatic cyst is also noted.

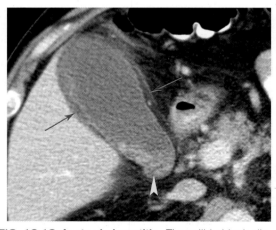

FIG. 12.18 **Acute cholecystitis.** The gallbladder is distended, its wall is shaggy and poorly defined, and edema *(red arrows)* extends from the gallbladder wall into pericholecystic tissues. Multiple small gallstones *(yellow arrow)* layer dependently within the gallbladder. Surgery confirmed uncomplicated acute cholecystitis.

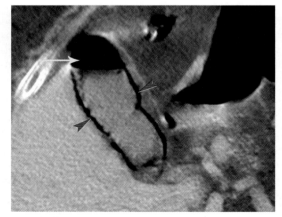

FIG. 12.19 **Emphysematous cholecystitis.** Gas infiltrates the wall *(red arrowheads)* of the gallbladder and forms an air-fluid level *(yellow arrow)* with bile in the gallbladder lumen.

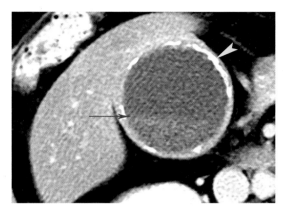

FIG. 12.20 **Porcelain gallbladder.** The wall of the gallbladder *(yellow arrowhead)* is thickened and partially calcified. A faint fluid level *(red arrow)* is seen in the gallbladder lumen, indicating chronic bile stasis.

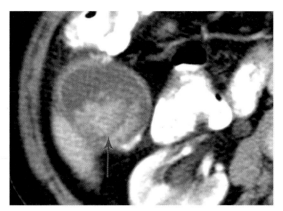

FIG. 12.21 **Gallbladder carcinoma.** An enhancing frond-like polypoid mass *(arrow)* within the gallbladder lumen is characteristic of gallbladder carcinoma. Gallstones were also present in the gallbladder (not shown).

are nearly always present. Gallbladder carcinoma may develop in 5% to 7% of patients with porcelain gallbladder. Cholecystectomy is often advocated even when the patient is asymptomatic.

Gallbladder Carcinoma

Gallbladder carcinoma is the most common malignancy of the biliary system. Most patients are aged 50 years or older. Because of the presence of gallstones and chronic cholecystitis, clinical and imaging evaluation commonly overlooks early disease. Because of advanced disease at diagnosis, the traditional 5-year survival rate is only 5%. Newer, more aggressive surgical techniques may increase the 5-year survival rate to 50%. Chronic cholelithiasis related to gallstones is the major risk factor for this tumor. CT demonstrates three major patterns of disease:

- A polypoid soft-tissue mass within the gallbladder lumen (~25% of cases) (Fig. 12.21). The cancerous polyps are usually larger than 1 cm and demonstrate early contrast enhancement and washout.
- Focal or diffuse thickening of the gallbladder wall, often more than 1 cm (~7% of cases).
- A mass containing gallstones replaces the gallbladder and invades the adjacent liver (~68% of cases).

Associated findings include gallstones; biliary dilatation; metastases in the liver; invasion of liver (Fig. 12.22), bowel, and adjacent structures; and calcification of the gallbladder wall.

Gallbladder Adenomyomatosis

Adenomyomatosis is a relatively common benign cause of thickening of the gallbladder wall. Wall thickening

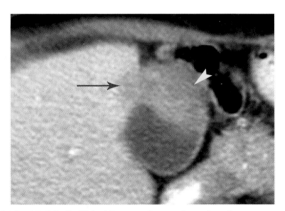

FIG. 12.22 **Gallbladder carcinoma invades the liver.** Adenocarcinoma *(yellow arrowhead)* arising within the gallbladder extends directly into the liver parenchyma *(red arrow)*.

is caused by hyperplasia of the muscularis propria and proliferation of the epithelium associated with development of epithelium lined pouches in the gallbladder wall. The thickened epithelium infolds to form bile-containing diverticula called *Rokitansky-Aschoff sinuses.* Stasis of bile within these diverticula may form cholesterol crystals that induce chronic inflammation. Gallstones may be present in 25% to 75% of patients. Most patients are asymptomatic, and the condition is discovered by imaging studies or from pathology specimens removed for symptomatic gallstones or cholecystitis. Adenomyomatosis has no malignant potential but may

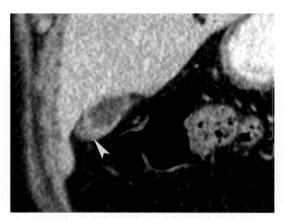

FIG. 12.23 Localized gallbladder adenomyomatosis.
Coronal postcontrast CT image showing focal thickening *(arrowhead)* of the gallbladder wall confined to the fundus. Low-attenuation areas within the thickened wall are Rokitansky-Aschoff sinuses.

be mistaken for gallbladder cancer. CT findings include four main patterns of disease:

- *Diffuse* adenomyomatosis involves the entire gallbladder, which is chronically contracted.
- *Localized* adenomyomatosis is usually confined to the gallbladder fundus, with the remainder of the gallbladder appearing normal (Fig. 12.23).
- *Segmental* disease involves the fundus and distal third of the body of the gallbladder. The diseased portion is contracted, while the proximal part of the gallbladder remains normal.
- *Annular* disease forms a ring of wall thickening, contracting the midportion of the gallbladder, creating an hour-glass shape. CT, especially with thin slices, effectively shows the wall thickening.

SUGGESTED READING

Bonatti, M., Vezzali, N., Lombardo, F., et al. (2017). Gallbladder adenomyomatosis: Imaging findings, tricks and pitfalls. *Insights Imaging, 8*, 243–253.

Castaing, D. (2008). Surgical anatomy of the biliary tract. *Healthcare Physiol Biochem Zool, 10*, 72–76.

Chung, Y. E., Kim, M.-J., Park, Y. N., et al. (2009). Varying appearances of cholangiocarcinoma: Radiologic-pathologic correlation. *Radiographics, 29*, 683–700.

Costi, R., Gnocchi, A., Di Mario, F., & Sarli, L. (2014). Diagnosis and management of choledocholithiasis in the golden age of imaging, endoscopy and laparoscopy. *World Journal of Gastroenterology, 20*, 13382–13401.

Hussain, H. M., Little, M. D., & Wei, S. (2013). Gallbladder carcinoma with direct invasion of the liver. *Radiographics, 33*, 103–108.

Joshi, A., Rajpal, K., Kakadiya, K., & Bansal, A. (2014). Role of CT and MRCP in evaluation of biliary tract obstruction. *Current Radiology Reports, 2*, 72–85.

O'Connor, O. J., O'Neill, S. O., & Maher, M. M. (2011). Imaging of biliary tract disease. *AJR. Am J Roentgenol, 197*, W551–W558.

Patel, N. B., Oto, A., & Thomas, S. (2013). Multidetector CT of emergent biliary pathologic conditions. *Radiographics, 33*, 1867–1888.

Ratanaprasatporn, L., Uyeda, J. W., Wortman, J. R., et al. (2018). Multimodality imaging, including dual-energy CT, in the evaluation of gallbladder disease. *Radiographics, 38*, 75–89.

Santiago, I., Loureiro, R., Curvo-Semedo, L., et al. (2012). Congenital cystic lesions of the biliary tree. *AJR. Am J Roentgenol, 198*, 825–835.

Woldenberg, N., Masamed, R., Petersen, J., et al. (2015). Murphy's law: What can go wrong in the gallbladder. *Radiographics, 35*, 1031–1032.

CHAPTER 13

Pancreas

WILLIAM E. BRANT

Multidetector CT is the imaging method of choice for evaluation of pancreatitis and competes with magnetic resonance imaging (MRI) for detection and staging of pancreatic tumors. Rapid CT acquisition times allow high-resolution multiphase scanning of the entire pancreas within a single breath hold in most instances.

CT TECHNIQUE

CT evaluation of pancreatitis is usually performed as a routine abdomen scan with extension of CT scanning of the pelvis if large fluid collections are present. Water may be substituted for oral contrast agents if stones in the distal part of the common bile duct are suspected. CT evaluation for a pancreatic mass is performed as a multiphase dynamic scan of the entire pancreas. Optimally each phase is performed during a single breath hold. Oral contrast agents are routinely given. CT without an intravenous contrast agent is performed from the liver dome through the iliac crest, reconstructing thin slices (1.25–3.0 mm) with sagittal and coronal reconstructions. A power injector is used to administer 120 to 150 mL of intravenous contrast agent at 4-5 mL per second. The arterial phase scan is obtained at 30 to 35 seconds following onset of injection. Both the liver and the pancreas show arterial opacification with minimal contrast enhancement of the portal vein. The venous phase scan of the entire abdomen is obtained at 60 to 70 seconds following initiation of contrast agent injection. Delayed scans may be obtained at 3 to 5 minutes after contrast agent injection through the liver and kidneys. Three-dimensional reconstructions may be performed as CT angiograms.

NORMAL ANATOMY OF THE PANCREAS

The pancreas lies within the anterior pararenal compartment of the retroperitoneal space, behind the left lobe of the liver and the stomach, and in front of the spine and great vessels (Fig. 13.1). The peritoneum-lined lesser sac forms a potential space between the stomach and the pancreas. The pancreas is divided anatomically into four parts: head, including the uncinate process, neck, body, and tail. The pancreas somewhat resembles a question mark turned on its left side, with the hook portion formed by the pancreatic head and uncinate process as they lie cradled in the duodenal loop. The portal vein fills the center of the hook. The uncinate process cradles the superior mesenteric vein (SMV) and tapers to a sharpened point directed leftward beneath the SMV. The neck is a slightly constricted portion of the pancreas just ventral to the portal vein confluence formed by the junction of the SMV and the splenic vein. The body and tail taper as they extend toward the splenic hilum. The pancreas is usually directed upward and to the left, although it may form an inverted-U shape with the tail directed caudad. Sequential CT slices must be mentally summated to assess the shape and size of the pancreas. The gland is 15 to 20 cm long. The maximum width is 3.0 cm for the head, 2.5 cm for the body, and 2.0 cm for the tail. The gland is larger in young people and progressively decreases in size with age. The CT attenuation is uniform and approximately equal to that of muscle. In young patients the pancreas resembles a slab of meat. Progressive infiltration of fat between the lobules of the pancreas gives it a feathery appearance with advancing age. The pancreatic duct is best visualized with thin slices (1.25–2.5 mm). It tapers smoothly to the tail, measuring a maximum of 3.5 mm in diameter in the head, 2.5 mm in the body, and 1.5 mm in the tail. The main duct (of Wirsung) joins the common bile duct at the sphincter of Oddi to enter the duodenum. The accessory duct (of Santorini) draining the anterior and superior portions of the pancreatic head drains into the duodenum via the minor papilla.

The complex vascular anatomy of the pancreas must be understood to correctly interpret pancreatic CT scans. The splenic vein runs a relatively straight course in the dorsum of the pancreas from the splenic hilum to its junction with the SMV just posterior to the neck of the pancreas. The plane of fat between the splenic vein and the pancreas must not be mistaken for the pancreatic duct. The splenic artery runs an undulating course through the pancreas from the celiac axis to the spleen. Atherosclerotic calcifications are common in the splenic artery and may be easily mistaken for pancreatic calcifications. The superior mesenteric artery (SMA) arises from the aorta dorsal to the pancreas and courses caudally, surrounded by a collar of fat. The SMV courses cranially, just to the right of the SMA, until it joins the splenic vein to form the portal vein. The pancreatic head entirely surrounds this junction, with the uncinate process extending beneath the SMV. The portal vein courses upward and rightward

with the hepatic artery and the common bile duct to the porta hepatis.

PANCREAS DIVISUM

The most common anomaly of the pancreatic ductal system is pancreas divisum, which is present in 4% to 10% of the population. In this anomaly, as a result of failure of fusion of the dorsal and ventral pancreas during embryologic development, the dorsal duct draining most of the pancreas empties into the minor papilla via the duct of Santorini rather than into the major papilla via the duct of Wirsung. Thin-section multidetector CT

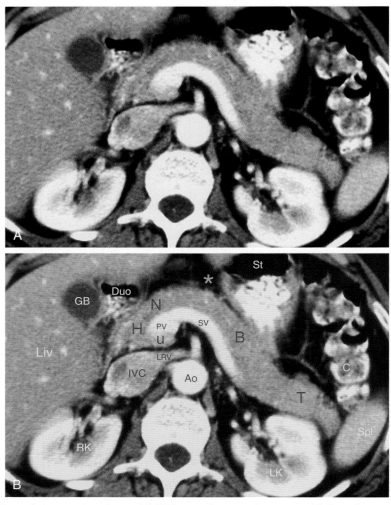

FIG. 13.1 **Normal pancreas anatomy.** (A) CT image of a normal pancreas. (B) Same image as in (A) with anatomic structures labeled.

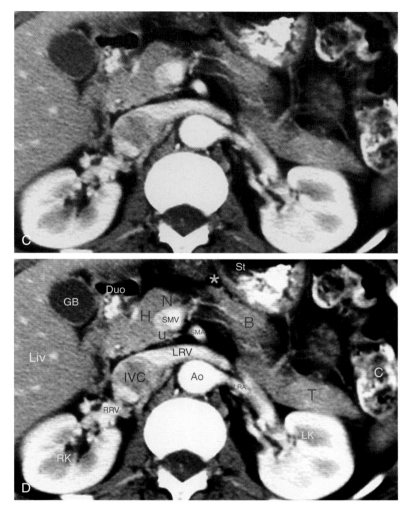

FIG. 13.1, cont'd (C) CT image of normal head and uncinate process of the pancreas. (D) Same image as in (C) with anatomic structures labeled. An asterisk indicates the location of the lesser sac. *Ao*, Aorta; *B*, body of pancreas; *C*, colon; *Duo*, duodenum; *GB*, gallbladder; *H*, head of pancreas; *IVC*, inferior vena cava; *Liv*, liver; *LK*, left kidney; *LRV*, left renal vein; *N*, neck of pancreas; *PV*, commencement of portal vein; *RK*, right kidney; *RRV*, right renal vein; *SMA*, superior mesenteric artery; *SMV*, superior mesenteric vein; *Spl*, spleen; *St*, stomach; *SV*, splenic vein; *T*, tail of pancreas; *u*, uncinate process of pancreatic head.

shows the dorsal pancreatic duct coursing posterior to the descending portion of the common bile duct cephalad to the sphincter of Oddi (Fig. 13.2). The distal portion of the dorsal pancreatic duct may be dilated at the junction with the duodenum, an anomaly known as a *santorinicele*. In most patients pancreas divisum is an incidental finding of no significance. However, the constriction of the dorsal duct at the minor papilla predisposes to recurrent pancreatitis in 25% to 38% of patients with pancreas divisum.

ANNULAR PANCREAS

Incomplete rotation of the embryologic ventral pancreas results in a segment of the pancreas encircling and often constricting the descending duodenum. Annular pancreas is rare, occurring as an isolated anomaly or in association with other congenital anomalies. It may present in the neonatal period with duodenal or biliary obstruction. In adults it may present with ulcer disease, duodenal obstruction, or pancreatitis. CT shows pancreatic tissue encircling the second portion of the

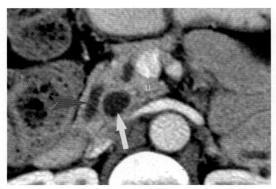

FIG. 13.2 Pancreas divisum. Magnified view from a contrast-enhanced axial CT image of the pancreatic head at the level of the uncinate process *(u)* showing a dilated pancreatic duct *(red arrowhead)* bypassing the common bile duct *(yellow arrow)*. The main (dorsal) pancreatic duct inserts into the more proximal minor papilla rather than joining the common bile duct to insert into the larger major papilla. This patient had a history of recurrent pancreatitis, likely related to low-grade obstruction at the minor papilla.

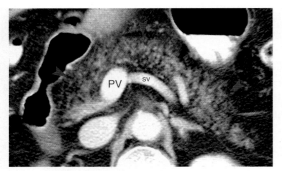

FIG. 13.4 Fatty infiltration of the pancreas. The pancreas *(arrowheads)* shows fat infiltrating between the atrophic lobules of parenchyma. Despite diffuse atrophy and fatty infiltration, the exocrine and endocrine functions of the pancreas were normal in this elderly patient. Note the vascular landmarks of the pancreas, the portal vein confluence *(PV)* and the splenic vein *(SV)*.

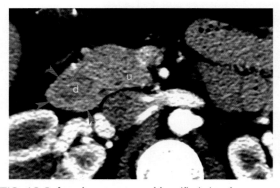

FIG. 13.3 Annular pancreas. Magnified view from a contrast-enhanced CT image of the pancreatic head at the level of the uncinate process *(u)* showing pancreatic tissue *(arrowheads)* completely encircling the slightly lower-attenuation second portion of the duodenum *(d)*. The duodenum is compressed and partially obstructed by the encircling pancreas.

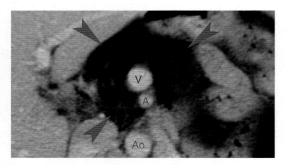

FIG. 13.5 Cystic fibrosis. Image of the pancreatic head in a patient with cystic fibrosis showing near complete atrophy of the pancreatic parenchyma *(arrowheads)* with replacement by fat. This is a common CT finding in patients with cystic fibrosis. *A,* Superior mesenteric artery; *Ao,* abdominal aorta; *V,* superior mesenteric vein.

duodenum (Fig. 13.3). Symptomatic cases warrant surgical correction.

FATTY INFILTRATION OF THE PANCREAS

Fatty infiltration of the pancreas occurs commonly with aging and obesity without affecting the function of the pancreas.

- Because the gland is not encapsulated, fatty infiltration between the lobules in older adult patients gives the pancreas a delicate, feathery appearance resembling a dust mop (Fig. 13.4).
- Fatty replacement may be diffuse or distributed unevenly throughout the pancreas. The head and uncinate process are common areas of focal sparing of fat infiltration. In some cases the head and uncinate process are involved and the remainder of the pancreas is spared.
- In advanced cystic fibrosis the pancreatic parenchyma is atrophic and is diffusely replaced by fat (Fig. 13.5), while exocrine function of the pancreas is severely impaired. The revised Atlanta classifica-

TABLE 13.1
Causes of Acute Pancreatitis
Gallstone passage/impaction (most common cause)
Alcohol abuse (dose-dependent increase in incidence and severity)
Smoking (independent risk and additive to alcohol risk)
Abdominal adiposity (waist circumference >105 cm)
Metabolic disorders
Diabetes mellitus
Hereditary pancreatitis (autosomal dominant)
Cystic fibrosis
Hypercalcemia
Hyperlipidemia, hypertriglyceridemia
Malnutrition
Trauma
Blunt abdominal trauma
Abdominal surgery
Endoscopic retrograde cholangiopancreatography
Autoimmune disease
Autoimmune pancreatitis
Celiac disease
Penetrating ulcer
Malignancy
Pancreatic cancers
Lymphoma
Drugs (corticosteroids, tetracycline, furosemide, many others)
Infection
Viral (mumps, hepatitis, infectious mononucleosis, acquired immunodeficiency syndrome)
Parasitic (ascariasis, clonorchiasis)
Structural
Choledochocele
Pancreas divisum
Idiopathic (20% of cases of acute pancreatitis)

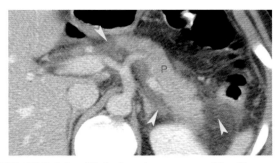

FIG. 13.6 **Interstitial edematous pancreatitis.** The pancreas *(P)* is mildly swollen, but all of the pancreatic parenchyma enhances normally. Edema and inflammation *(arrowheads)* infiltrate the peripancreatic tissues.

progress to recurrent acute pancreatitis then to chronic pancreatitis. The diagnosis of pancreatitis is made clinically by the presence of acute abdominal pain and elevated serum amylase and lipase levels. The role of CT is to document the presence and severity of disease and complications. Severity of CT findings correlates with prognosis. Demonstration of necrotic pancreatic tissue is associated with increased morbidity and mortality. Other prognostic factors associated with increased risk of complications include age, gallstone disease, and organ failure on admission. The 2012 revision of the Atlanta Classification for Acute Pancreatitis divides the disease into two distinct subtypes.

Interstitial edematous pancreatitis (IEP) accounts for 90-95% of cases of acute pancreatitis. Inflammation is present without necrosis.

- Post-contrast CT findings include diffuse or localized enlargement of the pancreas due to edema. The entire pancreatic parenchyma enhances (Fig. 13.6). Enhancement of the parenchyma may be homogeneous and normal or slightly heterogeneous. Peripancreatic inflammatory changes and fat stranding may be present associated with peripancreatic fluid of varying volumes.
- *Acute peripancreatic fluid collections* (Fig. 13.7) associated with IEP are defined as non-encapsulated, non-enhancing, low attenuation, liquefied collections without solid components shown on CT performed within 4 weeks of onset of symptoms. No necrotic tissue is present. Walls surrounding the collection are imperceptible.
- *Pseudocysts* associated with IEP are defined as homogeneous simple fluid collections with visible walls seen after 4 weeks from onset of symptoms (Fig. 13.8). Pseudocysts contain only fluid. The presence of any

tion also updates confusing terminology used to describe pancreatitis and peripancreatic fluid collection. It discourages the use of the terms *acute pancreatic pseudocyst* and *pancreatic abscess*.

ACUTE PANCREATITIS

Inflammation of the pancreas damages acinar tissue and leads to focal disruption of small ducts resulting in leakage of pancreatic juice. The absence of a capsule around the pancreas allows easy access of pancreatic secretions to surrounding tissues. Pancreatic enzymes digest through fascial layers to spread to multiple anatomic compartments. Acute pancreatitis in adults is most often caused by passage of a gallstone or by alcohol abuse (Table 13.1). The incidence of acute pancreatitis continues to increase. Acute pancreatitis may

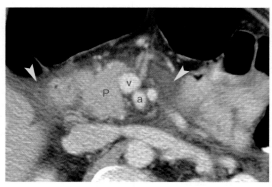

FIG. 13.7 **Acute peripancreatic fluid collection.** Post-contrast CT image of the pancreatic head *(P)* at 3 weeks following the onset of symptoms revealing unencapsulated non-enhancing peripancreatic fluid collections *(arrowheads)*. Vascular landmarks include the superior mesenteric vein *(v)* and superior mesenteric artery *(a)*.

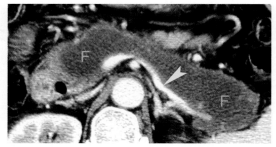

FIG. 13.9 **Necrotizing pancreatitis.** Liquefaction necrosis has completely destroyed the pancreas, replacing it with a loculated collection of fluid *(F)* in the pancreatic bed anterior to the splenic vein *(arrowhead)*.

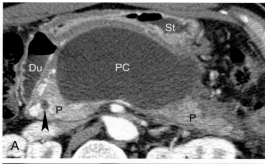

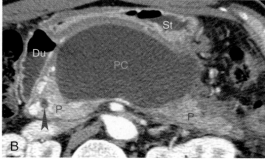

FIG. 13.8 **Pancreatic pseudocyst.** (A) Axial postcontrast CT at 6 weeks following the onset of symptoms shows a persisting fluid collection *(PC)* anterior to and compressing the pancreas *(P)*. The stomach *(St)* is compressed and displaced anteriorly, whereas the duodenum *(Du)* is displaced laterally. The common bile duct *(arrowhead)* is seen in the pancreatic head. (B) Sagittal reconstructed image from the same CT study providing better demonstration of the capsule *(arrows)* of the pseudocyst *(PC)*.

fat or soft tissue indicates the collection is walled-off necrosis (WON) not a pseudocyst.

- Fluid collections associated with IEP generally do not require drainage unless they become infected. The presence of gas within the collection is evidence of infection and the need for drainage.

Necrotizing pancreatitis accounts for 5-10% of cases of acute pancreatitis. CT shows three morphologic forms of acute pancreatic necrosis. Pancreatic necrosis is best assessed on early-phase post-contrast CT images performed at 40 seconds post injection. CT is most sensitive to necrosis at 72 hours following the onset of symptoms. The hallmark of necrosis is absence of enhancement of pancreatic parenchyma and/or surrounding tissues.

- *Pancreatic parenchymal necrosis with peripancreatic necrosis* accounts for 75-80% of cases (Fig. 13.9). CT shows lack of parenchymal contrast enhancement and heterogeneous non-liquefied areas of nonenhancement in the peripancreatic tissues, especially in the lesser sac and retroperitoneum.
- *Pancreatic necrosis alone* (5%) appears as focal or diffuse areas of absent parenchymal enhancement without associated collections.
- *Peripancreatic necrosis alone* (20%) appears on CT as non-enhancement of peripancreatic tissues with normal enhancement of all pancreas parenchyma. Peripancreatic collections contain liquefied and non-liquefied components.
- *Acute necrotic collections* (ANC) associated with necrotizing pancreatitis (Figs. 13.10 and 13.11) are defined as heterogeneous collections containing necrotic pancreatic parenchyma, hemorrhage, and necrotic fat seen on CT performed within 4 weeks of onset of symptoms. Collections may be within or surrounding pancreatic parenchyma or both.

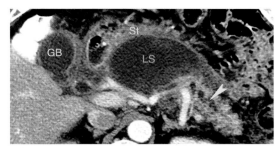

FIG. 13.10 **Acute necrotic collections.** Fluid collections resulting from acute pancreatitis extend from the necrotic pancreas into the lesser sac *(LS)*, compressing the stomach *(St)* and extending partially around the gallbladder *(GB)*. The distal part of the pancreatic duct *(arrowhead)* is dilated. The CT image was obtained at 3 weeks following the onset of symptoms.

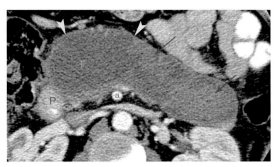

FIG. 13.12 **Walled-off necrosis.** CT image obtained at 6 weeks showing an encapsulated heterogeneous fluid collection *(F)* occupying the bed of the pancreas, which is completely necrotic except for the pancreatic head *(P)*. The thin enhancing wall *(yellow arrowheads)* is clearly visible. Necrotic debris *(red arrows)* is subtly higher in attenuation than the fluid in which it resides. The superior mesenteric artery *(a)* enhancing normally.

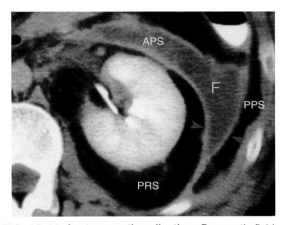

FIG. 13.11 **Acute necrotic collection.** Pancreatic fluid *(F)* and inflammation extend from the pancreas in the anterior pararenal space *(APS)* partially around the left kidney between the leaves of the posterior renal fascia *(arrowheads)*. Note that the perirenal space *(PRS)* and the posterior pararenal space *(PPS)* are spared.

- *Walled-off necrosis* (WON) is defined as an ANC that develops an enhancing wall and is seen on CT performed after 4 weeks from onset of symptoms (Fig. 13.12). WONs are heterogeneous and complex in appearance because of debris and variable amounts of necrotic tissue.
- Necrotic tissue is highly likely to become infected. CT demonstration of gas within a necrotic collection is strong evidence of infection. Percutaneous aspiration and drainage are needed to treat infected necrotic collections.

Organ failure and other complications commonly occur with acute pancreatitis. If no complications or organ failure is present the disease is defined as *mild*. Organ failure lasting less than 48 hours defines the disease as *moderate*. *Severe* disease is associated with single or multiple organ failure lasting 48 hours or longer. Organ failure includes impaired respiratory, cardiovascular, or renal function. Complications of acute pancreatitis include the following.

- *Secondary infection* occurs in 30-70% of patients with bacterial growth within necrotic tissues and fluid collections most commonly 2-3 weeks after onset of disease. Infection greatly worsens the prognosis with mortality rates of 20-30% for infected necrosis versus 5-10% for sterile necrosis. Fluid collections containing gas (Fig. 13.13) are suspicious for infection, but infected fluid collections may be indistinguishable from sterile fluid collections. Wall enhancement is not reliable as a sign of infection. CT, US, or endoscopic US-guided aspiration is needed to confirm diagnosis. Terms such as *pancreatic abscess, phlegmon, organized necrosis, necroma,* or *sequestration* are discouraged by the Atlanta Classification nomenclature.
- *Hemorrhage* is caused by erosion of blood vessels or bowel. It is seen as high attenuating fluid in retroperitoneum or peritoneal cavity. Hemorrhage commonly accompanies necrosis.
- *Pseudoaneurysms* are encapsulations of arterial hemorrhage with continued communication with eroded artery. Swirling and "to and fro" blood flow continue within the pseudoaneurysm. Risk of massive

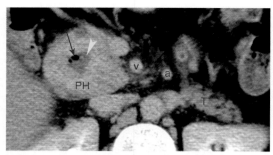

FIG. 13.13 Secondary infection. Marked enlargement of the pancreatic head *(PH)* caused by acute pancreatitis is complicated by a small fluid collection *(yellow arrowhead)* containing bubbles of gas *(red arrow)* indicating acute infection. Inflammatory edema partially envelops the superior mesenteric vein *(v)* and superior mesenteric artery *(a)*. *T,* tail of the pancreas.

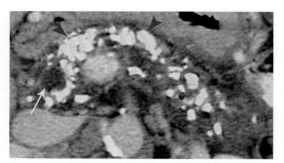

FIG. 13.15 Chronic pancreatitis: calcifications. Numerous coarse calcifications are seen throughout the pancreas *(red arrowheads)* in this patient with recurrent alcoholic pancreatitis. The common bile duct *(yellow arrow)* is mildly dilated because of a benign pancreatitis-associated stricture in the pancreatic head.

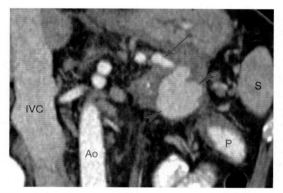

FIG. 13.14 Pseudoaneurysm. In a patient with acute pancreatitis, postcontrast coronal reconstruction CT shows a lobulated enhanced pseudoaneurysm *(arrowheads)* arising from the splenic artery *(arrow)*. Anatomic landmarks include the aorta *(Ao)*, the inferior vena cava *(IVC)*, the tail of the pancreas *(P)*, and the spleen *(S)*.

hemorrhage is high. A pseudoaneurysm must be excluded with contrast-enhanced CT (Fig. 13.14) or Doppler US prior to percutaneous puncture of pancreatic fluid collections. Pseudoaneurysms occur in 3-10% of patients with acute pancreatitis.

- *Thrombosis* of the splenic vein and other peripancreatic vessels occurs as a result of the inflammatory process. The thrombosed veins are distended with low attenuation thrombus and fail to enhance on venous phase scans.
- *Disconnection of the pancreatic duct* may occur as a result of necrosis resulting in a viable segment of pancreas, usually in the neck region, being disconnected from the intestinal tract. A fistula develops which continues to leak pancreatic fluid and enzymes into peripancreatic spaces.
- *Pancreatic ascites* is caused by leakage of pancreatic juice into the peritoneal cavity inducing secretion of fluid from peritoneal membranes. Pancreatic ascites contains a high level of amylase.
- *Recurrence* of acute pancreatitis occurs in half of the patients in whom the cause is alcohol abuse.

CHRONIC PANCREATITIS

Chronic pancreatitis is a chronic inflammatory disease of the pancreas characterized by progressive pancreatic damage with irreversible fibrosis. Affected patients have chronic abdominal pain, have frequent episodes of acute pancreatitis, and may develop impairment of the endocrine and exocrine functions of the pancreas. This process results in major structural abnormalities in various combinations, including parenchymal atrophy, calcifications, stricture and dilatation of the pancreatic duct, fluid collections, pseudomass formation, and alteration of peripancreatic fat. Although many patients with chronic pancreatitis have recurrent episodes of acute pancreatitis, chronic pancreatitis may also be a separate entity. The causes of chronic pancreatitis include alcoholism (60%), hereditary autosomal dominant disorder, autoimmune disease, tropical pancreatitis, nonalcoholic duct-destructive pancreatitis, and idiopathic causes (30%).

- Calcifications are commonly present (30%–50% of cases) in focal areas or spread diffusely throughout the pancreas (Fig. 13.15). Calcifications occur within the ductal system and range in appearance from finely stippled to coarse. Pancreatic calcifications oc-

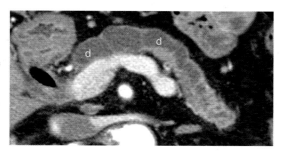

FIG. 13.16 **Chronic pancreatitis: dilated pancreatic duct.** The pancreatic duct *(d)* shows marked beaded dilatation. The pancreatic parenchyma is severely atrophied.

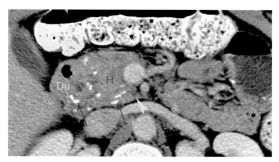

FIG. 13.17 **Chronic pancreatitis: mass.** Chronic pancreatitis causes enlargement of the pancreatic head *(H)* and blunting of the tip of the uncinate process *(yellow arrowhead)*. The mass partially encases the duodenum *(Du)*. A benign cause is suggested by the presence of calcifications *(red arrows)*, which are common with chronic pancreatitis and rare with pancreatic carcinoma. Compare this with Figs. 13.19 and 13.20.

cur most frequently in chronic pancreatitis because of alcoholism and in hereditary pancreatitis.
* The gland is focally or diffusely atrophic (54%) (Fig. 13.16). Atrophy may result in exocrine insufficiency and diabetes mellitus.
* The pancreatic duct has focal strictures and dilated segments (68%). This "beaded" dilatation is characteristic (Fig. 13.16).
* Focal areas of pancreatic enlargement caused by focal inflammation are common (30%) and must be distinguished from tumors (Fig. 13.17). The presence of calcifications within the mass strongly favors pancreatitis over tumor. Percutaneous biopsy, guided by ultrasonography or CT, or endoscopic ultrasound-guided biopsy is commonly needed to make an accurate diagnosis.

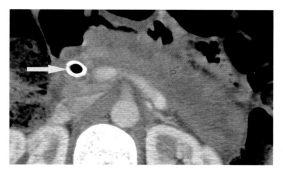

FIG. 13.18 **Autoimmune pancreatitis.** Postcontrast CT in a 70-year-old man shows the pancreas *(P)* to be diffusely enlarged and amorphous with well-defined margins but lacking the normal clefts of fat that separate lobules of the pancreas in patients of this age. A wall stent *(arrow)* has been placed in the common bile duct because of a distal biliary stricture associated with autoimmune pancreatitis.

* Bile ducts may be dilated because of inflammatory stricture of the common bile duct as it passes through the pancreas (Fig. 13-15).
* Fluid collections are caused by superimposed acute pancreatitis (30%).
* Pancreatic pseudocysts are found in 25% to 40% of patients.
* Peripancreatic tissues show inflammatory change with fascial thickening and stranding densities in peripancreatic fat. These changes result in poor definition of the pancreatic margins.

AUTOIMMUNE PANCREATITIS

Autoimmune pancreatitis is a variant of chronic pancreatitis characterized by periductal lymphoplasmacytic inflammation. Men aged 60 to 70 years are primarily affected. Patients present with abdominal pain, anorexia, weight loss, and obstructive jaundice. IgG4 levels are elevated, serving as a marker to distinguish this condition from neoplastic disease. Other associated conditions include panniculitis, sclerosing cholangitis, ulcerative colitis, fibrosing mediastinitis, and retroperitoneal fibrosis.
* CT reveals three morphologic patterns of disease: diffuse, focal, and multifocal.
* With diffuse disease the entire pancreas is enlarged with a characteristic smooth capsule-like rim, an appearance termed *sausage pancreas* (Fig. 13.18). The pancreas is featureless, with absence of the normal clefts of fat separating lobules. A hypoattenuating, hypoenhancing capsule is commonly present,

representing fibrous tissue or inflammatory fluid. Postcontrast images show weak and delayed enhancement of the parenchyma. The pancreatic duct appears diffusely and irregularly narrowed. The common bile duct is often narrowed with a thickened enhancing wall.

- Focal enlargement may mimic neoplasia, most commonly involving the head or uncinate process of the pancreas. Focal autoimmune pancreatitis shows slow progressive enhancement, whereas adenocarcinoma shows persistent low attenuation without notable enhancement. Pancreatic and peripancreatic blood vessels may be narrowed by either condition. Positron emission tomography with CT characteristically shows multifocal pancreatic and peripancreatic uptake in autoimmune pancreatitis that is lacking in adenocarcinoma.
- Multifocal disease appears as multiple nodules of focal enlargement.
- Enlarged lymph nodes are present near the portal vein and celiac axis as well as in peripancreatic areas in 21% of patients. The lymph nodes may show a characteristic low-attenuation halo similar to the halo that commonly surrounds the pancreas.
- Renal lesions associated with autoimmune pancreatitis are relatively common and include wedge-shaped hypodense lesions on postcontrast CT resembling pyelonephritis, multiple renal nodules resembling lymphoma, and mass-like lesions resembling renal cell carcinoma.
- Autoimmune pancreatitis characteristically demonstrates partial or complete resolution with corticosteroid treatment, a response not present in other forms of chronic pancreatitis.

TABLE 13.2
Solid Lesions of the Pancreas: Differential Diagnosis
Neoplastic solid tumors
Ductal adenocarcinoma
Pancreatic neuroendocrine tumor
Pancreatic lymphoma
Metastases to the pancreas
Solid pseudopapillary tumor
Pancreatoblastoma
Acinar cell carcinoma
Mesenchymal tumors (sarcoma, fibrous histiocytoma, etc.)
Nonneoplastic solid lesions
Focal chronic pancreatitis
Autoimmune pancreatitis
Groove pancreatitis
Focal sparing of diffuse pancreatic fatty infiltration
Intrapancreatic accessory spleen
Developmental pancreas lobulation
Sarcoidosis of the spleen

and small cysts in the wall of the duodenum. The inflammatory process forms a sheetlike mass. Enhancement is inhomogeneous and delayed.

- The common bile duct is smoothly narrowed.
- A variant form has fibrosis and inflammation only in the groove, sparing the pancreatic head.
- Differentiation from adenocarcinoma is difficult. Vascular invasion is strong evidence of tumor. Smooth tapering of the common bile duct on magnetic resonance cholangiopancreatography favors groove pancreatitis, whereas abrupt stricture favors carcinoma. Table 13.2 lists diagnostic considerations for solid lesions of the pancreas.

GROOVE PANCREATITIS

Groove pancreatitis is a rare form of chronic pancreatitis that characteristically involves the groove at the junction of the pancreatic head and the descending duodenum. The wall of the duodenum is thickened, is fibrotic, and contains cystic lesions. Most affected patients are men aged 30 to 50 years with a history of alcohol abuse. Duodenal obstruction results in severe abdominal pain, nausea, vomiting, and weight loss. The cause of groove pancreatitis is unknown but appears to be unrelated to gallstones or autoimmune pancreatitis.

- CT shows focal low-attenuation inflammation of the pancreatic head with inflammatory thickening

ADENOCARCINOMA OF THE PANCREAS

Pancreatic carcinoma is an aggressive and usually fatal tumor. Only 5% of afflicted patients survive for 5 years. The only realistic hope of cure is early detection and aggressive surgery (Whipple procedure). Most patients are in the age range of 60 to 80 years. Ductal adenocarcinoma accounts for 90% of pancreatic malignancies. Risk factors for pancreatic carcinoma are shown in Table 13.3. CT and MRI play equivalent pivotal roles in preoperative staging, separating those patients whose carcinoma is obviously *unresectable* from the 10% to 15% whose carcinoma is *potentially resectable*. Of those whose carcinoma is determined by CT to be potentially resectable 70% to 85% are able to undergo resection.

TABLE 13.3
Risk Factors for Pancreatic Cancer

Chronic pancreatitis
Alcohol abuse
Diabetes mellitus
Cigarette smoking
Hereditary pancreatitis
Infectious disease
    Chronic hepatitis B
    Helicobacter pylori infection

CT angiography is very helpful in determining vascular involvement by tumor. Unfortunately, most of those who undergo aggressive resection still eventually die of their disease.

- The tumor appears as a hypodense mass (96% of cases), which is enhanced minimally compared with normal pancreatic parenchyma. Because focal chronic pancreatitis may closely simulate malignancy in the pancreas, biopsy is frequently needed to confirm the diagnosis. Calcifications are rarely associated with adenocarcinoma but are common with mass-forming chronic pancreatitis. Tumors are localized in the head (60%), body (15%), and tail (5%), and are diffuse throughout the pancreas in 20% of cases. See Table 13.2 for differential diagnosis of solid lesions of the pancreas.
- The tumor may be subtle, appearing as focal enlargement of the pancreas with loss of surface lobulation.
- The pancreatic duct and/or common bile duct is commonly dilated proximal to the tumor.
- Atrophy of pancreatic tissue may occur proximal to the tumor.
- Signs of acute or chronic pancreatitis may be simultaneously present.

Signs of potential resectability include the following:
- Isolated pancreatic mass with or without dilatation of the bile and pancreatic ducts (Fig. 13.19).
- Combined bile duct–pancreatic duct dilatation without an identifiable pancreatic mass (pancreatic duct more than 5 mm in the head or more than 3 mm in the tail; common bile duct more than 9 mm). In 10% of cases the tumor is isoattenuating to pancreatic parenchyma. These patients may require MRI or endoscopic ultrasonography to define the mass.
- Detectable regional lymph nodes may or may not be involved with tumor. The size of the nodes is not a reliable criterion for tumor involvement. The presence of enlarged lymph nodes (>10 mm) does not preclude resectability.

- Clear fat planes around the celiac axis, SMA, and hepatic artery showing no evidence of tumor involvement are signs of resectability. Tumor abutment of the SMA not exceeding 180 degrees of the circumference of the vessel wall is borderline resectable.
- Absence of distortion of the SMV and portal vein is a sign of resectability. Venous involvement of the SMV or portal vein with tumor abutment but without narrowing of the vessel lumen may allow surgical resection of the tumor with vein reconstruction.

Signs of unresectability include the following:
- Involvement of major arteries, long segment involvement, or occlusion of major veins makes the tumor unresectable (Fig. 13.20).
- Encasement or invasion of the aorta or inferior vena cava, encasement of the SMA of more than 180 degrees, or abutment of the celiac axis is a sign that the tumor is unresectable. Signs include thickening of the vessels walls; soft-tissue involvement of perivascular fat abutting the vessels walls; narrowing, encasement, or distortion of the vessel lumen; the absence of vessel enhancement, implying occlusion; and dilatation of collateral vessels.
- Long-segment occlusion of the SMV or portal vein, precluding surgical reconstruction.
- Extension of tumor beyond the margins of the pancreas, the presence of liver or distant metastases, or metastases to lymph nodes outside the field of resection.
- Tumor tissue invasion of adjacent organs (spleen, stomach, duodenum).
- Ascites is presumptive evidence of peritoneal carcinomatosis, which may be confirmed by paracentesis.

NEUROENDOCRINE TUMORS

Neuroendocrine tumors (NETs) (formerly referred to as *islet cell tumors*) account for 10% of all pancreatic neoplasms. The tumors may be functioning, producing metabolically active hormones, with hypersecretion producing clinical symptoms, or they may be nonfunctioning, presenting as locally advanced disease with a mass effect, bowel obstruction, or metastases. Up to 25% of NETs are associated with multiple endocrine neoplasia type 1, neurofibromatosis type 1, von Hippel–Lindau syndrome, or tuberous sclerosis. Functioning NETs produce distinct clinical syndromes and usually present when the tumors are small. Nonfunctioning tumors (60%–80% of pancreatic NETs) are clinically silent until they present with symptoms of a large

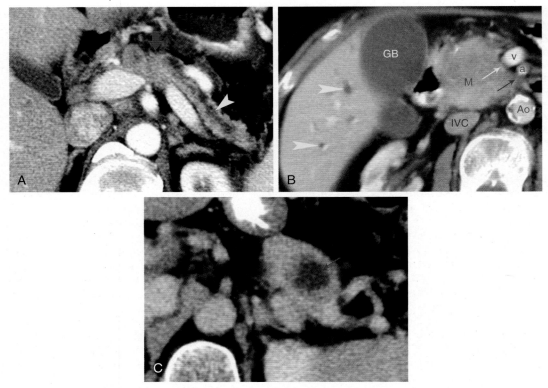

FIG. 13.19 **Potentially resectable pancreatic carcinomas in three patients.** (A) A subtle isoattenuating tumor *(red arrow)* in the pancreatic body is detected because it obstructs and dilates the pancreatic duct *(yellow arrowhead)*, resulting in atrophy of the pancreatic tail. (B) A mass *(M)* in the pancreatic head obstructs the common bile duct, resulting in dilatation of the intrahepatic bile ducts *(yellow arrowheads)* and distension of the gallbladder *(GB)*. The tumor abuts the superior mesenteric vein *(v)* *(yellow arrow)* and the superior mesenteric artery *(a)* *(red arrow)* but at less than 180 degrees, making the tumor potentially resectable. Clear fat margins separate the tumor from the inferior vena cava *(IVC)* and aorta *(Ao)*. (C) An isolated mass *(arrow)* in the pancreatic tail was discovered incidentally and showed no additional findings. All three lesions were completely resected at surgery.

growing mass. Functioning tumors range in malignant potential from 10% for insulinoma to 60% for gastrinoma, 70% for glucagonoma, and 75% for vipoma. Up to 90% of nonfunctioning tumors are malignant.

- Small tumors (1–2 cm) are homogeneous and usually isodense with the unenhanced pancreas. They enhance brightly and usually uniformly during the arterial phase of contrast agent administration (Fig. 13.21). Hormone-producing tumors are usually small.
- Large tumors (4–20 cm) are usually heterogeneous with calcification, cystic degeneration, necrosis, vascular invasion, and direct tumor extension into adjacent structures (Fig. 13.22). Nonfunctioning tumors are commonly large.

- Metastases (20%–40% of cases at diagnosis) occur to lymph nodes and the liver and to distant organs (lungs, bones, peritoneal cavity, brain, and breast). Metastases are usually hypervascular and enhance avidly.

PANCREATIC LYMPHOMA

Lymphoma must be differentiated from adenocarcinoma because the diagnosis and treatment are radically different. Lymphoma involves the pancreas most commonly by direct extension from peripancreatic lymphadenopathy. Most lymphomas are non-Hodgkin B-cell lymphomas with pancreatic involvement in 30% of patients. Primary pancreatic lymphoma is rare (less than 0.5% of pancreatic tumors).

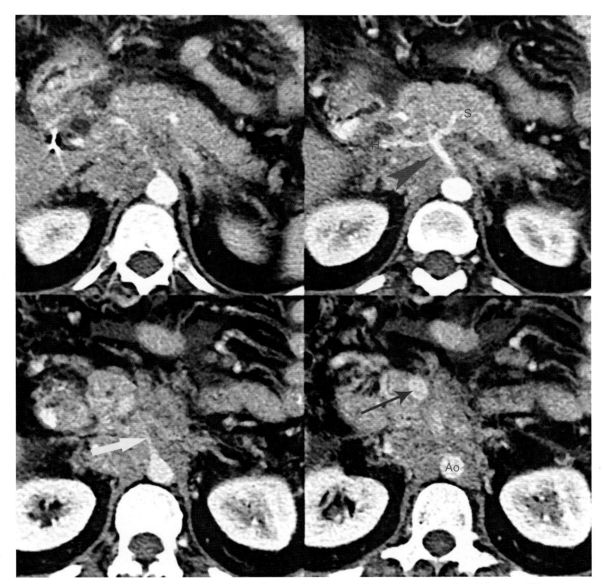

FIG. 13.20 **Unresectable pancreatic carcinoma.** Four images from a postcontrast multidetector CT examination demonstrating tumor encasement of the celiac axis *(red arrowhead)*, common hepatic artery *(H)* and splenic artery *(S)*, superior mesenteric artery *(yellow arrow)*, and superior mesenteric vein *(blue arrow)*. Tumor extensively infiltrates the retroperitoneal fat and partially encases the aorta *(Ao)*.

- Focal tumor that is well circumscribed with homogeneous attenuation less than that of muscle and that enhances weakly but uniformly is characteristic. In distinction with adenocarcinoma the main pancreatic duct is typically not dilated or is minimally dilated.

- Diffuse infiltration of the pancreas resembles pancreatitis but without clinical evidence of pancreatitis.
- Peripancreatic lymphadenopathy that extends into and displaces the pancreas is characteristic of secondary pancreatic lymphoma (Fig. 13.23).

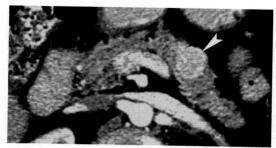

FIG. 13.21 Small neuroendocrine tumor: insulinoma.
A small insulin-producing neuroendocrine tumor *(arrow)* showing early enhancement during an arterial phase CT scan. The patient presented with episodes of hypoglycemia. Hormone-producing neuroendocrine tumors usually present clinically when they are still small.

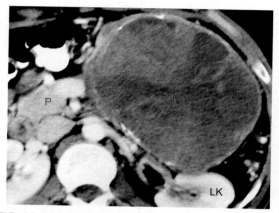

FIG. 13.22 Malignant nonfunctioning neuroendocrine tumor. A huge heterogeneous solid mass *(M)* arising from the body and tail of the pancreas *(P)* displaces the bowel and compresses the left kidney *(LK)*. Non–hormone secreting tumors may grow to a large size before presenting clinically.

- A bulky mass with no or minimal dilatation of the pancreatic duct strongly favors lymphoma over adenocarcinoma.
- Lymphadenopathy below the level of the renal veins is seen with lymphoma but not with pancreatic adenocarcinoma.
- Vascular invasion, tumor necrosis, and calcification are rare.

METASTASES TO THE PANCREAS

Metastases to the pancreas are unusual and are present in only 3% to 12% of patients with advanced malignancy. The most common primary tumors are

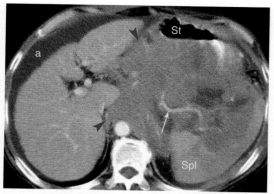

FIG. 13.23 Lymphoma. Massive confluent adenopathy (between *red arrowheads*) envelopes the pancreas, invades the spleen *(Spl)*, encases the aorta, and displaces the stomach *(St)*. Only the splenic artery *(yellow arrow)*, serving as a landmark for the location of the pancreas, is clearly visible within the mass of tumor. Ascites *(a)* is present.

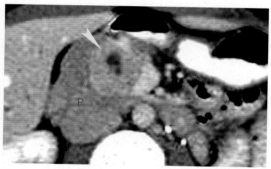

FIG. 13.24 Metastasis from renal cell carcinoma to the pancreas. The brightly enhanced tumor *(arrowhead)* in the head of the pancreas *(P)* proved to be a metastasis from renal carcinoma after nephrectomy years earlier. The tumor shows low-attenuation central necrosis.

melanoma and carcinomas of the kidney, lung, or breast. Metastases account for 2% to 4% of pancreatic masses.

- Most tumors are round or ovoid with smooth discrete margins.
- Metastases are found with equal frequency in all portions of the pancreas.
- Most (75%) demonstrate heterogeneous contrast enhancement.
- Renal cell carcinoma metastases are often uniformly hypervascular (Fig. 13.24) and resemble NETs.
- Tumors are commonly solitary (50%–79%) and simulate primary pancreatic adenocarcinoma.

TABLE 13.4
Cystic Lesions of the Pancreas: Differential Diagnosis

Pseudocyst
Serous cystadenoma
Mucinous cystic neoplasm
Intraductal papillary mucinous neoplasm
Solid and papillary epithelial neoplasm
True epithelial cyst
Duodenal diverticulum
Cystic neuroendocrine tumors
Ductal adenocarcinoma with cystic degeneration
Cystic metastases
Cystic degeneration of sarcoma, hemangioma, and
   paraganglioma

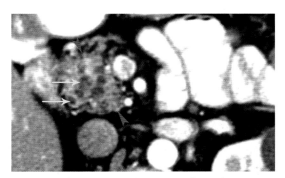

FIG. 13.25 **Serous cystadenoma: polycystic appearance.** Postcontrast CT reveals a polycystic mass (between *red arrows*) replacing the head of the pancreas. The mass consists of numerous small cysts *(yellow arrows)* separated by fibrous septations, a characteristic appearance of benign serous cystadenoma.

- Diffuse involvement (5%–44%) causes generalized pancreatic enlargement.
- Multiple nodules are found in 5% to 17% of cases.
- Involvement of pancreatic blood vessels is rare.
- Lesions in the head and neck may obstruct the main pancreatic duct (37%) or common bile duct.
- Metastases in other organs and at other sites are usually present.

CYSTIC LESIONS

Cystic lesions of the pancreas are being discovered with increased frequency. Although most are benign, many are malignant or potentially malignant and require accurate diagnosis to direct treatment (Table 13.4).

Pseudocysts

By far the most common cystic lesions in and around the pancreas, pseudocysts are collections of pancreatic fluid that have become encapsulated within fibrous walls. They result from episodes of acute pancreatitis. Although most patients with pancreatitis have abdominal pain, some do not. Pseudocyst must always be included in the differential diagnosis of cystic pancreatic lesions. Fluid aspirated from pseudocysts has high levels of amylase.

- Pseudocysts appear as low-attenuation collections of fluid (Fig. 13.8). The collections are unilocular or multilocular. Fluid attenuation may be higher than that of simple fluid because of the presence of hemorrhage or liquefied cellular debris.
- Distinct walls are well-defined and of variable thickness. There is no solid tissue or enhancing components. Calcifications are occasionally present in the cyst wall.

- Most are unilocular. Some contain a few septa.
- Signs of pancreatitis are usually present.

Serous Cystadenoma

Serous cystadenomas are benign cystic pancreatic tumors with no malignant potential. Most lesions are discovered incidentally as most patients are asymptomatic. These tumors are common in patients with von Hippel–Lindau disease. Most patients are older than 60 years and are predominantly female (female-to-male ratio 4:1). Serous cysts contain clear fluid. Endoscopic ultrasound-guided aspiration that yields clear rather than mucinous fluid helps confirm the diagnosis. These lesions occur in three morphologic forms:

- The polycystic (bunch of grapes) appearance (70%) is characterized by multiple cysts 2 cm or smaller separated by fibrous septa (Fig. 13.25). Most cysts are smaller than 1 cm.
- The honeycomb appearance (20%) is a well-circumscribed mass of innumerable tiny cysts producing a spongy solid–appearing low-attenuation mass on imaging (Fig. 13.26). The innumerable tiny cyst may appear as a solid mass of low attenuation.
- The macrocystic (oligocystic) (10%) appearance consists of a few cysts larger than 2 cm (Fig. 13.27). The oligocystic appearance closely mimics that of mucinous cystadenoma, from which it must be differentiated.

The more common unilocular form is 2 to 6 cm in size and may be indistinguishable from mucinous cystic neoplasms (MCNs). Lobulated contour, the absence of wall enhancement, and location in the pancreatic

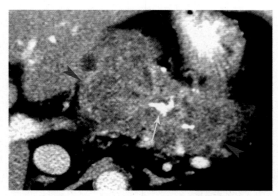

FIG. 13.26 **Serous cystadenoma: honeycomb appearance.** Although it consists of innumerable tiny cysts, this tumor (between *red arrowheads*) resembles a solid mass. The central calcification *(yellow arrow)* within a stellate scar is characteristic. This is a benign tumor arising from the neck of the pancreas.

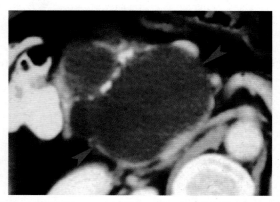

FIG. 13.27 **Serous cystadenoma: macrocystic appearance.** The pancreatic head is replaced by a cystic mass (between *red arrowheads*) consisting of two large cysts. This appearance is consistent with either a mucinous cystic neoplasm or a macrocystic serous cystadenoma. Compare this with Fig. 13.28. Endoscopic ultrasonography may be used to guide aspiration of the cyst fluid to determine if the fluid is serous or mucinous.

head favor serous cystadenoma. Serous cystadenomas are most common in the pancreatic head and do not communicate with the pancreatic duct. A central stellate scar, often with calcification (Fig. 13.26), may be present.

Mucinous Cystic Neoplasms

Cystic mucin-producing neoplasms of the pancreas are classified as *mucinous cystic neoplasms* (MCNs) and *intraductal papillary mucinous neoplasms* (IPMNs). These

tumors are characterized pathologically by mucin-producing epithelial tumor cells that form papillae and grow as cystic lesions. Both tumor types show pathologic progression from low-grade dysplasia (adenoma) to high-grade dysplasia (carcinoma in situ) to invasive carcinoma. Benign lesions are considered premalignant.

International consensus guidelines for management of mucinous tumors of the pancreas were revised in 2012 (Fukuoka guidelines). Radiologic features determine the classification of tumors. Invasive cancer is rare in asymptomatic cysts smaller than 10 mm. "Worrisome features" on imaging include cysts of 3 cm or more in diameter; enhancing thickened cyst walls; main pancreatic duct diameter of 5 to 9 mm; mural nodules without enhancement; abrupt narrowing of the main pancreatic duct with proximal atrophy of pancreatic parenchyma; and regional lymphadenopathy. "High-risk stigmata" on imaging include common bile duct obstruction with jaundice associated with cystic tumor in the pancreatic head; enhancement of solid components; and main pancreatic duct diameter of 10 mm or greater. The Fukuoka guidelines recommend resection without further testing for cystic lesions with high-risk stigmata. Cystic lesions with worrisome features and cysts larger than 3 cm without worrisome features should undergo endoscopic ultrasonography for further characterization. Cysts 3 cm or smaller should undergo routine surveillance with contrast-enhanced multidetector CT or MRI with magnetic resonance cholangiopancreatography.

MCNs are rare primary tumors of the pancreas found most commonly in middle-aged women (95% of cases). All are considered to be potential cystadenocarcinomas, although most are low grade. Low-grade MCNs have an excellent prognosis with surgical resection. High-grade invasive mucinous cystadenocarcinomas (6%–36% of cases) have a poor prognosis. Histologic identification of ovarian stroma distinguishes MCNs from other pancreatic tumors. Surgical resection recommendations follow international guidelines.

- Tumors appear as multiloculated cysts with thin (<2 mm) septa (Fig. 13.28). Six or fewer cysts larger than 2 cm are considered typical of the lesion. CT may not demonstrate the thin septa on unenhanced images, but the septa usually enhance and are well seen following contrast agent administration.
- Attenuation of fluid within the cyst tends to be heterogeneous and varies with content (watery to mucoid to hemorrhagic).
- Calcifications are seen in the capsule or septa in 10% of lesions. Peripheral calcifications are characteristic of MCN, whereas serous cystadenomas have only central calcifications.

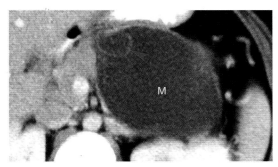

FIG. 13.28 **Mucinous cystic neoplasm.** A large cystic mass *(M)* arises from the body of the pancreas. A thin enhancing septation *(arrow)* is present. Differential diagnosis would include pseudocyst and the macrocystic form of serous cystadenoma.

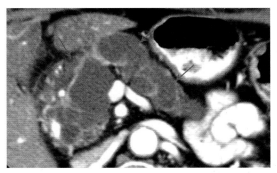

FIG. 13.30 **Intraductal papillary mucinous neoplasm: main-duct type.** The main pancreatic duct *(arrows)* is massively and diffusely dilated in a beaded pattern. Very little pancreatic parenchyma is visible.

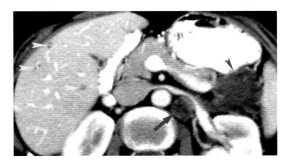

FIG. 13.29 **Mucinous cystic neoplasm: metastases.** A low-attenuation cystic mass (between *red arrowheads*) is evident at the tail of the pancreas. Small low-attentuation lesions *(yellow arrowheads)* in the liver and an enlarged lymph node *(red arrow)* behind the left renal vein represent metastatic spread of the malignant tumor.

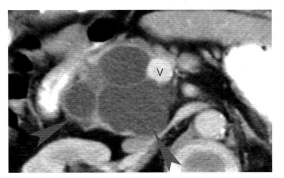

FIG. 13.31 **Intraductal papillary mucinous neoplasm: branch-duct type.** A multicystic mass *(arrowheads)* arises from the uncinate process of the pancreas and envelops the superior mesenteric vein *(V)*. Magnetic resonance cholangiopancreatography confirmed communication of the lesion with the pancreatic duct.

- Lesions range in size from 2 to 36 cm, with an average size of 6 to 10 cm.
- Tumors are most common in the distal body and tail of the pancreas.
- These tumors do not communicate with the ductal system of the pancreas.
- Metastases may be evident (Fig. 13.29).

IPMNs secrete mucin into the pancreatic ducts, producing progressive dilation of the ducts. IPMNs are divided into *main-duct* and *branch-duct* types. Branch-duct tumors have a better prognosis. The prevalence of cancer in branch-duct IPMNs is 15% to 20% compared with 60% to 92% for main-duct IPMNs. IPMNs arise from the epithelium lining the pancreatic ducts. IPMNs are differentiated histologically by the absence of ovarian stroma that characterized MCNs. Surgical resection recommendations follow international guidelines.

- IPMNs arising in the main pancreatic duct produce marked diffuse or segmental enlargement of the main pancreatic duct associated with atrophy of the pancreatic parenchyma (Fig. 13.30). Amorphous calcification may be evident within the dilated duct.
- IPMNs of branch ducts produce a bunch-of-grapes appearance that bulges the contour of the pancreas. Branch-duct IPMNs are most common in the uncinate process (Fig. 13.31).
- Intraductal papillary solid masses may be seen within the dilated pancreatic ducts and serve as strong evidence of malignancy. Dilatation of the main pancreatic duct to greater than 15 mm is also predictive of malignancy.

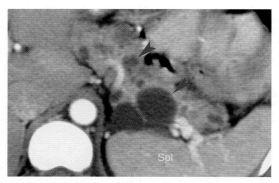

FIG. 13.32 **Von Hippel-Lindau Disease.** Multilocular and unilocular cysts *(arrowheads)* are seen throughout the body and tail of the pancreas in this patient with von Hippel-Lindau disease. *Spl,* Spleen.

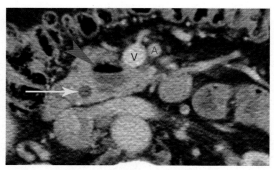

FIG. 13.33 **Duodenal Diverticulum.** A diverticulum *(red arrowhead)* arising from the second portion of the duodenum creates a mass with an air-fluid level in the uncinate process of the pancreas. Duodenal diverticula may mimic a cystic pancreatic neoplasm, or in the right clinical setting, an abscess. The common bile duct *(yellow arrow)* courses adjacent to the diverticulum. Occasionally the common bile duct may insert into the diverticulum instead of the duodenum. This may result in obstruction of the common bile duct. *A,* Superior mesenteric artery; *V,* superior mesenteric vein.

- Magnetic resonance cholangiopancreatography and endoscopic retrograde cholangiopancreatography show the characteristic communication between the IPMN and the pancreatic duct.

True Epithelial Cysts

True pancreatic cysts are rare and are seen far less frequently than pancreatic pseudocysts. Congenital epithelium-lined cysts are usually solitary. Multiple pancreatic cysts are seen with von Hippel–Lindau disease (50% of patients) and autosomal dominant polycystic disease (5% of patients). Rarely epithelial lined cysts are seen in patients with cystic fibrosis.

- Cysts appear as well-defined fluid-filled masses of various sizes with walls of variable thickness (Fig. 13.32). Internal septa and contrast enhancement are not present.
- In von Hippel–Lindau disease the pancreas is also involved with serous cystadenomas (12%) and NETs (7%–12%). A small number of the NETs are malignant. The cystic lesions in the pancreas are benign.

DUODENAL DIVERTICULUM

Duodenal diverticula are common lesions that may be entirely fluid filled and mimic a cystic neoplasm of the pancreas (Fig. 13.33). Duodenal diverticula are outpouchings of the wall of the duodenum and are most common protruding from the medial wall of the second portion of the duodenum.

SUGGESTED READING

Al-Hawary, M. M., Francis, I. R., Chari, S. T., et al. (2014). Pancreatic ductal adenocarcinoma radiology reporting template: Consensus statement of the Society of Abdominal Radiology and the American Pancreatic Association. *Radiology, 270,* 248–260.

Baker, M. E., Nelson, R. C., Rosen, M. P., et al. (2014). ACR appropriateness criteria – acute pancreatitis. *Ultrasound Quarterly, 30,* 267–273.

Borghei, P., Sokhandon, F., Shirkhoda, A., & Morgan, D. E. (2013). Anomalies, anatomic variants, and sources of diagnostic pitfalls in pancreatic imaging. *Radiology, 266,* 28–36.

Foster, B. R., Jensen, K. K., Bakis, G., et al. (2016). Revised Atlanta classification for acute pancreatitis: A pictorial essay. *Radiographics, 36,* 675–687.

Freeny, P. C., & Saunders, M. D. (2014). Moving beyond morphology: New insights into the characterization and management of cystic pancreatic lesions. *Radiology, 272,* 345–363.

Horger, M., Lamprecht, H.-G., Bares, R., et al. (2012). Systemic IgG4-related sclerosing disease: Spectrum of imaging findings and differential diagnosis. *AJR. American Journals Roentgenology, 199,* W276–W282.

Khandelwal, A., Shanbhogue, A. K., Takahashi, N., et al. (2014). Recent advances in the diagnosis and management of autoimmune pancreatitis. *AJR. Amrican Journals Roentgenology, 202,* 1007–1021.

Kim, K. W., Krajewski, K. M., Nishino, M., et al. (2013). Update on the management of gastroenteropancreatic neuroendocrine tumors with emphasis on the role of imaging. *AJR. Amrican Journals Roentgenology, 201,* 811–824.

Lee, E. S., & Lee, J. M. (2014). Imaging diagnosis of pancreatic cancer: A state-of-the-art review. *World Journal of Gastroenterology, 20,* 7864–7877.

Murphy, K. P., O'Connor, O. J., & Maher, M. M. (2014). Updated imaging nomenclature for acute pancreatitis. *AJR. Amrican Journals Roentgenology, 203,* W464–W469.

Qayyum, A., Tamm, E. P., Kamel, I. R., et al. (2017). ACR appropriateness criteria - staging of pancreatic ductal adenocarcinoma. *Journals of American College of Radiology, 14,* S560–S569.

Raman, S. P., Salaria, S. N., Hruban, R. H., & Fishman, E. K. (2013). Groove pancreatitis: Spectrum of imaging findings and radiology-pathology correlation. *AJR. Amrican Journals Roentgenology, 201,* W29–W39.

Seo, N., Byun, J. H., Kim, J. H., et al. (2016). Validation of the 2012 international consensus guidelines using computed tomography and magnetic resonance imaging: Branch duct and main duct intraductal papillary mucinous neoplasms of the pancreas. *Annals of Surgical, 263,* 557–564.

Tanaka, M., Fernandez-del Castillo, C., Adsay, V., et al. (2012). International consensus guidelines 2012 for the management of IPMN and MCN of the pancreas. *Official Journal of the International Association of Pancreatology, 12,* 183–197.

CHAPTER 14

Spleen

WILLIAM E. BRANT

With high-resolution multidetector CT and dynamic multiphase postcontrast protocols, an increasing number of splenic lesions are being detected. These require characterization by combination of imaging findings with clinical data. Many spleen lesions are nonspecific in appearance. At a minimum, splenic lesions should be characterized as benign or potentially malignant.

ANATOMY

The spleen occupies a relatively constant position in the left upper quadrant of the abdomen. It is a soft and pliable organ that conforms to the shape of adjacent structures (Fig. 14.1). The diaphragmatic surface is smooth and convex, conforming to the dome of the diaphragm, whereas the visceral surface has concavities for the stomach, kidneys, and colon. The splenic artery and vein course in close relationship with the pancreas to the splenic hilum, where each vessel divides into multiple branches. The normal spleen has lobulations, notches, and clefts that may be mistaken for abnormalities (Fig. 14.2). Lobulations in the splenic contour can generally be identified on serial slices as part of the spleen. They have sharply defined margins, have no perisplenic abnormalities, and have uniform attenuation equal to that of the remainder of the spleen. They show enhancement equal to that of the spleen.

The CT density of the normal spleen is less than or equal to the CT density of the normal liver. Attenuation of the normal unenhanced spleen is 40 to 60 Hounsfield units (HU), which is 5 to 10 HU less than that of the normal unenhanced liver. Most splenic lesions are seen best on contrast-enhanced CT scans.

A heterogeneous serpentine, cord-like enhancement of the spleen can be expected during the arterial phase (Fig 14.3). This pattern is caused by variable blood flow through the red pulp and white pulp of the normal spleen. Delayed images show uniform splenic parenchymal enhancement. Fast contrast medium injection rates, congestive heart failure, portal hypertension, and splenic vein thrombosis are associated with exaggeration and prolongation of the serpentine enhancement pattern.

TECHNICAL CONSIDERATIONS

The spleen is included on every CT scan of the abdomen as well as multiphase CT scans of the liver and pancreas. Typically, images are viewed at 2.5 to 5-mm thickness. Contrast medium is administered at 2 to 3 mL per second for a total dose of 120 to 150 mL. Routine scans are obtained at 50 to 60 seconds after contrast medium injection (essentially in the portal venous phase). To characterize a splenic lesion, aquisition of noncontrast images is followed by aquisition of dual-phase postcontrast images obtained at 30 and 60 seconds.

ANOMALIES
Accessory Spleen

Accessory spleens, also called *splenules*, are nodules of normal splenic tissue that are formed separately from the main spleen. They are present in 10% to 30% of individuals and may be solitary or multiple.
- Splenules appear as round or oval masses up to 2 to 3 cm in diameter, most commonly located near the hilum of the spleen (Fig 14.4).
- They have the same CT density, tissue texture, and enhancement patterns as the main spleen.
- Accessory spleens may hypertrophy after splenic resection.

Wandering Spleen

Wandering spleen refers to a normal spleen that is found outside the left upper quadrant of the abdomen. Congenital laxity of the ligaments, often associated with anomalies of intestinal fixation, allows the spleen to be freely mobile and to be located anywhere in the abdomen. Wandering spleens are usually asymptomatic but may be a cause of a palpable abdominal mass and are more susceptible to traumatic injury and torsion.
- Diagnosis is made by one noting the absence of a normal spleen in its typical location and that the ectopic mass has the attenuation, shape, and enhancement patterns of normal splenic tissue.
- Documentation of blood supply by splenic vessels is confirmatory.

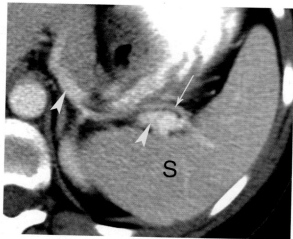

FIG. 14.1 **Normal spleen.** Delayed contrast CT shows the smooth contours and homogeneously enhanced parenchyma of the normal spleen (S). Contrast medium has washed out of the splenic artery (arrow) seen at the splenic hilum. The splenic vein (arrowheads) is enhanced and shown coursing through the pancreas and at the hilum of the spleen.

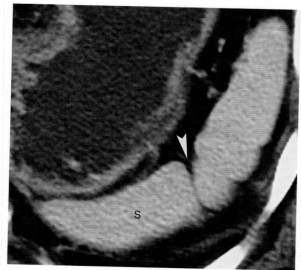

FIG. 14.2 **Normal cleft.** A prominent, but normal, cleft (arrowhead) is evident in the spleen (S).

Splenic Regeneration/Splenosis

Remnants of splenic tissue after splenic injury and remnant accessory spleens may hypertrophy after splenectomy, resulting in single or multiple left upper abdominal masses. The diagnosis is suggested clinically when a patient with a history of splenectomy has no Howell-Jolly bodies on peripheral blood smear. Howell-Jolly bodies are remnants of nuclear material in red blood cells that are routinely removed from the circulating blood by splenic tissue.

- Regenerative splenic remnants have the CT appearance of abnormally shaped, but otherwise normal-appearing, splenic tissue (Fig. 14.5). The presence of splenic tissue may be confirmed by technetium-99m sulfur colloid radionuclide imaging.
- Splenic remnants may be found in unusual locations: in the thorax (associated with traumatic rupture of the diaphragm), in the liver (splenic vein emboli), near the kidney mimicking a renal mass, and subcutaneously (associated with a surgical incision or traumatic wound).

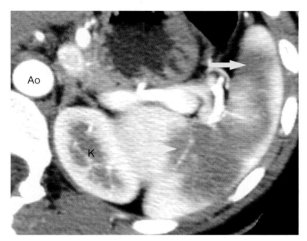

FIG. 14.3 **Normal splenic flow defects.** Inhomogeneous enhancement of the spleen produces a pseudomass effect *(arrows)* during the early stage of intravenous contrast medium administration with a power injector. The bright enhancement of the aorta *(Ao)* and enhancement of only the cortex of the kidney *(K)* indicate the early arterial stage of contrast enhancement. Images obtained a few minutes later demonstrated uniform density of the spleen as illustrated in Fig. 14.1.

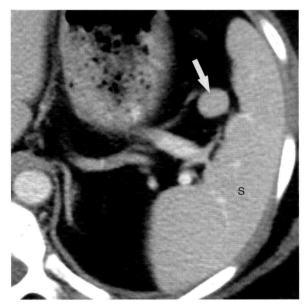

FIG. 14.4 **Accessory spleen.** An accessory spleen *(arrow)* is evident near the hilum of the spleen *(S)*.

Splenomegaly

Spleen size varies with age, body habitus, state of hydration, and nutrition. The spleen normally decreases in size with age. The causes of splenomegaly are exhaustive but can be classified into myeloproliferative, infectious, inflammatory, congestive, and infiltrative categories. Most conditions do not affect CT density of the spleen, so differentiation is based on other CT findings or clinical evaluation.

- Size greater than 12 to 14 cm in any dimension is a primary sign of splenomegaly in adults.
- Spleen length greater than 20 cm indicates massive splenomegaly.

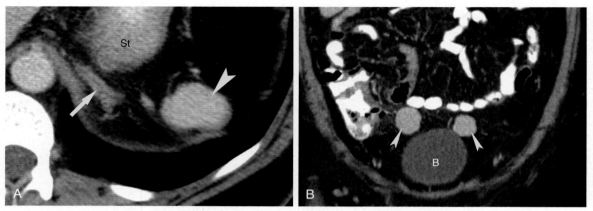

FIG. 14.5 Splenic regeneration. (A) In a patient after splenectomy for traumatic injury resulting in a severely shattered spleen, contrast-enhanced CT shows a uniformly enhanced rounded mass *(arrowhead)* in the splenic bed. Anatomic landmarks include the stomach *(St)* and left adrenal gland *(arrow)*. (B) Coronal image in the same patient showing similar enhanced rounded masses *(arrowheads)* near the bladder *(B)*. Technetium sulfur colloid radionuclide scan confirmed functioning splenic tissue that regenerated from remnants of the shattered spleen.

- Extension of the spleen tip inferior to the lower pole of the left kidney is an imaging sign of splenomegaly.

FOCAL LESIONS
Cysts
Cystic lesions of the spleen have a variety of causes. An accurate diagnosis can usually be made by correlation of CT findings with the medical history and clinical findings.

- *Posttraumatic cysts* are the most common splenic cyst, accounting for 80% of all splenic cystic lesions. They result from previous hemorrhage, infarction, or infection, and basically represent the end stage of an intrasplenic hematoma. They are false cysts without epithelial lining. The wall is fibrous tissue of variable thickness. Internal debris, fluid levels, and milk of calcium are common features. Calcification is found in the wall in 30% to 40% of cases (Fig 14.6).
- *Congenital epithelium-lined cysts* are true cysts with epithelium lining the cyst wall. Other terms for this entity include *epidermoid cyst* and *mesothelial cyst*. They are usually solitary and account for up to 20% of splenic cysts. CT shows a well-defined, spherical, and usually unilocular cyst with thin walls (Fig. 14.7). Cyst contents are of water density and do not show contrast enhancement. Internal debris is sometimes present. Calcification is found in the walls in about 5% of cases.

- *Echinococcal cysts* may be indistinguishable from traumatic and epithelial cysts but are rare, affecting less than 2% of patients with hydatid disease. Patients have abdominal pain, fever, and splenomegaly. Most patients with splenic involvement also have liver involvement. The CT appearance of a splenic echinococcal cyst is similar to that of those in the liver. The cysts may be homogeneous, with internal CT density of water, mimicking other splenic cysts. The lesion may show a larger mother cyst containing smaller daughter cysts near the periphery (Fig. 14.8). Ring-like calcification of the walls of the mother cyst and the internal daughter cysts is common. Hydatid sand appears as layering internal debris of higher CT density than the cyst fluid. Because of the risk of spontaneous or posttraumatic rupture, splenic echinococcal cysts are usually treated surgically.
- *Pancreatic pseudocysts* result from pancreatitis with fluid gaining access to the splenic parenchyma from the pancreas by dissection through the splenic hilum (Fig. 14.9). CT demonstrates a characteristically subcapsular fluid collection of water attenuation. Findings of pancreatitis are usually present.

Infarction
Splenic infarctions may be asymptomatic or present with left upper quadrant pain. The causes include involvement of splenic vessels by atherosclerosis, arteritis, tumor, or pancreatitis. Additional causes include systemic emboli and sickle disease. Splenomegaly is a

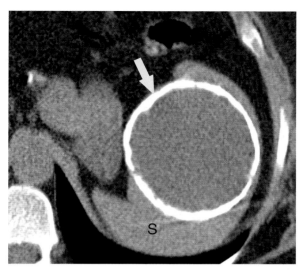

FIG. 14.6 **Posttraumatic cyst.** Liquefaction of an old hematoma in the spleen *(S)* resulted in formation of this cystic mass *(arrow)* with a densely calcified thickened wall.

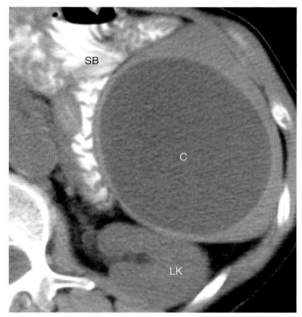

FIG. 14.7 **Epidermoid cyst.** A large cyst *(C)* expands the spleen, compressing the left kidney *(LK)* and displacing small bowel *(SB)* on this noncontrast CT image.

predisposing factor for infarction. Infarcts easily become infected if the patient develops bacteremia.

- The classic appearance of an acute infarction is a wedge-shaped low-attenuation defect that extends to the splenic capsule. Extension to the splenic cap-

sule is a characteristic finding as many splenic infarcts are not wedge-shaped (Fig. 14.10).

- Infarctions will atrophy over time, resulting in depressed areas and notching of the splenic contour. Calcifications may occur in the infarcted area.

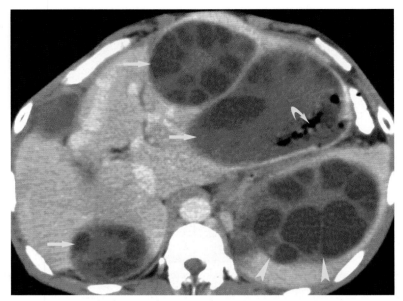

FIG. 14.8 **Echinococcal cysts** in the spleen *(arrowheads)* and liver *(straight arrows)* show a classic appearance of a mother cyst containing multiple daughter cysts. Air bubbles *(curved arrow)* in one of the liver lesions indicates secondary bacterial infection within the hydatid cyst.

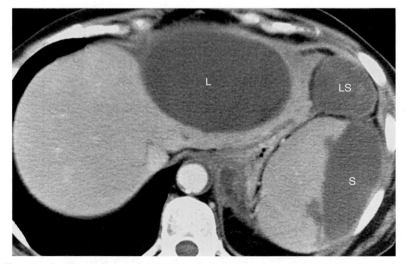

FIG. 14.9 **Pancreatic pseudocysts.** Subcapsular fluid collections associated with acute pancreatitis are present in the spleen *(S)* and liver *(L)*. Loculated fluid is also seen in a recess of the lesser sac *(LS)*. High amylase content of the fluid was confirmed by CT-guided aspiration and drainage.

Bacterial Abscesses

Bacterial abscesses occur uncommonly but are associated with high mortality when untreated. The signs and symptoms may be vague. Diseased spleens are particularly susceptible to abscess formation when organisms are delivered hematogenously from distant foci of infection. Abscesses may also result from spread of infection from adjacent organs or from suppuration in a traumatic hematoma. Patients are often debilitated by diabetes, immune system compromise, or intravenous drug abuse.

- Abscesses appear on CT as single or multiple low-density areas with ill-defined walls, which may be thickened and enhance with contrast medium. Internal attenuation is 20 to 40 HU. Abscesses may

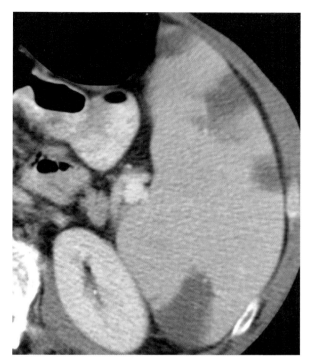

FIG. 14.10 **Infarction.** The spleen shows multiple low-attenuation lesions extending to the splenic capsule in this patient with splenomegaly related to chronic lymphocytic leukemia. Although some lesions are wedge-shaped, others are not. Extension to the splenic capsule is the most characteristic finding of splenic infarction.

contain gas (20%) or demonstrate fluid levels. Gas within the splenic fluid collection is considered to be diagnostic of abscess (Fig. 14.11). Percutaneous aspiration of infected fluid confirms the diagnosis. Treatment is by catheter drainage or splenectomy.

Microabscesses

Patients who are immunocompromised because of AIDS, chemotherapy, lymphoma, leukemia, or organ transplantation may develop microabscesses caused by opportunistic infections. Most microabscesses in the spleen are caused by fungal infection (*Candida, Pneumocystis jiroveci, Aspergillus, Cryptococcus, Histoplasma*). Less common causes include cytomegalovirus and Mycobacterium tuberculosis.

- Multiple low-density defects in the spleen are 2 to 10 mm in size (Fig. 14.12).
- Differential diagnosis of multiple, small, low-density splenic defects includes lymphoma, Kaposi sarcoma (Fig. 14.13), sarcoidosis, and metastases.

Lymphoma

The spleen is the largest lymphoid organ in the body, so it is hardly surprising that involvement by lymphoma is common. Primary splenic lymphoma is rare, but secondary involvement of the spleen by systemic lymphoma is common. Approximately one-third of all patients with lymphoma have involvement of the spleen. Lymphoma is the most common malignant tumor of the spleen. CT is not reliable in the detection of lymphomatous involvement. The spleen may be normal yet involved, or may be enlarged and not involved. Focal lesions are a reliable sign of disease.

- Diffuse infiltration may result in homogeneous enlargement without masses.
- Multiple lesions are the most characteristic. They range from the miliary pattern of tiny lesions up to lesions of 2 to 10 cm. The lesions are not enhanced with intravenous contrast medium administration. Necrosis is rare.
- A solitary large mass may represent a confluent deposit of lymphomatous tissue (Fig. 14.14).
- Enlarged nodes are usually seen in the splenic hilum, along the splenic vessels, and elsewhere in the abdomen.
- Lymphoma predisposes the spleen to infarction.

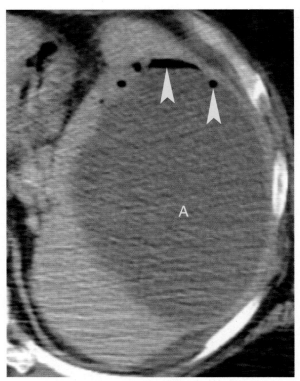

FIG. 14.11 Abscess. CT image of a patient with leukemia showing a large fluid collection *(A)* within the enlarged spleen. Gas bubbles *(arrowheads)*, which rise nondependently within the fluid, are strong evidence of abscess.

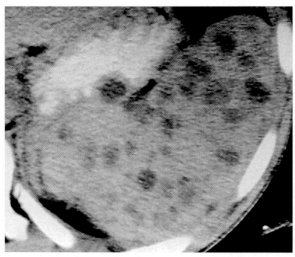

FIG. 14.12 Microabscesses. Many ill-defined low-attenuation lesions are seen in the spleen in this patient with acute myelogenous leukemia. The lesions were as a result of *Candida albicans* sepsis.

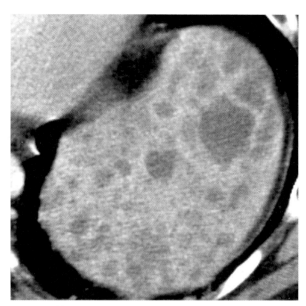

FIG. 14.13 Kaposi sarcoma. CT of the spleen in a patient with AIDS and cutaneous lesions of Kaposi sarcoma shows innumerable low-attenuation lesions throughout the spleen indistinguishable from the microabscesses of opportunistic infection.

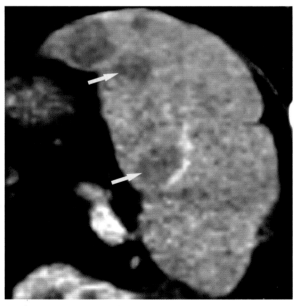

FIG. 14.14 Lymphoma. Coronal CT image of the spleen showing multiple ill-defined low-attenuation lesions *(arrows)* that proved to be non-Hodgkin lymphoma.

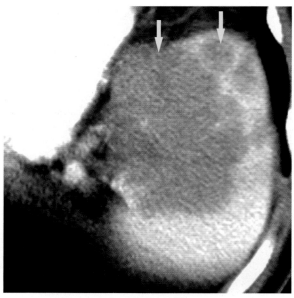

FIG. 14.15 Metastases. Metastases *(arrows)* from malignant melanoma cause multiple homogeneous low-attenuation lesions of various sizes in the spleen.

Metastases

Melanoma and lung, breast, and ovarian carcinoma are the most common sources of splenic metastases. Metastases are surprisingly uncommon and are seen in only 2% to 9% of patients with widespread malignancy. Melanoma is the source of 50% of the splenic metastases detected in imaging studies. Lesions appear late in the course of the disease.

- Most appear as ill-defined low-density, but not water-density, nodules with some degree of peripheral enhancement (Fig. 14.15). They may be solitary or multiple.
- Melanoma commonly causes well-defined cystic metastases.
- Isolated splenic lesions seen in patients with known malignancy are usually not metastases unless widespread metastatic disease is present.

Sarcoidosis

Sarcoidosis is a systemic granulomatous disease that involves many abdominal organs particularly the liver and spleen, which are involved in 5% to 15% of patients. About 60% of patients with sarcoidosis have involvement of the spleen. Liver involvement is even more common but is often not detectable with CT.

- Sarcoidosis of the spleen may cause splenomegaly or may be evident as single or multiple low-attenuation nodules with indistinct margins (Fig. 14.16). Abdominal lymphadenopathy may be present.

Hemangioma

Although unusual, hemangiomas are the most common benign neoplasm of the spleen. As in the liver, the lesion consists of endothelium-lined blood-filled spaces of various sizes. Most are asymptomatic, but very large hemangiomas may cause pain and splenomegaly. Confident diagnosis may be difficult because of the wide variation in appearance.

- Lesions may appear cystic or solid on unenhanced CT. They may be solitary or multiple. The size ranges from 1 to 15 cm. Klippel-Trénaunay-Weber syndrome is associated with multiple splenic hemangiomas that appear strikingly cystic. Punctate calcifications may be present.
- Following contrast medium administration, splenic hemangiomas may demonstrate characteristic nodular enhancement from the periphery very similar to the enhancement pattern of liver hemangiomas (Fig. 14.17). However, atypical patterns of enhancement are common.
- Some may remain hypodense, whereas others enhance uniformly on arterial phase images.
- Central punctate or peripheral curvilinear calcifications may be present.

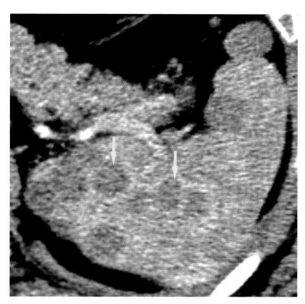

FIG. 14.16 **Sarcoidosis.** Multiple ill-defined low-attenuation lesions *(arrows)* of the spleen represent the noncaseous granulomas of sarcoidosis. The appearance overlaps that of microabscess, metastases, lymphoma, and Kaposi sarcoma.

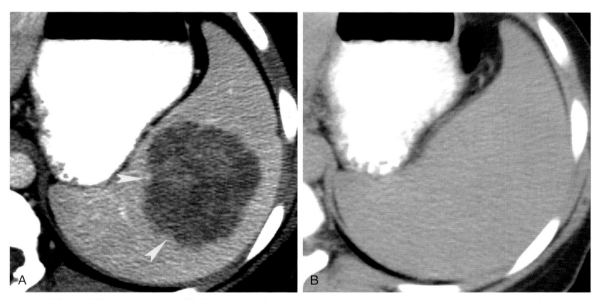

FIG. 14.17 **Hemangioma.** (A) Relatively early postcontrast image showing small nodules of peripheral enhancement *(arrowheads)*. (B) Delayed postcontrast scan showing that the lesion has become isodense with the splenic parenchyma and is no longer evident.

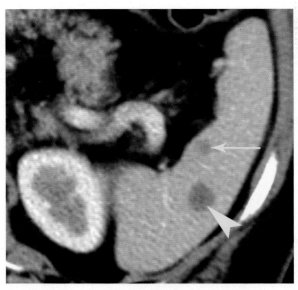

FIG. 14.18 **Lymphangioma.** Early postcontrast CT reveals a homogeneous low-attenuation lesion *(arrowhead)* in the spleen. A second, similar lesion is partially visualized *(arrow)*. A total of three lesions were present. None showed contrast enhancement. Percutaneous CT-guided biopsy confirmed lymphangioma.

Lymphangioma

Lymphangiomas are uncommon splenic tumors that are usually small and asymptomatic. They are benign and slow growing.

- On CT they are usually small, multiple, homogeneous, and cystic in appearance with internal attenuation of 15 to 35 HU (Fig. 14.18). They demonstrate no contrast enhancement and are typically subcapsular in location. Occasionally thin calcification of the wall is present.

Hamartoma

Hamartomas are rare lesions consisting of a mixture of normal elements of splenic tissue. They may be single or multiple and are associated with tuberous sclerosis.

- The CT appearance may be similar to that of splenic hemangioma. However, differentiation is usually not important as both are benign lesions.
- The lesions are of low attenuation or isointense to spleen on noncontrast CT (Fig. 14.19) and show slow enhancement after contrast medium administration, usually becoming isointense on delayed postcontrast images. The lesion typically bulges the contour of the spleen. Central punctate or peripheral curvilinear calcifications may be present. Necrotic and cystic areas may also be present.

Angiosarcoma

Angiosarcoma is a rare primary malignancy of the spleen arising from the endothelium of blood vessels in the spleen. The tumor is aggressive, usually presenting with widespread metastases to lung, bone, and especially the liver. Most patients die of their disease within 12 months. The tumor may spontaneously rupture and hemorrhage into the peritoneal cavity.

- Multiple enhancing nodules with irregular and poorly defined contours are the most common CT appearance.
- Angiosarcoma may also appear as a complex mass of cystic and solid components that enhance irregularly (Fig. 14.20). Hemorrhage of various stages is commonly present.
- The spleen is usually enlarged.

Splenic Calcifications

Splenic calcifications are a frequent CT finding;

- Multiple small focal calcifications (Fig. 14.21) in an otherwise normal-appearing spleen are the result of previous histoplasmosis or tuberculosis.

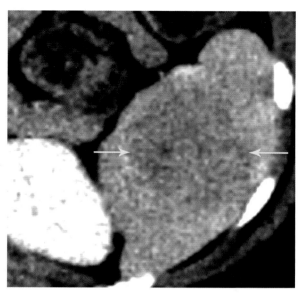

FIG. 14.19 **Hamartoma.** A large but subtle, poorly defined lesion *(arrows)* in the spleen proved on biopsy to be a splenic hamartoma.

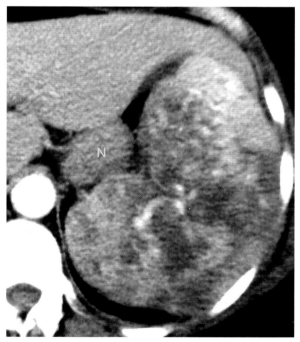

FIG. 14.20 **Angiosarcoma.** A complex mass of low- and high-density components with tangled enhancing vessels replaces most of the splenic parenchyma. Metastatic tumor causes enlargement of a lymph node *(N)* in the splenic hilum.

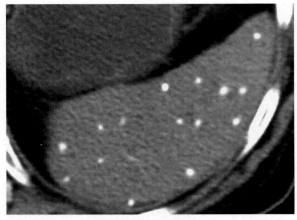

FIG. 14.21 **Calcified granulomas.** Calcified granulomas without associated mass are seen in the spleen on this noncontrast CT image. These were most likely caused by histoplasmosis.

- Larger, coarser calcifications result from previous infarction, infection, or trauma.
- Sickle hemoglobinopathy alone or in combination with thalassemia or hemoglobin C disease can result in infarction and calcification of the entire spleen, which atrophies and becomes functionless.

SUGGESTED READING

Ahmed, S., Horton, K. M., & Fishman, E. K. (2011). Splenic incidentalomas. *Radiologic clinics of North America, 49,* 323–347.

Chapman, J., & Bhimji, S. (2017). Splenomegaly National Center for Biotechnology Information Bookshelf. *Treasure Island: StatPearls Publishing.*

Dhyani, M., Anupindi, S. A., Ayyala, R., et al. (2013). Defining an imaging algorithm for noncystic splenic lesions identified in young patients. *AJR American journal of roentgenology, 201,* W893–W899.

Kaza, R. K., Azar, S., Al-Hawary, M. M., & Francis, I. R. (2010). Primary and secondary neoplasms of the spleen. *Cancer Imaging, 10,* 173–182.

Lake, S. T., Johnson, P. T., Kawamoto, S., et al. (2012). CT of splenosis: Patterns and pitfalls. *AJR American journal of roentgenology, 199,* W686–W693.

Mortele, K. J., Mortele, B., & Silverman, S. G. (2004). CT features of the accessory spleen. *AJR American journal of roentgenology, 183,* 1653–1657.

Saboo, S. S., Krajewski, K. M., O'Regan, K. N., et al. (2012). Spleen in haematological malignancies: Spectrum of imaging findings. *The British journal of radiology, 85,* 81–92.

Singh, A. K., Shankar, S., Gervais, D. A., et al. (2012). Image-guided percutaneous splenic interventions. *Radiographics, 32,* 523–534.

Thipphavong, S., Duigenan, S., Schindera, S. T., et al. (2014). Nonneoplastic, benign, and malignant splenic diseases: Cross-sectional imaging findings and rare disease entities. *AJR American journal of roentgenology, 203,* 315–322.

Urritia, M., Mergo, P. J., Ros, L. H., et al. (1996). Cystic lesions of the spleen: Radiologic-pathologic correlation. *Radiographics, 16,* 107–129.

CHAPTER 15

Kidneys and Ureters

WILLIAM E. BRANT

KIDNEYS

Anatomy of the Retroperitoneal Space

A detailed understanding of the retroperitoneal fascial planes and compartments is a prerequisite for accurate interpretation of abdominal CT. The retroperitoneum is the anatomic compartment between the posterior parietal peritoneum and the transversalis fascia extending from the diaphragm to the pelvic brim. It is divided into three distinct compartments—anterior pararenal, perirenal, and posterior pararenal spaces—by the anterior renal fascia and posterior renal fascia (Fig. 15.1).

The *anterior pararenal space* extends between the posterior parietal peritoneum and the anterior renal fascia. It is bounded laterally by the lateroconal fascia, which is the continuation of the posterior layer of the posterior renal fascia. The pancreas, duodenal loop, and ascending and descending portions of the colon are enveloped by fat within the anterior pararenal space. This compartment is continuous across the midline, allowing spread of fluid processes and gas.

The anterior renal fascia and posterior renal fascia encompass the kidney, renal pelvis, proximal part of the ureter, adrenal gland, renal and perirenal blood vessels, and lymphatics invested by perirenal fat within the *perirenal space*. The perirenal space is an inverted cone shape extending from the diaphragmatic fascia to the iliac fossa. The anterior renal fascia (Gerota fascia) is thin and consists of one layer of connective tissue. The posterior renal fascia (Zuckerkandl fascia) is thicker and consists of two layers of connective tissue. The anterior layer of the posterior renal fascia is continuous with the anterior renal fascia. The posterior layer of the posterior renal fascia is continuous with the lateroconal fascia, forming the lateral boundary of the anterior pararenal space. The anterior and posterior layers of the posterior renal fascia may be separated by inflammatory processes, such as pancreatitis, extending from the anterior pararenal space. The perirenal space is discontinuous across the midline owing to fusion of the renal fascial layers with connective tissues surrounding the aorta and inferior vena cava. The perirenal space on the right abuts the bare area of the liver, allowing spread of inflammatory and neoplastic processes from the right kidney to the liver. On the left the perirenal space abuts the left subphrenic space. The ureter passes through the apex of the cone of the perirenal space as it courses to the pelvis.

The *posterior pararenal space* is a potential space, occupied only by fat, blood vessels, and lymphatics, extending from the posterior renal fascia to the transversalis fascia. The posterior pararenal fat continues into the flank as the properitoneal fat stripe seen on conventional radiographs of the abdomen. Air and fluid processes in this compartment may extend to the anterior abdominal wall. This compartment does not extend across the midline, limited medially by the lateral edge of the psoas and quadratus lumborum muscles.

The kidneys are covered by a tight fibrous capsule that produces a sharp margin defined by perirenal fat on CT. The perirenal fat extends into the renal sinus, outlining blood vessels and the renal collecting system. Connective tissue septa extend between the fibrous capsule of the kidney and the renal fascia. These septa divide the perirenal space into multiple compartments and may be seen as prominent stranding densities in the perirenal fat when they are thickened by inflammation, hemorrhage, or ischemia. Inflammatory fluid or hemorrhage in the perirenal space is not free flowing but is compartmentalized by these bands of fascia. Collections of fluid or blood beneath the fibrous capsule of the kidney will compress and distort the renal parenchyma, often without affecting the perirenal fat.

The renal arteries and veins can be identified from the great vessels to the kidneys. The right renal artery courses behind the vena cava. The right renal vein extends anterior to the right renal artery directly from the right kidney to the vena cava. The left renal vein crosses between the aorta and the superior mesenteric artery, passing anterior to the left renal artery, which extends directly from the aorta to the left kidney. The aorta, inferior vena cava, and their branches are invested by fascial layers that usually, but not always, prevent communication with the pararenal and perirenal spaces.

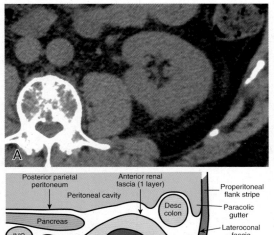

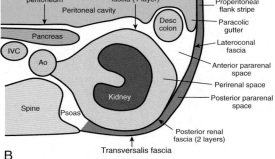

FIG. 15.1 **Retroperitoneal anatomy.** CT image of the left kidney without intravenous contrast medium (A) and a corresponding diagram (B) demonstrating the fascial planes and compartments of the retroperitoneum. *Ao,* Abdominal aorta; *Desc,* descending; *IVC,* inferior vena cava.

Technical Considerations

Because the kidneys actively concentrate contrast medium within the parenchyma, most renal abnormalities are best seen on CT after intravenous contrast medium administration. Unenhanced CT is performed to demonstrate calcifications and calculi that may be obscured by contrast medium administration. Multidetector CT (MDCT) is optimal for renal evaluation and is the current technique of choice. The sensitivity for detection of renal masses differs considerably with the imaging modality: 67% for traditional excretory urography, 79% for sonography, and at least 95% for MDCT.

- The *CT urogram* (CT intravenous pyelogram - also known as the CT-IVP) has evolved as the imaging method of choice to provide the most comprehensive evaluation of the urinary tract, often used in the setting of hematuria:
    - No bowel preparation or oral contrast medium is needed. A noncontrast CT scan is obtained from the kidneys through the bladder to document the presence of calculi or parenchymal calcifications.
    - Between 125 and 150 mL of 60% iodine nonionic contrast medium is injected intravenously at 3 to 4 mL per second.
    - A nephrogram phase scan is obtained at 80-second scan delay with 2.5-mm or thinner collimation and a single breath hold.
    - A pyelogram phase scan is obtained at 5 to 8 minutes after contrast medium injection with thin slices (1.25 mm) through the full length of kidneys, ureters, and bladder. Images are reconstructed in axial, coronal, and sagittal planes (Fig. 15.2).
- *CT for renal masses.* We use MDCT with contiguous thin slices with a single breath hold at identical locations before and after bolus contrast medium administration.
    - A precontrast scan is performed through both kidneys (Fig. 15.3A) to document the presence of calculi and calcifications and to serve as a baseline to assess lesion enhancement.
    - Between 100 and 150 mL of 60% iodine nonionic contrast medium is given intravenously by a power injector at 2.5 to 3.0 mL per second.
    - A corticomedullary phase scan is obtained with a 30-second scan delay (Fig. 15.3B and C). This scan extends from the dome of the diaphragm through the bottom of the kidneys. Scanning during this phase is used to evaluate other abdominal organs for metastatic disease and to evaluate the renal arteries and veins.
    - A nephrogram phase scan is obtained at 80 to 90 seconds after contrast medium administration (Fig. 15.3D). The scan extent includes only the kidneys from top to bottom.
    - A pyelogram phase scan is added at 3 to 5 minutes after injection of contrast medium.
    - The scan may be continued through the pelvis to evaluate the retroperitoneum, ureters, and bladder.
- *Corticomedullary phase scans.* When one is scanning the abdomen for reasons other than renal mass characterization, renal images are commonly obtained with contrast enhancement limited to the renal cortex (Fig. 15.3B and C). The corticomedullary phase is usually seen at about 30 to 50 seconds after contrast medium injection into an arm vein. This phase is of limited use for detection of renal masses because only the renal cortex is enhanced and the medullary portions of the kidney remain unenhanced. The corticomedullary phase defines the renal artery and vein better than the nephrogram phase.

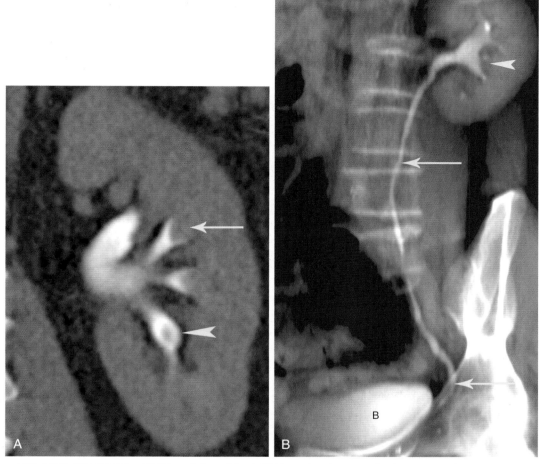

FIG. 15.2 **CT urogram.** (A) Coronal view of the left kidney showing normal calyces appearing as cup-shaped *(arrow)* or circular *(arrowhead)* structures depending on the plane of the CT section. (B) An oblique view of the left kidney, collecting system *(arrowhead)*, ureter *(arrows)*, and bladder *(B)* was created from a series of thin-slice axial CT images. It nicely demonstrates the course and size of the ureter. Portions of the normal ureter may be nonopacified because of ureteral peristalsis.

- *Stone protocol CT.* Renal stone CT (sometimes called CT-KUB - CT of the kidneys, ureters, and bladder) is a noncontrast helical MDCT of the urinary tract used to diagnose the presence of urinary tract calculi and to detect acute urinary tract obstruction caused by stones.
  - No oral or intravenous contrast medium is administered.
  - Data acquisition is continuous from the top of the kidneys through the base of the bladder (mid-T12 level through the pubic symphysis) with use of 0.625- to 2.5-mm collimation.

Images may be viewed at 1.25- to 2.5-mm slice thickness. Thin slices allow identification of very small stones that may be overlooked with thicker slices.
  - Turning the patient to the prone position will allow differentiation of stones impacted at the ureterovesical junction from stones that have already passed into the bladder.
  - Whenever the noncontrast renal stone CT findings are equivocal, intravenous contrast medium may be given to clarify the diagnosis.

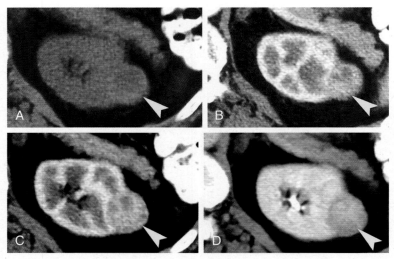

FIG. 15.3 **CT of renal mass.** Noncontrast (A), corticomedullary phase (B and C), and nephrogram phase (D) images from a helical CT study demonstrating a small renal carcinoma *(arrowheads)* arising from the left kidney. The tumor is nearly isointense with the renal parenchyma in the noncontrast study. Early arterial enhancement of the tumor coincides with enhancement of the renal cortex on the corticomedullary phase images. The tumor is mildly hypointense compared with the renal parenchyma during the nephrogram phase.

Congenital Anomalies

Horseshoe Kidney

Congenital fusion of the lower poles of the kidneys is a relatively common (1 in 400 births) congenital anomaly.

- The isthmus extends across the aorta just below the origin of the inferior mesenteric artery, which prevents the normal ascent of the kidneys to the renal beds (Fig. 15.4). The tissue connecting the lower poles of the kidneys may be functioning renal parenchyma or fibrous bands
- The fused kidneys are low in position and malrotated, with the renal pelvis directed anteriorly and the lower poles converging instead of diverging. Malposition is associated with multiple renal arteries of anomalous origin and urinary stasis often resulting in stone formation and recurrent infection. Venous drainage is also usually aberrant.
- In one-third of cases other congenital anomalies of the urologic, skeletal, neurologic, and gastrointestinal systems are also present.
- Transitional cell carcinoma (TCC) is three to four times more common in individuals with horseshoe kidneys than in the general population.

Renal Masses

The features that must be evaluated to characterize a renal mass are the presence and type of calcification,

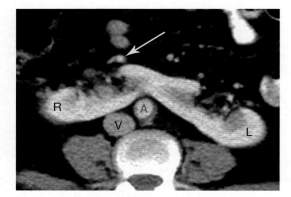

FIG. 15.4 **Horseshoe kidney.** The lower poles of the right kidney *(R)* and the left kidney *(L)* are fused across the midline anterior to the aorta *(A)* and inferior vena cava *(V)*. The fused kidney is held low in position within the abdomen because its ascent to its normal location is impaired by the origin of the inferior mesenteric artery *(arrow)*.

attenuation of the mass before and after contrast medium administration, the margin of the mass with the kidney and with surrounding tissues, and the presence and thickness of septa and the thickness of the wall of cystic masses. Artifactual pseudoenhancement, related to a beam-hardening effect from iodinated contrast medium, may increase attenuation of lesions

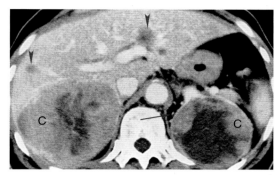

FIG. 15.5 **Bilateral clear cell renal cell carcinomas.** Renal cell carcinomas *(C)* arise from the upper poles of both kidneys. The low-attenuation regions within the tumors are areas of necrosis and hemorrhage. Enhanced tumor vessels *(arrow)* are seen in the perirenal fat. Metastases are present in the liver *(arrowheads)*.

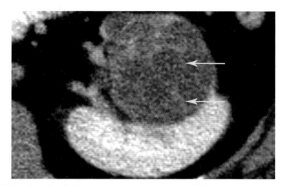

FIG. 15.6 **Multilocular cystic renal cell carcinoma.** Nephrogram phase CT image showing a low-attenuation heterogeneous mass projecting from the left kidney. Enhanced septa *(arrows)* are faintly demonstrated.

by up to 10 Hounsfield units (HU). Attenuation must increase by a minimum of 20 HU following bolus intravenous contrast medium administration to be considered enhancement. An increase in attenuation of less than 10 HU is not considered enhancement. An increase in attenuation of 10 to 20 HU is equivocal enhancement.

Renal Cell Carcinoma

Renal cell carcinoma (RCC) accounts for 90% of solid tumors of the kidney. Most large lesions can be easily diagnosed by CT. Small lesions are commonly indeterminate. About 15% to 20% of small solid renal tumors are benign. Histologic subtypes of RCC have distinctive imaging findings and differ in treatment response and prognosis:

- Clear cell, also called conventional, RCC accounts for 70% of RCCs. Tumors are typically heterogeneous with mixtures of solid tissue, cysts, and foci of hemorrhage and necrosis (Fig. 15.5). Tumors arise from the renal cortex and show expansile growth with hypervascularity. Tumor enhancement is greatest, typically exceeding 84 HU, in the corticomedullary phase and remains high in the nephrogram and excretory phases. Multicentric and bilateral tumors are rare (<5%). Clear cell RCC has the least favorable prognosis.
- Multilocular cystic RCC is a variant of clear cell RCC. Clusters of cysts of variable size are bound by a thin fibrous capsule and have septa of variable thickness that are lined with clear cell RCC (Fig. 15.6). About 20% have calcification in the wall or septa. Cystic RCCs show slower growth and have lower

propensity for metastases and tumor recurrence than solid tumors.
- Papillary (chromophil) RCCs account for 10% to 15% of RCCs. They occur most commonly in end-stage failed kidneys arising from distal convoluted tubules. On CT they appear as hypovascular homogeneous solid tumors (Fig. 15.7). Enhancement is far less prominent than with clear cell RCC. Bilateral and multicentric tumors are more common than with other cell types. As the tumors become large they may develop hemorrhage, necrosis, and calcification. Very rarely tumors may contain macroscopic fat because of the presence of cholesterol-filled macrophages. Cystic papillary RCCs have enhancing nodules or papillary projections that project from the cyst wall (Fig. 15.8). On discovery, 70% of papillary RCCs are confined to the kidney, resulting in a good prognosis with surgical removal.
- Chromophobe RCCs account for 5% of RCCs. This tumor arises from collecting duct cells. On ultrasound imaging, small chromophobe RCCs appear homogeneously hyperechoic, mimicking the appearance of small angiomyolipoma (AML). This finding necessitates the performance of CT or MRI to differentiate the two lesions. Characteristically chromophobe RCCs show homogeneous enhancement, even when large. However, a variety of appearances are reported, including central scar, necrosis, and calcifications. A spoke-wheel pattern of enhancement of some tumors mimics oncocytoma. Most tumors (86%) are stage 1 or stage 2 at the time of discovery, resulting in a relatively good prognosis.

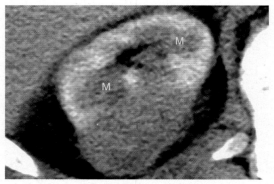

FIG. 15.7 Papillary renal cell carcinoma. Postcontrast CT image during corticomedullary phase showing low-grade enhancement within a poorly defined mass arising from the right kidney. During the corticomedullary phase the tumor *(T)* is difficult to distinguish from unenhanced renal medulla *(M)*.

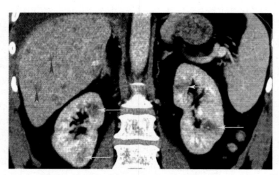

FIG. 15.8 Metastasis to the kidney. Coronal plane CT image of a patient with colon cancer showing numerous ill-defined low-attenuation lesions in both kidneys *(yellow arrows)* and in the liver *(red arrowheads)*.

- Hereditary cancer syndromes account for 5% of RCCs and are associated with early development of multicentric and bilateral RCCs. Von Hippel–Lindau syndrome is associated with clear cell RCC (Fig. 15.9), whereas Birt-Hogg-Dubé syndrome is associated with chromophobe RCC.
- Other rare cell types each account for less than 1% of RCCs. Renal medullary carcinoma is associated with sickle cell trait occurring in patients younger than 40 years. The tumor arises in the medulla and is infiltrative and heterogeneous in appearance. Collecting duct RCC is highly aggressive, with an infiltrative growth pattern. Mucinous tubular and spindle cell RCCs are found predominantly in women. Translocation (juvenile) RCCs occur in children and young adults.

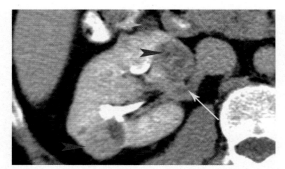

FIG. 15.9 Renal cell carcinoma in von Hippel–Lindau syndrome. CT in a patient with von Hippel–Lindau syndrome reveals the development of two renal cell carcinomas *(red arrowheads)* in the right kidney. Tumor thrombus *(yellow arrow)* extends into the right renal vein. Both kidneys contained multiple cysts *(green arrow)* and angiomyolipomas. The patient had a history of partial nephrectomy on the left for renal cell carcinoma.

- On unenhanced CT, RCCs contain noncalcified solid areas measuring 20 to 70 HU. Homogeneous lesions with attenuation outside this range tend to be benign. This finding is of increasing importance as current practice favors the obtaining of increasing numbers of unenhanced abdominal CT scans.
- Small solid renal lesions (<3 cm) are being discovered with increased frequency by CT, MRI, or ultrasound imaging. Benign and malignant lesions overlap in appearance, with 15% to 20% of these small lesions being benign. Differential diagnosis includes RCC, oncocytoma, AML without visible fat, papillary adenoma, and metanephric adenoma. Percutaneous biopsy is used to diagnose these lesions before percutaneous ablation procedures or surgery.

CT Staging of Renal Cell Carcinoma

RCC responds poorly to all types of radiation therapy and chemotherapy despite many innovative new therapy attempts. The only completely effective therapy remains surgical excision or percutaneous ablation of all tumor. CT is highly accurate in assisting the urologist in planning surgery or ablation procedures. Nephron-sparing surgery with partial nephrectomy performed laparoscopically or with robotics, or procedures such as radiofrequency ablation or cryoablation, decrease the morbidity of treatment of small tumors. Immunotherapy shows promise in the treatment of advanced disease. (See the internet link to TMN staging of renal carcinoma).

- Extension of tumor through the renal capsule into the perinephric fat is not accurately demonstrated

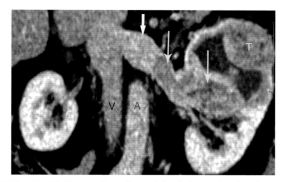

FIG. 15.10 **Tumor invasion of the left renal vein.** Coronal plane CT clearly shows tumor *(yellow arrows)* extending from the left upper pole renal carcinoma *(T)* into the left renal vein. A segment *(white arrow)* of the left renal vein near the inferior vena cava *(V)* is spared, allowing the urologist space to clamp the left renal vein and avoid venous spread of tumor during surgery. *A,* Aorta.

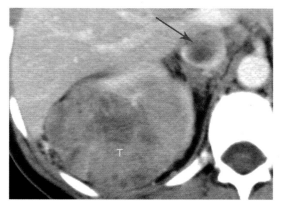

FIG. 15.11 **Tumor invasion of the inferior vena cava.** An infiltrative renal cell carcinoma *(T)* largely replaces the parenchyma of the right kidney. Tumor thrombus is seen as a filling defect *(arrow)* in the inferior vena cava.

by CT. However, this differentiation does not affect the surgical approach to the lesion.

- Tumor may grow into the main renal vein (20%–35%) (Fig. 15.10) and inferior vena cava (IVC) (4%–10%) (Fig. 15.11). Venous invasion consists of tumor growing within the vein often associated with variable amount of bland thrombus. Involved veins are usually enlarged. Tumor thrombus is seen as nodular low density within the vein. Enhancement of the thrombus within the vein is evidence that the thrombus consists of growing tumor. Determining the presence or absence of venous involvement is essential to surgical planning (Fig. 15.10). CT is 95% accurate in the determination of venous involvement.
- Filling defects within the collecting system on the pyelographic phase of CT is reliable evidence of tumor invasion of the collecting system.
- Regional lymph nodes greater than 2 cm in short axis nearly always contain metastatic tumor. Involved lymph nodes are most common in renal hilum, pericaval, and periaortic regions.
- Lymph nodes 1 to 2 cm in short axis are indeterminate, hyperplastic versus metastatic, and should always be removed at surgery to determine prognosis. Lymphadenectomy does not improve prognosis.
- Lymph nodes smaller than 1 cm in short axis are usually benign.
- Hematogenous metastases are most common in lung, liver, and bone.
- Adrenalectomy is optional if the adrenal gland appears normal on CT.

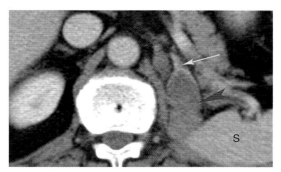

FIG. 15.12 **Renal cell carcinoma recurrence.** CT performed 1 year after left-sided nephrectomy for renal cell carcinoma reveals a recurrent mass *(red arrowhead)* in the left renal bed involving the left adrenal gland *(yellow arrow)* and the spleen *(S)*.

Recurrence of Renal Cell Carcinoma

CT is highly accurate for surveillance of recurrent disease after surgery. Recurrence of RCC usually occurs in the first 6 years after surgery. The median time for appearance of detectable recurrent disease is 15 to 18 months after nephrectomy. The risk of recurrence increases with the stage of the tumor at the time of the initial surgery. Occasionally the tumor will recur after the patient has apparently been disease-free for 10 years or more.

- Local recurrence in the renal fossa occurs in 5% of patients (Fig. 15.12). Recurrent tumor appears as an irregularly enhancing mass that commonly involves the psoas or quadratus lumborum muscles. Adjacent structures, including bowel, which usually occupies the renal fossa after nephrectomy, are displaced.

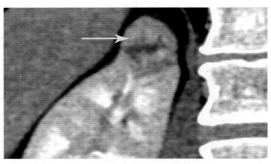

FIG. 15.13 **Oncocytoma.** Coronal plane CT during the nephrogram phase shows a small heterogeneous mass *(arrow)* arising from the upper pole of the right kidney. Although pathology revealed a benign oncocytoma, on CT the mass is indistinguishable from a renal carcinoma.

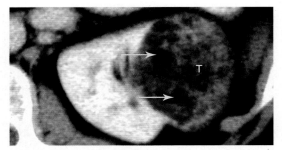

FIG. 15.14 **Solitary angiomyolipoma.** Foci of distinct fat density *(arrows)* define this renal tumor *(T)* as an angiomyolipoma. Compare the fat density within the lesion with the fat surrounding the kidney. Areas of soft-tissue density, representing smooth muscle and enhanced blood vessels, are also evident within the mass.

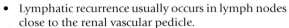

- Lymphatic recurrence usually occurs in lymph nodes close to the renal vascular pedicle.
- Distant metastases develop in 20% to 30% of patients. The most common sites are the lungs (50%–60%), mediastinum, bone, liver, contralateral kidney or adrenal gland, and brain.
- Late metastases (>10 years after surgery) are most common to lung, pancreas, bone, skeletal muscle, and bowel. Surgical resection of isolated late metastases may be curative.

Oncocytoma

Oncocytoma is a benign solid tumor that arises from the proximal renal tubule. Most tumors are found in men in their 60s. They account for about 5% of renal neoplasms. Unfortunately, no imaging test can reliably differentiate these benign tumors from RCC. Treatment is surgical. Exploration with limited tumor excision may be attempted if CT findings suggest the possibility of oncocytoma.

- The "classic" CT features of oncocytoma, which unfortunately can also be seen with RCC, are homogeneous attenuation after contrast medium administration and a central, sharply marginated, stellate, low-attenuation scar (~33% of tumors). Most are solitary, well-defined, homogeneous tumors arising in the renal cortex. Features more characteristic of RCC, such as heterogeneous attenuation, necrosis, and hemorrhage, may also be seen with oncocytoma (Fig. 15.13).

Angiomyolipoma

Angiomyolipoma (AML) is the most common benign tumor of the kidney. It is composed of blood vessels *(angio)*, smooth muscle *(myo)*, and fat *(lipoma)*. Tumor arteries have thicker than normal, but abnormally weak, vessel walls and are predisposed to aneurysm formation. Larger tumors and larger aneurysms have a higher rate of rupture, making hemorrhage the most common complication. AML occurs in two distinct clinical settings. The sporadic and usually solitary tumor (80%–90%) is most common in middle-aged women (female-to-male ratio 4:1; average age 43 years). Multifocal and bilateral tumors occur in patients with tuberous sclerosis. Many tumors are discovered incidentally during CT, MRI, or ultrasound imaging for other reasons. The presence of distinct pockets of fat allows a specific CT diagnosis of AML.

- The proportion of each tissue element present within the tumor determines the imaging appearance.
- CT typically shows a well-marginated predominantly fat-containing lesion arising from the cortex (Fig. 15.14). Most tumors are smaller than 5 cm. Vascular and smooth muscle portions of the tumor appear of soft-tissue density on noncontrast CT and enhance with contrast medium administration.
- The diagnostic feature of AML on CT is the presence of fat (CT density <–10 HU) (Fig. 15.14). Compare low-attenuation areas within the tumor with perirenal and subcutaneous fat. Soft-tissue density elements are often dispersed throughout the background of distinctly fatty tissue. At other times soft-tissue density predominates and diagnosis is made by the presence of small discrete pockets of fat. Thin-section CT (1–3-mm collimation) is recommended for confident diagnosis. Use of intravenous contrast medium is not necessary to confirm the presence of fat within the lesion. Approximately 95% of tumors can be characterized by the presence of fat within the lesion.
- Sonography characteristically demonstrates AML as small (<3 cm) well-defined echogenic tumors.

Unfortunately, up to 32% of small (<3 cm) RCCs also appear as echogenic masses. Therefore CT characterization of all small echogenic renal mass lesions is recommended.

- Hemorrhage is common with AML because of the characteristically weak wall of the tumor blood vessels. Hemorrhage commonly extends into the perirenal space, may obscure fat density within the tumor, and often makes tumor margins indistinct (Fig. 15.15). The risk of hemorrhage is increased when tumors exceed 4 cm in size.

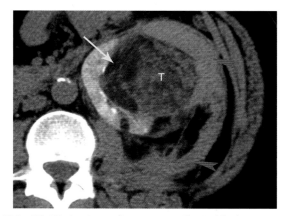

FIG. 15.15 **Angiomyolipoma complicated by hemorrhage.** Postcontrast CT reveals an infiltrative renal tumor *(T)* with hemorrhage *(red arrowheads)* within the tumor and extending to the perirenal space. Although much of the tumor is obscured by hemorrhage, distinct foci of fat density *(yellow arrow)* are present to characterize the tumor as an angiomyolipoma.

- Approximately 5% of AMLs are lipid-poor and show no areas of distinct fat attenuation on CT. Lipid-poor AMLs have attenuation values higher than −10 HU on unenhanced CT. These tumors may be indistinguishable from RCC. Some of these lesions may show a loss of signal intensity on opposed-phase MRI. However, some clear cell RCCs may show similar signal loss on opposed-phase MRI. The presence of fat in RCC has been attributed to osseous metaplasia of stromal portions of the tumor with growth of fatty marrow, or the presence of fat-laden macrophages in chromophobe RCCs. Calcifications are usually present in association within fat deposits arising from bone marrow. Intratumoral calcifications are virtually never present with AML. Fat-containing RCCs often show other signs of malignancy. AML is suggested if the lesions show homogeneous high attenuation on unenhanced CT and show homogeneous increased attenuation on enhanced CT (Fig. 15.16). Biopsy is usually required to differentiate lipid-poor AML from RCC.
- In patients with tuberous sclerosis, multiple AMLs are usually found in both kidneys (80% of patients). Up to 50% of patients have multiple renal cysts. AMLs are often large, and the risk of hemorrhage is increased (Fig. 15.17). Approximately 2% to 3% of patients develop RCC at a young age (average 28 years).
- Tumors may grow extensively into the perirenal space. Tumor margins are commonly indistinguishable from perirenal fat. These lesions resemble retroperitoneal liposarcomas. A distinct defect in the kidney from which AMLs arise is a distinguishing

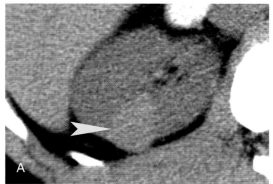
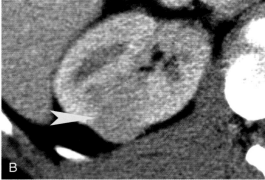

FIG. 15.16 **Lipid-poor angiomyolipoma.** (A) Noncontrast CT reveals a faintly visualized high-attenuation lesion *(arrowhead)* within the right kidney. CT attenuation of the lesion was measured at 41 Hounsfield units (HU). (B) Early postcontrast CT shows enhancement of the lesion *(arrowhead)* to 85 HU. Biopsy was required to confirm benign angiomyolipoma.

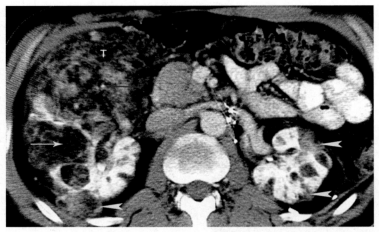

FIG. 15.17 **Tuberous sclerosis: bilateral angiomyolipomas.** Both kidneys, in this patient with tuberous sclerosis, are extensively replaced by angiomyolipomas. The tumor *(T)* arising anteriorly from the right kidney extends all the way to the anterior abdominal wall. Low-attenuation areas *(yellow arrow)* within the tumor are nearly identical in density to subcutaneous and intra-abdominal fat, confirming the diagnosis of angiomyolipoma. Soft-tissue density nodules and strands correspond to smooth muscle components of the tumor. Bright dots *(red arrow)* represent blood vessels within the highly vascular tumor. Multiple angiomyolipomas *(yellow arrowheads)* distort the parenchyma of both kidneys. Functioning renal parenchyma enhances brightly with contrast medium. Despite extensive renal involvement by tumor, this patient had normal renal function.

feature. AMLs characteristically increase in size when they spread outside the renal capsule. Liposarcomas may displace or compress the kidney but usually do not invade the kidney.

Transitional Cell Carcinoma

Transitional cell carcinoma (TCC) may arise anywhere along the uroepithelium lining the intrarenal collecting system, renal pelvis, ureter, or bladder. Most tumors (90%) arise in the bladder, with only 5% to 10% arising within the upper tracts (intrarenal collecting system, renal pelvis, ureter). A characteristic of TCC is that additional TCC may be present synchronously, or may arise subsequently elsewhere in the uroepithelium. A concurrent bladder cancer has been reported in 17% of cases of upper tract TCC. Most cases present with gross or microscopic hematuria. CT urography has replaced intravenous urography as the imaging method of choice for detection of upper tract urothelial carcinoma as it has a higher diagnostic accuracy (95% vs. 85%). CT is also preferred for tumor staging. For optimal distension of the collecting system and ureter, injection of a diuretic during a CT urogram has been recommended. Several patterns of disease have been described:

- On unenhanced CT, TCC is typically of the same attenuation as the renal parenchyma. With contrast

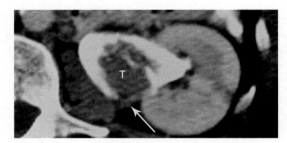

FIG. 15.18 **Transitional cell carcinoma: renal pelvis.** Pyelogram phase CT of the left kidney demonstrates a transitional cell carcinoma appearing as a soft-tissue attenuation mass *(T)* surrounded by high-attenuation contrast agent within the renal pelvis. The tumor extends through the wall of the renal pelvis into the perirenal fat *(arrow)*. The tumor is papillary in nature with contrast outlining its irregular border.

medium, TCC shows variable, but usually poor, enhancement.

- *Single or multiple filling defects* in the renal pelvis (35%) have a smooth surface or a stippled papillary pattern (Fig. 15.18) with tracking of contrast medium into the interstices of the tumor. Renal sinus fat may be compressed or invaded by the tumor.

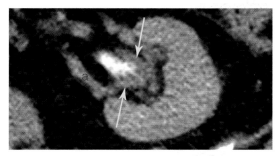

FIG. 15.19 **Transitional cell carcinoma: renal pelvis.** Pyelogram phase CT in a patient with hematuria reveals irregular thickening *(arrows)* of the walls of the renal pelvis. *a,* Left renal artery.

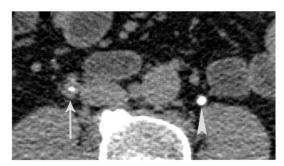

FIG. 15.20 **Transitional cell carcinoma: ureter.** In a transverse image from a CT urogram the right ureter *(arrow)* shows irregular circumferential wall thickening with narrowing of the contrast-filled lumen. The tumor extends into the periureteral fat. The left ureter *(arrowhead)* is contrast filled and normal in appearance.

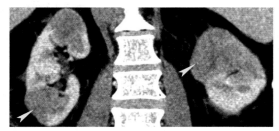

FIG. 15.21 **Renal lymphoma: multiple masses.** Coronal plane CT shows multiple low-attenuation ill-defined masses *(arrowheads)* in both kidneys, proven by percutaneous biopsy to be lymphoma.

- *Filling defects within dilated calyces* (26%) may obstruct at the infundibulum. A "phantom" calyx fails to opacify and may be associated with a focal delayed or increasing dense lobar nephrogram.
- *Thickening of the wall of the renal pelvis* (Fig. 15.19) may be relatively subtle.
- *Absent or decreased contrast medium excretion* (13%) is caused by long-standing obstruction at the ureteropelvic junction.
- *Diffuse hydronephrosis with renal enlargement* (6%) is seen with tumor obstruction at the ureteropelvic junction.
- Most ureteral uroepithelial tumors (>70%) occur in the distal part of the ureter. Tumors appear as small filling defects in the contrast-filled ureter or as circumferential thickening of the wall of the ureter on CT urography (Fig. 15.20). The part of the ureter proximal to the tumor may be dilated. Calcified

ureteral TCC may be mistaken for calculi. The location of the calcified tumor at a position atypical for impacted calculi may be a clue to diagnosis. Calculi typically impact at the ureteropelvic junction, pelvic brim, or ureterovesical junction.
- Large tumors invade the renal sinus fat and infiltrate into the parenchyma. Differentiation from RCC may be difficult. TCCs center on the renal pelvis. RCCs center on the renal parenchyma.
- Advanced disease shows extrarenal extension, regional lymph node involvement, and distant metastases to lungs and bone. TCC may rarely invade the renal vein and inferior vena cava.
- Calcification occurs in up to 5% of tumors. It may appear coarse, punctate, linear, granular, or stippled and indistinct. Calcified tumors, especially in the ureter, may be mistaken for calculi.

Renal Lymphoma

Renal involvement with lymphoma almost always occurs in the setting of systemic disease. Although autopsy studies show the kidneys are involved in 34% to 68% of patients with lymphoma, CT shows renal involvement in only 3% to 8%. B-cell non-Hodgkin lymphoma and Burkitt lymphoma are the most common lymphoma types to involve the kidney. Multiple characteristic patterns of involvement have been described. Atypical patterns of involvement present a diagnostic challenge:
- On unenhanced CT, lymphoma is homogeneous and typically of lower attenuation than renal cortex. Margins with the renal parenchyma are usually indistinct.
- Following contrast enhancement, lymphoma remains homogeneous and is always hypodense compared with enhanced renal parenchyma.
- *Multiple bilateral renal masses* are the most common (60%) CT appearance of lymphoma (Fig. 15.21).

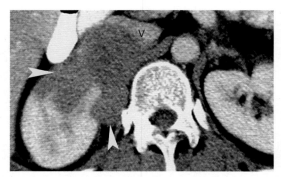

FIG. 15.22 **Renal lymphoma: contiguous invasion.** A homogeneous, minimally enhancing mass *(arrowheads)* envelops and obscures the right renal vein, invades the right kidney, and distorts and anteriorly displaces the inferior vena cava *(V)*.

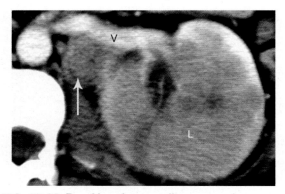

FIG. 15.23 **Renal lymphoma: solitary mass.** Lymphoma replaces parenchyma in the midportion of the left kidney, appearing as a large mass *(L)* with ill-defined borders. An enlarged lymph node *(arrow)* is seen posterior to the left renal vein *(V)*. The renal vein is uninvolved. Renal cell carcinoma commonly invades the renal vein, whereas renal lymphoma rarely does. Compare this with Fig. 15.9.

Occasionally, the multiple masses may affect only one kidney. The lesions typically have a size of 1 to 3 cm. Necrosis and calcification are rare. Retroperitoneal adenopathy is often not present.

- *Contiguous invasion from the retroperitoneum* is seen in 35% to 60% of cases. Bulky retroperitoneal adenopathy extends along the renal vessels into the renal sinus and then into the renal parenchyma (Fig. 15.22). Tumor encasement of the renal artery and vein hardly ever results in thrombosis, a finding highly characteristic of lymphoma.
- A *solitary renal mass* (10%–20%) may highly resemble RCC. However, the mass is routinely very homogeneous and shows minimal enhancement (Fig. 15.23). Tumor invasion of the renal vein is exceedingly rare.
- *Perirenal lymphoma* most often accompanies contiguous invasion from the retroperitoneum. Bulky disease surrounds the kidney but usually does not compress the parenchyma or interfere with its function. Perirenal disease patterns include multiple perirenal masses, soft-tissue nodules and plaques, curvilinear soft-tissue mass separate from the kidney (Fig. 15.24), and thickened renal fascia.
- *Diffuse infiltration* (~20%) enlarges the kidney without altering its reniform shape. In nearly all cases both kidneys are involved. Contrast enhancement is typically limited, patchy, and associated with poor contrast medium excretion.
- Absence of involvement of retroperitoneal nodes is relatively common (up to 43% of all cases) and excludes lymphoma as a cause of renal masses.
- Atypical manifestations include spontaneous hemorrhage, necrosis, heterogeneous attenuation, cystic

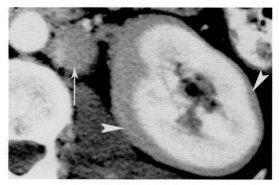

FIG. 15.24 **Renal lymphoma: perirenal.** The enhanced parenchyma of the left kidney is completely encased by nonenhancing homogenous soft tissue *(arrowheads)* representing lymphomatous tissue. An enlarged lymph node *(arrow)* is present between the kidney and the aorta. The renal contour is not compressed or distorted.

change, and calcification. Atypical findings are most common after treatment. Usually with successful therapy the CT appearance of the kidney eventually returns to normal.
- Whenever imaging findings suggest renal lymphoma, image-guided biopsy of the lesions should be recommended so that unnecessary surgery can be avoided and proper treatment instituted.

Metastases to the Kidneys

Metastases to the kidneys are present in 7% to 13% of patients with extrarenal cancers in autopsy series.

The most common primary tumors to metastasize to the kidneys are lung, breast, and gastrointestinal adenocarcinomas. Lesions are identified on CT usually only in patients with advanced widespread metastatic disease.

- Multiple bilateral low-attenuation renal nodules are the most common CT pattern (Fig. 15.8).
- Isolated solitary metastasis is seen most commonly with colon cancer and melanoma.
- Diffusely infiltrative metastases are uncommon.
- Occasionally the kidney may be the only site of metastatic disease.

Papillary Adenoma

Papillary adenomas by pathologic definition are small (<5 mm) solid renal masses that arise from the epithelium of the renal tubules. They are solitary and subcapsular in location. Most are discovered incidentally in surgical specimens (7% of nephrectomy, 10% of autopsies). They are also found in association with long-term hemodialysis and acquired renal cystic disease. Lesions larger than 5 mm are considered carcinomas. Some consider papillary adenoma a precursor of papillary RCC.

- CT shows a tiny solid renal mass smaller than 5 mm indistinguishable from papillary RCC.

Metanephric Adenoma

Metanephric adenomas are very rare benign tumors of the kidneys histogenetically related to Wilms tumor and nephroblastomatosis. The tumors doe not have malignant potential. No treatment is needed.

- The typical appearance is a solitary well-defined solid mass with attenuation higher than that of renal parenchyma on noncontrast CT. Metanephric adenomas are hypovascular and show limited enhancement. The mean size is 5 cm. Larger masses are heterogeneous with an area of hemorrhage, necrosis, and calcification (20%). Differentiation from malignant tumor usually requires pathologic diagnosis.

Cystic Renal Masses

Cystic renal masses are an extremely common finding on abdominal CT. The challenge is to separate the ubiquitous simple cyst and other benign cysts from a host of potentially malignant cystic lesions.

Bosniak Classification of Cystic Renal Masses

In 1986 Morton Bosniak described a classification system for cystic renal masses that became widely used. The classification scheme was modified in 1993 and is

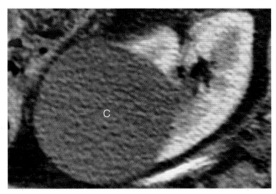

FIG. 15.25 **Simple renal cyst: Bosniak category I.** A large cyst *(C)* arising from the left kidney demonstrates the classic CT features of a simple renal cyst with sharp definition, no discernible wall, homogeneous internal attenuation near that of water, and no enhancement. This lesion is benign, and no further evaluation or follow-up is necessary.

currently in common use by radiologists and urologists. Cystic lesion classification is based on CT findings:

- *Bosniak category I: benign simple cyst.* CT shows homogeneous internal attenuation of water density, a hairline thin wall, no enhancement with intravenous contrast medium, and no septa, calcifications, or solid components (Fig. 15.25).
- *Bosniak category II: benign complicated cyst.* Cysts become complicated by developing internal hemorrhage or becoming infected, causing minor alterations in CT appearance (Fig. 15.26). CT shows a benign-appearing cyst that may contain fine septa, thin calcification in the cyst wall, a short segment of minimally thickened and smooth calcification in the cyst wall, or uniform high internal attenuation in a sharply marginated cyst smaller than 3 cm. No lesions show enhancement. High-attenuation fluid within cysts represents old hemorrhage.
- *Bosniak category IIF: follow-up.* This category was added in 1993 for lesions that are almost certainly benign but for which follow-up is recommended because the findings are more pronounced than for category II lesions (Fig. 15.27). CT shows multiple septa, minimal enhancement of the cyst wall or septa, thick or nodular calcification without enhancement, or totally intrarenal non-enhancing high-attention renal lesions of 3 cm or larger. No enhancing solid tissue components are seen in these lesions. Follow-up CT is generally recommended at 6 months and 1 year and then annually for 5 years. Absence of change supports benignity, whereas

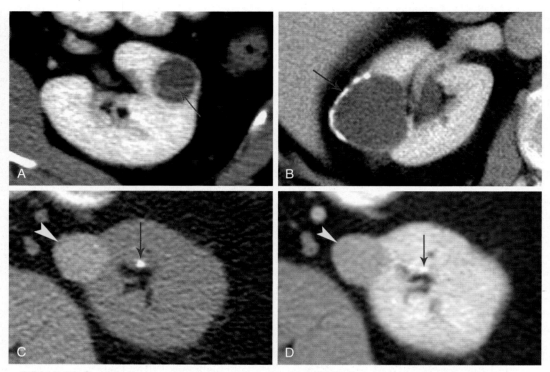

FIG. 15.26 Complicated renal cysts: Bosniak category II. (A) A single thin septation *(arrow)* is present in this otherwise simple left-sided renal cyst. (B) The wall of this cyst extending from the right kidney has foci of thin smooth calcification *(arrow)* in its wall. (C) CT without contrast medium demonstrates a uniformly high attenuation (64 Hounsfield units) mass *(yellow arrowhead)* arising from the left kidney. A renal calculus *(red arrow)* is also evident. (D) Contrast-enhanced CT at the same location as in (C) shows no enhancement of the renal mass *(yellow arrowhead)*. The findings are indicative of a Bosniak II high-density renal cyst. Note how contrast enhancement of the renal parenchyma obscures visualization of the renal calculus *(red arrow)*. High attenuation of fluid within a simple cyst represents old hemorrhage.

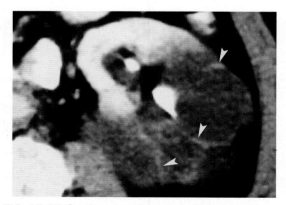

FIG. 15.27 Cystic mass with enhancing septa: Bosniak category IIF. A complex cystic mass arising from the left kidney has enhancing septations *(arrowheads)*. Serial CT scans over 3 years showed no change in this mass.

increase in septal thickness or solid components indicates that neoplasm is likely.

- *Bosniak category III: indeterminate cystic lesions.* These lesions have thickened walls, nodularity (Fig. 15.28), and septa in which enhancement can be seen (Fig. 15.29). Thick nodular calcification may be seen in the cyst wall or septa. Lesions may be benign or malignant, and include such entities as multilocular cystic nephroma, localized cystic renal disease, and multicystic RCC. Category III lesions may require surgical exploration. The risk of malignancy has been reported as 30% to 100%

- *Bosniak category IV: malignant cystic tumors.* CT shows findings seen in category III lesions, but with enhancing soft-tissue components adjacent to or within the wall of the cystic lesion (Fig. 15.30). Category IV lesions are considered to be malignant until proven otherwise.

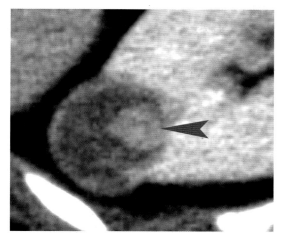

FIG. 15.28 Cystic mass with an enhancing nodule: Bosniak category III. A cystic mass arising from the right kidney has a mildly enhancing nodule *(arrowhead)* that makes the mass indeterminate and possibly malignant. Surgical exploration was recommended. This lesion proved to be a papillary renal carcinoma.

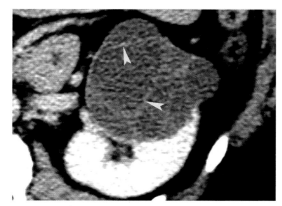

FIG. 15.29 Multilocular cystic renal tumor: Bosniak category III. Nephrogram phase CT of the left kidney in a 48-year-old woman shows a cystic mass with enhancing septations *(yellow arrowheads)* and an enhancing nodule *(red arrow)*. These finding led to surgical removal. Pathology confirmed benign multilocular cystic nephroma.

Simple Cyst

Simple renal cysts are benign, nonneoplastic, fluid-filled masses that are present in half the population older than 55 years. Small cysts are asymptomatic incidental findings. Large cysts (>4 cm) occasionally cause hypertension, hematuria, pain, or ureteral obstruction. Multiple and bilateral cysts are common. Strict criteria

that allow confident CT diagnosis of a renal mass as a simple cyst (Bosniak category I) (Fig. 15.25) include:

- Sharp margination with the renal parenchyma.
- No perceptible wall.
- Homogeneous attenuation near water density (-10 to 20 HU) on unenhanced CT. Homogeneous attenuation values may be up to +30 HU (pseudoenhancement) on postcontrast CT. Homogeneous RCCs have attenuation values no lower than +42 HU on postcontrast CT. Pseudoenhancement is defined as an artifactual increase of 10 HU or more on postcontrast nephrogram phase images compared with unenhanced images. Pseudoenhancement is seen with increased frequency with cysts smaller than 1 cm and central location of the cyst. Pseudoenhancement occurs in 19% of cysts with a size of 10 to 15 mm. It rarely occurs with cysts larger than 15 mm.
- No significant enhancement after intravenous contrast medium administration.
- On follow-up, simple cysts commonly slowly increase in size (~6% per year).

Renal Abscess

Pyelonephritis complicated by suppuration and liquefaction of renal parenchyma may result in the formation of an abscess. Alternatively preexisting cysts may become infected. On CT, abscesses appear as thick-walled, low-attenuation fluid collections within the renal parenchyma (Fig. 15.31). Gas is sometimes seen within the pus collection. The wall commonly enhances with contrast medium administration. Septations may be thick and irregular. Multiple locules of pus are common. Extension of infection into the perirenal space is common.

Cystic or Multicystic Renal Cell Carcinoma

Some clear cell RCCs are composed of multiple fluid-filled noncommunicating cystic spaces (see Fig. 15.6). Malignant tumor cells line the loculations. Rarely, RCC may arise within or adjacent to a simple renal cyst. Cystic forms of papillary RCC appear as a cystic mass with enhancing papillary projections or enhanced solid components (see Fig. 15.28).

Mixed Epithelial and Stromal Tumor

Mixed epithelial and stromal tumor is rare recently described entity presenting as complex cystic and solid masses. Histologically, stromal elements resemble ovarian stroma. Cystic components are lined by normal epithelium. Most patients are perimenopausal women, outnumbering men by 11 to 1. On CT, mixed epithelial and stromal tumors are indistinguishable from cystic RCC.

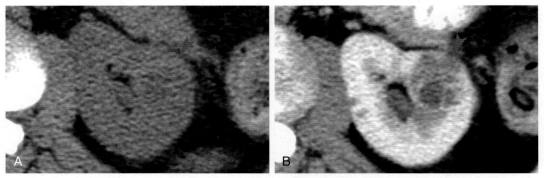

FIG. 15.30 Cystic mass with marked enhancement: Bosniak category IV. CT reveals a poorly marginated cystic mass *(arrowheads)* in the left kidney that showed enhancement from 18 Hounsfield units (HU) on noncontrast CT (A) to 48 HU on nephrogram phase CT (B). Nephrectomy confirmed a clear cell renal cell carcinoma.

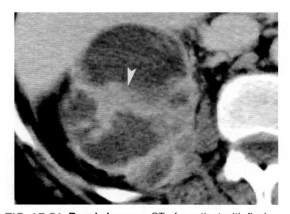

FIG. 15.31 Renal abscess. CT of a patient with flank pain and fever shows a large fluid collection extending from the upper pole of the right kidney. Irregular thick septations *(arrowhead)* are present. The abscess resolved with catheter drainage and antibiotics.

Multilocular Cystic Renal Tumor

Multilocular cystic nephroma, or currently called simply *cystic nephroma*, is an uncommon benign renal neoplasm composed of cysts of various sizes separated by connective tissue septa. Two-thirds of these tumors occur in males between 2 months and 4 years of age. The remainder occur in women aged 40 to 60 years. The treatment is surgical excision.

- The mass is solitary and unilateral, and most commonly arises from the upper pole.
- The multiple fluid-filled locules range in size from a few millimeters to 2.5 cm.
- The septa enhance moderately but less than RCC (see Fig. 15.29).

- Small locules and high-density fluid with the locules may make portions of the mass appear solid.
- Calcification, hemorrhage, and necrosis are rare.

Localized Renal Cystic Disease

Localized renal cystic disease is a benign condition that resembles multilocular cystic nephroma. The lesion consists of multiple cysts of various sizes separated by normal or atrophic renal parenchyma (see Fig. 15.27). The disease is not hereditary and is not associated with renal insufficiency. Most patients are asymptomatic.

- Multiple simple cysts of various sizes are separated by normally enhancing renal parenchyma.
- No discrete encapsulation is present.
- Other, clearly separate, benign cysts are often found nearby.
- The lesion most commonly affects a portion of one kidney.
- Occasionally an entire kidney is affected by localized renal cystic disease and resembles unilateral autosomal dominant polycystic kidney disease.
- Localized renal cystic disease is not associated with the presence of cysts in other organs.

The Small Indeterminate Renal Mass

High-quality cross-sectional imaging has resulted in the increased detection of small renal masses. The prognosis for cure of RCC is best when the lesions are small and are completely removed surgically before metastatic spread occurs. Currently 25% to 40% of RCCs are discovered on imaging studies as an "incidental" renal mass. Before the age of widespread cross-sectional imaging, only 10% of RCCs were discovered incidentally. Improved detection of small tumors has

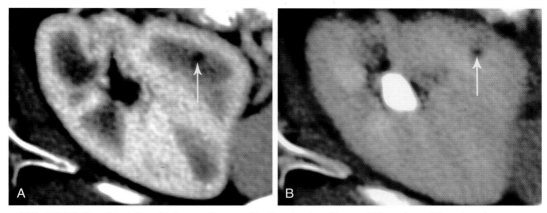

FIG. 15.32 **Small indeterminate renal mass.** Postcontrast corticomedullary phase (A) and pyelogram phase (B) images showing a tiny nonenhancing low-attenuation renal mass *(arrows)*. This most likely represents a tiny renal cyst.

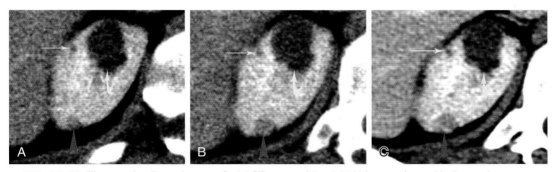

FIG. 15.33 **Tiny renal cell carcinoma.** Serial CT scans of the right kidney performed in the nephrogram phase showing three renal lesions: (A) initial scan, (B) scan at 1 year, and (C) scan at 2 years. The posterior lesion *(red arrowheads)* is most concerning as it is only slightly lower in attenuation than the enhanced renal parenchyma. Over time the lesion shows slow, but progressive, growth. Percutaneous biopsy before radiofrequency ablation confirmed renal cell carcinoma. The larger lesion *(curved yellow arrows)* shows low attenuation, but its interface with the renal parenchyma is not well defined. However, serial CT shows no change in the lesion and no enhancement. The small lesion seen laterally *(straight yellow arrows)* is indeterminate because of its small size but also shows no change on follow-up.

resulted in improved overall prognosis. Unfortunately, improved techniques also result in the detection of a large number of small renal lesions that are benign. The challenge to radiologists is to accurately differentiate benign lesions from malignant lesions. Accurate characterization requires high-quality CT. Despite optimal imaging evaluation, a considerable number of renal masses, especially small ones, remain indeterminate. A number of strategies have been recommended:

- Most small renal masses are simple cysts (Fig. 15.32). Volume averaging of small cysts complicates assessment of lesion attenuation and contrast enhancement. Bright enhancement of surrounding renal parenchyma during the corticomedullary and nephrogram phases may increase the apparent attenuation of a simple cyst by 5 to 10 HU. Ultrasound imaging is useful in characterizing small simple cysts that show this pseudoenhancement.
- In asymptomatic low-risk patients, lesions smaller than 10 mm are assumed to be benign cysts.
- In high-risk patients (von Hippel–Lindau disease, strong family history of RCC, acquired renal cystic disease of dialysis), the urologist may choose surgical excision.
- CT follow-up at 3- or 6-month intervals for at least 1 year is an option. Small RCCs tend to grow slowly (mean 0.36 cm per year) and are not an immediate threat to the patient's life (Fig. 15.33). Evidence of

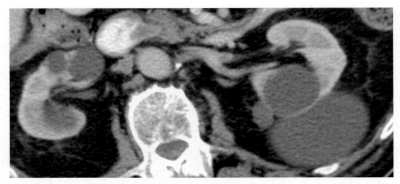

FIG. 15.34 Multiple simple cysts. CT demonstrates multiple simple cysts of various sizes throughout both kidneys. These are incidental findings.

lesion growth or the appearance of more aggressive features is indicative of RCC.

- Historically image-guided biopsy of a renal mass was rarely used. More recently, advances in biopsy and cytology techniques have confirmed the utility of percutaneous image-guided renal mass biopsy, especially for small lesions with uncertain imaging diagnosis. Confirmation of a benign renal lesion obviously contributes significantly to limiting patient morbidity.

Multiple Renal Cysts

When multiple renal cysts are encountered, the following conditions should be considered.

Multiple Simple Cysts

Simple cysts increase in frequency with age and are commonly multiple and bilateral (Fig. 15.34). Patients older than 50 years with no cysts in other organs and who have no family history of renal cystic disease and normal renal function are most likely to have multiple simple cysts.

Autosomal Dominant Polycystic Kidney Disease

The cortex and medulla of both kidneys are progressively replaced by multiple noncommunicating cysts of various sizes in this common hereditary disorder. Although this disease may be detected in childhood and may even be evident in the fetus, most cases present clinically with hypertension and renal failure at the age of 30 to 50 years. The renal cysts are commonly complicated by bleeding or infection, which causes thickening of the cyst walls and an increase in attenuation of cyst fluid (Fig. 15.35). Berry aneurysms are present in the circle of Willis in 10% to 15% of patients. CT findings

become more pronounced as the disease progresses. Autosomal dominant ("adult") polycystic disease is differentiated from other conditions by the presence of cysts in other organs, most commonly the liver; a family history; and the presence of renal failure and hypertension. Diagnostic CT findings include the following:

- Progressive replacement of renal parenchyma with cysts of various sizes associated with progressive bilateral increase in renal volume (Fig. 15.35).
- Cysts are often present in other organs, most commonly the liver (30%–50%) and pancreas (10%).
- Cysts in the kidneys may have calcified walls and high internal attenuation because of previous hemorrhage, infection, inflammation, or ischemia.
- Renal stones are common (20%–40% of patients).

Autosomal Recessive Polycystic Kidney Disease

Autosomal recessive polycystic kidney disease is characterized by ectasia and cystic dilation of the renal tubules involving both kidneys. It most often presents at birth with severe renal function impairment. Infants with less severe renal disease develop congenital hepatic fibrosis, portal hypertension, bile duct ectasia, and bile duct cysts (Caroli disease).

- Ultrasound imaging is the imaging method of choice and can usually detect the presence of this disease in utero. Older children may undergo CT.
- The kidneys are massively enlarged, with innumerable 1- to 2-mm microcysts expanding the renal medullas and compressing the renal cortex (Fig. 15.36). As the child ages, the cysts enlarge and become more visible on imaging. A striated appearance results from dilatation of the collecting tubules.
- CT shows the associated finding of hepatic fibrosis and portal hypertension.

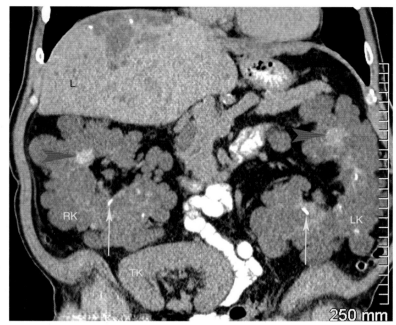

FIG. 15.35 Autosomal dominant polycystic kidney disease. CT image in the coronal plane from a noncontrast scan showing the native right kidney *(RK)* and left kidney *(LK)* to be markedly enlarged with the parenchyma replaced by innumerable cysts of variable size. Some of the renal cysts are high in attenuation *(red arrowheads)*, indicating previous hemorrhage. Some of the cysts contain calcification in the cyst wall *(yellow arrows)*. The liver *(L)* also shows the presence of multiple cysts. The findings are characteristic of autosomal dominant polycystic disease. Because of advanced renal failure, the patient has received a transplant kidney *(TK)*.

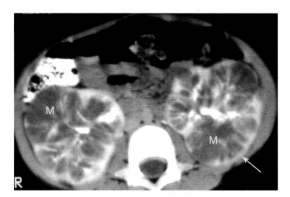

FIG. 15.36 Autosomal recessive polycystic kidney disease. Postcontrast CT performed on a 5-year-old shows massive enlargement of both kidneys. The medullary regions *(M)* of both kidneys are greatly enlarged by dilatation of the collecting tubules. Enhancement of the medulla is poor. The enhanced renal cortex *(arrow)* is markedly thinned by the expanded medulla.

Multicystic Dysplastic Kidney

This is a nonhereditary renal dysplasia in which the kidney consists of multiple, thin-walled cysts held together by connective tissue. Renal dysplasia results from high-grade urinary tract obstruction during embryogenesis. The involved kidney is functionless. The imaging appearance depends on the age of the patient. At birth the involved kidney is greatly enlarged. In childhood and through early adulthood the affected kidney appears as a nonfunctioning multiloculated cystic mass that may be confused with a cystic renal neoplasm. With advancing age the kidney progressively shrinks and often becomes calcified. Rarely, only a portion of one kidney may be involved. Bilateral multicystic dysplastic kidneys occur but are fatal at birth. The opposite kidney is affected by ureteropelvic junction obstruction, vesicoureteral reflux, or another anomaly in 30% of cases.

Von Hippel-Lindau Disease

Von Hippel-Lindau disease is a rare autosomal dominant disorder characterized by cerebellar, spinal cord,

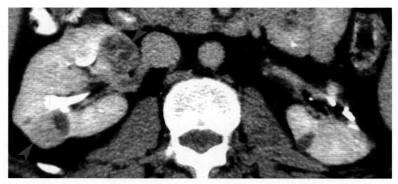

FIG. 15.37 Von Hippel–Lindau disease. Two partially cystic renal cell carcinomas *(arrowheads)* are seen in the right kidney. A partial nephrectomy had been performed on the left to remove a renal cell carcinoma. The complete CT scan showed numerous cysts in both kidneys.

and retinal hemangioblastomas, renal and pancreatic cysts, RCC, and pheochromocytoma.
- Multiple bilateral renal cysts are present in 50% to 75% of patients. Over time cysts may gradually enlarge or involute.
- RCC occurs in 28% to 45% of patients (Fig. 15.37). Tumors are most often solid, multicentric, and bilateral. Some appear as complex cysts with enhancing septa. Most are clear cell RCCs.
- Pheochromocytoma is seen in 30% of cases. It is bilateral in 50% of cases and malignant in 10% to 15% of cases.

Tuberous Sclerosis
This autosomal dominant syndrome combines multiple renal cysts and multiple and bilateral renal AMLs (see Fig. 15.17) with seizures, mental retardation, adenoma sebaceum, and cutaneous, retinal, cardiac, and cerebral hamartomas. In up to 60% of patients the condition occurs sporadically without a family history. Up to 40% of patients die by the age of 35 years of brain tumors, renal failure, or lung disease. Up to 75% of patients with tuberous sclerosis have renal AMLs. About 20% of patients with renal AML have tuberous sclerosis. Up to 50% of patients with tuberous sclerosis have renal cysts. Compared with sporadic occurrence of AMLs, the AMLs seen in association with tuberous sclerosis are multiple, bilateral, and larger and grow. Rupture of AML is a significant risk especially when females become pregnant. The renal cysts in tuberous sclerosis are multiple and bilateral and occur in younger patients. RCC occurs with the same incidence as in the general population but occurs at an earlier age in patients with tuberous sclerosis (average age of 28 years). Retroperitoneal lymphangioleiomyomatosis

may also occur, appearing as multiple retroperitoneal thin-walled or thick-walled cysts representing dilated lymphatic channels.

Acquired Renal Cystic Disease
Patients receiving long-term hemodialysis commonly develop innumerable cysts in their native kidneys. More than 90% of patients who are receiving dialysis for 5 to 10 years are affected. Many of the cysts are lined by hyperplastic and dysplastic epithelium. The condition is complicated by hemorrhage from the cysts and the development of RCC (in 3%–7% of patients).
- The affected kidneys are end-stage failed kidneys affected by conditions other than hereditary renal cystic disease. As such the kidneys are smaller than normal.
- The renal parenchyma is progressively replaced by myriad tiny cysts (<6 mm) (Fig. 15.38). Some cysts are up to 2 cm in size. The kidney slowly enlarges over time as cysts develop. Fluid within the cysts is often of high attenuation because of the presence of blood products and calcium oxalates. Calcification of the wall of cysts is common.
- The cysts usually regress within months of renal transplantation.

Infection
CT is indicated when complications of renal infection are suspected. Predisposing conditions, including urinary calculi, neurogenic bladder, immune system compromise, diabetes, intravenous drug abuse, or chronic debilitating disease, increase the risk of complications that require intervention. Most urinary tract infections are caused by gram-negative bacilli, but the incidence of fungal and tuberculous infections is increasing.

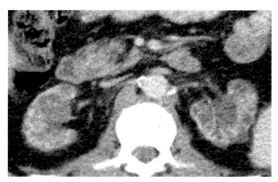

FIG. 15.38 **Acquired renal cystic disease.** CT scan of a patient with a 12-year history of hemodialysis revealed numerous small cysts in both kidneys. The kidneys are of low normal size. No solid masses were detected.

Acute Bacterial Pyelonephritis

Acute pyelonephritis is a multifocal infection of one or both kidneys. In patients with uncomplicated pyelonephritis, all symptoms usually resolve within 72 hours of institution of appropriate antibiotic therapy. Patients who fail to improve should undergo imaging to detect complications. CT signs of acute bacterial infection of the kidneys include the following:

- Wedge-shaped areas of mottled decreased parenchymal enhancement are seen (Fig. 15.39). The CT appearance is very similar to that of renal infarction. Decreased enhancement is the result of decreased blood flow caused by edema and inflammation within the parenchyma confined by the renal capsule.
- A striated pattern of linear alternating increased and decreased attenuation on enhanced scans is particularly characteristic.
- High-attenuation areas of parenchyma on unenhanced scans indicate parenchyma hemorrhage caused by inflammation and ischemia.
- Stranding densities in the perirenal fat and thickening of the renal fascia occur as a result of inflammation and edema in the perirenal space.
- Severe localized infection (variously called· *focal pyelonephritis, acute focal bacterial nephritis, lobar nephronia,* etc.) produces a poorly defined mottled low-attenuation mass without distinct liquefaction. These phlegmons may evolve into an abscess, resolve completely, or result in a scar.
- *Emphysematous pyelonephritis* is a severe life-threatening necrotizing type of diffuse pyelonephritis that occurs in people with diabetes (90%), immuno-compromised patients, and patients with urinary tract obstruction. Gas is produced by metabolism of

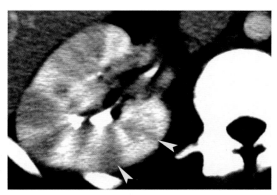

FIG. 15.39 **Acute pyelonephritis.** The right kidney shows the wedge-shaped areas of decreased parenchymal enhancement *(arrowheads)* characteristic of acute pyelonephritis. Severe edema in affected regions of the kidney results in diminished blood flow, producing the enhancement defects. The left kidney (not shown) was normal.

glucose by gram-negative bacteria. CT shows gas in the renal parenchyma in addition to signs of renal inflammation (Fig. 15.40). Emergency nephrectomy may be required.
- *Emphysematous pyelitis* refers to gas confined to the renal pelvis and calyces. This finding may be found with infection, trauma, instrumentation, or fistula, and lacks the dire implications of gas within the renal parenchyma. CT reveals dilatation of the collecting system containing bubbles of gas or gas-fluid levels without gas present in the renal parenchyma.
- *Abscess* refers to a collection of pus and liquefied tissue within the kidney (see Fig. 15.31) or with spread into the perirenal space (Fig. 15.41). CT demonstrates a fluid collection (10–30 HU) with an enhancing rim. Gas may be present within the collection, especially in patients with diabetes. Large abscesses usually require catheter or surgical drainage.

Pyonephrosis

Pyonephrosis is an acute infection with pus within an obstructed collecting system. Renal destruction is rapid, and urgent drainage of the collecting system is required.
- The collecting system is dilated, and the fluid contained within it is of high attenuation with layering sometimes evident.
- The wall of the collecting system is thickened (>2mm).
- The renal parenchyma is often thinned. Intraparenchymal abscesses may be present.
- Inflammatory changes surround the kidneys and collecting structures.

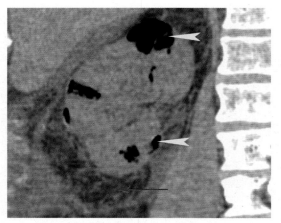

FIG. 15.40 **Emphysematous pyelonephritis.** Coronal plane image from noncontrast CT in a septic patient with right flank pain showing multiple gas collections *(yellow arrowheads)* within the renal parenchyma. Stranding *(red arrow)* within the perirenal fat is further evidence of inflammation.

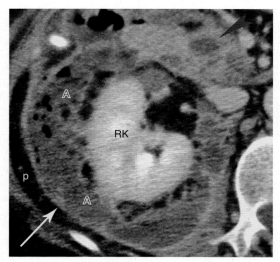

FIG. 15.41 **Perirenal abscess.** A bacterial abscess *(A)* complicating acute pyelonephritis in a patient with diabetes has spread through the renal capsule into the perirenal space, appearing as a loculated collection of fluid and gas. The margins of the right kidney *(RK)* are indistinct because of inflammation with stranding and thickening of fibrous sheets in the perirenal space. The renal fascia *(yellow arrow)* is thickened by inflammation but serves as a barrier preventing spread of infection to the posterior perirenal space *(p)*. The purulent process has spread anteriorly to involve the head of the pancreas *(red arrowhead)* in the anterior perirenal space.

Renal Tuberculosis

Tuberculosis remains the leading cause of death from infectious disease in the world. The urinary tract is the most common extrapulmonary site of infection and is involved in 15% to 20% of cases. The urinary tract may be involved even though chest radiographs do not show evidence of tuberculosis. Multiple caseous granulomas form in the renal cortex because of its favorable blood supply. These may remain dormant or may reactivate, spreading organisms to the tubules, resulting in papillary necrosis. Progressive infection will eventually destroy the kidney.

- Disease is often unilateral with a predilection for the poles of the kidney.
- Calcifications are a hallmark of disease shown by CT in 40% to 70% of cases. Calcifications are typically within the renal parenchyma and may be coarse, globular, curvilinear, or granular. Extensive calcification of a nonfunctioning kidney (putty kidney) is characteristic of end-stage renal tuberculosis.
- Fibrotic strictures with wall thickening of the infundibula, pelvis, and ureter are characteristic.
- Calyces are often dilated because of strictures of the collecting system. The dilated calyces are filled with clear fluid, debris, or calculi.
- Cortical thinning, caused by focal or diffuse parenchymal scarring, is usually present.

Xanthogranulomatous Pyelonephritis

Xanthogranulomatous pyelonephritis results from a combination of chronic renal obstruction and chronic infection. The renal parenchyma is progressively destroyed and replaced by lipid-filled macrophages. A staghorn calculus results in involvement of the entire kidney. A solitary calculus or infundibular stricture may result in focal involvement.

- CT reveals low-attenuation enlargement of the entire kidney or the affected area, with multiple low-attenuation masses representing dilated calyces. The kidney may enhance but fails to excrete contrast medium (Fig. 15.42).
- The obstructing calculus is seen within the renal pelvis or calyces.
- Obstructed calyces and intrarenal abscesses may be filled with pus and debris.
- Extension of the infective process into the perirenal tissues is common.

URETER
Anatomy

The ureter is a muscular tube approximately 30 cm long that lies on the psoas muscle. At the pelvic brim

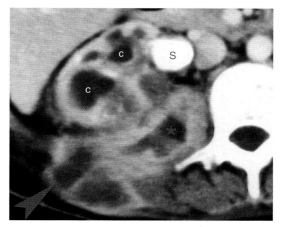

FIG. 15.42 **Xanthogranulomatous pyelonephritis.** A large stone *(S)* fills the renal pelvis and causes obstruction, resulting in dilatation of the collecting system *(c)*. The chronic infective process extends from the kidney through the perirenal space *(asterisk)* and into the subcutaneous soft tissues *(arrowhead)*. A nephrectomy was performed and yielded *Proteus* organisms on bacterial culture.

it courses medially to the sacroiliac joint then laterally near the ischial spine before it turns medially to enter the bladder through a submucosal tunnel (the ureterovesical junction) in the wall of the bladder. The ureter is lined by transitional epithelium, has a muscular wall consisting of circular and longitudinal muscle bundles, and has an outer adventitia that is continuous with the renal capsule and adventitia of the bladder. On unenhanced CT, 3 mm is the upper limit of normal cross-sectional diameter. Peristalsis of the ureter occurs approximately six times per minute in well-hydrated patients. Peristalsis may result in short segments of dilated ureter without other evidence of obstruction.

Ureteral Duplication

Duplication of the ureters is the most common anomaly of the urinary tract, affecting about 1% of the population. Complete duplication is associated with ectopic insertion of the ureter, ectopic ureteroceles, and vesico-ureteral reflux, and is more common in females.

- The ureter draining the upper pole of the kidney typically has fewer calyces, inserts into the bladder medially and inferiorly into the lower pole ureter (Weigert-Meyer rule), and is more likely to be ectopic, obstructed, and end in a ureterocele. With high-grade obstruction the upper pole of the kidney is atrophic and replaced by a cyst representing the dilated upper pole pelvis (Fig. 15.43).

- The ureter draining the lower pole of the kidney typically inserts into the bladder at the normal location. The lower pole system is prone to reflux if an ectopic ureterocele from the upper pole system distorts the lower pole ureterovesical junction.

- An increased frequency of ureteropelvic junction obstruction is seen in the lower pole system.

- When duplication is incomplete, the ureters typically fuse at a variable distance from the kidney, resulting in a single ureteral insertion into the bladder. Yo-yo reflux of urine occurs between the two ureters induced by peristalsis of one ureter then the other.

Transitional Cell Carcinoma of the Ureter

TCC (uroepithelial carcinoma) accounts for 90% of ureteral tumors. About 75% occur in the distal part of the ureter. More than 50% are associated with the presence or development of bladder TCC. Tumor growth patterns include papillary appearing as a filling defect in the dilated lumen of the ureter or infiltrating appearing as irregular wall thickening and stricture.

- Tumors appear as a soft-tissue mass, higher in attenuation than unopacified urine, expanding and obstructing the ureter (Fig. 15.44). When contrast medium is present, the lesion appears as an irregular filling defect within high-attenuation urine. Irregular thickening of the ureteral wall is seen with stricturing lesions (Fig. 15.45). Enhancement of the tumor with intravenous contrast medium is minimal.

Renal Stone Disease

MDCT has forever changed the imaging of renal stone disease. CT is the imaging method of choice to detect renal stones and to diagnose the complications of renal stone disease. Conventional radiographs have a specificity for stones of only 77%. Conventional radiographs and intravenous pyelograms have been replaced by MDCT. CT for stones requires no contrast medium and no patient preparation. With MDCT the study is routinely completed in seconds. CT may also provide an alternative diagnosis of the patient's symptoms, including other urinary disease, acute appendicitis, diverticulitis, pancreatitis, adnexal masses, or leaking aneurysms.

CT Appearance of Urinary Stones

Although only about 85% of urinary stones are seen as calcific densities on conventional radiographs, CT detects nearly all calculi. Calcium oxalate and calcium phosphate stones are most common (73%) and typically have a CT attenuation of 1200 to 2800 HU.

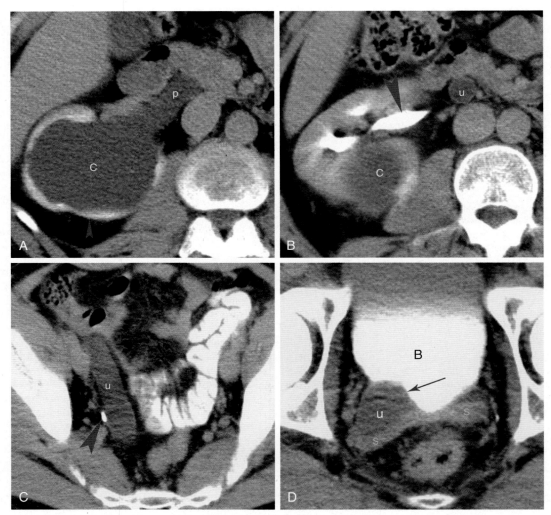

FIG. 15.43 **Obstructed ureteral duplication.** (A) A cystic structure *(C)* at the upper pole of the right kidney communicates with a dilated pelvis *(p)*. The cystic structure represents the obstructed collecting system of the upper pole of the kidney. Absence of contrast medium excretion into the obstructed collecting system is evidence of absent renal function of the upper pole. The parenchyma *(arrowhead)* of the chronically obstructed upper pole system is markedly atrophic. (B) CT image obtained inferior to the image in (A) showing the caudal portion of the obstructed upper pole system *(C)* and the functioning lower pole system excreting contrast medium into a separate renal pelvis *(arrowhead)*. The dilated ureter *(u)* continuing from the upper pole system is also evident. (C) Lower in the pelvis the greatly dilated upper pole ureter *(u)* resembles a fluid-filled sausage. The lower pole ureter *(arrowhead)* is normal in size and is filled with contrast medium. (D) The dilated ureter *(u)* of the upper pole terminates in the bladder *(B)* as a bulging ectopic ureterocele *(arrow)*. The bladder shows a contrast-urine fluid level with the contrast agent excreted from the normally functioning lower pole system layering dependently. The normal lower pole ureter inserted into the bladder at a higher level. The seminal vesicles *(s)* are distorted and displaced by the dilated upper pole ureter.

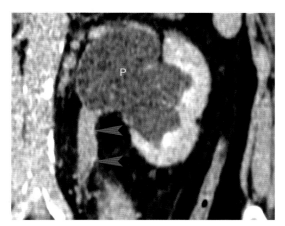

FIG. 15.44 **Transitional cell carcinoma of the ureter obstructing the left kidney.** Coronal plane postcontrast CT image showing marked dilatation of the pelvis of the left kidney *(P)* and the collecting system associated with delayed contrast medium excretion from the left kidney. The proximal part of the left ureter *(red arrowheads)* is dilated and of uniform soft-tissue attenuation, replacing internal fluid attenuation. Transitional cell carcinoma was confirmed by ureteroscopic biopsy.

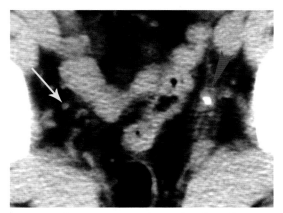

FIG. 15.46 **Stone in ureter: tissue rim sign.** Noncontrast CT of the pelvis shows a stone impacted in the distal part of the left ureter *(red arrowhead)* seen as an irregularly shaped high-attenuation focus. The wall of the ureter produces a rim of soft-tissue density around the stone (the "tissue rim sign"). The normal right ureter *(yellow arrow)* is identified by scrolling through sequential CT images, keeping track of the course of the ureter.

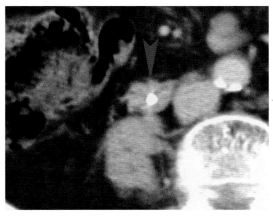

FIG. 15.45 **Transitional cell carcinoma of the ureter.** The wall of the ureter *(arrowhead)* is markedly and irregularly thickened with soft-tissue strands extending into the adjacent fat. CT-guided percutaneous biopsy confirmed transitional cell carcinoma. A stent, seen as a high-density structure within the ureter, was placed because the ureter was severely strictured.

Struvite stones (magnesium aluminum phosphate; 15% of renal stones) are seen with chronic infection. Struvite attenuation ranges from 600 to 900 HU. Uric acid stones (8%), which are radiolucent on conventional radiographs, have an attenuation of 200-450 HU

and are well shown on CT. Cystine stones (1%–4%) are moderately radiopaque on radiography because of their sulfur content. Calcium may be present in some cystine stones. Cystine stones have attenuation values of 200 to 1100 HU depending on the calcium content. High CT attenuation makes stones easy to differentiate from other urinary tract lesions such as tumors, hematoma, fungus balls, or sloughed papilla.

- Virtually all stones, even those that are radiolucent on conventional radiographs, are identified as high-attenuation foci on CT images viewed on soft-tissue windows (Fig. 15.46, see also Fig. 15.42). The threshold size for stone detection by CT is approximately 1 mm.
- Ureteral calculi are usually geometric or oval in shape (Figs. 15.46 and 15.47). They are seldom completely round. This feature is useful in differentiating stones from phleboliths. The positive predictive value of geometric shape in identifying a calculus has been reported to be as high as 100%.
- Phleboliths are small calcifications within thrombosed veins. They are most often seen in the pelvis. They are of no clinical importance unless they are mistaken for urinary calculi. Phleboliths are nearly always round or cylindrical and well defined. They are present in about 35% of the population older than 40 years.

- The single exception to stones being of high attenuation on CT is crystalline stones in the urine related to use of protease inhibitors (indinavir, Crixivan) in the treatment of human immunodeficiency virus disease. These stones are of soft-tissue attenuation on CT scans but may cause acute ureteral obstruction. Contrast-enhanced CT demonstrates these stones as tiny filling defects in the collecting system or ureter.
- The burden of stones in the kidneys is easily determined by CT. Stones are seen in the region of the minor calyces or medullary pyramids. The stone burden is defined as the number and size of stones present. Stone burden is used to determine therapy, such as lithotripsy.
- The tips of the renal pyramids are of high attenuation when the patient is dehydrated (Fig. 15.48). This normal finding of "white pyramids" should not be interpreted as representing renal stones.

Acute Ureteral Obstruction

Noncontrast MDCT has a reported sensitivity of 94% to 98% and specificity of 96% to 98% for acute ureteral obstruction caused by an impacted stone. CT evidence of acute ureteral obstruction caused by stones includes the following:

- A stone is demonstrated in the ureter (Figs. 15.46, 15.47, and 15.49B). The most common locations for stone impaction are at the ureteropelvic junction, where the ureter crosses the pelvic brim, and at the ureterovesical junction. The ureter is followed on consecutive slices until a stone is identified. Scrolling on the CT monitor is the easiest way to follow the course of the ureter. Knowledge of the anatomy of the course of the ureter and of adjacent vessels is crucial for accurate interpretation.
- The size of the stone is measured, and its location is precisely reported. The probability of spontaneous stone passage is related to the size and location of the ureteral stone. Stones smaller than 4 mm nearly always pass spontaneously. Stones of 6 mm pass about half of the time. Stones larger than 8 mm rarely pass spontaneously. The size and location of the stone are important factors used to determine the treatment of stones that do not pass spontaneously. Stones larger than 5 mm and located in the proximal two-thirds of the ureter are more likely to require lithotripsy or endoscopic removal.

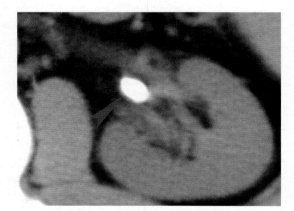

FIG. 15.47 **Stone at the ureteropelvic junction.** A large stone is impacted at the left ureteropelvic junction *(arrowhead)*. Bloom artifact from the high-attenuation stone obscures the tissue rim sign. The stone is confirmed to be located at the ureteropelvic junction by careful inspection of serial CT images. Even though the obstruction is high grade, the degree of hydronephrosis is slight because the obstruction is acute.

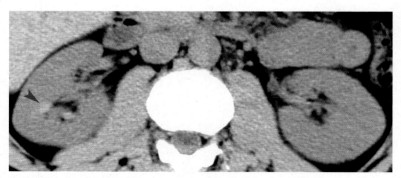

FIG. 15.48 **Unilateral absence of white pyramids.** The tips of the medullary pyramids in the right kidney show high attenuation *(arrowhead)*, indicating that this patient with left flank pain is dehydrated. On the symptomatic left side, no white pyramids are seen. The unilateral absence of white pyramids is a subtle sign of acute obstruction. A stone was demonstrated at the left ureterovesical junction.

- To confirm a stone in the ureter, look for a tissue rim sign (present in approximately 76% of cases). The *tissue rim sign* (Fig. 15.46) describes a halo of soft tissue that surrounds stones in the ureter. The soft-tissue rim is the wall of the ureter. The tissue rim sign may be absent because of a bloom effect artifact or a very thin ureteral wall (Fig. 15.47).
- The CT scout scan is useful for detection of stones and other abnormalities. Examination of the scout scan should be included in every CT interpretation. If the stone is visible on the scout scan, then conventional radiographs can be used to monitor its passage. Calculi not visible on conventional radiographs can be followed, when necessary, with unenhanced CT.
- Secondary findings of urinary obstruction are common but often subtle (Fig. 15.50). Comparison with the opposite side is highly useful in differentiating preexisting findings from acute obstruction. The presence of multiple secondary findings increases the confidence and accuracy of diagnosing acute obstruction. The frequency of visualization of secondary signs increases with the duration of symptoms.
- The obstructed kidney may be enlarged and slightly decreased in CT density because of edema. A 5-HU attenuation decrease is significant as evidence of edema in an obstructed kidney.
- Periureteral and perinephric fat stranding occurs secondary to edema produced by acute obstruction.

The amount of edema present correlates with the severity of the obstruction. Many patients, particularly older ones, may have preexisting stranding in the perinephric fat. Look for asymmetry of stranding on the involved side.
- The pelvicalyceal system is at most mildly dilated with acute stone obstruction. Dilated calyces are best seen at the poles of the kidney as rounded fluid-filled structures that displace renal sinus fat. Comparison with the opposite kidney is always helpful. Profound dilatation of the collecting system is evidence of chronic, rather than acute, obstruction.
- Unilateral absence of "white pyramids" on the affected side has been described as a subtle sign of obstruction (Fig. 15.48). Edema and swelling resulting from acute ureteral obstruction counteract the urine concentration effect of systemic dehydration.
- The ureter is mildly dilated to the level of the stone. Normal ureteral peristalsis produces transient focal areas of dilatation and narrowing that must be differentiated from diffuse dilatation to the level of obstruction. The ureter below the obstructing calculus is not dilated.
- Focal perinephric fluid collections (Fig. 15.49) may occur secondary to rupture of the collecting system at the fornix of a calyx caused by obstruction and high urine output.
- Axial plane CT images may be reformatted into coronal and sagittal plane images in problematic cases.

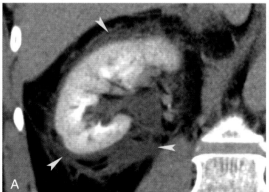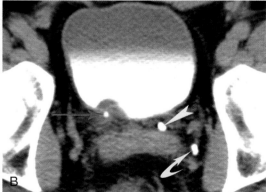

FIG. 15.49 **Obstruction: ruptured calyx.** (A) Postcontrast CT image shown in the coronal plane revealing delayed contrast medium excretion from the right kidney and fluid *(yellow arrowheads)* representing unopacified urine infiltrating the perirenal space. Acute high-grade obstruction of the kidney in a well-hydrated patient with good kidney function may result in rupture of the collecting system at the calyceal fornix. The diuretic effect of intravenous contrast medium administration may even precipitate the rupture. (B) Axial CT image in the same patient revealing the obstructing stone *(red arrow)* impacted at the swollen ureterovesical junction. The normal contrast-filled left ureter *(yellow arrowhead)* is also demonstrated. A phlebolith *(curved yellow arrow)* is present posteriorly on the left.

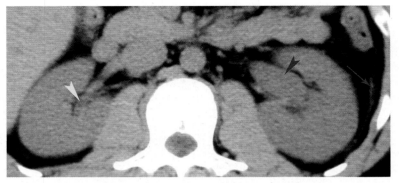

FIG. 15.50 **Acutely obstructed kidney.** CT image of a patient with left flank pain demonstrating subtle swelling and decreased density of the left kidney with mild dilatation of the pelvis of the left kidney *(red arrowhead)* and calyces. Compare this with the size of the pelvis of the right kidney *(yellow arrowhead)*. The margin of the left kidney with perirenal fat is indistinct. The left renal fascia *(red arrow)* is mildly thickened. This constellation of subtle findings is suggestive of left ureteral obstruction. A stone impacted at the left ureterovesical junction was seen on CT images through the pelvis.

Pitfalls in Diagnosis of Stones in the Ureter

No imaging test is perfect. A wide variety of pitfalls complicate interpretation of renal stone CT:

- An extrarenal pelvis may mimic pelviectasis. A normal renal pelvis tucked into the hilum of the kidney is restricted in size by surrounding tissue. A normal renal pelvis that extends outside the renal hilum is surrounded only by compressible fat and may dilate to a moderate degree. An extrarenal pelvis is not associated with dilation of the calyces.
- Peripelvic cysts may simulate hydronephrosis (Fig. 15.51), especially on CT performed without contrast medium. Cysts adjacent to calyces may mimic dilated calyces.
- Many patients, especially older ones, have preexisting stranding in the peripelvic fat. Comparison with the opposite side is critical to detect asymmetric stranding.
- Preexisting postobstructive changes are difficult to differentiate from acute obstruction.
- Phleboliths commonly mimic stones (Fig. 15.52). Phleboliths are calcifications that originate in thrombi within pelvic veins. Most phleboliths are found in perivesical veins, in periprostatic veins in men, and in periuterine and perivaginal veins in women. Occasionally phleboliths are seen in the gonadal veins that parallel the course of the ureters. Most phleboliths are round. They are seldom oval and are never geometric in shape. Visualization of a central lucency is highly characteristic of phleboliths but is less often evident on CT than on conventional radiographs. The *tail sign* describes a tail of noncalcified thrombosed vein extending from the phlebolith. A tail sign has been reported to be associated with 21% to 65% of phleboliths. Phleboliths are of lower attenuation than most stones, with a mean attenuation of 160 HU and a range of 80 to 278 HU. The probability that a calcification represents a phlebolith is 0.03% when the mean attenuation is 311 HU or more.
- Atherosclerotic calcifications may be mistaken for ureteral stones. Differentiation is made by careful examination of serial slices and determination of whether the calcification is vascular or ureteral.
- When signs of ureteral obstruction are present yet no stone is evident, consider a recently passed stone, pyelonephritis, stricture or tumor, or protease inhibitor treatment–related stone.
- Stones passed from the ureter may be identified in the bladder or urethra, or may not be seen.
- Always look for evidence of nonurinary causes of flank pain. Unenhanced CT has been reported to be 94% accurate in the diagnosis of appendicitis. Adnexal masses, such as hemorrhagic ovarian cysts, are usually easily detected.
- A subsequent contrast-enhanced CT scan may be needed in up to 20% of cases to provide an unequivocal diagnosis.

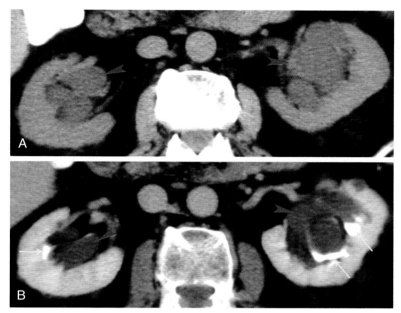

FIG. 15.51 Peripelvic cysts. (A) Noncontrast CT reveals bilateral cystic structures *(red arrowheads)* in the renal sinuses that resemble hydronephrosis. (B) Postcontrast CT in the pyelogram phase shows no contrast filling of the cystic structures *(red arrowheads)*, indicating that they are peripelvic cysts. Contrast medium does opacify the collecting systems *(yellow arrows)*, which are compressed by the cysts within the renal sinuses of both kidneys. The clue to diagnosis is inspection of serial images that reveal no connection of the peripelvic cysts with a dilated renal pelvis.

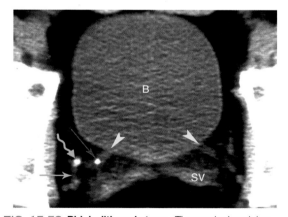

FIG. 15.52 Phlebolith and stone. The seminal vesicles *(SV)* serve as an anatomic landmark for the level of the ureterovesical junctions *(yellow arrowheads)*. The right and left ureterovesical junctions are always located at the same axial level on CT. A stone *(red arrow)* is impacted in the distal part of the right ureter. An adjacent phlebolith *(squiggly green arrow)* is identified by the tail sign, representing the thrombosed vein *(straight green arrow)*. The bladder *(B)* is filled with urine, making identification of the ureterovesical junctions easier.

SUGGESTED READING

American Cancer Society. (2018). Kidney Cancer Staging. https://www.cancer.org/cancer/kidney-cancer/detection-diagnosis-staging/staging.html.

Bai, X., & Wu, C.-L. (2012). Renal cell carcinoma and mimics: Pathologic primer for radiologists. *AJR. American Journal of Roentgenology, 198*, 1289–1293.

Bosniak, M. A. (2011). The Bosniak renal cyst classification: 25 years later. *Radiology, 282*, 781–785.

Cheng, P. M., Moin, P., Dunn, M. D., et al. (2012). What the radiologist needs to know about urolithiasis: Part 1 – pathogenesis, types, assessment, and variant anatomy. *AJR. American Journal of Roentgenology, 198*, W540–W547.

Cheng, P. M., Moin, P., Dunn, M. D., et al. (2012). What the radiologist needs to know about urolithiasis: Part 2 – CT findings, reporting, and treatment. *AJR. American Journal of Roentgenology, 198*, W548–W554.

Das, C. J., Ahmad, Z., Sharma, S., & Gupta, A. K. (2014). Multimodality imaging of renal inflammatory lesions. *World Journal of Radiology, 6*, 865–887.

Dillman, J. R., Trout, A. T., Smith, E. A., & Towbin, A. J. (2017). Hereditary renal cystic disorders: Imaging of the kidneys and beyond. *Radiographics, 37*, 924–946.

Ganeshan, D., Morani, A., Ladha, H., et al. (2014). Staging, surveillance, and evaluation of response to therapy in renal cell carcinoma: Role of MDCT. *Abdom Imaging, 39,* 66–85.

Krishna, S., Murray, C. A., McInnes, M. D., et al. (2017). CT imaging of solid renal masses: Pitfalls and solutions. *Clinical Radiology, 72,* 708–721.

Park, B. K. (2017). Renal angiomyolipoma: Radiologic classification and imaging features according to the amount of fat. *AJR. American Journal of Roentgenology, 209,* 1–10.

Potenta, S. E., D'Agostino, R., Sternberg, K. M., et al. (2015). CT urography for evaluation of the ureter. *Radiographics, 35,* 709–726.

Prasad, S. R., Humphrey, P. A., Catena, A. D., et al. (2006). Common and uncommon histologic subtypes of renal cell carcinoma: Imaging spectrum with pathologic correlation. *Radiographics, 26,* 1795–1810.

Raman, S. P., & Fishman, E. K. (2017). Upper and lower tract urothelial imaging using computed tomography urography. *Radiologic Clinics of North America, 55,* 225–241.

Sheth, S., Ali, S., & Fishman, E. (2006). Imaging of renal lymphoma: Patterns of disease with pathologic correlation. *Radiographics, 26,* 1151–1168.

Tappouni, R., Kissane, J., Sarwani, N., & Lehman, E. B. (2012). Pseudoenhancement of renal cysts: Influence of lesion size, lesion location, slice thickness, and number of MDCT detectors. *AJR. American Journal of Roentgenology, 198,* 133–137.

Tirkes, T., Sandrasegaran, K., Patel, A. A., et al. (2012). Peritoneal and retroperitoneal anatomy and its relevance for cross-sectional imaging. *Radiographics, 32,* 437–451.

Wolin, E. A., Hartman, D. S., & Olson, J. R. (2013). Nephrographic and pyelographic analysis of CT urography: Differential diagnosis. *AJR. American Journal of Roentgenology, 200,* 1197–1203.

Wolin, E. A., Hartman, D. S., & Olson, J. R. (2013). Nephrographic and pyelographic analysis of CT urography: Principles, patterns, and pathophysiology. *AJR. American Journal of Roentgenology, 200,* 1210–1214.

Wood, C. G., III, Stromberg, L. J., III, Harmath, C. B., et al. (2015). CT and MR imaging for evaluation of cystic renal lesions and diseases. *Radiographics, 35,* 125–141.

CHAPTER 16

Adrenal Glands

WILLIAM E. BRANT

The adrenal glands are the primary focus of diagnostic attention in three clinical circumstances. A patient may be referred for imaging because a clinical diagnosis of adrenal hormone hyperfunction has been made. CT is then used to identify and characterize the lesion. The adrenal glands are commonly imaged to detect suspected metastatic disease, especially when the primary tumor, such as lung carcinoma, commonly metastasizes to the adrenal glands. Adrenal lesions are frequently detected incidentally on imaging studies performed for other indications (about 5% of all abdominal CT scans). The significance of the finding must be assessed radiographically and clinically. CT remains the imaging method of first choice for evaluation of the adrenal glands.

NORMAL ADRENAL GLANDS
The adrenal glands have an outer cortex and an inner medulla that are functionally independent and anatomically distinct. The cortex secretes steroid hormones, including cortisol, aldosterone, androgens, and estrogens. The medulla produces the catecholamines epinephrine and norepinephrine. The adrenal glands lie in the perirenal space surrounded by retroperitoneal fat. The glands are usually triangular, or shaped like an inverted V or an inverted Y (Fig. 16.1). The right adrenal gland lies above the right kidney posterior to the inferior vena cava between the right crus of the diaphragm and the right lobe of the liver. The left adrenal gland lies adjacent to the upper pole of the left kidney, posterior to the pancreas and splenic vessels and lateral to the left crus of the diaphragm. The limbs of the adrenal gland are 4 to 5 cm long and normally do not exceed 10 mm in thickness. Limb thickness is uniform, and the margins are straight or concave. Normal adrenal glands are about equal to muscle in CT attenuation on precontrast scans. Moderate enhancement is evident after contrast medium administration.

CT TECHNIQUE FOR ADRENAL LESIONS
Noncontrast scans are obtained to document adrenal anatomy and to measure the precontrast attenuation of any lesions to serve as baseline attenuation for contrast enhancement. A slice thickness of 0.625 to 2.5 mm is used. The attenuation of any adrenal nodule or mass lesion is measured in the region of interest (ROI) that encompasses most of the lesion. If the average attenuation of the lesion is below 10 Hounsfield units (HU), the lesion is highly likely to be a benign adrenal adenoma. If the average attenuation of the lesion is above 10 HU, a contrast-enhanced study should be performed. Routinely 100 to 120 mL of nonionic contrast agent with an iodine concentration of 350 mg/mL is administered intravenously at 3.0 mL per second. Repeated thin-section scans (optimally 0.625 mm) through both adrenal glands are obtained at 60 seconds after contrast medium injection for the adrenal cortical phase and again at 15 minutes after contrast medium injection for the delayed phase.

ADRENAL LESIONS WITH A SPECIFIC IMAGING APPEARANCE
Myelolipoma
Myelolipoma is an uncommon benign adrenal tumor consisting of mature fat with interspersed hematopoietic bone marrow elements. The lesion is not associated with endocrine abnormalities and has no malignant potential. The tumor is most often discovered as an incidental finding. Occasionally tumors present with acute spontaneous painful hemorrhage. Tumors may also arise outside the adrenal gland.
- The presence of fat is characteristic. CT demonstrates large deposits of fat interspersed with higher-density soft tissue (Fig. 16.2). The average fat attenuation within the tumor is −74 HU on unenhanced CT. The soft-tissue components are relatively low in CT attenuation (20–30 HU), reflecting the mixture of fat with the myeloid tissue.

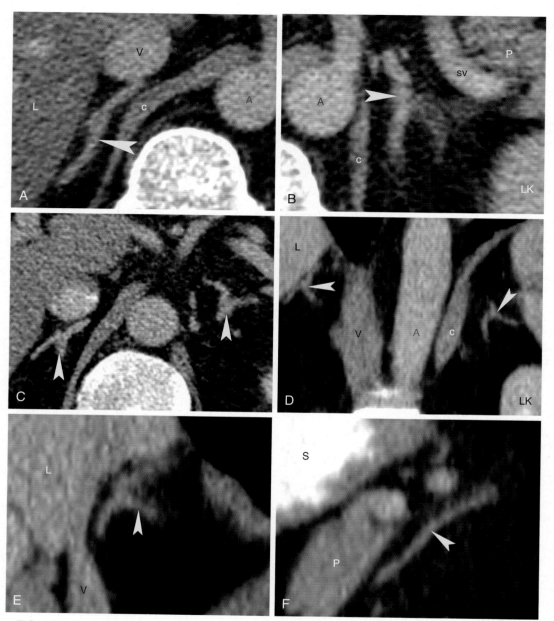

FIG. 16.1 Normal adrenal glands. (A) Axial CT image showing a linear appearance of a right adrenal gland *(arrowhead)*. Note the anatomic landmarks used to identify the right adrenal gland. (B) Axial CT image showing an inverted-Y appearance of a left adrenal gland *(arrowhead)*. Note the anatomic landmarks used to identify the left adrenal gland: (C) Axial CT image showing bilateral normal adrenal glands *(arrowheads)*. Note the anatomic landmarks and the variable shape of the normal glands. (D) Coronal CT image showing bilateral normal adrenal glands *(arrowheads)*. (E) Sagittal CT image showing a normal right adrenal gland *(arrowhead)*. (F) Sagittal CT image showing a normal left adrenal gland *(arrowhead)*. *A,* Aorta; *c,* right crus of the diaphragm in (A), left crus of the diaphragm in (B), crus of the diaphragm in (C); *L,* liver; *LK,* left kidney; *P,* pancreas; *S,* stomach containing oral contrast medium; *sv,* splenic vein; *V,* inferior vena cava.

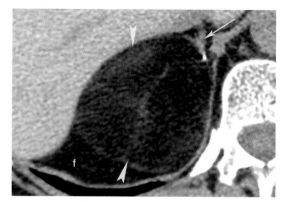

FIG. 16.2 **Myelolipoma.** A fat-density tumor (between *arrowheads*) arises from the right adrenal gland. The streaks of soft-tissue density within the tumor represent hematopoietic bone marrow elements. A remnant of normal-appearing right adrenal gland *(arrow)* is evident. Note the low density of the lesion is the same as that of retroperitoneal fat *(f)*.

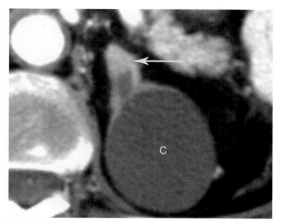

FIG. 16.3 **True adrenal cyst.** A purely cystic *mass (C)* arises from the left adrenal gland *(arrow)*. No discernible cyst wall is evident. The internal density is homogeneously low and near to that of water in attenuation.

- Small calcifications may be present (24%).
- Hemorrhage alters the imaging appearance. CT shows acute hemorrhage as foci of high attenuation within the fatty mass. Size greater than 7 cm is associated with increased risk of hemorrhage. Surgical removal is recommended.
- Tumors range in size from 1 to 2 cm up to 17 cm. Growth of the lesion is reported in 50% of cases.
- Extra-adrenal myelolipomas are most common in the presacral space and retroperitoneum, occurring less commonly in the mediastinum, abdomen, and muscle fascia.

Cysts

True cysts of the adrenal gland are lined with endothelium or epithelium. Most lesions are asymptomatic and are discovered incidentally. They may produce symptoms because of hemorrhage.
- Cysts are well-marginated, thin-walled (<3 mm), nonenhancing, homogeneous, fluid-containing masses (Fig. 16.3). Thin internal septations are sometimes present.
- The size may be up to 20 cm. The size of benign cysts may increase over time.
- The wall may have thin peripheral calcification if hemorrhage has previously occurred.
- Cyst contents have the characteristics of simple fluid (<20 HU) unless hemorrhage has occurred.
- Very rare parasitic cysts are usually caused by *Echinococcus granulosus* infection.

Pseudocysts

Pseudocysts account for about 40% of adrenal cysts. They occur as a sequela of previous adrenal hemorrhage. Pseudocysts have fibrous walls without a cellular lining.
- Pseudocyst appears as a hypodense mass with a thin or thick wall and, commonly, internal septations.
- Cyst contents are usually of higher attenuation than simple fluid, but cyst contents are not enhanced. Fluid-fluid levels may be present.
- Calcification in the wall is commonly present (56%) (Fig. 16.4).

Adrenal Hemorrhage

Adrenal hemorrhage is common in the newborn and is caused by hypoxia, birth trauma, or septicemia. In older children and adults, hemorrhage is induced by blunt abdominal trauma, coagulopathy, or underlying tumor.
- On unenhanced CT, acute adrenal hemorrhage appears round or oval and hyperdense (50–90 HU) (Fig. 16.5). Stranding is commonly present in the periadrenal fat.
- Posttraumatic adrenal hemorrhage has a marked predisposition to be unilateral on the right side as the right adrenal gland is compressed between the liver and the spine.
- With evolution and liquefaction of the blood clot, the adrenal mass shrinks and decreases in attenuation. Calcification of the hemorrhagic area may occur.
- Chronic changes of hemorrhage may be difficult to differentiate from other adrenal masses.

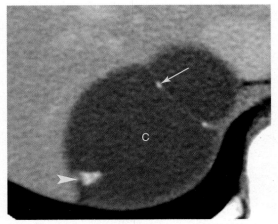

FIG. 16.4 Adrenal pseudocyst. This cystic right adrenal gland mass *(C)* has calcification in a thin septation *(arrow)* and contains a coarse dense calcium deposit *(arrowhead)*. This appearance is characteristic of a posthemorrhage adrenal pseudocyst.

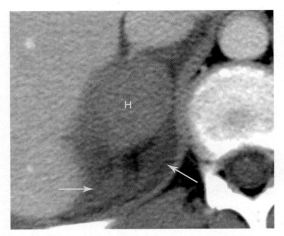

FIG. 16.5 Adrenal hemorrhage. Postcontrast CT in a patient injured in a motor vehicle collision shows hemorrhage expanding the right adrenal gland *(H)* producing a homogeneous mass. Additional hemorrhage *(arrows)* is seen in the perirenal space. Follow-up CT 4 months later confirmed complete resolution of the adrenal hemorrhage.

Pseudolesions

A variety of nonadrenal structures may simulate adrenal masses. Differentiation is made by having a high index of suspicion for pseudolesions and by performing appropriate correlative imaging tests. Accurate imaging diagnosis should obviously be made before adrenal biopsy. Pseudolesions are much more common on the left side because of the larger number of structures in the region of the left adrenal gland. Optimal CT technique with oral and intravenous contrast agents and multiplanar reconstructions makes confusion of pseudolesions with real adrenal lesions less likely.

- Unopacified portions of the stomach or small bowel are differentiated from an adrenal mass by administering oral contrast medium and repeating the CT scan (Fig. 16.6).
- Tortuous blood vessels are identified by contrast-enhanced CT or Doppler ultrasound imaging. Splenic artery aneurysms often have a calcified wall and mimic a pseudocyst.
- An accessory spleen or a splenic lobulation is recognized by its smooth margin and by CT attenuation and enhancement identical to those of splenic tissue.

Adrenocortical Carcinoma

Primary carcinoma of the adrenal gland is rare, occurring in people aged 30 to 70 years. Adrenal carcinoma is associated with adrenal hyperfunction in 50% of cases.

Cushing syndrome is most common. Other tumors present with abdominal pain or an abdominal mass. Most primary carcinomas are easily differentiated from adenomas by their imaging findings. The tumor is aggressive and highly lethal, with a strong propensity to invade blood vessels.

- The adrenal mass is usually large (>5–6 cm, average 12 cm) and markedly heterogeneous (Fig. 16.7). A non–fat containing adrenal mass larger than 6 cm has an 85% chance of being malignant. Tumors usually replace the adrenal gland. Tumors are bilateral in 10% of cases.
- Central necrosis is common, and irregular calcification (Fig. 16.8) is present in 30% of cases.
- Tumors enhance heterogeneously and have washout characteristics of malignant lesions (Fig. 16.9). On unenhanced CT, tumor attenuation is greater than 10 HU.
- Tumor thrombus in the renal vein or inferior vena cava (Fig. 16.10) is a frequent complication that carries a significant risk of pulmonary embolus.
- Direct invasion of adjacent structures and metastases to regional lymph nodes, liver, bone, and lung are common findings at presentation.
- Focal fat deposits are sometimes present in adrenal carcinomas. However, all fat-containing tumors reported have had other evidence of malignancy.
- Rarely, large degenerated benign adrenal adenomas have an appearance similar to that of adrenal carcinoma.

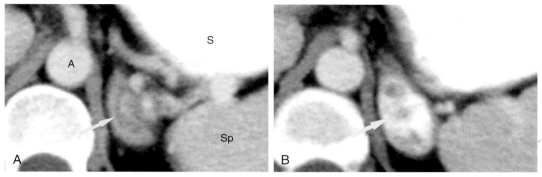

FIG. 16.6 **Adrenal pseudolesion.** (A) Initial CT scan revealing an apparent mass *(arrow)* in the region of the left adrenal gland. (B) Subsequent CT scan after administration of additional oral contrast medium showing contrast medium filling a gastric diverticulum *(arrow)*. *A,* Aorta; *S,* stomach filled with oral contrast medium; *Sp,* spleen.

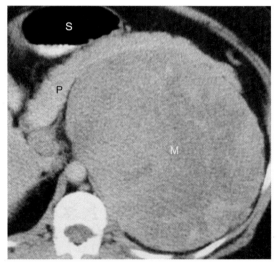

FIG. 16.7 **Adrenal carcinoma.** A huge solid heterogeneous mass *(M)* replaces the left adrenal gland. The pancreas *(P)* and stomach (S) are anteriorly displaced by the mass, confirming that the origin of the tumor is in the retroperitoneum.

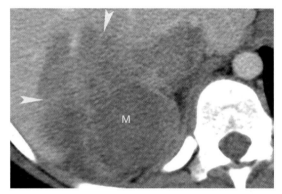

FIG. 16.8 **Adrenal carcinoma with necrosis.** Postcontrast CT reveals a solid mass *(M)* arising from the right adrenal gland and invading the liver *(arrowheads)*. Extensive low attenuation within the mass is evidence of necrosis.

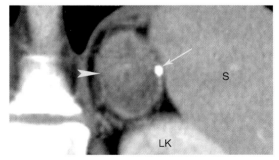

FIG. 16.9 **Adrenal carcinoma.** Coronal CT image showing a heterogeneously enhancing mass *(arrowhead)* arising from the left adrenal gland. A coarse calcification is present. The heterogeneous contrast enhancement and calculated relative percentage washout of 28% are characteristic of malignancy. *LK,* Left kidney; *S,* spleen.

Lymphoma

The adrenal gland is involved in approximately 4% of patients with non-Hodgkin lymphoma. Primary lymphoma arising in the adrenal gland is extremely rare.

- Most common is total encasement of the adrenal gland by retroperitoneal adenopathy (Fig. 16.11). The adrenal gland is often not visible.
- Other imaging appearances include small discrete focal or multifocal adrenal masses and diffuse adrenal enlargement. Both glands are involved in half of cases.
- Postcontrast washout is characteristic of malignant diseases.

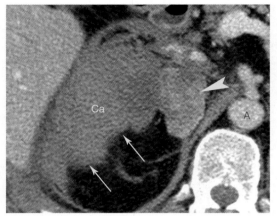

FIG. 16.10 **Adrenal carcinoma invading the inferior vena cava.** A large solid tumor *(Ca)* replaces the right adrenal gland and invades the retroperitoneal fat *(arrows)*. The tumor extends into and enlarges the inferior vena cava *(arrowhead)*. *A,* Aorta.

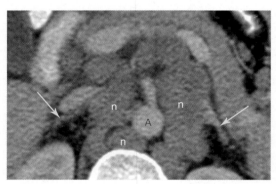

FIG. 16.11 **Lymphoma.** Enlarged lymphomatous nodes *(n)* surround the aorta *(A)* and partially engulf both adrenal glands *(arrows)*.

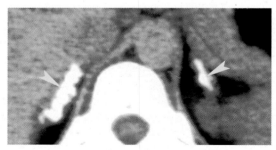

FIG. 16.12 **Adrenal calcifications.** Both adrenal glands *(arrowheads)* are densely calcified, probably the result of remote hemorrhage.

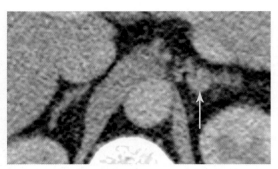

FIG. 16.13 **Adrenal cortical hyperplasia.** Both adrenal glands *(arrows)* show diffuse thickening of their limbs.

Adrenal Calcifications

Most adrenal calcifications in both children and adults are sequelae of adrenal hemorrhage. Tuberculosis and histoplasmosis cause adrenal calcifications and may be associated with Addison disease.

- Coarse punctate calcification in one or both glands without a mass being evident is characteristic of remote adrenal hemorrhage (Fig. 16.12).
- Adrenal tumors in children that calcify include neuroblastoma and ganglioneuroma.
- Adrenal tumors in adults that calcify include adrenal carcinoma, pheochromocytoma, ganglioneuroma, and metastases.
- Wolman disease is a rare autosomal recessive condition associated with enlarged calcified adrenal glands, hepatomegaly, and splenomegaly.

HYPERFUNCTIONING ADRENAL LESIONS
Adrenal Cortical Hyperplasia

Adrenal hyperplasia is usually associated with adrenal endocrine hyperfunction, especially Cushing syndrome, associated with excess secretion of adrenocorticotropic hormone (ACTH) from the pituitary gland or an ectopic site.

- The adrenal glands most commonly are uniformly enlarged but maintain their normal adrenal shape (Fig. 16.13). The thickness of the limbs of the gland exceeds 10 mm.
- A multinodular pattern of adrenal hyperplasia may also occur. The appearance may be indistinguishable from that of multiple small adrenal metastases.
- Biochemical hyperplasia may be associated with a normal size and normal imaging appearance of the adrenal glands.

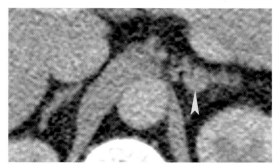

FIG. 16.14 **Aldosterone-secreting adenoma.** A tiny left adrenal gland nodule *(arrowhead)* was proven by adrenal vein sampling and surgical resection to be a benign aldosterone-secreting adenoma.

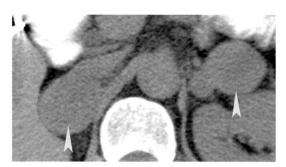

FIG. 16.15 **Bilateral pheochromocytomas.** Noncontrast CT shows homogeneous well-defined adrenal masses *(arrowheads)* slightly lower in attenuation than the normal liver. Surgery confirmed bilateral pheochromocytomas.

Cushing Syndrome

Cushing syndrome is produced by excess secretion of glucocorticoids, producing symptoms of weight gain, hypertension, acne, muscle weakness, diabetes, and deposits of fatty tissue in the face, back, and neck. About 70% of patients have bilateral adrenal hyperplasia, 20% have a benign hyperfunctioning adrenal adenoma, and 10% have adrenocortical carcinoma. Cushing syndrome may also be caused by iatrogenic administration of glucocorticoids. *Cushing disease* is caused by an ACTH-secreting pituitary adenoma, which stimulates the adrenal gland. MRI of the pituitary gland is often definitive in identifying the causative pituitary adenoma:

- Benign hyperfunctioning adenomas are round or oval and are usually less than 2 cm in diameter.
- Hyperfunctioning adenomas are indistinguishable from nonhyperfunctioning adenomas.
- Adrenal hyperplasia is usually diffuse, smooth, and bilateral. About 3% of patients with Cushing syndrome have nodular adrenal hyperplasia.

Conn Syndrome

Primary hyperaldosteronism is caused by a benign hyperfunctioning adenoma (40%) or by bilateral adrenal hyperplasia (60%), and is characterized clinically by hypertension with or without hypokalemia. Adrenal carcinoma is rarely a cause of hyperaldosteronism.

Adrenogenital Syndrome

Excess secretion of androgens may be a congenital or an acquired condition. Congenital adrenogenital syndrome results from an autosomal recessive enzyme deficiency and is associated with bilateral adrenal hyperplasia. Acquired adrenogenital syndrome is usually caused by a hyperfunctioning benign adrenal adenoma (80%) (Fig. 16.14), but 20% are associated with adrenal cortical carcinoma.

Pheochromocytoma

Pheochromocytoma is a catecholamine-secreting tumor that arises from chromaffin cells of the sympathetic nervous system. Most (90%) arise in the adrenal medulla and are benign and unilateral. About 10% ("rule of 10s") are extra-adrenal, with the most common location being the organ of Zuckerkandl near the origin of the inferior mesenteric artery. About 10% are bilateral, and 10% are associated with syndromes including multiple endocrine neoplasia type 2, von Hippel–Lindau syndrome, tuberous sclerosis, Sturge–Weber syndrome, and neurofibromatosis.

- Occasionally pheochromocytomas are detected before the patient presents with symptoms. Typical symptoms include episodic headache, sweating, and tachycardia associated with hypertension, dyspnea, tremor, and pallor.
- CT most often shows a round homogeneous 3 to 5-cm mass with precontrast attenuation about equal to that of normal liver (Fig. 16.15). However, the lesion is characterized by having a broad range of appearance on CT.
- Cystic change, central necrosis, and calcifications may be present, especially in larger lesions (Fig. 16.16).
- Contrast enhancement with the old ionic contrast agents has been reported to precipitate a hypertensive crisis in some patients. Nonionic contrast agents appear to be safe to administer. Most lesions show avid enhancement. The washout characteristics following contrast agent administration are similar to those of malignant adrenal lesions for most pheochromocytomas, whether they are benign or malignant. Uncommonly, pheochromocytomas enhance poorly or show washout characteristic of benign lesions.

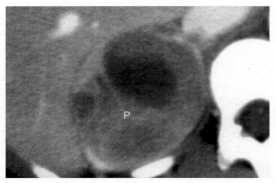

FIG. 16.16 **Pheochromocytoma: necrotic.** An unsuspected pheochromocytoma is seen as a heterogeneous mass (P) arising from the right adrenal gland. Necrosis and cystic change are present. Nonionic contrast medium was administered by intravenous bolus without an adverse effect. Hypertensive crisis has been precipitated by intravenous injection of ionic contrast agents in patients with pheochromocytoma, but the incidence of serious adverse reaction is negligible with nonionic contrast agents.

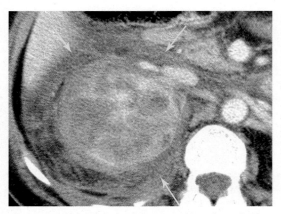

FIG. 16.17 **Pheochromocytoma: spontaneous hemorrhage.** A large right-sided pheochromocytoma (P) presented with sudden onset of right flank and abdominal pain shown by CT to be hemorrhage (arrows) extending into the perirenal space.

- Some pheochromocytomas present with spontaneous hemorrhage (Fig. 16.17).
- Metaiodobenzylguanidine or indium-111 pentetreotide scintigraphy may be used to locate extra-adrenal pheochromocytoma not identified by CT.

PROBLEMATIC ADRENAL MASSES

Benign nonhyperfunctioning adrenal adenomas are common incidental findings on cross-sectional imaging examinations. Up to 5% of CT scans obtained for other reasons demonstrate an adrenal lesion. Adrenal masses discovered incidentally in patients without known malignant disease are almost never malignant. Even in patients with known malignancy, benign adrenal masses as common as metastases to the adrenal glands. Accurate tumor staging requires definitive diagnosis of adrenal lesions.

Imaging differentiation of benign adenomas from metastases is based on the increased intracellular fat content found within most functioning adrenocortical adenomas. Cholesterol is a precursor of adrenocortical hormones, and cholesterol, fatty acids, and neutral fats are stored within functioning adrenal cells. CT and chemical shift MRI accurately demonstrate the increased intracellular fat content of benign adenomas.

It should be remembered that the lipid in benign adenomas is intracytoplasmic within adrenal cortical cells, whereas the lipid in myelolipomas is macroscopic and within fat cells. Thus myelolipomas have fat density on CT, whereas adenomas have low density but usually not as low as subcutaneous fat.

General Features of Benign Adrenal Adenomas

Patients with benign nonhyperfunctioning adenomas have no symptoms related to adrenal function and have normal adrenal hormone levels. Adenomas are found in 9% of individuals at autopsy.

- Adrenal adenomas typically are sharply defined, homogeneous, round masses of 3 cm (Fig. 16.18). On noncontrast CT scans, adenomas are hypodense compared with normal liver. Lipid-rich adenomas (~70% of benign adenomas) have noncontrast CT attenuation of –2 to 10 HU. Lipid-poor adenomas (~30% of benign adenomas) have noncontrast CT attenuation of 20 to 25 HU.
- Contrast enhancement tends to be moderate in intensity and relatively uniform throughout the tumor. Washout of contrast medium is significantly more rapid with benign adenomas than with metastases. This important feature is used to characterize benign adenomas that are low in intracellular fat content (lipid-poor adenomas).
- Because of the variability in contrast medium administration and the timing of routine CT imaging, adenomas cannot be definitively characterized as benign on a single postcontrast CT scan.

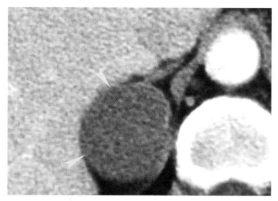

FIG. 16.18 **Benign adrenocortical adenoma.** Even though this CT scan was performed following intravenous contrast medium administration, the uniform low attenuation of this lipid-rich benign adrenal adenoma *(arrowheads)* is easily appreciated. Note the sharp outline and homogeneous attenuation of the mass characteristic of benign adenomas.

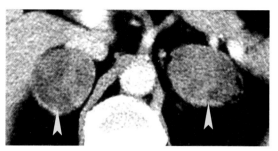

FIG. 16.19 **Bilateral adrenal metastases.** Adrenal metastases *(arrowheads)* from lung carcinoma replacing both adrenal glands are relatively well defined but heterogeneous in attenuation. Compare this with the uniform low attenuation of the benign adenoma in Fig. 16.18.

- A small adrenal mass with the characteristics described that remains stable in size and appearance on follow-up examination for 6 months or more is very likely to be benign, making it important to search for prior CT or MRI studies that include the adrenal glands.

General Features of Metastases to the Adrenal Glands

Metastases to the adrenal glands are found in 27% of patients with epithelial malignancies in autopsy studies. The most common primary tumors are lung, breast, and colon adenocarcinoma, and melanoma.

- Larger metastases (>3–4 cm) tend to be heterogeneous and lobulated in contour with less-well defined margins. Hemorrhage and calcification are common. Enhancement is nonuniform (Fig. 16.19). These large, heterogeneous, irregular lesions should not be confused with benign adrenal adenomas. Most adrenal masses larger than 5 cm are malignant (metastasis or adrenal carcinoma).
- Cystic changes may be present. Cystic metastases have thick irregular walls that enhance with contrast medium.
- Smaller metastases (<3 cm) tend to be homogeneous, round, and relatively well defined. These lesions may be indistinguishable from benign adenomas on routine imaging. Size alone is not a useful criterion for distinguishing benign adenomas from metastases (Fig. 16.20).

- Metastases are more commonly bilateral than unilateral. Masses that exceed 43 HU on unenhanced CT are very likely to be metastases.

Features that Characterize Benign Adenomas and Adrenal Metastases

CT differentiation of benign adenomas from malignant lesions is based on high intracellular lipid content and/or rapid contrast medium washout that characterizes benign adrenal adenomas:

- *Unenhanced CT attenuation.* On unenhanced CT, a mean attenuation of less than 10 HU is indicative of a benign adenoma (specificity 98%, sensitivity 71%). A threshold value of less than 2 HU yields specificity of 100% with sensitivity of 47%. This criterion defines "lipid-rich" benign adrenal adenomas (Fig. 16.21). Approximately 70% of benign adenomas are lipid rich and can be characterized by unenhanced CT attenuation. The remaining 30% of benign adenomas are "lipid poor" and will not be characterized as benign by this criterion.
- *Setting the ROI.* To use threshold values of CT attenuation, the ROI cursor must be properly placed within the central half to two-thirds of the mass (Fig. 16.22). Any regions of calcification or necrosis should be excluded from the cursor measurement. Lesions with large areas of necrosis or cystic change cannot be characterized by calculations of contrast medium washout.
- *Enhanced CT attenuation.* Attenuation values of benign adenomas and metastases on routine contrast-enhanced CT scans show too much overlap to be clinically useful in differentiation. Unfortunately many adrenal masses are discovered

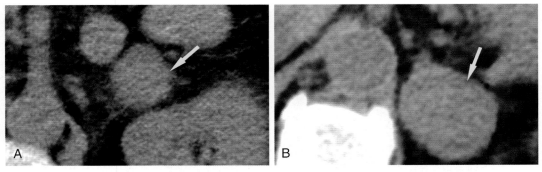

FIG. 16.20 **Problematic adrenal lesions.** (A) This well-defined adrenal nodule *(arrow)* is a benign adenoma. (B) This well-defined adrenal nodule *(arrow)* is a metastasis from lung carcinoma.

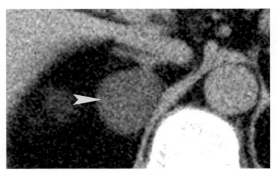

FIG. 16.21 **Benign lipid-rich adenoma.** A well-defined 2.5-cm mass *(arrowhead)* arising from the right adrenal gland measures – 2 Hounsfield units in CT attenuation. These CT characteristics define a benign lipid-rich adrenal adenoma.

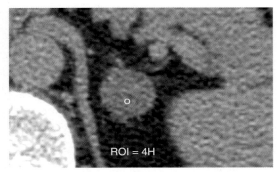

FIG. 16.22 **Standardized region-of-interest measurement.** The region-of-interest cursor is placed on the central half to two-thirds of an adrenal lesion. Any areas of calcification or necrosis are excluded from the measurement.

incidentally on postcontrast CT scans. In such cases repeated imaging is usually required to accurately characterize the lesions. The CT protocol for measuring lesion washout includes obtaining unenhanced images, early postcontrast images at 1 minute, and delayed postcontrast images usually at 15 minutes.

- *Contrast medium washout.* Although absolute attenuation values after contrast agent administration have not been proven to be diagnostic, benign adenomas show a characteristic brisk washout of the contrast agent that can be used to characterize the lesions as benign. Metastases and other malignant lesions show a characteristically slow washout of contrast agent.

- *Percentage enhancement washout.* Two formulas are in use to determine percentage enhancement washout, relative percentage washout (RPW) and absolute percentage washout (APW):

$$\text{RPW} = \frac{E - D}{E} \times 100,$$

$$\text{APW} = \frac{E - D}{E - U} \times 100,$$

where E is the enhanced attenuation value, D is the delayed attenuation value, and U is the unenhanced attenuation value.

The *unenhanced attenuation value* is determined on a midlesion precontrast image with use of an ROI that encompasses half to two-thirds of the lesion. The *enhanced attenuation value* is determined by ROI measurement performed in the same manner at the same location on the immediate postcontrast image of the lesion. *The delayed attenuation value* is determined by ROI measurement in the same manner and at the same location on the 15-minute delayed image of the lesion.

RPW greater than 40% is highly indicative of benign adenoma, and RPW less than 40% indicates a likely

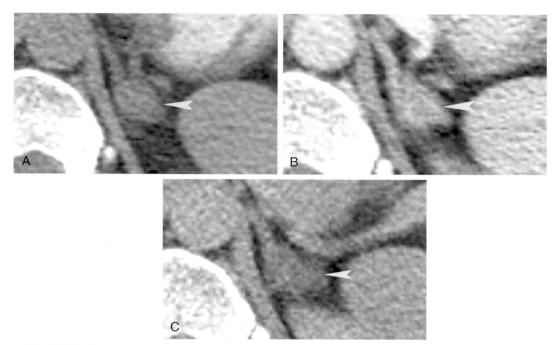

FIG. 16.23 **Contrast agent washout: lipid-poor adenoma.** (A) Small left adrenal mass *(arrowhead)* that measures 26 Hounsfield units (HU) on unenhanced CT. This attenuation is not compatible with a lipid-rich adenoma. A decision was made to proceed with intravenous contrast agent administration following the CT technique for the adrenal mass protocol outlined at the beginning of this chapter. (B) The immediate post-contrast scan demonstrates that the mass avidly enhancing to 94 HU. (C) The 15-minute-delay postcontrast scan shows rapid washout of contrast agent, with attenuation of the mass now measuring 30 HU. The relative percentage washout is 68%, considered diagnostic of a lipid-poor adenoma.

malignant lesion. APW greater than 60% is highly indicative of a benign adenoma, and APW less than 60% indicates a likely malignant lesion. These values have a reported sensitivity and specificity near 100%.

As an example, CT of an adrenal lesion performed according to the adrenal mass protocol yielded the following data (Fig. 16.23):

- Unenhanced attenuation: 26 HU.
- Enhanced attenuation (immediate): 94 HU.
- Delayed attenuation (15 minutes): 30 HU.
- RPW = 64/94 × 100 = 68%.
- APW = 64/68 × 100 = 94%.

This lesion is characterized as a benign adrenal adenoma.

- *Chemical shift MRI.* Chemical shift MRI may be used to accurately characterize lipid-rich adenomas. Fat and water protons precess at different frequencies. Gradient echo image sequences can be obtained so that fat and water proton signals can be separated within an imaged voxel. At 1.5-T fat and water protons are out of phase at an echo time of 2.3 milliseconds

and in phase at an echo time of 4.6 milliseconds. Fat-containing adenomas show a distinct drop in signal intensity on out-of-phase images (the signals from water and fat cancel out each other) compared with in-phase images (additive signal of water and fat) (Fig. 16.24). Lipid-poor and malignant lesions show no loss of signal intensity on out-of-phase images (Fig. 16.25). Subjective assessment of signal loss is sufficient and is equivalent to quantitative measurements of signal loss. Although MRI is as accurate as noncontrast CT for characterization of lipid-rich adenomas, it offers no advantage over CT. Only the lipid-rich adenomas that can be definitively characterized by noncontrast CT can be characterized by in-phase/out-of-phase MRI. Attempts to assess gadolinium washout on MRI have so far not been successful.

- *Biopsy.* Lesions that are not adequately characterized by CT or MRI may require image-guided percutaneous biopsy. This procedure has been shown to be safe and effective. CT is routinely used to guide the biopsy procedure.

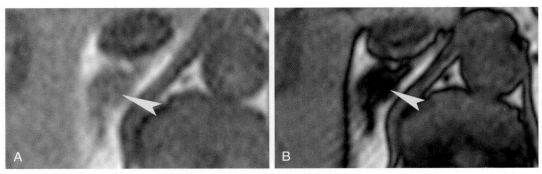

FIG. 16.24 MRI of benign adrenal adenoma. (A) In-phase magnetic resonance image showing a right adrenal gland mass *(arrowhead)* that is near to liver in signal intensity. (B) Out-of-phase magnetic resonance image showing a marked drop in signal intensity of the mass *(arrowhead)*, indicating the high intracellular lipid content of a benign lipid-rich adenoma.

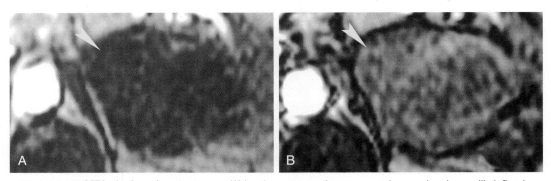

FIG. 16.25 MRI of adrenal metastases. (A) In-phase magnetic resonance image showing an ill-defined left adrenal gland mass *(arrowhead)* of low signal intensity. (B) Out-of-phase magnetic resonance image showing an increase rather than a decrease in signal intensity of the mass *(arrowhead)*. This patient has metastatic sarcoma.

SUGGESTED READING

Boland, G. W. L. (2010). Adrenal imaging: Why, when, what, and how? Part 1. Why and when to image. *AJR. American Journal of Roentgenology, 195,* W377–W381.

Boland, G. W. L. (2011). Adrenal imaging: Why, when, what, and how? Part 2. What technique? *AJR. American Journal of Roentgenology, 196,* W1–W5.

Boland, G. W. L. (2011). Adrenal imaging: Why, when, what, and how? Part 3. The algorithmic approach to definitive characterization of the adrenal incidentaloma. *AJR. American Journal of Roentgenology, 196,* W109–W111.

Ganeshan, D., Bhosale, P., & Kundra, V. (2012). Current update on cytogenetics, taxonomy, diagnosis, and management of adrenocortical carcinoma: What radiologists should know. *AJR. American Journal of Roentgenology, 199,* 1283–1293.

Lattein, G. E., Jr., Sturgill, E. D., Tujo, C. A., et al. (2014). Adrenal tumors and tumor-like conditions in the adult: Radiologic-pathologic correlation. *Radiographics, 34,* 805–829.

Sargar, K. M., Khanna, G., & Bowling, R. H. (2017). Imaging of nonmalignant adrenal lesions in children. *Radiographics, 37,* 1648–1664.

Schieda, N., & Siegelman, E. S. (2017). Update on CT and MRI of adrenal nodules. *AJR. American Journal of Roentgenology, 206,* 1206–1217.

Wagner-Bartak, N. A., Baiomy, A., Habra, M. A., et al. (2017). Cushing syndrome: Diagnostic workup and imaging features, with clinical and pathologic correlation. *AJR. American Journal of Roentgenology, 209,* 19–32.

CHAPTER 17

Gastrointestinal Tract

WILLIAM E. BRANT

BASIC PRINCIPLES

CT complements endoscopy and barium examination of the gastrointestinal (GI) tract by demonstration of intramural and extraintestinal components of GI disease, including disease in the mesentery, peritoneal cavity, lymph nodes, and liver. CT is used to diagnose the presence of GI disease, evaluate its nature and extent, and demonstrate complications such as abscess, phlegmon, fistula, and perforation. CT is excellent for determining the extent of GI disease but is less often specific for its nature.

The GI tract is shown on every CT of the abdomen. The intestinal lumen should be distended and opacified for routine abdominal CT by administration of 700 to 800 mL of 2% to 3% iodinated, or barium, contrast agent at least 1 hour before routine scanning. Water is an excellent contrast agent for the lumen of the stomach and upper intestinal tract and can be used whenever disease in the upper abdomen is suspected. Intravenous contrast medium is used to assess enhancement of the GI mucosa and of lesions, to demonstrate blood vessels, and to evaluate the solid organs of the abdomen. Thin-section scans improve lesion definition. The short scan times of multidetector CT (MDCT) improve image quality by limiting motion artifact. Collapsed bowel loops without intraluminal contrast enhancement may mimic adenopathy and mass lesions. However, when scans are obtained during the arterial phase of bolus contrast medium enhancement, identification of enhanced bowel wall confirms the nature of nondistended bowel.

A CT hallmark of intestinal disease is thickening of the bowel wall. When fully distended, the bowel wall is 1 to 2 mm thick. When collapsed, the bowel wall should not exceed 3 to 4 mm, except in the stomach near the esophageal junction, where the normal stomach wall may be 2 cm thick when collapsed. The CT appearance of wall thickening is helpful in differentiating benign wall thickening from malignant wall thickening (Table 17.1). Benign wall thickening usually does not exceed 1 cm, is homogeneous in attenuation, and is circumferential, symmetric, and segmental

in distribution. The *double halo and target* appearance of the intestine in cross section is caused by inflammation, edema, and hyperemia and is best demonstrated on contrast-enhanced scans. Neoplastic wall thickening is thicker (1–2 cm), asymmetric, nodular, lobulated, or spiculated in contour and tends to narrow the intestinal lumen. Benign wall thickening is caused by inflammatory bowel disease, intestinal ischemia, and intramural hemorrhage. Neoplastic wall thickening is produced by adenocarcinoma, lymphoma, and GI stromal tumors (GISTs).

CT ENTEROGRAPHY

CT enterography using MDCT is a first-line modality for examination of small bowel disease. CT enterography differs from routine CT of the abdomen and pelvis by use of large volumes of low-attenuation intraluminal contrast agent to optimally distend the bowel

TABLE 17.1
Benign Versus Malignant Bowel Wall Thickening

Benign	Malignant
Homogeneous attenuation	Heterogeneous attenuation
Symmetric	Asymmetric
Circumferential	Eccentric
Thickening <1 cm	Thickening >1–2 cm
Segmental or diffuse involvement	Focal mass
"Double-halo sign"	Abrupt transition
Dark inner ring	Lobulated contour
Bright outer ring	Spiculated contour
"Target sign"	Narrowed bowel lumen
Bright inner ring	Enlarged lymph nodes
Dark middle ring	Liver metastases
Bright outer ring	

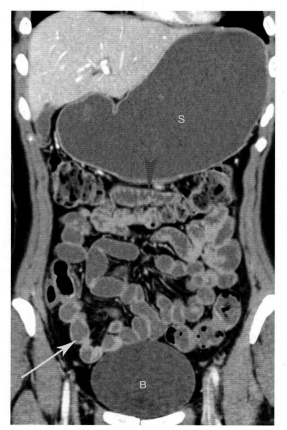

FIG. 17.1 CT enterography. Coronal image from a CT enterography examination using a low-attenuation intraluminal contrast agent as well as an intravenous contrast agent showing the normal fold pattern of the jejunum *(red arrowhead)* and the normal absence of folds of the ileum *(yellow arrow)*. The stomach *(S)* is well distended with intraluminal contrast agent. The bladder *(B)* is also filled.

lumen, matched with thin-slice collimation and routine high-detail coronal and sagittal reformations. Low-attenuation intraluminal contrast agent paired with intravenous contrast agent administration optimally displays both the lumen and the wall of the small bowel (Fig. 17.1). The advantages of CT enterography over traditional barium-based small bowel follow-through examination include demonstration of the entire thickness of the bowel wall and disease in the mesentery, as well as display of bowel loops without superimposition. The indications for CT enterography include Crohn disease and other suspected inflammatory bowel diseases, intermittent small-bowel obstruction, obscure GI bleeding, and suspected tumors of

small bowel. A typical protocol for CT enterography includes:

- A minimum 4-hour fast.
- Administration of low-attenuation (20 Hounsfield units [HU]) oral contrast agent, typically VoLumen, a low-concentration barium sulfate suspension, 0.1% w/v (Bracco E-Z-EM). A total volume 1400 mL is given in divided doses: 450 mL 60 minutes before scanning, 450 mL 40 minutes before scanning, 250 mL 20 minutes before scanning, and 250 mL 10 minutes before scanning. Glucagon (0.5 mg) may be given intramuscularly to inhibit bowel motion.
- Administration of 125 mL of 60% iodine intravenous contrast agent at 3 to 4 mL per second provides enhancement of the bowel wall as well as of any lesions.
- MDCT scanning is performed from the dome of diaphragm through the ischial tuberosities with 0.625-mm collimation with reconstructions at 2.5-mm slice thickness.
- For inflammatory bowel disease or other diffuse bowel disease, images are obtained after contrast agent administration only in the portal venous phase with an 80-second delay.
- For occult GI bleeding or suspected GI malignancy, scans are obtained in the arterial phase (30-second scan delay), portal venous phase (80-second scan delay), and delayed phase (3-minute scan delay).
- Images are reconstructed in axial, coronal, and sagittal planes.

CT ENTEROCLYSIS

CT enteroclysis is performed on patients with small-bowel obstruction to find the level and cause of obstruction (Fig. 17.2). For CT enteroclysis, contrast medium for small-bowel distention is injected into the small bowel through a nasojejunal tube rather than given orally as for CT enterography. A nasojejunal tube is positioned at the duodenojejunal junction under fluoroscopic guidance. A total of 1200 to 1600 mL of low-attenuation oral contrast medium is injected into the small bowel at 60 to 120 mL per minute. Glucagon, or other antispasmodic medication, is administered. Intravenous contrast agent is used, and MDCT scanning is performed with the same parameters as for CT enterography.

CT COLONOGRAPHY

CT colonography is used to investigate the colon for colorectal polyps and cancers. CT colonography

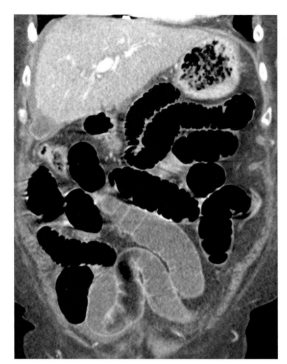

FIG. 17.2 CT enteroclysis: distal small-bowel obstruction. Coronal image from a CT enteroclysis examination showing diffuse dilatation of the small bowel with a low-attenuation intraluminal contrast agent and air. An adhesion was the cause of distal small-bowel obstruction.

is now the radiologic examination of choice for the diagnosis of colorectal malignancy. Numerous studies have shown that CT colonography is nearly equal to traditional optical colonoscopy for detecting cancer and precancerous lesions. Many patients prefer CT colonography over colonoscopy because of perceived safety and convenience. The obvious disadvantage of CT colonography is for that lesions that require biopsy, the patient will have to undergo subsequent colonoscopy.

- Standard bowel preparation, similar to that used for colonoscopy, is begun the day before the examination.
- Barium sulfate and iodinated contrast medium solutions are given orally to tag remaining stool and colonic fluid.
- For the examination a catheter is placed in the rectum and the colon is insufflated with an automated carbon dioxide system that provides pressure and volume regulation.

- MDCT scanning is performed with 1.25-mm collimation and a low-radiation dose protocol with the patient in both the prone and the supine position.
- Images are reviewed on a workstation that provides three-dimensional volume rendering with endoluminal display and "fly-through" capability (Fig. 17.3).

ESOPHAGUS

Anatomy

The esophagus is a muscular tube that extends from the cricopharyngeus muscle at the level of the cricoid cartilage to the stomach. The major portion of its length is within the middle mediastinum. The cervical portion extends from the level of the C6 vertebral body to the thoracic inlet. A short abdominal segment extends below the diaphragm to the gastroesophageal junction. The esophagus is lined by squamous epithelium to the gastric junction, where the mucosa abruptly changes to columnar epithelium. The lack of serosal covering allows early invasion by esophageal tumors into periesophageal tissues. The musculature of the esophageal wall is striated in the upper third, striated and smooth muscle in the middle third, and solely smooth muscle in the distal third.

On CT the esophagus appears as an oval of soft-tissue density often containing air or contrast material within its lumen (Fig. 17.4). When distended, the wall of the esophagus should not exceed 3 mm in thickness. In the neck and upper thorax the esophagus courses between the trachea and the spine. In the lower thorax the esophagus courses to the right of the descending aorta between the left atrium and the spine. The esophagus enters the abdomen through the esophageal hiatus and courses to the left to join the stomach. The edges of the diaphragmatic crura forming the esophageal hiatus are seen as often prominent, teardrop-shaped structures partially surrounding the esophagus. Air columns in the esophagus longer than 10 to 15 cm may be evidence of stricture or impaired peristalsis. Air-fluid levels in the esophagus are always abnormal.

Esophageal Carcinoma

Because of the lack of serosal covering, carcinoma spreads beyond the esophagus early in its course, resulting in a poor prognosis. Ninety percent of tumors are squamous cell carcinoma, with the remaining 10% being adenocarcinoma arising in Barrett esophagus in the distal esophagus. The CT findings in esophageal carcinoma may be duplicated by benign disease. Diagnosis depends on biopsy. CT is performed to assess the extent of disease and to identify those patients whose

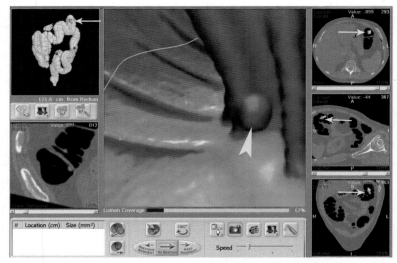

FIG. 17.3 **CT colonography.** Image from a three-dimensional work station used for interpretation of CT colonography examinations showing the location of a polyp *(yellow arrowhead)* in the splenic flexure of the colon 121.6 cm from the anal verge. Accurate landmarks *(yellow arrows* and *blue markers)* allow rapid localization of the polyp for removal by colonoscopy.

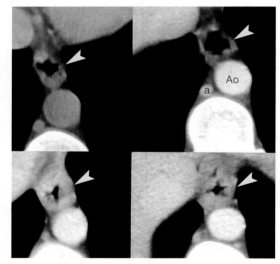

FIG. 17.4 **Normal esophagus.** Sequential axial CT slices demonstrate the normal appearance of the esophagus *(arrowheads)*. The descending thoracic aorta *(Ao)* and azygos vein *(a)* are evident.

disease cannot be surgically resected. The CT findings in esophageal carcinoma include the following:

- Irregular thickening of the wall of the esophagus of more than 3 mm (Fig. 17.5).
- Intraluminal polypoid mass.
- Eccentric narrowing of the lumen.

- Dilatation of the esophagus above the area of narrowing with air or fluid.
- Invasion of periesophageal tissues: fat, aorta, trachea.
- Tumor invasion of the trachea or bronchi is suggested by tumor that displaces or indents the posterior airway wall (90% accurate).
- Tumor invasion of the aorta is suggested by an arc of contact between the tumor and aorta of greater than 90 degrees. An arc less than 45 degrees indicates no invasion, and an arc between 45 and 90 degrees is indeterminate. These findings are about 80% accurate.
- Metastases to lymph nodes, liver, and other organs.
- Esophageal carcinoma spreads to paraesophageal, other mediastinal, gastrohepatic ligament, and left gastric nodal chains (Fig. 17.6). Microscopic disease in normal-sized nodes, and lymph node enlargement as a result of benign conditions, limits the CT accuracy of nodal involvement by esophageal carcinoma to 39% to 85%.
- Tumor recurrence after esophagectomy is well demonstrated by CT. Tumors may recur anywhere within the mediastinum, in distant lymph nodes in the neck or abdomen, and in the liver, lung, pleural space, adrenal glands, or peritoneal cavity.

Esophageal Mesenchymal Tumors

Leiomyoma is the most common benign tumor of the esophagus. Most smooth muscle tumors of the

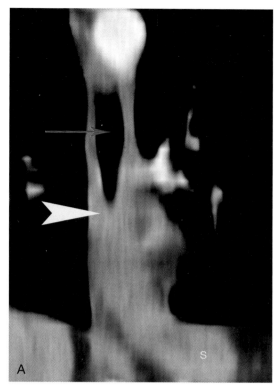

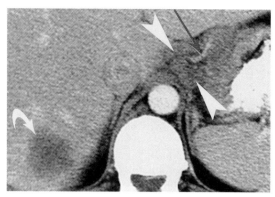

FIG. 17.6 **Carcinoma of the gastroesophageal junction.** Carcinoma arising near the gastroesophageal junction has spread to the liver *(curved yellow arrow)* and to lymph nodes *(yellow arrowheads)* surrounding the celiac axis *(straight red arrow)*.

esophagus are true leiomyomas. GISTs are rare tumors of the esophagus, occurring more commonly in the stomach and small intestine. Immunohistologic studies differentiate the two tumors. Most esophageal mesenchymal tumors are asymptomatic until they become very large and cause dysphagia. Endoscopy demonstrates a submucosal mass, usually easily differentiated from carcinoma.

- On CT, leiomyoma appears as a smooth, well-defined 2- to 8-cm mass of uniform soft-tissue attenuation. The esophageal wall is eccentrically thickened, and the lumen is deformed. A large, well-defined mass is much more likely to be a leiomyoma than a carcinoma. Leiomyomas occurs multiply in about 4% of cases.
- Leiomyomas, and rarely GISTs, are the only tumors of the esophagus that may have coarse calcifications (Fig. 17.7).
- Compared with leiomyomas, GISTs appear more heterogeneous, tend to be larger, and enhance more avidly on CT. GISTs are markedly avid for ^{18}F-fludeoxyglucose (FDG) on positron emission tomography. Esophageal leiomyomas are infrequently FDG avid.
- Both leiomyomas and GISTs have malignant potential. Leiomyosarcomas tend to grow intraluminally, are usually large (>5 cm), have heterogeneous attenuation, and may ulcerate.

Esophageal Varices

Esophageal varices are most often caused by portal hypertension but may occur with superior vena cava obstruction. The major complication is hemorrhage.

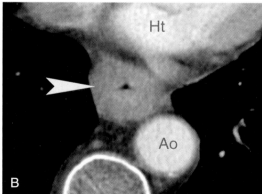

FIG. 17.5 **Adenocarcinoma: esophagus.** (A) Coronal reconstruction CT image showing distension of the normal upper esophagus *(red arrow)* with air caused by abrupt narrowing *(yellow arrowhead)* of the lumen of the mid esophagus. The stomach *(S)* is evident below the diaphragm. (B) Axial CT image at the level of the stricture showing circumferential thickening of the wall of the esophagus *(arrowhead)*, with narrowing of its lumen marked by a small pocket of air. Biopsy revealed adenocarcinoma in a long segment of Barrett esophagus. *Ao,* Thoracic aorta; *Ht,* heart.

- Varices are clearly recognized on postcontrast CT as well-defined enhancing nodular and tubular densities adjacent to the esophagus and within its wall (Fig. 17.8).
- Varices cause scalloped thickening of the esophageal wall that may be indistinguishable from tumor or inflammation without the use of contrast enhancement.
- Signs of cirrhosis, portal hypertension, and other portosystemic collateral vessels are usually present.

Esophagitis

The causes of esophagitis include gastroesophageal reflux, corrosive ingestion, long-term intubation, radiation, and infection. Infectious esophagitis is most commonly seen in immunosuppressed patients. Causative organisms include *Candida*, herpes simplex virus, cytomegalovirus, and Mycobacterium tuberculosis.

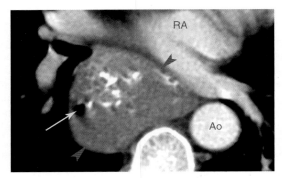

FIG. 17.7 **Leiomyoma of the esophagus.** Axial CT in a patient with dysphagia reveals a large tumor (between *red arrowheads*) with coarse calcifications eccentrically narrowing and markedly displacing the lumen *(yellow arrow)* of the esophagus. Surgical removal confirmed a benign leiomyoma. *Ao*, Thoracic aorta; *RA*, right atrium of the heart.

- The major CT finding of severe esophagitis is a relatively long segment of circumferential symmetric wall thickening (>5 mm) (Fig. 17.9), often with mucosal enhancement.
- The presence of a target sign, indicating submucosal edema, helps to differentiate esophagitis from other causes of wall thickening.
- Strictures are seen as areas of luminal narrowing with dilatation of the esophagus above the lesion.
- Severe esophagitis may lead to deep ulcers, perforation, mediastinitis, and abscess.

Esophageal Injury and Perforation

Esophageal perforation may be traumatic, may be iatrogenic after instrumentation, or may result from neoplasm or inflammation. Boerhaave syndrome is spontaneous rupture of the esophagus associated with violent vomiting. Because it may be lethal, prompt recognition of esophageal perforation is essential. Underlying esophageal disease is often present.

- Wall thickening, high-attenuation intramural hematoma, and mediastinal inflammation are signs of esophageal injury.
- Periesophageal fluid or contrast medium and extraluminal mediastinal air are the most specific findings of esophageal perforation (Fig. 17.10).
- Pleural effusions are common.

STOMACH
Anatomy

The posteriorly located gastric fundus is seen on CT sections through the level of the dome of the diaphragm. The esophagus joins the stomach a short distance

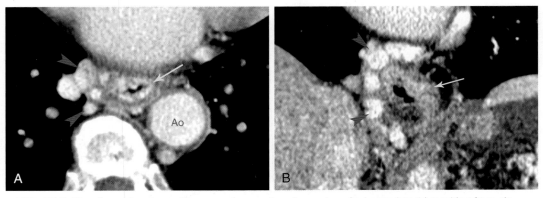

FIG. 17.8 **Esophageal varices.** Numerous large enhancing varices *(red arrowheads)* resulting from cirrhosis and portal hypertension surround and indent the distal esophagus *(yellow arrow)*. (A) Axial postcontrast CT. (B) Coronal postcontrast CT in the same patient. *Ao*, Descending thoracic aorta.

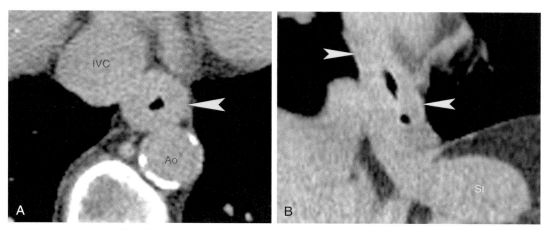

FIG. 17.9 **Esophagitis.** Reflux esophagitis causes circumferential thickening of the wall of the distal esophagus *(arrowheads)*. (A) Axial noncontrast CT. (B) Coronal noncontrast CT in the same patient. *Ao,* Descending thoracic aorta; *IVC,* inferior vena cava; *St,* stomach.

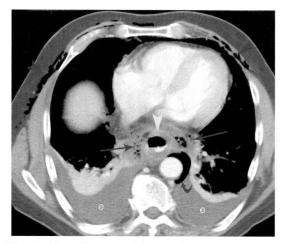

FIG. 17.10 **Perforation of the esophagus.** Perforation of the distal esophagus during a stenting procedure for esophageal stricture is evidenced by extensive air in the mediastinum *(straight red arrows)*, around the aorta *(curved red arrow)*, and in the subcutaneous tissues of the chest *(red arrowheads)*. The esophagus *(yellow arrowhead)* has a thickened wall. Bilateral pleural effusions *(e)* are evident.

below the fundus. A prominent pseudotumor, caused by thickening of the gastric wall as a result of incomplete distention, is often seen near the gastroesophageal junction. Additional distention with more air or contrast agent will eliminate this pseudotumor. The body of the stomach sweeps toward the right. The antrum crosses the midline of the abdomen between the left lobe of the liver and the pancreas to join the duodenal bulb in the region of the gallbladder.

The normal gastric wall should not exceed 5 mm in thickness when the stomach is well distended. Rugal folds are commonly visualized even with good distention. As for the esophagus, benign and malignant conditions produce similar CT findings. CT is performed to document the extent of extraluminal disease.

Technical Considerations

The stomach must be filled with positive contrast medium or distended with air or water for optimal assessment by CT. Oral contrast agent or water (200–300 mL) is routinely given to fill the stomach just before the patient lies down on the CT couch. Alternatively, distention of the stomach with air may be achieved by the giving of gas-producing crystals (4–6 g of citrocarbonate granules with 16–30 mL of water) instead of the opaque contrast agent. A nasogastric tube may also be used to distend the stomach. The patient can be repositioned, in the prone or decubitus position, to optimize distention of the different portions of the stomach with air or contrast agent.

Hiatus Hernia and Gastric Volvulus

Hiatus hernia is a protrusion of any portion of the stomach into the thorax. A major reason to recognize a hiatus hernia is to avoid mistaking it for a tumor. Large hiatus hernias are associated with gastric volvulus.

• On CT, a sliding hiatus hernia (95% of hiatus hernias) is identified by recognition of gastric folds appearing above the esophageal hiatus (Fig. 17.11). The herniated stomach may create an air- or contrast-filled mass contiguous with the esophagus above and the remainder of the stomach below.

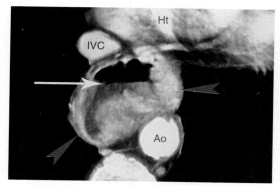

FIG. 17.11 **Hiatus hernia.** Axial CT image showing a portion of the stomach extending through the esophageal hiatus to form a hiatal hernia *(red arrowheads)*. Gastric folds are evident. Fluid retained within the herniated stomach forms an air-fluid level *(yellow arrow)*. *Ao,* Thoracic aorta; *Ht,* heart; *IVC,* inferior vena cava.

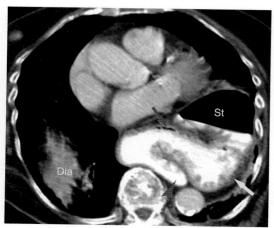

FIG. 17.12 **Paraesophageal hiatus hernia with organoaxial rotation of the stomach.** Axial postcontrast CT shows the stomach *(St)* in the left chest cavity above the left hemidiaphragm. The stomach has rotated on its long axis so that the greater curvature *(red arrow)* of the stomach is anterior and to the patient's right, whereas the lesser curvature *(yellow arrow)* of the stomach is posterior and to the patient's left. The gastroesophageal junction *(red arrowhead)* is just above the esophageal hiatus. A portion of the right hemidiaphragm *(Dia)* is shown.

- The edges of the esophageal hiatus are often widely separated, exceeding 15 mm in width.
- With a paraesophageal hernia the gastric cardia and gastroesophageal junction are below the esophageal hiatus and the fundus of stomach is above the hiatus adjacent to the distal esophagus. A variant of paraesophageal hernia is coexistence of a sliding hiatal hernia with the paraesophageal intrathoracic fundus.
- In organoaxial rotation (Fig. 17.12) the stomach rotates around its long axis, resulting in the convex greater curvature of the stomach being positioned in the chest anteriorly, superiorly, and to the right of the concave lesser curvature.
- In the much less common mesenteroaxial rotation the stomach turns upside down. The antrum and pylorus are superior and in the chest, whereas the fundus is near the diaphragm.
- The term *gastric volvulus* refers to abnormal gastric rotation associated with strangulation and obstruction. Patients have acute abdominal pain, nausea, and vomiting. Complete gastric obstruction occurs with twisting greater than 180 degrees. CT shows gastric distention with retained contrast medium, air, and food. Emergency surgical repair is needed to avoid ischemia.

Thickened Gastric Wall

Thickening of the gastric wall, either focal or diffuse, is an important but nonspecific sign of gastric disease. With good technique, which includes aggressive distention of the stomach with air or contrast agent, wall thickening greater than 5 mm can be considered abnormal. The causes include carcinoma, lymphoma, gastric inflammation (peptic or Crohn disease), perigastric inflammation (pancreatitis), and radiation. CT may show gastric ulcers as collections of contrast agent within a thickened wall. Penetrating ulcers appear as a sinus tract, marked by contrast agent or air, extending to adjacent structures.

Gastritis

Gastritis is a very common disease with numerous causes. Erosive gastritis is caused by nonsteroidal antiinflammatory drugs, aspirin, alcohol, radiation, and ischemia. Nonerosive gastritis is caused most commonly by *Helicobacter pylori* infection.

- Thickened gastric folds are the best CT sign of gastritis. Wall thickening is often focal and most common in the antrum.
- When gastritis is erosive, the mucosa may enhance brightly during the arterial phase because of hyperemia, causing a three-layer wall appearance that differentiates this benign condition from malignant wall thickening.
- *Emphysematous gastritis* is a rare life-threatening condition characterized by air within the thickened gastric wall (Fig. 17.13). It is caused by invasion of

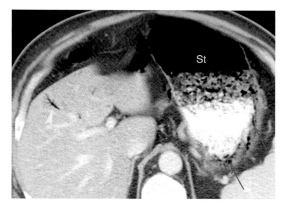

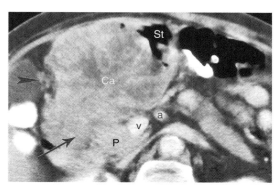

FIG. 17.13 **Emphysematous gastritis.** CT performed following oral and intravenous contrast medium administration shows gas in the wall *(red arrows)* of the stomach *(St)* as well as within the portal vein *(yellow arrowhead)* in the liver. The wall of the stomach is thickened.

FIG. 17.15 **Large gastric carcinoma.** Adenocarcinoma of the distal stomach *(St)* produces a large heterogeneous mass *(Ca)* containing low-attenuation areas of necrosis and hemorrhage. The tumor has extended through the stomach wall into the perigastric fat *(red arrowhead)*, has obliterated the fat plane *(red arrow)* between the stomach and the pancreas, and has invaded the pancreas *(P)*. *a*, Superior mesenteric artery; *v*, superior mesenteric vein.

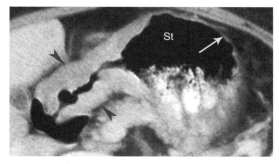

FIG. 17.14 **Gastric carcinoma.** Nodular thickening of the wall of the distal stomach *(St)* and gastric antrum *(red arrowheads)* is striking in comparison with the normal wall of the gastric body *(yellow arrow)*.

- Diffuse wall thickening with irregular narrowing of the lumen is indicative of scirrhous carcinoma (linitis plastica).
- Extension of tumor into the perigastric fat is nearly always present when the wall thickness exceeds 2 cm (Fig. 17.15). The serosal surface is blurred, and strands and nodules of tumor are seen in the adjacent fat.
- Perigastric lymph nodes are considered to be involved when the short axis diameter is more than 6 mm. A round shape and heterogeneous or marked enhancement are additional signs of nodal involvement. Nodes near the celiac axis and in the gastrohepatic ligaments are most likely to be involved.
- Hematogenous metastases go first to the liver then to the lungs, adrenal glands, kidneys, bones, and brain.
- Peritoneal carcinomatosis may occur.
- Local recurrence of gastric carcinoma appears as focal wall thickening at the anastomosis or in the remaining stomach. Nodal recurrence is most common along the course of the hepatic artery or in the para-aortic region. Peritoneal recurrence is seen in the cul-de-sac, on parietal peritoneal surfaces, or on the surface of bowel.

the gastric wall by gas-producing *Escherichia coli* or *Staphylococcus aureus*, accompanying inflammation associated with caustic ingestion or alcohol abuse. The gas may extend into the portal venous system.

Gastric Carcinoma

Adenocarcinoma is the cause of 95% of gastric malignancy. Risk factors include age of 50 to 70 years, chronic atrophic gastritis, pernicious anemia, familial adenomatous polyposis, and Ménétrier disease. CT is used to stage disease and identify patients whose disease is not surgically resectable.

- The primary tumor appears as focal, nodular, or irregular thickening of the gastric wall (Fig. 17.14), or as a polypoid intraluminal mass of soft-tissue attenuation.

Gastric Lymphoma

The stomach is the most common site of involvement for primary GI lymphoma. Most cases (90%–95%) are non-Hodgkin lymphoma of B-cell origin. Mucosa-associated lymphoid tissue lymphoma is an indolent form of lymphoma with a significantly better prognosis.

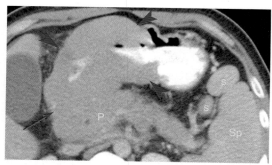

FIG. 17.16 Gastric lymphoma. B-cell lymphoma causes a large mass (between *red arrowheads*) that massively thickens the wall of the distal stomach. Compare this with Fig. 17.15. Note the homogeneous attenuation of lymphoma compared with the large adenocarcinoma. Lymphoma also obliterates the fat plane *(red arrow)* between the stomach and the pancreas *(P)*. The spleen *(Sp)* and two splenules *(s)* are enlarged.

- Gastric lymphoma may cause a polypoid mass, diffuse wall infiltration with featureless walls, or markedly thickened walls with nodular thickened folds.
- CT features that favor lymphoma over carcinoma include more dramatic thickening of the stomach wall (>3 cm), involvement of more than one region of the GI tract, transpyloric spread of tumor (occurs in 30% of gastric lymphoma), and more widespread adenopathy above and below the level of the renal hilum (Fig. 17.16). Luminal narrowing is typical of carcinoma but rare with lymphoma.
- Low-grade mucosa-associated lymphoid tissue lymphomas are superficial spreading lesions that are seen as mucosal nodularity, shallow ulcers, and minimal fold thickening.
- High-grade lymphomas tend to be seen as bulky mass lesions or marked fold and wall thickening.

Gastrointestinal Stromal Tumors

The belief that GI mesenchymal tumors arise from a common precursor cell (the Cajal cell) led to the term *gastrointestinal stromal tumor* (GIST). Most GISTs arise in the muscularis propria throughout the GI tract, with 60% to 70% of these arising in the stomach and 20% to 30% arising in the small bowel. Lesions are rare in the colon, rectum, and esophagus. Other primary sites of origin include the omentum, mesentery, and retroperitoneum. Gastric tumors previously identified as leiomyomas, leiomyosarcomas, and leiomyoblastomas are now mostly classified as GISTs. Approximately 10% to 30% of GISTs are malignant. GISTs are differentiated from true leiomyomas and leiomyosarcomas by the

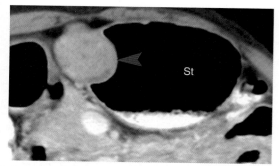

FIG. 17.17 Gastric gastrointestinal stromal tumor: benign. A wall mass *(arrowhead)* of uniform attenuation and enhancement projects both into the lumen of the stomach *(St)* and into the abdominal cavity.

presence of the protein KIT (CD117), a tyrosine kinase growth factor receptor that is tested for by immunohistochemical stain. Only in the esophagus are leiomyomas more common than GISTs. In other portions of the GI tract, GISTs are the most common mesenchymal tumor. Most tumors present with GI bleeding resulting from mucosal ulceration. GISTs are rarely seen in patients younger than 40 years.

- Tumors arise from the bowel wall and grow away from the gut lumen to project into the abdominal cavity. The size ranges from millimeters to 30 cm. Small lesions that are homogeneous in attenuation are usually benign (Fig. 17.17).
- Ulceration of the luminal surface is seen in 50% of lesions.
- Cystic degeneration, hemorrhage, and necrosis are common especially in large lesions (Fig. 17.18). The tumor cavity may communicate with the gut lumen and may contain air or oral contrast medium. Calcification in the tumor is rare.
- Contrast enhancement is seen in viable tumor, most commonly in the periphery of the mass.
- The risk of malignancy is increased in tumors that arise outside the stomach or are larger than 5 cm. Metastases are most common in the liver and the peritoneal cavity.

Gastric Varices

Gastric varices occur as a result of portal hypertension or splenic vein thrombosis.

- Varices appear as well-marginated clusters of rounded and tubular densities in, or adjacent to, the wall of the stomach, most commonly in the fundal region. Bright enhancement with intravenous contrast medium administration clinches the diagnosis (Fig. 17.19).

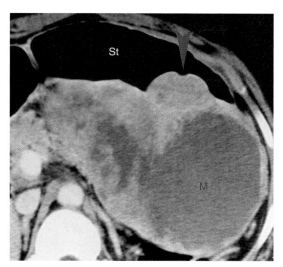

FIG. 17.18 **Gastric gastrointestinal stromal tumor: malignant.** A huge heterogeneous mass *(M)* arises from the posterior wall of the stomach *(St)*. Large low-density areas within the mass correspond to hemorrhage and necrosis. An ulcer crater *(arrowhead)* is identified within a nodular tumor projection into the gastric lumen.

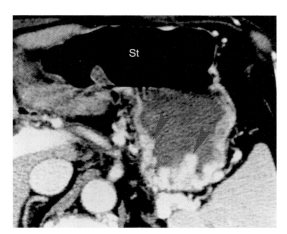

FIG. 17.19 **Gastric varices.** Bolus intravenous contrast medium administration causes bright enhancement of varices *(arrowheads)* in the wall of the gastric fundus in this patient with alcoholic liver disease and portal hypertension. *St,* Stomach.

- CT signs of liver disease and other portosystemic collateral vessels are often present.
- Gastric varices without esophageal varices is a hallmark finding associated with splenic vein thrombosis.

SMALL BOWEL
Anatomy

The duodenum extends from the pylorus to the ligament of Treitz, forming the familiar C loop. The duodenum becomes retroperitoneal at the right free edge of the hepatoduodenal ligament, closely related to the neck of the gallbladder. The descending duodenum passes to the right of the pancreatic head to just below the uncinate process, where the duodenum turns to the left. The horizontal portion crosses anterior to the inferior vena cava and aorta and posterior to the superior mesenteric vein and artery. The fourth portion ascends just left of the aorta to the ligament of Treitz, where the bowel becomes the intraperitoneal jejunum.

The jejunum occupies the left side of the upper abdomen, whereas the ileum lies in the right side of the lower abdomen and right pelvis. Jejunal loops are feathery with distinct folds. Ileal loops are featureless with thin walls. Distention of the lumen with oral contrast medium is essential to adequately evaluate the bowel. Unopacified small bowel may mimic adenopathy and abdominal masses. The small-bowel mesentery contains many vessels that are easily visualized when outlined by fat. The normal luminal diameter of the small bowel does not exceed 2.5 cm. The normal wall thickness is less than 3 mm.

Normal small bowel shows uniform mural enhancement with intravenous contrast medium administration. With full luminal distension the enhancing wall is thin, measuring 1 to 2 mm. Enhancement is best appreciated with the low-attenuation contrast agents routinely used with CT enterography. Absence of mural enhancement is indicative of ischemia. A target appearance of mural enhancement with high-attenuation mucosa and serosa separated by low-attenuation submucosa is indicative of a benign process such as Crohn disease, infection, angioedema, hemorrhage, or radiation enteritis. Heterogeneous enhancement is typical of small-bowel tumors. Mild wall thickening (3–4 mm) is most characteristic of hypoalbuminemia, infectious enteritis, or mild Crohn disease. Moderate wall thickening (5–9 mm) is seen with ischemia caused by mesenteric vein thrombosis, intramural hemorrhage, vasculitis, radiation (Fig. 17.20), and moderate Crohn disease. Marked wall thickening (>10 mm) is associated with lymphoma and other neoplasms, vasculitis, and intramural hemorrhage. Infectious enteritis seldom causes this degree of wall thickening. Mural thickening of more than 20 mm is almost always neoplastic. Benign conditions generally cause symmetric thickening along the circumference of the wall. Asymmetric wall thickening suggests neoplastic disease. Lymphoma is an exception, commonly causing symmetric wall thickening.

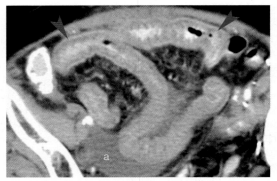

FIG. 17.20 **Wall thickening caused by radiation enteritis.** Small-bowel loops in the pelvis demonstrate characteristic benign diffuse circumferential wall thickening *(arrowheads)*. In this case the benign wall thickening is associated with radiation enteritis. Ascites *(a)* is present.

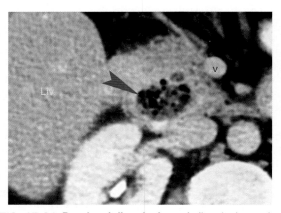

FIG. 17.21 **Duodenal diverticulum.** A diverticulum, arising from the second portion of the duodenum, is seen as a mass *(arrowhead)* containing bubbles of air and fluid that displaces the superior mesenteric vein *(v)*. *Liv*, Liver.

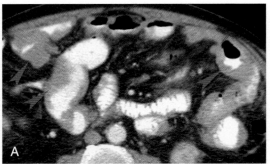

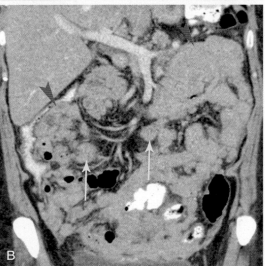

FIG. 17.22 **Small-bowel lymphoma.** (A) Axial CT shows small-bowel loops in the central abdomen with asymmetric nodular wall thickening *(red arrowheads)*. (B) Coronal CT in a different patient reveals diffuse involvement of the small bowel and mesentery with nodular thickening of the wall of the small bowel *(red arrowheads)* and enlarged lymph nodes in the mesentery *(yellow arrows)*.

Small-Bowel Diverticula

Small-bowel diverticula may cause unusual collections of fluid, air, contrast material, or soft-tissue nodules in the fat and tissues adjacent to the bowel. These must not be mistaken for abscesses, pancreatic pseudocysts, or tumors. Rescanning the patient will often demonstrate a significant change in the appearance of diverticula.

- Typically diverticula appear as mucosal sacs without folds and containing air or contrast medium located adjacent to a loop of bowel (Fig. 17.21).

Small-Bowel Neoplasms

Both benign and malignant small-bowel tumors are uncommon. CT enterography is the optimal imaging technique for demonstrating small-bowel tumors,

which appear as a soft-tissue mass or wall thickening. CT excels in demonstrating extraluminal tumor growth, involvement of adjacent structures, adenopathy, and complications such as fistulas or necrosis.

- *Lymphomas* appear as single or multiple, often large (9 cm), soft-tissue masses, a discrete polyp that may be the lead point of intussusception, or as focal or diffuse nodular wall thickening with or without aneurysmal distention of the bowel lumen (Fig. 17.22). Wall thickening is usually symmetric around the lumen but may be asymmetric, resembling adenocarcinoma. Ulceration is common. The ileum is the most common location. Mesenteric or bulky retroperitoneal adenopathy is seen in half of cases.

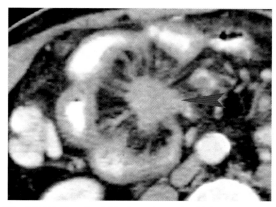

FIG. 17.23 **Carcinoid tumor.** A carcinoid (neuroendocrine) tumor arising in the ileum causes a mass *(arrow)* in the small-bowel mesentery. Characteristic thick fibrotic strands radiate from the mass to the adjacent bowel, which shows wall thickening.

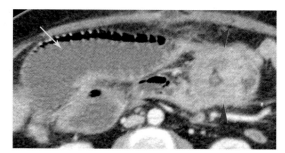

FIG. 17.24 **Adenocarcinoma of the jejunum.** An irregular solid mass (between *red arrowheads*) that caused obstruction of the proximal small bowel *(yellow arrow)* proved to be an adenocarcinoma arising in the jejunum.

- *Carcinoid* (neuroendocrine) tumors occur most commonly in the appendix (50%) and mesenteric small bowel (20%). They are the second most common small-bowel malignancy. All tumors have the potential to metastasize and are considered malignant, although some may have an indolent course. The primary tumor tends to be small and difficult to detect on CT. Carcinoid tumors appear as a brightly enhancing wall mass. Aggressive tumors tend to be larger than 2 cm and have necrosis and ulceration. Tumor invasion of the bowel wall induces a dramatic fibrosing reaction in the mesentery that is the hallmark of CT diagnosis (Fig. 17.23). Linear strands of fibrosis radiate into the mesenteric fat from the soft-tissue mass or focal wall thickening of the primary tumor. Carcinoid syndrome (cutaneous flushing and diarrhea) is associated with release of vasoactive amines by the tumor. The syndrome occurs only in the presence of liver metastases because the liver will metabolize amines released into the portal venous system. Metastases are hypervascular and are best seen on arterial phase postcontrast CT images.
- *Adenocarcinoma* of the small bowel is a rare lesion that is most common in the duodenum (50%), especially near the ampulla. Tumors appear as a constricting annular mass with abrupt irregular margins and overhanging edges, as a distinct polypoid nodule, or as an ulcerative mass. Postcontrast CT shows only mild enhancement of the tumor rather than the hyperenhancement characteristic of carcinoid. Only a short segment of bowel is involved. Partial or complete bowel obstruction may be present (Fig. 17.24).

- *GISTs* are most commonly solitary benign tumors that occur anywhere in the small bowel. Malignant GISTs are most common in the distal small bowel. Small GISTs appear homogeneous, whereas large GISTs are heterogeneous, necrotic, and often ulcerated (Fig. 17.25).
- *Metastases* to the small bowel occur as serosal implants with peritoneal carcinomatosis or with hematogenous spread of tumor as intramural masses (Fig. 17.26). Metastases closely resemble the primary tumor in CT appearance. The most common primary tumors are malignant melanoma and breast, lung, and renal cell carcinoma. Lesions from melanoma are small and round and may cause intussusception. Metastases may be single or multiple, flat or polypoid, submucosal or ulcerative, producing a "target" appearance.
- *Multiple small-bowel polyps* are found with Peutz-Jeghers syndrome and other polyposis syndromes. Polyps associated with Peutz-Jeghers syndrome are hamartomatous.

Crohn Disease
Crohn disease is characterized by inflammation of the bowel mucosa, bowel wall, and mesentery with marked submucosal edema. These features are nicely reflected in the CT appearance, especially on CT and magnetic resonance enterography, which have become the small-bowel imaging methods of choice for patients with Crohn disease.
- The small bowel, especially the terminal ileum, is affected in 80% of cases, and the colon is affected in 50% of cases.
- Circumferential thickening of the bowel wall (>3mm) is a hallmark of disease (Fig. 17.27). Thickening can be up to 3 cm. Wall thickening may be homogeneous or may have a stratified "target" or "double-halo" appearance caused by bands of

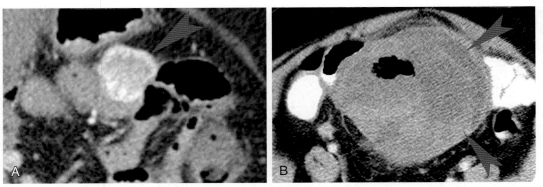

FIG. 17.25 **Small-bowel gastrointestinal stromal tumor.** (A) A small benign gastrointestinal stromal tumor *(arrowhead)* arising in the jejunum shows marked enhancement on this axial postcontrast CT image. (B) Postcontrast CT in a different patient shows a very large gastrointestinal stromal tumor *(arrowheads)* arising from distal small bowel in the pelvis. This tumor shows weak enhancement, necrosis, and ulceration. It proved to be malignant.

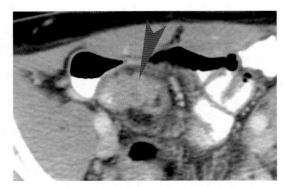

FIG. 17.26 **Metastasis to small bowel.** An irregular nodular mass *(arrowhead)* extending from the wall of the ileum into the mesentery is a hematogenous metastasis from breast cancer. The patient had widespread metastatic disease.

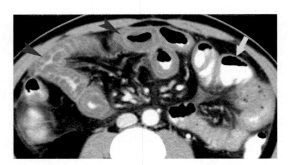

FIG. 17.27 **Crohn disease: wall thickening.** Many loops of small bowel show circumferential wall thickening *(red arrowheads)*, whereas others *(yellow arrow)* are unaffected, representing skip lesions.

edema. Wall thickening is measured only in bowel loops well distended by enteric contrast agents. Wall thickening is considered mild at 3 to 5 mm, moderate at 5 to 9 mm, and severe at 10 mm or more.

- Acutely inflamed bowel demonstrates wall thickening with marked wall enhancement after intravenous contrast medium administration. The degree of enhancement correlates with the intensity of inflammation and is the best indicator of active disease.
- The "comb sign" produced by hyperemic thickening of the vasa recta is a sign of active disease (Fig. 17.28). The swollen blood vessels produce a comblike appearance extending from the thickened bowel wall into the mesenteric fat.
- Wall hyperenhancement without wall thickening is a nonspecific finding that may indicate early inflammation or other processes, including fibrosis or chronic mesenteric venous occlusion.
- Wall thickening results in strictures narrowing the bowel lumen in advanced disease.
- "Skip areas" of normal bowel intervening between diseased segments are characteristic of Crohn disease.
- Ulcerations are evidence of severe inflammation. Ulcerations appear as small breaks in the luminal surface of the bowel associated with extension of air or contrast agent into inflamed, thickened bowel wall.
- Diffuse haziness and increased density of the mesenteric fat is evidence of mesenteric inflammation.

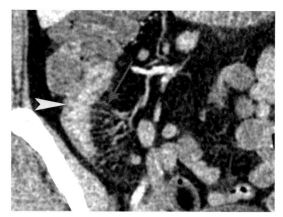

FIG. 17.28 **Crohn disease: comb sign of active disease.** CT enterography image in the coronal plane showing wall thickening and enhancement of the terminal ileum *(yellow arrowhead)*. Thickening of the vasa recta *(red arrow)* in the mesentery produces the comb sign of active inflammation.

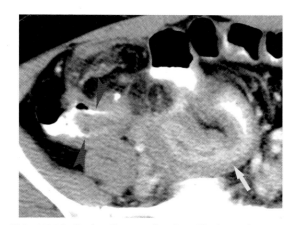

FIG. 17.29 **Crohn disease: fistulas.** The ileum *(yellow arrow)* in the right lower quadrant demonstrates marked wall thickening and matting of bowel loops caused by inflammation of the mesentery on this axial CT image. A double-tract bowel lumen *(red arrowheads)* is seen, indicating the formation of an ileoileal fistula.

- Fistulas and sinus tracts between bowel loops (Fig. 17.29), or to the bladder, adjacent muscle, or the skin surface, are characteristic of Crohn disease. Fistulas appear as linear tracts often containing fluid that extend extraluminally between bowel loops, bladder, or skin. Fistulas usually show enhancement.
- Extramural abscesses appear as fluid collections in the mesentery. Mesenteric lymph nodes may be enlarged. Mesenteric abscesses contain fluid, air, or contrast material.

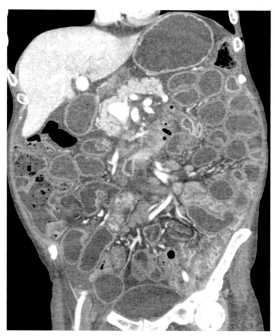

FIG. 17.30 **Celiac disease.** Coronal image from a CT enterography examination showing findings of advanced celiac disease with diffuse dilatation of small-bowel loops from the duodenum to the ileum, diffuse thinning of the wall of the small bowel, and ascites. Chronic malnutrition has resulted in weight loss and the presence of very little subcutaneous or mesenteric fat.

Celiac Disease

Celiac disease is a chronic autoimmune-related inflammation of the small bowel caused by ingestion of gluten in patients who are susceptible to gluten's irritative properties. Although some patients are asymptomatic, others have abdominal pain and malabsorption.

- The chronic inflammatory process results in dilated and fluid-filled small-bowel loops (Fig. 17.30). The duodenum, jejunum, and ileum are involved. Wall thickening is present early in the disease, followed by atrophy and wall thinning in chronic cases. Fat deposition in the wall is stimulated by chronic inflammation.
- Affected small-bowel loops are dilated and fluid filled. Malabsorption in the small bowel leads to excess nutrients being delivered to the colon. Metabolism by colon bacteria results in chronic excess production of gas, distending the colon and decreasing its tone. Fluid excess is seen in the ascending colon, with increased gas present throughout the colon. Disease leads to flatulence and constipation as weak colon peristalsis cannot move stool along.

- Jejunization of the ileum is a characteristic finding seen as a decrease in folds in the jejunum with an increase in folds in the ileum. The jejunum appears atrophic.
- Flocculation occurs when barium is administered as an oral contrast agent. The term *flocculation* refers to precipitation of small high-attenuation flecks of barium distributed throughout the dilated small bowel, occurring as a result of progressive dilution of enteric barium.
- Patients are prone to transient small-bowel intussusception.
- Additional findings include increased vascularity of the mesentery and mesenteric and retroperitoneal adenopathy.

Mesenteric Ischemia

Mesenteric ischemia may be classified as acute or chronic. Arterial causes of acute mesenteric ischemia are most common and include occlusion of the superior mesenteric artery caused by thrombosis or emboli (60%–70% of cases) and low-flow states related to cardiac malfunction. Thrombosis of the superior mesenteric vein accounts for 5% to 15% of cases. *Intestinal angina* refers to chronic mesenteric ischemia usually related to atherosclerosis.

- Findings of bowel ischemia caused by venous occlusion include circumferential wall thickening as a result of edema or hemorrhage, mural hyperenhancement if arterial supply is intact or mural hypoenhancement if arterial supply is impaired, venous engorgement in the mesentery, and visible thrombus in the superior mesenteric vein.
- With exclusive arterial occlusion the bowel wall becomes thinner, lacking in edema or hemorrhage. Mural enhancement is absent. Thrombi or emboli may be evident in the mesenteric arteries. Infarction may result in perforation.
- Acute ischemia may result in pneumatosis and portal venous gas (Fig. 17.31).

Small-Bowel Obstruction

CT is reported to be up to 95% sensitive for detecting small-bowel obstruction and up to 73% sensitive in identifying its cause. CT enteroclysis is useful in the evaluation of equivocal cases.

- If the bowel is significantly distended on a conventional radiograph, administration of oral contrast medium is not needed. Intravenous contrast medium is recommended because it provides enhancement of the bowel wall, detects ischemia, and provides better visualization of pathologic processes.

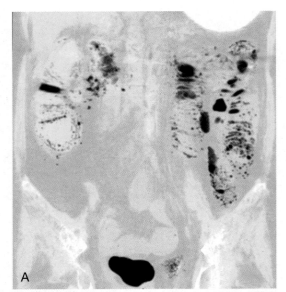

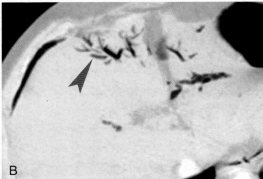

FIG. 17.31 **Mesenteric ischemia: pneumatosis.** (A) Coronal CT image shown with an air window revealing diffuse pneumatosis (bubbles of gas in the wall) of small and large bowel. (B) Axial CT image in the same patient also shown with lung windows demonstrating gas *(arrowhead)* in the portal veins within the liver.

Oral contrast medium may obscure assessment of small-bowel mural enhancement.
- *Complete mechanical small-bowel obstruction* appears as dilatation of proximal small bowel (>2.5 cm), with a distinct transition zone to the collapsed distal small bowel (Fig. 17.32). No oral contrast medium passes the transition zone. The colon is not dilated (>6 cm in diameter), is often completely collapsed, and contains minimal fluid or gas.
- *Paralytic ileus* appears as dilatation of both proximal and distal small bowel without a transition zone. The colon is distended with fluid and gas and may

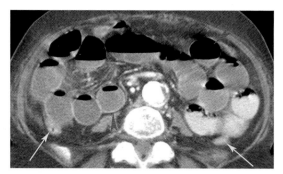

FIG. 17.32 **Small-bowel obstruction.** CT demonstrates diffuse dilatation of small bowel without wall thickening. Most loops *(red arrowheads)* contain air-fluid levels. The colon *(yellow arrows)* is collapsed. The findings indicate distal small-bowel obstruction.

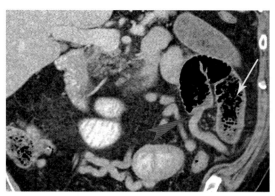

FIG. 17.33 **Small-bowel obstruction: abrupt transition.** Coronal CT nicely demonstrates an abrupt transition *(red arrowhead)* between dilated proximal small bowel and nondilated small bowel. This finding is indicative of an adhesion causing proximal small-bowel obstruction. The obstructed dilated proximal small bowel demonstrates "the small bowel feces sign" *(yellow arrow)*.

contain oral contrast medium. However, a totally collapsed descending colon is common in nonobstructive ileus and should not be mistaken for evidence of a transition zone.

- *The appearance of partial mechanical small-bowel obstruction* falls between that of complete small-bowel obstruction and ileus. The proximal bowel is less dilated, and the transition zone is less distinct. The bowel distal to the obstruction is not completely collapsed. The colon is normal or slightly dilated and contains moderate amounts of fluid and gas. The "small-bowel feces sign" (Fig. 17.33) is uncommon but highly indicative of partial small-bowel obstruction. Intestinal transit is slowed, resulting in increased water absorption, causing small-bowel content to resemble feces.

- Adhesions cause 50% to 75% of small-bowel obstructions but are not directly visualized by CT. Abrupt transition from dilated to nondilated bowel without other findings suggests adhesions as the cause (Fig. 17.33). Beak-like narrowing at the transition zone is characteristic of adhesions but is not common.

- Tumor, abscess, intussusception, inflammation, endometriosis, and hernia causing obstruction are identified by characteristic signs. Hernias are the second most common cause of small-bowel obstruction, accounting for 10% of cases.

- *Closed loop obstruction* has higher morbidity and mortality than simple obstruction. *Closed loop obstruction* refers to a loop of bowel occluded at two adjacent points along its course, usually as a result of adhesions or internal hernia. The obstructed loop may twist, resulting in volvulus. The "beak" or "whirl"

sign may be seen at the obstruction and volvulus. Dilated bowel loops with stretched and prominent mesenteric vessels converging on a site of obstruction suggest closed loop obstruction. *Strangulation* refers to closed loop obstruction with intestinal ischemia. Strangulation is suggested by associated mild circumferential thickening of the bowel wall, with the low-density concentric rings indicative of wall edema ("target" and "halo" signs). Poor or absent enhancement of the bowel wall is indicative of ischemia.

- *Midgut volvulus* is most common in children but may occur in adults. Most cases are associated with congenital malrotation of the small bowel with abnormal fixation of the small bowel mesentery and a short mesenteric root. Small bowel twists around its mesentery, resulting in closed loop obstruction. Intermittent volvulus causes intermittent abdominal pain that may be difficult to diagnose. CT shows swirling of the mesenteric vessels, reversed position of the superior mesenteric artery and vein, ectopic location of small-bowel loops, and abnormal position of the ligament of Treitz.

- *Intussusception* is an uncommon cause of small-bowel obstruction in adults (~5% of cases). The causes include lipoma and other benign submucosal tumors, carcinoma, metastatic disease, and lymphoma. CT demonstrates characteristic findings of bowel within bowel (Fig. 17.34). The distal receiving segment (intussuscipiens) is markedly dilated and has a thickened wall. Its lumen contains the entering loop (intussusceptum), appearing as an eccentric, soft-tissue mass with

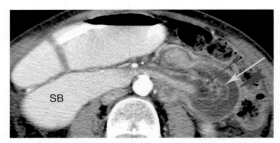

FIG. 17.34 **Intussusception.** A metastasis from melanoma to the ileum served as a lead mass for enteroenteric intussusception. This image shows the target appearance characteristic of intussusception with the receiving loop *(red arrowhead)*, the invaginating loop *(yellow arrow without tail)* and the eccentric mesentery *(red arrow with tail)*. The upstream small bowel *(SB)* is dilated and obstructed.

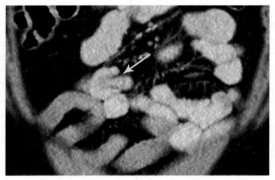

FIG. 17.35 **Transient intussusception.** Coronal post-contrast CT image showing a transient intussusception *(arrow)*. Serial images showed the intussusception involved only a short segment. The patient remained asymptomatic. The intussuscipiens is only slightly dilated. The small bowel proximal to the intussusception is not dilated.

an adjacent crescent of fat that represents the invaginated mesentery. The mass causing the intussusception can often be identified at the leading end of the intussusceptum.

- *Transient intussusception* is sometimes observed (Fig. 17.35). It is not associated with any symptoms and does not cause bowel obstruction. Most cases are of a jejunojejunal invagination. The appearance is similar to that of obstructing intussusception, with an intraluminal soft-tissue mass with eccentric intraluminal mesentery. The segment of involved bowel is short (a few centimeters), the intussuscipiens is only slightly dilated, and no upstream bowel obstruction is present.

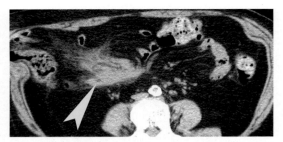

FIG. 17.36 **Sclerosing mesenteritis.** CT without intravenous contrast medium reveals an ill-defined mass *(arrowhead)* with stranding densities extending into the mesentery. This elderly patient has undergone several abdominal surgical procedures and reported continuing abdominal pain.

MESENTERY
Misty Mesentery

The term *misty mesentery* refers to a vaguely defined area of increased attenuation in mesenteric fat. Misty mesentery may be caused by mesenteric edema (hypoproteinemia, portal hypertension, mesenteric vein thrombosis, etc.), hemorrhage (trauma, ischemia, blood clotting disorders), inflammation (pancreatitis, inflammatory bowel disease), early-stage lymphoma or primary mesenteric neoplasms, or sclerosing mesenteritis.

- An ill-defined focus of mesenteric fat shows increased attenuation. This should be correlated with clinical and other imaging findings to determine the likely cause.
- *Sclerosing mesenteritis* refers to an inflammatory disorder of unknown cause affecting the mesentery. It usually involves the small-bowel mesentery but may also affect the mesocolon. Early-stage disease involves infiltration of fat with foamy macrophages (mesenteric lipodystrophy), followed by infiltration of fat with plasma cells, leukocytes, and foamy macrophages (mesenteric panniculitis). The final stage is fat necrosis with fibrosis and tissue retraction (retractile mesenteritis) (Fig. 17.36). Patients may present with abdominal pain. The cause is unknown, but sclerosing mesenteritis has been associated with abdominal surgery, trauma, autoimmune diseases, vasculitis, infection, and various malignancies.
- Continuing inflammation may coalesce into a soft-tissue mass that envelops the mesenteric vessels. Preservation of fat around enveloped vessels (the "fat halo sign") is characteristic. Retractile mesenteritis is more fulminant, with development of irregular fibrotic soft-tissue masses within the mesentery. Calcification may develop in areas of fat necrosis. The appearance may be indistinguishable from carcinoid tumor in the mesentery.

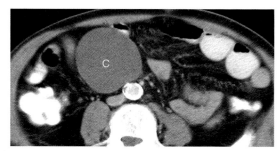

FIG. 17.37 **Mesenteric cyst.** A thin-walled completely cystic homogeneous nonenhancing mass *(C)* within the mesentery is characteristic of a mesenteric cystic lymphangioma (mesenteric cyst).

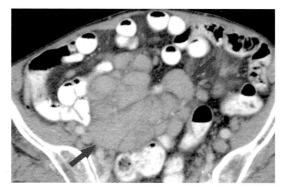

FIG. 17.38 **Mesenteric lymphoma.** Multiple bloated lymphomatous lymph nodes coalesce into a bulky mesenteric mass *(arrows)*.

Cystic Mesenteric Masses

Cystic lesions primary to the mesentery are more common than primary mesenteric neoplasms.

- *Mesenteric and omental cysts* can be classified as cystic lymphangiomas. Lymphangiomas are congenital malformations of the lymphatic system. They are thin walled, contain chylous or serous fluid, and may be unilocular or multilocular (Fig. 17.37). Internal hemorrhage may occur, increasing the attenuation of contained fluid. Large cysts may cause partial bowel obstruction.
- *Enteric duplication cysts* are thick-walled unilocular cysts that duplicate the normal bowel wall. The contents are usually serous. They may be attached to normal bowel or may be free within the mesentery. The thick wall enhances with intravenous contrast medium administration.
- *Enteric cysts* are similar but with thinner walls as they are lined by GI tract mucosa and do not contain the muscle layers of bowel wall. Most are unilocular with low-attenuation serous contents. Occasionally thin septations may be present.
- *Cystic mesothelioma* is a rare benign tumor that presents as a multilocular cystic mesenteric mass. Most are found in middle-aged women.
- *Cystic teratomas* contain cystic and solid components, fat, and calcifications. Most are discovered in pediatric patients.
- Complications of mesenteric tumors include intratumoral hemorrhage, fistula to small bowel, abscess, small-bowel ischemia or infarction, and mesenteric vein or artery thrombosis.

Mesenteric Neoplasms

A wide variety of lesions may produce solid masses within the mesentery:

- *Lymphoma* is the most common malignancy seen in the mesentery. Lymphoma of the small bowel appears as a discrete solitary mass, multiple masses, or focal nodular or circumferential wall thickening. Mesenteric involvement may consist of enlarged individual mesenteric nodes or large confluent masses (Fig. 17.38). Lymphomatous masses characteristically sandwich mesenteric vessels between thin layers of spared mesenteric fat (the *sandwich sign*). Retroperitoneal adenopathy is commonly present.
- *Metastases* to the mesentery are far more common than primary tumors arising in the mesentery. Metastatic spread to the mesentery may occur by direct extension (carcinoid and small-bowel adenocarcinoma), lymphatic flow (lymphoma and leukemia), hematogenous spread to bowel wall (melanoma and breast and lung cancer), and peritoneal seeding (ovarian and colon cancers).
- *Desmoid tumor* (mesenteric fibromatosis) arises most commonly in the mesentery of the small bowel. Most (75%) occur in patients who have undergone abdominal surgery. With Gardner syndrome (familial adenomatous polyposis) tumors are also found in the abdominal wall. The lesion consists of bland fibroblastic cells suspended in collagenous stroma. This produces a well-defined homogeneous solid mass without hemorrhage, necrosis, or cystic change (Fig. 17.39).
- *GISTs* that arise in the mesentery or omentum tend to be large (>10 cm) and demonstrate prominent hemorrhage, necrosis, and cystic change.
- *Sarcomas* that arise in the mesentery or omentum are indistinguishable from GISTs. Tissue types include leiomyosarcoma, fibrosarcoma, malignant fibrous histiocytoma, and liposarcoma.

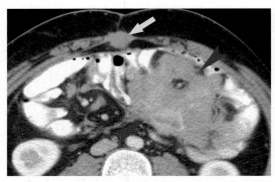

FIG. 17.39 **Mesenteric fibromatosis.** In a patient with Gardner syndrome after total colectomy, mesenteric fibromatosis (desmoid tumor) causes a homogeneous soft-tissue mass *(red arrowheads)*. A desmoid tumor is also seen in the anterior abdominal wall *(yellow arrow)*.

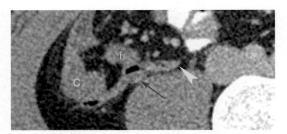

FIG. 17.40 **Normal appendix.** The wormlike normal appendix *(red arrows)* is visualized as it extends from the cecum *(C)* all the way to its tip *(yellow arrowhead)*. The peri-appendiceal fat provides sharp definition of the wall with no inflammatory infiltration. Bubbles of gas are present within it lumen. *i,* Ileum.

APPENDIX

Anatomy

The normal appendix can be seen on CT as a thin-walled tubular structure surrounded by mesenteric fat. It may be collapsed or filled with gas (60%), fluid, or contrast material. The normal appendix does not exceed 6 mm in diameter and has a sharp outer contour defined by homogeneous low-attenuation fat (Fig. 17.40). The origin of the appendix is between the ileocecal valve and the cecal apex, always on the same side of the cecum as the valve. Approximately one-third of appendixes course inferomedially from the cecum, whereas two-thirds are retrocecal.

Appendicitis

Acute appendicitis is the most common cause of acute abdominal pain, affecting 6% of the population. CT has 95% to 98% sensitivity in its diagnosis.

- The CT findings diagnostic of acute appendicitis are a distended appendix (>6 mm in diameter), thickened walls that enhance, and periappendiceal inflammatory changes with stranding in the fat (Fig. 17.41).
- The presence of an appendicolith, appearing as a ring-like or homogeneous calcification within, or adjacent to, a phlegmon or abscess is diagnostic of appendicitis. Appendicoliths may be seen in 28% of adult patients with acute appendicitis. Examination of CT images with bone windows aids in the detection of appendicoliths.
- Appendicitis confined to the distal tip is more difficult to diagnose. The proximal appendix may be collapsed or filled with air or contrast material. The inflamed distal appendix is distended

(average 13 mm), with thickened enhancing wall and periappendiceal fat stranding. A transition zone between normal thin appendiceal wall and the thickened wall with a narrowed lumen is seen.

- Appendicitis may recur in the stump of a residual appendix after previous laparoscopic or open appendectomy. CT findings include dilatation of the appendix stump and periappendiceal inflammatory changes.
- Complications associated with perforated appendicitis include phlegmon, seen as a periappendiceal soft tissue mass (>20 HU), and abscess, seen as a fluid collection (<20 HU). Phlegmons and abscesses smaller than 3 cm generally resolve on antibiotic treatment, whereas abscesses larger than 3 cm usually require surgical or catheter drainage.
- Additional complications that may be demonstrated by CT include small-bowel obstruction, hepatic abscess, and mesenteric vein thrombosis.
- Alternative diagnoses that may be demonstrated by CT in patients referred for suspected appendicitis include Crohn disease, cecal diverticulitis, perforated cecal carcinoma, ureteral stone, mesenteric adenitis, hemorrhagic ovarian cyst, and pelvic inflammatory disease.

Mucocele of the Appendix

Mucocele refers to a distended appendix filled with mucus. The causes include simple chronic obstruction, hyperplasia of the appendiceal mucosa, or most commonly obstructing benign or malignant neoplasms of the appendix.

- On CT, a mucocele appears as a well-encapsulated, cystic mass with thin walls that may be calcified (Fig. 17.42). The size is variable and ranges up to 15 cm. Mucoceles smaller than 2 cm in diameter are likely

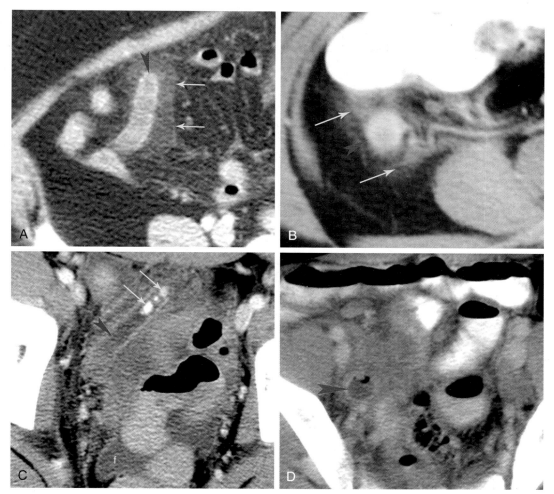

FIG. 17.41 Acute appendicitis. Four different examples of acute appendicitis. (A) The swollen appendix, measuring 9-mm in diameter, is identified by its bulbous tip *(red arrowhead)*. The periappendiceal fat is infiltrated by inflammation and edema *(yellow arrows)*. (B) The inflamed appendix *(red arrowhead)* is shown in cross section. The wall of the appendix enhances markedly, and extensive inflammation *(yellow arrows)* is present in the surrounding fat. (C) A row of high-attenuation appendicoliths *(yellow arrows)* is seen occluding the proximal appendix *(red arrowhead)*, which is dilated with an enhancing wall. Fluid *(f)* in the cul-de-sac is indicative of perforation, confirmed during surgery. (D) The appendix *(red arrowhead)* is difficult to identify because of the surrounding fluid and inflammation. Examination of serial images is needed to identify its origin from the cecum and its bulbous tip.

to be caused by a simple retention cyst near the appendix origin. Those larger than 2 cm are usually caused by a mucin-producing neoplasm
- Curvilinear calcification is seen in the wall in 50% of patients.

Neoplasms of the Appendix

Neoplasms of the appendix may present with acute appendicitis (30%–50% of cases), intussusception, GI bleeding, or mucocele.

- *Carcinoid tumors* are most common, accounting for 80% of appendiceal neoplasms. Most tumors are in the distal third of the appendix and cause no symptoms. Many are small and overlooked on CT. Tumors obstruct the appendix in 25% of cases. They appear as small irregular nodules, sometimes calcified, mimicking an appendicolith. Some appear as diffuse wall thickening.
- *Adenomas and adenocarcinomas* are usually mucin-producing tumors often producing a mucocele.

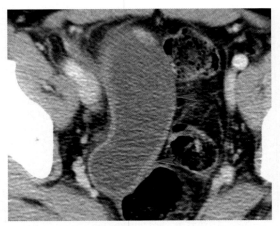

FIG. 17.42 **Mucocele of the appendix.** Postcontrast CT shows a sausage-shaped cystic structure *(arrowheads)* in the pelvis. Serial images confirmed this structure was the appendix markedly dilated and filled with fluid. Additional images showed flecks of calcification within its thickened wall. Wall calcifications are strong CT evidence of a mucocele. During surgery the appendix was filled with mucin and a small obstructing benign mucinous cystadenoma was discovered.

The findings include soft-tissue mass, often with calcification, and irregular wall thickening (Fig. 17.43). Peritoneal spread of tumor may result in pseudomyxoma peritonei.

- *Lymphoma* of the appendix may cause diffuse wall thickening, with dilatation of the appendiceal lumen associated with regional adenopathy.

COLON AND RECTUM
Anatomy

The colon is easily identified by its location and its haustral markings when it is distended by air or contrast agent. Mottled fecal material serves as a marker of the colon and rectum. The CT scout view of the abdomen should be inspected to determine the general outline and course of the colon. The cecum generally occupies the right iliac fossa, although, because of its variably long mesentery, it may be found almost anywhere in the abdomen or pelvis. Its identity is confirmed by recognition of the ileocecal valve or appendix. The ascending colon occupies a posterior and lateral position in the right flank. The hepatic flexure makes one or more sharp bends near the undersurface of the liver and gallbladder. The transverse colon sweeps across the abdomen on a long and mobile mesentery. Because of its anterior position, the transverse colon is usually filled with air when patients are supine

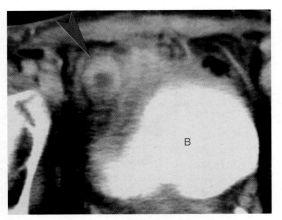

FIG. 17.43 **Carcinoma of the appendix.** The appendix *(arrowhead)* is dilated and has irregular wall thickening with associated infiltration of the periappendiceal fat. Surgical resection confirmed adenocarcinoma of the appendix. *B,* Bladder.

for CT. The splenic flexure makes one or more tight bends near the spleen. The descending colon extends caudad down the left flank. Remember that the ascending colon and the descending colon are retroperitoneal. The peritoneum sweeps over their anterior surfaces and extends laterally to form the paracolic gutters, which distend with fluid when ascites is present. The sigmoid colon begins in the left iliac fossa and extends a variable distance craniad before it dives toward the rectum. The sigmoid colon becomes the rectum at the level of the third sacral segment. The rectum distends to form the rectal ampulla and then abruptly narrows to form the anal canal. Fat around the colon is normally of uniform low attenuation. Soft-tissue stranding densities in the pericolic fat are indicative of inflammatory changes or neoplastic invasion.

The peritoneum covering the anterior surface of the rectum extends to the level of the vagina, forming the rectovaginal pouch of Douglas. In males the peritoneum extends to the seminal vesicles, 2.5 cm above the prostate, forming the rectovesical pouch. Three anatomic compartments are important to recognize when one is staging rectal carcinoma: (1) the peritoneal cavity above the peritoneal reflections, (2) the extraperitoneal compartment between the peritoneum and the levator ani muscle that forms the pelvic diaphragm, and (3) the perineum identified by the triangular ischiorectal fossa below and lateral to the levator ani. The lower two-thirds of the rectum are extraperitoneal. On CT the thickness of the wall of the normal distended colon does not exceed 3 mm.

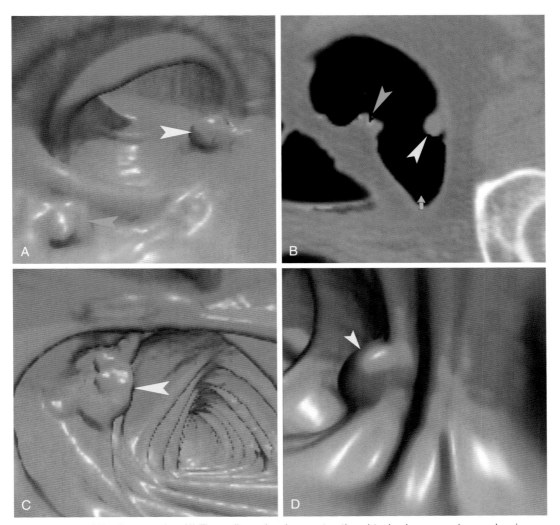

FIG. 17.44 **CT colonography.** (A) Three-dimensional reconstruction virtual colonoscopy image showing two polyps *(arrowheads)* projecting into the colon lumen. Several colonic folds are visible. (B) Source CT image showing the same two polyps *(arrowheads)* as in (A). (C) A villous polyp *(arrowhead)* with a lobulated contour is demonstrated. (D) A well-defined polyp *(arrowhead)* projects off a fold.

Technical Considerations

For routine scanning the rectum and colon can usually be adequately opacified by the giving of contrast agents orally. Scanning is then performed through the entire abdomen and pelvis. Demonstration of subtle findings is improved by thin slices (1.25–2.5 mm) through a defined area of abnormality. Enhancement with intravenous contrast medium is optional but usually helpful. CT colonography is generally used to screen patients for colorectal neoplasia (Fig. 17.44).

Colorectal Carcinoma

Colon cancer is the second leading cause of cancer death in the United States. Most colon cancers (70%) occur in the rectosigmoid region. The remainder are scattered fairly evenly throughout the rest of the colon. Colon cancer spreads by (1) direct extension with penetration of the colon wall, (2) lymphatic drainage to regional nodes, (3) hematogenous routes through portal veins to the liver, and (4) intraperitoneal seeding. CT has become routine for preoperative staging and

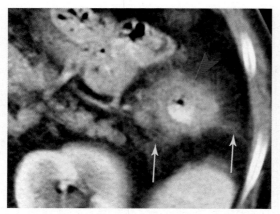

FIG. 17.45 **Colon carcinoma: wall thickening.** A carcinoma of the descending colon near the splenic flexure causes thickening of the colon wall *(red arrowhead)* and narrowing of the lumen. Stranding densities *(yellow arrows)* extending into the pericolonic fat suggest tumor extension through the bowel wall.

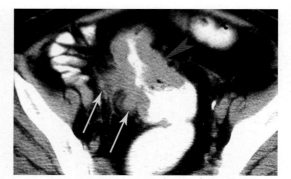

FIG. 17.46 **Rectal carcinoma – apple core lesion.** The rectum is involved with marked circumferential wall thickening *(red arrowhead)* associated with severe and irregular narrowing of the lumen. Spread of tumor into perirectal fat is evident *(yellow arrows)*.

surgical planning. The accuracy of CT staging of colon cancer ranges from 90% for tumor invasion beyond the bowel wall (T3–T4 lesions), to 77% for tumor invasion depth of 5 mm or greater (Tcd–T4 lesions), to 71% for nodal involvement (N+ lesions).

- The primary tumor may be a colon polyp. Polyps are seen as well-defined oval or round intraluminal projections usually seen best in profile (Fig. 17.44). Polyps of 5 mm or smaller are nearly all hyperplastic and are considered by most to be clinically insignificant (99% hyperplastic, 1% adenomatous). Polyps in the 6- to 9-mm range may contain dysplasia or very rarely cancer (<1%); however, 50% of lesions in this size range are adenomas and precancerous. Polyps with a size of 10 to 15 mm an 80% risk of being an adenoma and a 1% to 5% risk of being a cancer. Polyps larger than 2 cm have a 40% risk of being cancerous.
- Cancers appear as larger intraluminal masses with nodular contours and irregular mucosal surfaces, or as a soft-tissue mass that narrows the lumen of the colon (Fig. 17.45). Central low attenuation represents hemorrhage or necrosis. Air within the tumor indicates ulceration.
- Flat lesions appear as focal, lobulated, thickening of the bowel wall (>3 mm). Flat adenomas and annular constricting lesions are the major sources of interpretation error on CT colonography.
- "Apple core" lesions demonstrate irregular bulky circumferential wall thickening with marked and irregular narrowing of the bowel lumen (Fig. 17.46).

- Linear soft-tissue strands extending from the colonic mass into pericolic fat suggest extension of tumor through the bowel wall. Edema may cause stranding in the pericolic fat and thickening of the wall of the colon proximal to the tumor.
- Loss of fat planes between the tumor and adjacent structures suggests local invasion.
- Regional lymph nodes larger than 1 cm are considered positive for metastatic disease. However, some nodes smaller than 1 cm may contain tumor and some nodes larger than 1 cm may not contain tumor, limiting the value of CT.
- Distant metastases are seen in the liver (75%), lung (5%–50%), adrenal glands (14%), and elsewhere.
- Complications of colon malignancy include bowel obstruction (Fig. 17.47), perforation (Fig. 17.48), and fistula formation (Fig. 17.47). Obstructing colon cancers may cause ischemic colitis proximal to the tumor.
- Calcifications in the primary tumor and metastases occur with mucinous adenocarcinoma.

Colorectal Cancer Recurrence

CT is valuable in the detection of colorectal cancer recurrence as well as for initial staging. One-third of patients who have undergone a colorectal cancer resection will develop recurrent disease, most (70%–80%) within 2 years. About half of the colon cancer recurrences occur at the site of the original tumor, whereas the remainder recur at distant sites, especially in the liver. Multiple sites of tumor recurrence are more common than a solitary site of recurrence.

- Recurrences appear as irregular masses, often with a low-density necrotic center and an enhancing

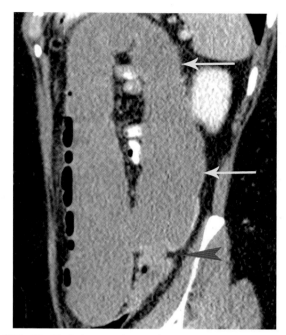

FIG. 17.47 **Colon carcinoma: large-bowel obstruction.** CT in the sagittal plane shows the colon *(yellow arrows)* to be diffusely dilated to the level of a constricting colon cancer *(red arrow)*.

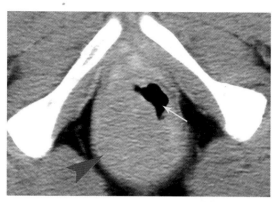

FIG. 17.49 **Lymphoma rectum.** In a patient with AIDS, non-Hodgkin lymphoma causes a bulky rectal mass *(red arrowhead)* that distorts the rectal lumen *(yellow arrow)*.

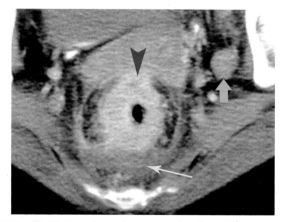

FIG. 17.48 **Rectal carcinoma: perforation.** The rectal wall *(red arrowhead)* is markedly and circumferentially thickened with an ill-defined outer margin. Low-attenuation fluid in the presacral area *(yellow arrow)* suggests focal perforation. An enlarged metastatic internal iliac lymph node *(green arrow)* is evident.

periphery. The bowel anastomosis marking the location of the original tumor may be identified by high-attenuation metallic bowel clips.

- Presacral soft-tissue densities, seen in patients who have undergone abdominoperineal resection, may be recurrent tumor or fibrosis. Recurrent tumor tends to be nodular, tends to be convex anteriorly, and enlarges over time. Fibrosis tends to be more uniform, tends to be concave anteriorly, and remains stable or shrinks over time. Percutaneous biopsy is generally required for confirmation.

Colon Lymphoma

Colon lymphoma is less common than gastric or small-bowel lymphoma but has a striking and fairly characteristic CT appearance. It occurs more commonly in association with ulcerative colitis or Crohn disease. Patients with the acquired immunodeficiency syndrome (AIDS) or who have had an organ transplant have a much higher incidence of colon involvement with lymphoma than the general population. B-cell lymphomas are most common.

- Marked thickening of the bowel wall often exceeds 4 cm. Wall thickening may involve a long segment and may be associated with loss of haustral markings.
- Multiple intraluminal nodules or focal intramural mass (Fig. 17.49) are additional appearances.
- The soft-tissue mass is homogeneous without calcification or necrosis.
- Minimal to no enhancement of the mass occurs with intravenous contrast medium.
- Regional and diffuse adenopathy is often massive.
- Lymphoma characteristically causes much larger soft-tissue masses than does carcinoma. The absence

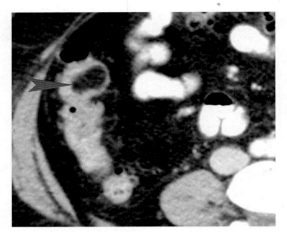

FIG. 17.50 **Lipoma colon.** Axial CT reveal a fat-attenuation mass *(arrowhead)* within the colon lumen. Note that the density of the lesion is identical to that of intra-abdominal fat.

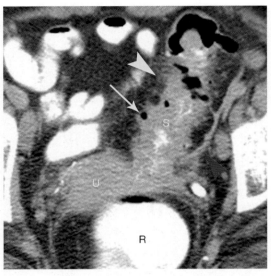

FIG. 17.51 **Acute diverticulitis: uncomplicated.** The sigmoid colon *(S)* shows wall thickening and luminal narrowing. Pericolonic inflammation is manifest by fascial thickening *(red arrowhead)* and stranding in the pericolic fat *(yellow arrowhead)*. Several diverticula *(yellow arrow)* are evident in the inflamed portion of the colon. *R*, Rectum; *U*, uterus.

of desmoplastic reaction is typical, and the colon lumen is commonly dilated or normal, rather than constricted at the site of tumor involvement. Bowel obstruction is uncommon.

Lipoma

CT can be used to make a specific noninvasive diagnosis of GI lipoma by demonstrating homogeneous fat density (–80 to –120 HU) within a sharply defined tumor (Fig. 17.50). Most lipomas are 2 to 3 cm, are round or ovoid, and are clinically silent. Some may bleed or be a cause of intussusception. Lipomas occur most commonly in the colon (65%–75%) and small bowel (20%–25%) and uncommonly in the stomach (5%), esophagus, and pharynx. They are often pedunculated lesions.

Acute Diverticulitis

Diverticulosis refers to small saclike outpouchings of mucosa and submucosa through the muscular layers of the wall of the colon. Diverticula are most common in the sigmoid colon but may occur throughout the colon. The incidence of diverticulosis increases with age, affecting more than 80% of the population older than 85 years. Obstruction of the neck of a diverticulum by feces, undigested food particles, or inflammation results in acute diverticulitis. Microperforation of the diverticulum causes pericolic inflammation. The inflammatory process commonly spreads to adjacent diverticula to affect a usually long segment of colon.

- Diverticula are easily visualized on CT as small, rounded collections of air, feces, or contrast material outside the lumen of the colon. The size ranges from 1 mm to 2 cm. Thickening of the muscular wall of the colon is commonly associated with the presence of diverticula.
- Acute diverticulitis demonstrates on CT a long colon segment (often 5 cm or more) with wall thickening, hyperemic contrast enhancement, and inflammatory changes that extend into the pericolic fat (Fig. 17.51). Identification of diverticula in the involved segment confirms the diagnosis of acute diverticulitis.
- Because most diverticula occur along the mesenteric surface of the colon, perforation as a result of diverticulitis is confined initially to between the leaves of the mesocolon. The inflammatory mass that forms is extraluminal and extraperitoneal. CT is well suited to document this extraluminal disease.
- Sinus tracts and fistulas may extend to adjacent organs or the skin and are represented by linear fluid or air collections. Air in the bladder suggests the possibility of colovesical fistula.
- Abscess formation may be extensive (Fig. 17.52). Obstruction of the colon or urinary tract may result from the inflammatory process.

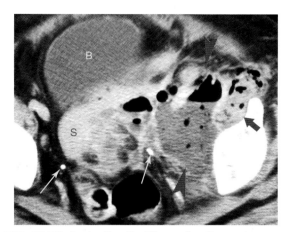

FIG. 17.52 **Acute diverticulitis: perforation and abscess.** A diverticulum arising in the sigmoid colon *(S)* has ruptured and caused a large pelvic abscess (between *red arrowheads*) containing air bubbles and fluid. The left iliopsoas muscle *(red arrow)* is involved by the abscess. Note the proximity of the ureters *(yellow arrows)* to the inflammatory process. They can easily become involved and obstructed. *B,* Bladder.

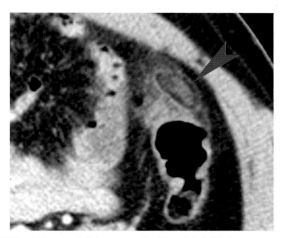

FIG. 17.53 **Epiploic appendagitis.** Axial CT shows a pericolonic focus of inflammation enveloping a focus of fat *(arrowhead).* This finding is characteristic of epiploic appendagitis.

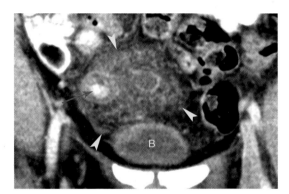

FIG. 17.54 **Meckel diverticulitis.** CT image in the coronal plane showing a large area of inflammation (between *yellow arrowheads*) in the pelvis. In the center of the ring-enhanced wall of a Meckel diverticulum is a high-attenuation structure *(red arrow)* that proved to be a fecalith obstructing the diverticulum.

- Diverticulitis of the ascending colon may be confused with acute appendicitis or Crohn disease.
- The CT appearance of diverticulitis overlaps that of colon cancer. Fluid in the sigmoid mesentery with engorgement of mesenteric vessels favors diverticulitis. Enlarged lymph nodes in the mesentery and the presence of an intraluminal mass favors cancer. Equivocal cases require biopsy.
- *Epiploic appendagitis* commonly mimics acute diverticulitis or acute appendicitis. Epiploic appendages are fat-containing peritoneum-bounded sacs containing fat and blood vessels that extend from the serosa of the colon. They range in size from 5 mm to 5 cm, occurring throughout the colon but are most numerous in the sigmoid colon. Normal epiploic appendages are usually not evident on CT. The sacs may undergo torsion, causing acute ischemia, inflammation, and pain. Although the disease is self-limited, acute pain may be severe. CT shows an oval fat-attenuation lesion of 2 to 5 cm with surrounding inflammatory changes abutting the wall of the colon (Fig. 17.53). Symptoms generally resolve within 2 weeks, but CT findings may persist for 6 months.
- *Meckel diverticulitis* may also mimic acute colonic diverticulitis. Meckel diverticulum is the most common congenital anomaly of the GI tract, occurring as a failure of obliteration of the omphalomesenteric duct that connects the yolk sac to the GI tract during embryonic

life. Meckel diverticulum extends from the ileum about 100 cm proximal to the ileocecal valve. The diverticulum may become obstructed and inflamed, similar to acute appendicitis. When inflamed the diverticulum appears as a blind-ending pouch with thickened wall, mural enhancement, and inflammation of surrounding fat usually located in the central abdomen or pelvis near the midline (Fig. 17.54).

Colitis

Patients with colitis commonly present with vague abdominal symptoms. CT is often the first imaging

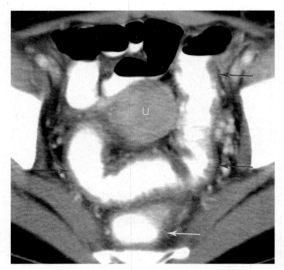

FIG. 17.55 Ulcerative colitis. The findings of ulcerative colitis on CT are often not dramatic. This scan demonstrates characteristic contiguous wall thickening from the rectum *(yellow arrow)* through the sigmoid colon *(red arrows)*. The wall thickening is symmetric around the lumen and is associated with pericolic inflammatory changes These findings are indicative of colitis and suggestive of ulcerative colitis but are not specific for the cause. *U*, Uterus.

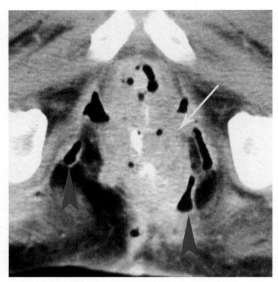

FIG. 17.56 Crohn colitis of the rectum: perianal fistulas. CT shows marked irregular thickening of the wall of the rectum *(yellow arrow)*, infiltration of the perirectal fat, and perianal fistulas extending into the ischiorectal fossa *(red arrowheads)*. The presence of fistulas is typical of Crohn colitis.

study that is performed. Thickening of the colon wall is the CT hallmark of colitis. Wall thickness greater than 3 mm when the colon is distended represents abnormal thickening. Bowel with mural thickening commonly demonstrates homogeneous mural enhancement or a "target" or "halo" appearance. The target or halo appearance is highly indicative of an inflammatory or infectious process rather than a neoplasm.

- *Ulcerative colitis* is characterized by inflammation and diffuse ulceration of the colon mucosa. The disease starts in the rectum and extends contiguously proximally to involve part or all of the colon. The CT hallmarks of ulcerative colitis are wall thickening with lumen narrowing (Fig. 17.55). The inflammatory changes are symmetric and circumferential around the lumen. The disease is characteristically continuous from the rectum, diffuse, and confluent. The inflammatory pseudopolyps that result from extensive mucosal ulceration are sometimes seen on CT. Mural thickening is usually in the range of 7 to 8 mm and commonly demonstrates the target or halo appearance. Narrowing of the rectal lumen with thickening of the rectal wall and widening of the presacral space are characteristic. Edematous stranding and mildly enlarged lymph nodes may be seen in the pericolic fat and mesocolon. Ulcerative colitis predominantly involves the colon but may extend to the terminal ileum as *backwash ileitis*. Complications include colon carcinoma, fibrous strictures, toxic megacolon, and massive hemorrhage. Associated diseases include sacroiliitis, cholangitis, uveitis, and iritis.

- *Crohn colitis* is characterized by transmural inflammation that usually affects the terminal ileum and proximal colon and then extends distally. Bowel wall thickening in Crohn colitis is typically 10 to 20 mm compared with the 7 to 8 mm in ulcerative colitis. With Crohn colitis the outer wall is irregular, whereas with ulcerative colitis the outer wall is smooth. Acute active disease shows layering of the colon wall (target and halo signs), whereas chronic disease with fibrosis show homogeneous enhancement of the colon wall. Fibrous and fat proliferation in the mesentery ("creeping fat") separates bowel loops with extensive fat-containing fibrous strands. Lymph nodes up to 1 cm in size are seen in the mesentery and mesocolon. Fistulas and sinus tracts are additional characteristics of Crohn disease (Fig. 17.56). These may lead to intra-abdominal abscesses, which occur in 15% to 20% of patients. Phlegmons are poorly defined inflammatory masses that occur in the mesentery or omentum.

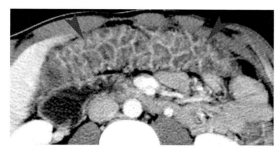

FIG. 17.57 **Pseudomembranous colitis.** The transverse colon *(arrowheads)* demonstrates the "accordion pattern" of irregular wall thickening characteristic of *Clostridium difficile* colitis.

- *Pseudomembranous colitis* results from overgrowth of *Clostridium difficile* in the colon as a complication of antibiotic therapy. A cytotoxic enterotoxin produced by the bacillus ulcerates the mucosa and creates pseudomembranes of mucin, fibrin, inflammatory cells, and sloughed mucosal cells. A pancolitis or segmental colitis with irregular wall thickening (up to 30 mm) and shaggy endoluminal contour is characteristic. Submucosal edema is marked, resulting in the "accordion pattern" of disease that is characteristic of pseudomembranous colitis on CT (Fig. 17.57).
- *Typhlitis,* or *neutropenic colitis,* refers to a potentially fatal infection of the cecum and ascending colon in patients who are neutropenic and severely immunocompromised. It is classically seen in patients with leukemia who are undergoing chemotherapy. CT demonstrates marked circumferential symmetric wall thickening (10–30 mm), low-attenuation edema within the cecal wall, and pericecal fluid and inflammation (Fig. 17.58). Colon wall ischemia leads to pneumatosis, necrosis, and perforation.
- *Ischemic colitis* occurs most commonly in the setting of low cardiac output in a patient with extensive but nonocclusive vascular disease. Most patients are older than 70 years. CT features include mild to moderate circumferential thickening of the colon wall in a segment of colon corresponding to an anatomic vascular distribution. Watershed areas at the splenic flexure and rectosigmoid are most commonly affected. Submucosal edema produces the target or halo sign on postcontrast scans. Stranding and inflammation are seen in the pericolic fat. Hemorrhage and pneumatosis may occur in the bowel wall (Fig. 17.59).
- *Radiation colitis* occurs only within the area treated by radiation. CT in the acute phase demonstrates

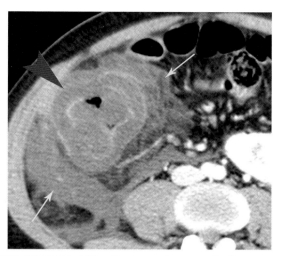

FIG. 17.58 **Typhlitis.** The ascending colon *(red arrowhead)* and cecum demonstrate dramatic wall thickening, poor enhancement, and pericolic fluid collections *(yellow arrows)* and edema. The transverse colon and descending colon were unaffected. This patient was neutropenic as a result of chemotherapy.

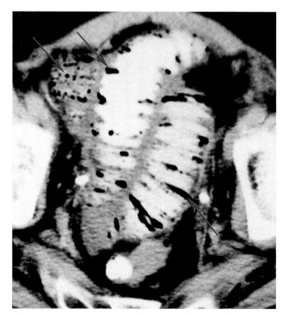

FIG. 17.59 **Pneumatosis: bowel ischemia.** In an acutely ill patient, CT reveals gas *(arrows)* in the wall and folds of the small bowel and large bowel. Wall thickening and pericolic edema are present. This patient died of acute bowel infarction.

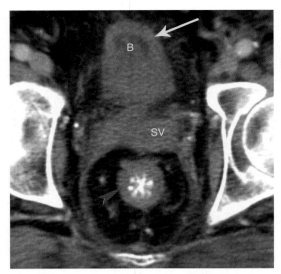

FIG. 17.60 **Chronic radiation proctitis.** CT without intravenous contrast medium reveals circumferential thickening of the wall *(red arrowhead)* of the rectum. The rectum was in the radiation field for treatment of prostate cancer. The wall *(yellow arrow)* of the bladder *(B)* is also thickened, reflecting chronic bladder outlet obstruction caused by enlargement of the prostate. *SV,* Seminal vesicles.

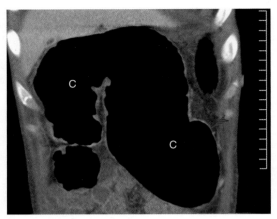

FIG. 17.61 **Toxic megacolon.** In a young patient with severe ulcerative colitis, coronal CT demonstrates marked dilatation of the colon *(C)* with thinning of its walls *(red arrowheads)*. The diameter of the lumen of the colon exceeded 7 cm. This finding places the patient at high risk of colon perforation.

mild wall thickening and pericolic stranding confined to the radiation port. Chronic radiation injury is seen 6 to 24 months following treatment and appears as mural thickening with prominent stranding in expanded pericolic fat. These findings are seen most often in the rectum (Fig. 17.60) and sigmoid colon in patients who have undergone pelvic radiation therapy.

- *Infectious colitis* may be caused by bacteria (*Shigella, Salmonella, Campylobacter, Yersinia, Staphylococcus*), fungal disease (histoplasmosis, mucormycosis, actinomycosis), viruses (herpesvirus, cytomegalovirus), parasitic disease (amebiasis), or tuberculosis. Differentiation is based on clinical findings because the CT findings are nonspecific. Circumferential wall thickening with homogeneous enhancement or wall edema affects all or portions of the colon. Inflammatory stranding and edema are seen in pericolic fat. Air-fluid levels may be seen in the colon because of increased volumes of fluid mixed with feces.

- *Enterohemorrhagic colitis* is caused by a specific strain of *Escherichia coli* most commonly acquired from undercooked ground beef. Patients present with cramps and watery diarrhea that progresses to bloody diarrhea. CT demonstrates wall thickening to 20 mm of segments of the colon with submucosal edema (target sign) and stranding of the pericolic fat.

- *Toxic megacolon* is a potentially fatal complication of many types of colitis. Severe inflammation damages the mucosa and muscular layers of the colon wall, paralyzing segments of the colon, resulting in dilatation, loss of peristalsis, hemorrhage, and fluid and fecal accumulation in the colon lumen. Complications include sepsis, shock, and colon perforation. The CT hallmarks are dilatation of the colon (>5 cm) with thinning of the colon wall, pneumatosis, and air in the peritoneal cavity or retroperitoneum, reflecting colon perforation (Fig. 17.61).

Pneumatosis Intestinalis and Ischemic Bowel

Pneumatosis intestinalis is the term applied to all cases of intramural intestinal gas. This is an imaging sign not a diagnosis. At least 58 causative factors ranging from life threatening to insignificant have been reported. The major causes can be grouped into four categories. *Bowel necrosis* is the most important because it is life threatening. Bowel necrosis may occur with any cause of bowel ischemia, volvulus, necrotizing enterocolitis, typhlitis, or sepsis. *Mucosal disruption* related to peptic ulcers, endoscopy, enteric tubes, trauma, child abuse, ulcerative colitis, or Crohn disease may cause pneumatosis. *Increased mucosal permeability* is associated with

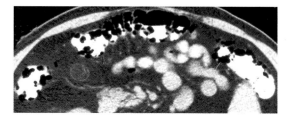

FIG. 17.62 Pneumatosis coli: benign. CT reveals well-defined bubbles of air in the dependent wall *(arrowheads)* and nondependent wall of the transverse colon. The colon wall is not thickened. No pericolic inflammation is present. The patient was not acutely ill. These findings are indicative of benign pneumatosis.

immunosuppression in AIDS, organ transplantation, chemotherapy, steroid therapy, or graft-versus-host disease. In *pulmonary conditions* such as chronic obstructive pulmonary disease, asthma, cystic fibrosis, chest trauma, or mechanical ventilation, air from disrupted alveoli may dissect along the bronchopulmonary interstitium to the mediastinum and retroperitoneum to extend along the visceral vessels to the bowel wall. The key is to differentiate patients with pneumatosis indicative of significant disease from those in whom pneumatosis is an incidental finding. The clinical condition of the patient is key. Patients who are asymptomatic can be safely observed. Those who are critically ill with clinical and imaging evidence of bowel ischemia require urgent surgery. Patients with bowel ischemia usually have predisposing conditions such as hypotension, congestive heart failure, cardiac arrhythmias, sepsis, or dehydration.

- *Cystic pneumatosis* appears as well-defined blebs or grapelike clusters of spherical air collections in the subserosal region of the bowel wall. Surrounding tissue is usually normal, and the cause is usually benign (Fig. 17.62). The air cysts may rupture, resulting in *benign pneumoperitoneum.*
- *Linear pneumatosis* appears as streaks of gas within and parallel to the bowel wall. This may be associated with either benign or ischemic causes. Turning the patient from the supine to the prone or lateral decubitus position may be needed to confirm that gas is in the bowel wall rather than in the bowel lumen.
- Findings of bowel ischemia that may be seen in addition to pneumatosis include intestinal dilatation, thickening of the bowel wall with submucosal edema or hemorrhage that may appear as thumbprinting or the target sign, engorgement of mesenteric vessels, thrombosis of mesenteric vessels, and gas in mesenteric or portal veins (Fig. 17.59).

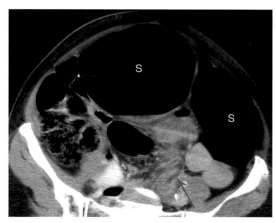

FIG. 17.63 Sigmoid volvulus. Axial CT of the lower abdomen shows two portions of the sigmoid colon *(S)* are markedly dilated and adjacent to each other. Serial images showed convergence of the dilated loops toward the left lower quadrant. Twisting of the mesocolon *(arrow)* is evident. Sigmoid volvulus was confirmed by sigmoidoscopy.

Colonic Volvulus

Volvulus of the large bowel involves a twisting or folding of an intraperitoneal segment of the colon. Diagnosis is usually made by conventional radiographs of the abdomen, but CT is used to confirm the diagnosis and to detect evidence of ischemia.

- *Sigmoid volvulus* involves the sigmoid colon twisting on its mesocolon approximately 15 cm above the anal verge. CT scout scan or conventional radiographs demonstrate the distended sigmoid colon appearing like a bent inner tube with the apex pointing toward the left lower quadrant (Fig. 17.63). Axial CT shows the distended colon with the mesenteric twist appearing as a whirl. Signs of bowel ischemia include wall thickening, infiltration of pericolic fat, and pneumatosis. Sigmoid volvulus accounts for 60% to 75% of colonic volvulus.
- *Cecal volvulus* characteristically has the dilated gas-filled cecum twisted into the left upper quadrant or central abdomen with the apex of the distended colon pointed toward the right lower quadrant and the whirl of cecal mesentery in the right abdomen. The axis of torsion is in the ascending colon above the ileocecal valve. The small bowel is more commonly dilated in association with cecal volvulus (Fig. 17.64). The distal colon is decompressed. Ischemic changes are also more common. Cecal volvulus accounts for 25% to 40% of colonic volvulus.

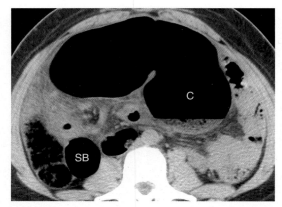

FIG. 17.64 Cecal volvulus. CT demonstrates a markedly dilated cecum *(C)* transposed to the left upper quadrant of the abdomen. The distal small bowel *(SB)* was also dilated.

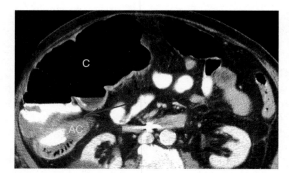

FIG. 17.65 Cecal bascule. The cecum *(C)* is dilated and displaced into the central abdomen. A fold *(arrow)* separates the dilated cecum and proximal ascending colon from the nondilated distal ascending colon *(AC)*.

- *Cecal bascule* refers to a folding rather than a twisting of a mobile cecum. The cecum folds over on itself like folding the toe of a sock. The cecum is markedly distended and is displaced into the central abdomen (Fig. 17.65). The small bowel is often not obstructed.

Acute Gastrointestinal Bleeding

Acute GI bleeding is typically initially evaluated with upper GI tract endoscopy and colonoscopy. If these fail to identify a cause of bleeding, multiphase contrast-enhanced CT enterography performed with arterial, portal venous, and delayed phase scans may be helpful.
- Active bleeding appears as a gradual accumulation of intravenous contrast material within the bowel lumen.

- Angiodysplasia, the most common cause of occult GI bleeding, appears as a markedly enhancing nodule or plaque that fades in enhancement on delayed phase images.
- Other causes of GI bleeding include neoplasms, Meckel diverticulum, and vascular malformations.

SUGGESTED READING

Almeida, A. T., Melao, L., Viamonte, B., et al. (2009). Epiploic appendagitis: An entity frequently unknown to clinicians - diagnostic imaging, pitfalls, and look-alikes. *AJR. American Journal of Roentgenology, 193,* 1243–1251.

Baxi, A. J., Chintapalli, K., Katkar, A., et al. (2017). Multimodality imaging findings in carcinoid tumors: A head-to-toe spectrum. *Radiographics, 37,* 516–536.

Bruning, D. H., Zimmerman, E. M., Loftus, E. V., Jr., et al. (2018). Consensus recommendations for evaluation, interpretation, and utilization of computed tomography and magnetic resonance enterography in patients with small bowel Crohn's disease. *Radiology, 286,* 776–799.

Childers, B. C., Cater, S. W., Horton, K. M., et al. (2015). CT evaluation of acute enteritis and colitis: Is it infectious, inflammatory, or ischemic? *Radiographics, 35,* 1940–1941.

Chin, C. M., & Lim, K. L. (2015). Appendicitis: Atypical and challenging CT appearances. *Radiographics, 35,* 123–124.

Dane, B., Hindman, N., Johnson, E., & Rosenkrantz, A. B. (2017). Utility of CT findings in the diagnosis of cecal volvulus. *AJR. American Journal of Roentgenology, 209,* 762–766.

Elsayes, K. M., Al-Hawary, M. M., Jagdish, J., et al. (2010). CT enterography: Principles, trends, and interpretation of findings. *Radiographics, 30,* 1955–1974.

Hong, S. J., Kim, T. J., Nam, K. B., et al. (2014). New TMN staging system for esophageal cancer: What chest radiologists need to know. *Radiographics, 34,* 1722–1740.

Kiyosue, H., Ibukuro, K., Maruno, M., et al. (2013). Multidetector CT anatomy of drainage routes of gastric varices: A pictorial review. *Radiographics, 33,* 87–100.

Leonards, L. M., Pahwa, A., Patel, M. K., et al. (2017). Neoplasms of the appendix: Pictorial review with clinical and pathologic correlation. *Radiographics, 37,* 1059–1083.

Levsky, J. M., Den, E. I., DuBrow, R. A., et al. (2010). CT findings of sigmoid volvulus. *AJR. American Journal of Roentgenology, 194,* 136–143.

Lewis, R. B., Mehrotra, A. K., Rodriquez, P., et al. (2014). Gastrointestinal lymphoma: Radiologic and pathologic findings. *Radiographics, 34,* 1934–1953.

Maddu, K. K., Mittal, P., Shuaib, W., et al. (2014). Colorectal emergencies and related complications: A comprehensive imaging review – imaging of colitis and complications. *AJR. American Journal of Roentgenology, 203,* 1205–1216.

Marini, T., Desai, A., Kaproth-Joslin, K., et al. (2017). Imaging of the esophagus: Beyond cancer. *Insights Imaging, 8,* 365–376.

Mc Laughline, P. D., Filippone, A., & Maher, M. M. (2013). The "misty mesentery": Mesenteric panniculitis and its mimics. *AJR. American Journal of Roentgenology, 200,* W116–W123.

McLaughlin, P. D., & Maher, M. M. (2013). Nonneoplastic diseases of the small intestine: Differential diagnosis and Crohn disease. *AJR. American Journal of Roentgenology, 201,* W174–W182.

McLaughlin, P. D., & Maher, M. M. (2013). Primary malignant diseases of the small intestine. *AJR. American Journal of Roentgenology, 201,* W9–W14.

Nerad, E., Lahaye, M. J., Maas, M., et al. (2016). Diagnostic accuracy of CT for local staging of colon cancer: A systematic review and meta-analysis. *AJR. American Journal of Roentgenology, 207,* 984–995.

Nougaret, S., Lakhman, Y., Reinhold, C., et al. (2016). The wheel of the mesentery: Imaging spectrum of primary and secondary mesenteric neoplasms – how can radiologist help plan treatment? *Radiographics., 36,* 412–413.

Olpin, J. D., Sjoberg, B. P., Stilwill, S. E., et al. (2017). Beyond the bowel: Extraintestinal manifestations of inflammatory bowel disease. *Radiographics, 37,* 1135–1160.

Paulsen, E. K., & Thompson, W. M. (2015). Review of small-bowel obstruction: The diagnosis and when to worry. *Radiology, 275,* 332–342.

Sandrasegaran, K., Rajesh, A., Rydberg, J., et al. (2005). Gastrointestinal stromal tumors: Clinical, radiologic, and pathologic features. *AJR. American Journal of Roentgenology, 184,* 803–811.

Scholz, F. J., Afnan, J., & Beht, S. C. (2011). CT findings in adult celiac disease. *Radiographics, 31,* 977–992.

Spada, C., Stoker, J., Alarcon, O., et al. (2015). Clinical indications for computed tomographic colonography: European Society of Gastrointestinal Endoscopy (ESGE) and European Society of Gastrointestinal and Abdominal Radiology (ESGAR) guideline. *European Radiology, 25,* 331–345.

Winant, A. J., Gollub, M. J., Shia, J., et al. (2014). Imaging and clinicopathologic features of esophageal gastrointestinal stromal tumors. *AJR. American Journal of Roentgenology, 203,* 306–314.

CHAPTER 18

Pelvis

WILLIAM E. BRANT

ANATOMY

The *true (lesser) pelvis* is divided from the *false (greater) pelvis* by an oblique plane extending across the pelvic brim from the sacral promontory to the symphysis pubis. The true pelvis contains the rectum, bladder, pelvic ureters, and prostate and seminal vesicles in males, or vagina, uterus, and ovaries in females. The false pelvis is open anteriorly and is bounded laterally by the iliac fossae. It contains small-bowel loops and portions of the ascending colon, descending colon, and sigmoid colon.

Muscle groups form prominent anatomic landmarks on CT. The psoas muscles extend from the lumbar vertebrae through the greater pelvis to join with the iliacus muscles arising from the iliac fossa. The iliopsoas muscles exit the pelvis anteriorly to insert on the lesser trochanters of the femurs. The obturator internus muscles line the interior surface of the lateral walls of the true pelvis. Involvement of these muscles by pelvic tumors generally precludes surgical resection of the tumor. The piriformis muscles arise from the anterior sacrum and exit the pelvis through the greater sciatic foramen to insert on the greater trochanter of the femur. The piriformis forms a portion of the lateral wall of the true pelvis. The pelvic diaphragm, composed of the levator ani anteriorly and the coccygeus posteriorly, stretches across the pelvis to separate the pelvic cavity from the perineum. The pelvic diaphragm is penetrated by the rectum, urethra, and vagina.

The pelvis is divided into three major anatomic compartments (Figs. 18.1 and 18.2). It is important to understand these because anatomic compartments allow determination of the origin and spread of disease. The *peritoneal cavity* extends to the level of the vagina, forming the pouch of Douglas in females, or to the level of the seminal vesicles, forming the rectovesical pouch in males. The *extraperitoneal space* of the pelvis is continuous with the retroperitoneal space of the abdomen. Pathologic processes from the extraperitoneal space of the pelvis may spread preferentially into the retroperitoneal compartments of the abdomen. The retropubic space (of Retzius) is continuous with the posterior pararenal space and the extraperitoneal fat of the abdominal wall. Fascial planes also allow communication with the scrotum and labia. The presacral space between the sacrum and the rectum normally contains only fat. Any soft-tissue density in this space is abnormal and must be explained. The *perineum* lies below the pelvic diaphragm. On CT the most obvious portion of the perineum is the ischiorectal fossa. This fossa is seen as a triangular area of fat density extending between the obturator internus laterally, the gluteus maximus posteriorly, and the anus and urogenital region medially.

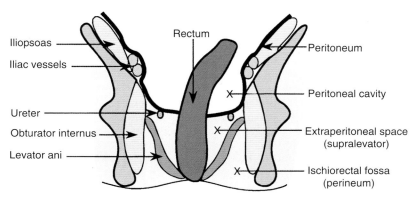

FIG. 18.1 **Anatomic compartments of the pelvis.** Posterior coronal section at the level of the rectum demonstrating the major anatomic compartments of the pelvis.

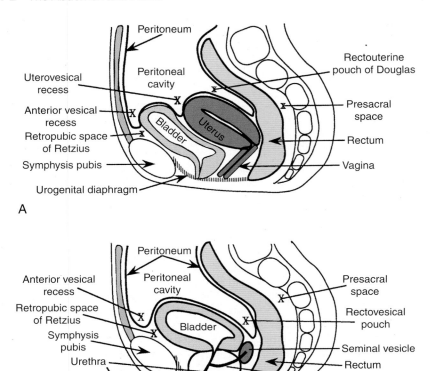

FIG. 18.2 **Anatomic compartments of the pelvis.** Midline sagittal planes through a female pelvis (A) and a male pelvis (B) demonstrating the pelvic compartments and peritoneal recesses and their relationships to pelvic organs.

The arteries and veins define the location of the major lymphatic node chains in the pelvis (Fig. 18.3). The aorta and inferior vena cava divide to form the common iliac vessels at the level of the top of the iliac crest. The common iliac vessels divide at the pelvic brim, marked on CT by the transition between the convex sacral promontory and the concave sacral cavity. The internal iliac (hypogastric) vessels course posteriorly across the sciatic foramen, dividing rapidly into smaller branches. The external iliac vessels course anteriorly adjacent to the iliopsoas to exit the pelvis at the inguinal ligament. Pelvic lymph nodes are classified with their accompanying vessels and are correspondingly named the *common iliac, internal iliac,* and *external iliac nodal chains.* The obturator nodes are satellites of the external iliac chain and course along the midportion of the obturator internus. Inguinal nodes in the subcutaneous tissue near the common femoral vessels drain the perineum but not the true pelvis. Pelvic lymph nodes are considered pathologically enlarged on CT when they exceed 10 mm in short axis.

The bladder is best appreciated on CT when filled with urine or contrast agent. The normal bladder wall does not exceed 5 mm in thickness when the bladder is distended. The dome of the bladder is covered by peritoneum, whereas its base and anterior surface are extraperitoneal. The ureters course anterior to the psoas, cross over the common iliac vessels at the pelvic brim, pass on either side of the cervix, and insert into the bladder trigone. In males the ureters insert into the bladder just above the prostate at the level of the seminal vesicle.

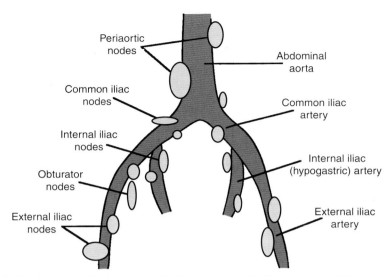

FIG. 18.3 **Pelvic lymph node chains.** Aortic bifurcation and the iliac arteries and the classification and naming of pelvic lymph nodes.

The vagina is seen in cross section as a flattened ellipse of soft tissue between the bladder and rectum. An inserted tampon will outline the cavity of the vagina with air density and is useful in marking the vagina for pelvic CT. The level of the cervix is recognized by the transition from the elliptic shape of the vagina to the rounded shape of the cervix. Contrast-filled ureters are frequently identified in close proximity to the cervix. The uterus is seen as a homogeneous, smooth-outlined oval of soft-tissue density. The myometrium is highly vascular, causing the uterus to enhance more than most pelvic organs. Assessment of the uterus on CT is made difficult by variation in the position and flexion of the uterus and the amount of bladder filling. The broad ligament is a sheetlike fold of peritoneum that drapes over the uterus and extends laterally to the pelvic sidewalls. Between the leaves of the broad ligament is the *parametrium*, which is loose connective tissue and fat through which pass the fallopian tubes, uterine and ovarian blood vessels and lymphatics, the pelvic ureters, and the round ligament. Determination of tumor extension into the parametrium is an important part of gynecologic tumor staging. The fallopian tube forms the superior free edge of the broad ligament, best seen when outlined by ascites. The fallopian tube with its covering broad ligament is rather like a sheet folded over a clothes line with the parametrium between the folds of the sheet. The cardinal ligaments extend laterally from the cervix to the obturator internus muscles, forming the base of the broad ligament. The cardinal ligaments

appear on CT as triangular densities extending laterally from the cervix. The round ligaments extend from the uterine fundus through the internal inguinal ring to terminate in the labia majora. Uterosacral ligaments extend in an arc from the cervix to the anterior sacrum. Uterine arteries branch from the hypogastric trunk and course in the parametrium just superior to the cardinal ligaments. Enhanced parametrial blood vessels are commonly prominent on contrast-enhanced CT scans obtained with bolus contrast medium administration. Normal ovaries are sometimes difficult to identify on CT. Because they are mobile, they may be anywhere in the pelvis, but they are most commonly seen adjacent to the uterine fundus. They appear as oval soft-tissue densities, approximately 2 × 3 × 4 cm. The presence of cystic follicles allows positive identification of the ovaries.

The normal prostate gland is seen at the base of the bladder as a homogeneous, rounded soft-tissue organ up to 4 cm in maximal diameter. Prostate zonal anatomy, well shown by magnetic resonance imaging, is not demonstrated by CT. A well-defined plane of fat separates the prostate from the obturator internus. This fat plane may be invaded by carcinoma. Denonvilliers fascia provides a particularly tough barrier between the prostate and the rectum, usually preventing spread of tumors from one organ to the other. The paired seminal vesicles produce a characteristic bow tie–shaped soft-tissue structure in the groove between the bladder base and the prostate. Normal testes are easily identified in the scrotum as homogeneous oval structures 3 to 4 cm in diameter. The spermatic cord can be recognized in the inguinal canal as a thin-walled oval structure of fat density containing small dots representing the vas deferens and spermatic vessels.

TECHNICAL CONSIDERATIONS

The ideal technique for CT of the pelvis requires optimal bowel opacification. A typical procedure involves the giving of 500 mL of dilute contrast agent orally the evening before the examination and a repeated dose 45 to 60 minutes before the examination. The colon and rectum can be distended by placement of a tube in the rectum and insufflation with 20 puffs of air, or to the limit of patient comfort. Patients are asked to avoid urination for 30 to 40 minutes before the examination to allow bladder filling. Intravenous contrast medium is routinely given by a mechanical injector at 2 to 3 mL per second for a total dose of 150 mL of 60% contrast agent. CT images through the pelvis are viewed as contiguous 2.5- to 5-mm-thick slices. The abdomen should also be in patients with known or suspected pelvic malignancy. To optimize contrast enhancement of pelvic organs, the pelvis can be scanned first, then the abdomen. Coronal and sagittal plane reconstructions are often helpful.

BLADDER
Bladder Carcinoma

Bladder cancer may be superficial and confined to the mucosa. However, with invasion of the bladder wall musculature, the risk of spread to regional and distant nodes increases. As the number and size of nodal metastases increases, so does the risk of hematogenous spread to bone and lung. CT is useful for the staging of advanced disease but is not accurate in defining early-stage disease. Patients are generally referred for CT staging after muscle invasive disease is suspected on cystoscopy. The key elements of staging are the depth of tumor invasion into the bladder wall and the involvement of adjacent and distant sites by tumor. Most malignant bladder tumors (95%) are uroepithelial (transitional cell) carcinomas that carry a risk of multiple synchronous tumors in the ipsilateral ureter and renal collecting system. Squamous cell carcinomas (4%–5%) are usually associated with chronic inflammation. Adenocarcinomas account for less than 2% of bladder tumors. The CT findings are as follows:

- The primary tumor appears as a focal thickening of the bladder wall or as a soft-tissue mass projecting into the bladder lumen (Fig. 18.4). Early postcontrast scans

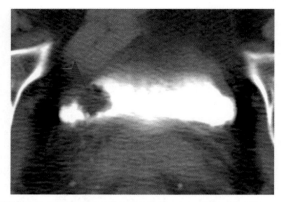

FIG. 18.4 **Transitional cell carcinoma of the bladder: polypoid.** Bone windows provide the best visualization of a polypoid frond-like mass *(arrowhead)* projecting into the bladder lumen and seen as a filling defect within the intraluminal contrast material layering within the bladder.

may demonstrate a weakly enhancing mural nodule on a background of low-attenuation urine. Delayed scans show a soft-tissue filling defect on a background of high-attenuation contrast-opacified urine. Masses may be plaque-like, polypoid, or papillary.
- Multicentric tumors occur in 30% to 40% of cases, with tumors in the upper tracts in 2% to 5% of cases. One should always look for additional tumors.
- The bladder must be well distended or subtle tumors, especially small flat lesions, can easily be overlooked. Bladder tumors enhance maximally at 60 seconds after contrast medium injection, stressing the need to scan the pelvis during this time frame.
- Calcifications are seen in 5% of transitional cell carcinomas
- Perivesical spread is seen as soft-tissue density in the perivesical fat (Fig. 18.5). Extension to the pelvic sidewall musculature precludes complete surgical resection.
- Pelvic lymph nodes larger than 10 mm in short axis are considered positive for metastatic disease. Smaller nodes are unlikely to be involved.
- Hematogenous metastases are most common in the liver, lungs, bones, and adrenal glands.
- Rare bladder tumors to be considered in the differential diagnosis include pheochromocytoma, leiomyoma, lymphoma (Fig. 18.6), sarcoma, and metastases.

Bladder Diverticulum

Bladder diverticula are seen as a cystic pelvic mass. Identification of communication with the bladder lumen is the key to correct diagnosis (Fig. 18.7).

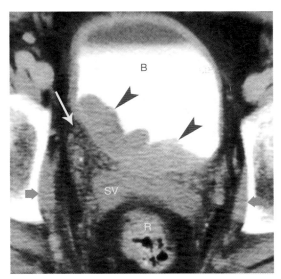

FIG. 18.5 **Transitional cell carcinoma of the bladder: wall thickening.** Spreading tumor *(red arrowheads)* thickens the bladder wall and projects into the bladder lumen *(B)* near the trigone. Tiny nodules and strand-like densities *(yellow arrow)* infiltrate the normally clear fat triangle between the bladder and the seminal vesicles *(SV)*. In this case the tumor penetrated the bladder wall and infiltrated the perivesical fat; however, this finding is not always a reliable indication of tumor spread. The obturator internus muscles *(green arrows)* are clearly not involved, indicating that this tumor is potentially resectable. Clear fat separates these muscles from the perivesical tumor nodules. *R*, Rectum.

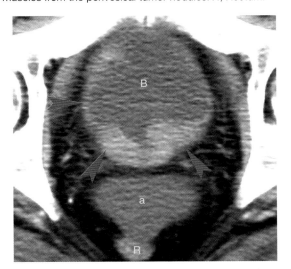

FIG. 18.6 **Lymphoma of the bladder.** Lymphoma *(arrowheads)* causes nodular thickening extending into the bladder lumen *(B)* mimicking transitional cell carcinoma. Ascites *(a)* is present, distending the rectovesical pouch of Douglas. *R*, Rectum.

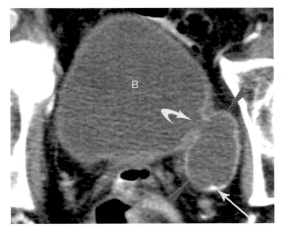

FIG. 18.7 **Bladder diverticulum.** A bladder diverticulum (between *red arrowheads*) extends from the lateral wall of the bladder *(B)*, maintaining communication with the bladder lumen through a large ostium *(curved yellow arrow)*. Small stones *(straight yellow arrow)* layer dependently in the diverticulum. Bladder diverticula serve as a site for urinary stasis, predisposing to urinary infection and stone formation.

Bladder diverticula provide a site for urine stasis, which commonly results in stone formation and recurrent infection.

Cystitis

Cystitis refers to inflammation of the bladder wall. It is a common condition affecting patients of all ages. It is most common in women.

- *Acute bacterial cystitis* is most common and usually caused by *Escherichia coli* infection. The diagnosis is made clinically, and imaging is usually not required. Bullous mucosal edema may thicken the bladder wall and give it a cobblestone appearance. Chronic cystitis usually related to poor bladder emptying caused by neurogenic bladder or chronic bladder outlet obstruction may result in a fibrotic contracted bladder with a thick wall (Fig. 18.8).
- *Cystitis cystica and cystitis glandularis* are inflammatory disorders that result from chronic irritation of the bladder wall caused by recurrent bacterial cystitis or bladder stones. CT shows multiple hypervascular enhancing polypoid masses of variable size.
- *Interstitial cystitis* is an uncommon idiopathic disease characterized by fibrosis of the bladder wall. Bladder volume is restricted, and the bladder wall ultimately becomes thinned.

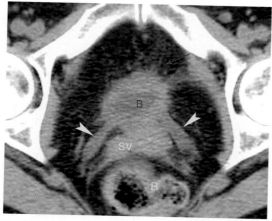

FIG. 18.8 Chronic cystitis. CT in the axial plane without intravenous contrast medium shows the bladder *(B)* to be contracted and thick walled in a paraplegic patient with neurogenic bladder and chronic cystitis. The ureters *(yellow arrowheads)* are seen entering the bladder. Inflammatory stranding *(red arrow)* extends into the pericystic fat. *R,* Rectum; *SV,* seminal vesicles.

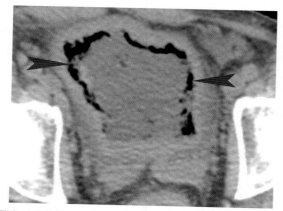

FIG. 18.9 Emphysematous cystitis. Gas *(arrowheads)* is present in the wall of the bladder in this diabetic patient with urinary sepsis.

- *Emphysematous cystitis* refers to the presence of gas in the bladder wall and lumen caused by bacterial infection in glucose-laden urine. The disease occurs in patients with diabetes mellitus who have bladder dysfunction related to neurogenic bladder, bladder diverticula, or chronic bladder outlet obstruction. CT shows thickening and streaks and bubbles of gas in the bladder wall (Fig. 18.9). Gas in the bladder lumen forms air-fluid levels.
- *Tuberculosis* of the bladder is an extension of renal tuberculosis. CT findings in the acute stage include

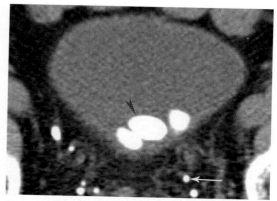

FIG. 18.10 Bladder stones. Three calculi *(red arrowhead)* are seen as oval high-attenuation masses within the bladder lumen. Numerous phleboliths *(yellow arrow)* are present in the pelvis, seen as high-attenuation foci within thrombosed veins.

bladder wall thickening, trabeculation, and irregular mucosal masses representing tubercles. In the chronic stage the bladder becomes contracted and the wall is commonly calcified.
- *Schistosomiasis* is caused by infestation with the parasite *Schistosoma haematobium,* which is most commonly found in Africa. Eggs laid in the bladder wall produce nodular wall thickening in the acute phase and result in a fibrotic contracted bladder with wall and distal ureteral calcification in the chronic phase.

Bladder Stones

Bladder stones are much less common than kidney stones. Bladder stones may form primarily within the bladder, from foreign bodies within the bladder, or from kidney stones that are retained within the bladder. Most occur in the setting of urinary stasis within the bladder caused by neurogenic bladder, an enlarged prostate, recurrent urinary infections, or a bladder diverticulum.
- CT is sensitive for detection of even very small stones in the bladder. Stones appear as foci of high attenuation (Fig. 18.10).

UTERUS
Leiomyoma

Leiomyomas (fibroids) are found in up to 40% of women older than 30 years. As frequent findings, their CT features should be recognized.
- Leiomyomas appear as homogeneous or heterogeneous masses that may be hypodense, isodense,

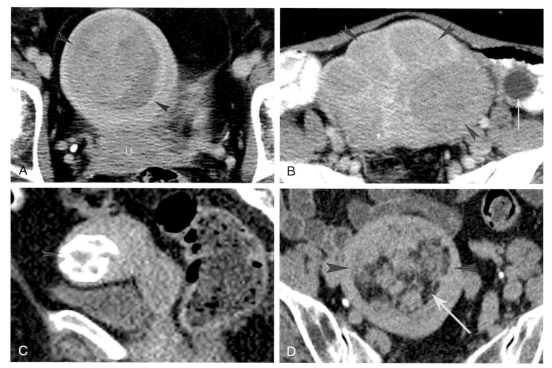

FIG. 18.11 **Leiomyoma uterus.** (A) Axial CT shows a large leiomyoma (between *red arrowheads*) extending anteriorly from the uterus *(U)*. (B) Axial postcontrast CT image of another patient showing multiple leiomyomas *(red arrowheads)* enlarging the uterus and deforming its contour. The left ovary *(yellow arrow)* contains a physiologic cyst. (C) Sagittal CT image demonstrating the coarse "popcorn" calcification *(arrow)* characteristic of degenerated leiomyomas. (D) Axial postcontrast CT shows a large heterogeneous leiomyoma (between *red arrows*) with areas that are clearly of fat attenuation *(yellow arrow)*. Compare this with adjacent pelvic fat. This finding is characteristic of lipoleiomyoma.

or hyperdense relative to enhanced myometrium (Fig. 18.11). Diffuse enlargement of the uterus and lobulation of its contour are common (Fig. 18.11B).

- Coarse dystrophic mottled calcifications within the mass are common and characteristic (Fig. 18.11C).
- Cystic degeneration produces interior low density and may convert the mass into a large cavity.
- Pedunculated leiomyomas may appear as adnexal masses rather than uterine masses. Parasitic leiomyomas are separate from the uterus, having undergone torsion and detached from the uterine pedicle and implanted on the peritoneum.
- Lipoleiomyomas are variant tumors consisting of smooth muscle, fibrous tissue, and mature fat. CT shows foci of fat attenuation (below −30 Hounsfield units) within the tumor (Fig. 18.11D).
- Rare leiomyosarcomas cannot be accurately differentiated from leiomyomas by CT appearance alone. Rapid growth of a uterine mass in a postmenopausal woman

suggests malignancy. Leiomyosarcomas appear as large masses with prominent irregular low-attenuation areas of necrosis and hemorrhage (Fig. 18.12). The appearance of leiomyosarcoma overlaps that of benign leiomyoma with extensive degeneration.

Carcinoma of the Cervix

Although CT has been used to stage cervical carcinoma, MRI is preferable in most instances. CT is useful to stage advanced disease and to detect recurrence. Unsuspected cervical cancers may also be detected by CT performed for other indications. Cervical malignancies are squamous cell carcinomas (85%) and adenocarcinomas (15%) that spread primarily by direct extension to adjacent organs and tissues. Lymphatic spread to regional nodes is common. Hematogenous spread to lung, bone, and brain is uncommon and occurs late in the course of disease. The accuracy of CT staging is in the range of 65%, compared with 90% reported for MRI. The CT findings include the following:

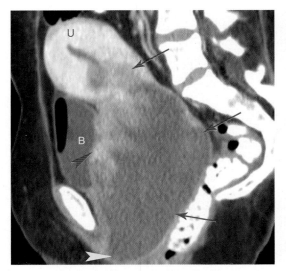

FIG. 18.12 **Leiomyosarcoma uterus.** Postcontrast CT image in the sagittal plane showing a large heterogeneous hemorrhagic tumor *(red arrows)* arising from the lower uterine segment and invading the cervix and vagina. The tumor mass presents at the introitus *(yellow arrowhead)*. The posterior wall of the bladder *(B)* is invaded by tumor *(red arrowhead)*. The bladder contains air from previous catheterization. *U,* Fundus of the uterus.

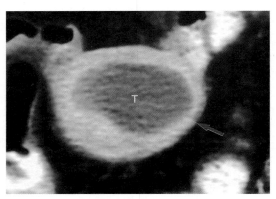

FIG. 18.13 **Cervical carcinoma confined to the cervix.** Postcontrast axial CT through the cervix demonstrates a squamous cell carcinoma of the cervix as a low-attenuation tumor *(T)* confined within the enhancing cervix. The cervical tissue is asymmetrically thinned on the left *(arrow)* but the paracervical tissues are not invaded.

- The normal cervix enhances variably on early post-contrast scans but is uniformly enhanced on scans obtained with several minutes' delay. The primary tumor may be of low attenuation (50%) or isoat-

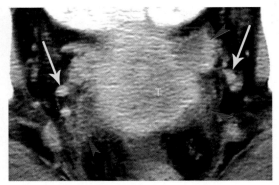

FIG. 18.14 **Cervical carcinoma invading the parametrium.** Axial CT through the cervix shows that the cervical tumor *(T)* is slightly lower in attenuation than the enhancing cervix. The borders of the tumor are indistinct. However, extension of the tumor into the parametrium *(red arrowheads)* is apparent. Soft-tissue density of the tumor approaches the ureters *(yellow arrows)* but does not involve them. The proximity of the ureters to the cervix places them at risk of obstruction by tumor spread.

tenuating (50%) compared with normal cervix (Fig. 18.13). Low attenuation is caused by reduced vascularity, necrosis, or ulceration. The primary tumor may enlarge the cervix (>3.5 cm diameter).

- Fluid collections in the uterine cavity, representing serous fluid, blood, or pus, are common because of tumor obstruction of the cervix.
- Spread of tumor by direct extension (Figs. 18.14 and 18.15) is seen as thick, irregular tissue strands or masses fanning out from the cervix into the parametrium often encasing the ureters, extending into the vagina, or extending to the pelvic sidewalls. Normal broad, round, cardinal, and uterosacral ligaments should not be mistaken for tumor extension. Encasement of the ureter is a specific sign of parametrial invasion.
- Extension to the pelvic sidewall is indicated when tumor nodules are seen within 3 mm of the obturator internus or piriformis muscles. Tumor invasion is seen as an enhancing mass within enlarged muscles.
- Invasion of the bladder or rectum is indicated by loss of the perivesical or perirectal fat plane, nodular thickening of the wall of the bladder or rectum, or a mass within the bladder or rectum. Air within the bladder suggests fistula formation.
- Enlarged lymph nodes (>10 mm in short axis) are strong evidence of metastatic involvement, but cervical carcinoma will commonly involve nodes without enlarging them. These small but involved nodes cannot be differentiated from benign nodes by CT. Necrotic lymph nodes are likely involved by tumor.

- Recurrences appear as soft-tissue masses anywhere in the pelvis but most commonly at the top of the vaginal cuff in patients who have undergone hysterectomy. Enlarged nodes are also suggestive of recurrence. Biopsy is usually needed to confirm the diagnosis.

Endometrial Malignancy

Carcinoma of the endometrium is the most common invasive gynecologic malignancy. Peak incidence occurs at the age of 55 to 65 years. Most tumors (90%) are endometrioid adenocarcinomas. Clear cell and papillary serous subtypes are more aggressive. Müllerian mixed tumor is a sarcoma of the endometrium. Tumors spreads first by invasion of the myometrium, then by lymphatic channels to regional nodes, or by direct extension through the uterine wall to parametrial tissues. When the uterine serosa is penetrated, diffuse peritoneal spread may occur. Hematogenous spread to lung, bone, liver, and brain is much more common with endometrial cancer than with cervical cancer. As with cervical carcinoma, MRI is preferred for preoperative imaging staging of known tumors. CT is generally not used for initial diagnosis or local staging, although unsuspected tumors may be encountered. CT staging is reported to be on the order of 60% accurate compared with 90% for MRI. Surgical staging is the method of choice. Imaging staging is useful in patients with advanced disease or who are difficult to examine clinically.

- Endometrial cancers are isoattenuating with uterine tissue on unenhanced CT, and therefore cannot be reliably differentiated from myometrium.
- On postcontrast CT the primary tumor appears as diffuse thickening of the endometrium or as a hypodense polypoid mass within the endometrial cavity (Fig. 18.16). The uterine cavity is frequently fluid filled owing to tumor obstruction. Fluid may assist in outlining mural implants of tumor in the expanded uterine cavity. The uterus may be greatly enlarged. The tumor typically enhances heterogeneously and less so than the surrounding myometrium.

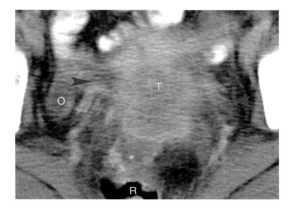

FIG. 18.15 **Cervical carcinoma invading the parametrium and obstructing the ureter.** An ill-defined tumor mass *(T)* of squamous cell carcinoma of the cervix shows extensive nodular stranding *(arrowheads)* in the parametrium, indicating tumor invasion. The left ureter was obstructed at this level. The rectum *(R)* was also invaded. *O*, Right ovary.

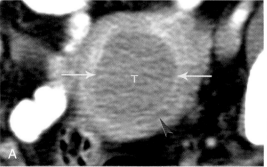
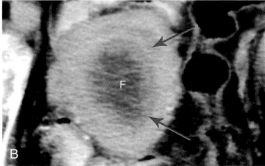

FIG. 18.16 **Endometrial carcinoma.** (A) A low-attenuation tumor mass *(T)* of endometrial carcinoma fills the uterine cavity (between *yellow arrows*) of this postmenopausal woman. A few millimeters of posterior myometrium *(red arrowhead)* was invaded by this neoplasm. (B) In another postmenopausal patient, bloody fluid *(F)* distends the uterine cavity. Endometrial tumor *(arrows)* is intermediate in attenuation between the dark fluid and the enhancing myometrium. This tumor also invades less than 50% thickness of the myometrium.

- Myometrial invasion may be recognized as hypodense infiltrating tumor within the more enhanced normal myometrium. CT is less than 60% accurate in evaluating the depth of myometrial invasion.
- Cervical invasion is indicated by heterogeneous enlargement of the cervix.
- Irregular uterine margins and strands and nodules of soft tissue extending into adjacent fat are evidence of parametrial invasion.
- Enlarged pelvic lymph nodes (>1 cm) indicate tumor involvement. However, as with other pelvic tumors, CT will miss microscopic nodal metastases that do not enlarge the nodes. CT can be used to guide percutaneous biopsy of suspicious lymph nodes.
- Müllerian mixed tumor is suggested by massive enlargement of the uterus, large areas of necrosis and hemorrhage within the tumor, and rapid growth of metastases.
- Tumor recurrences appear as pelvic soft-tissue masses or nodal enlargement. Most recurrences happen within 2 years.

OVARIES
Ovarian Cancer

Ovarian malignancy encompasses a wide range of histologic tumor types, but most share a common pattern of spread and similar range of CT appearances. Two-thirds of ovarian cancers are cystic, 25% are bilateral, and 15% are endocrinologically functional. The primary route of tumor spread is diffusion throughout the peritoneal cavity, present in 70% of cases at the time of diagnosis. Direct extension to pelvic organs, lymphatic spread to nodes, and hematogenous spread to lung, liver, and bone also occur. Most patients are directly referred for surgery for initial staging, hysterectomy, salpingo-oophorectomy, omentectomy, and tumor debulking without preoperative imaging. CT is, however, the imaging method of choice for documenting residual tumor and response to therapy and for detection of postoperative recurrence. MRI remains inferior to CT, primarily because of the difficulty in differentiating intraperitoneal tumor from bowel. The staging accuracy of CT is about 80%. The CT findings of ovarian malignancy include the following:

- The primary tumor is usually cystic with thick irregular walls, internal septations, and prominent soft-tissue components (Fig. 18.17). Uniformly solid tumors and mixed cystic/solid tumors also occur. Calcifications may be evident in both the primary tumor and metastases.

- Direct tumor extension commonly involves the uterus, colon, small bowel, and bladder. Tumor extension to adjacent pelvic organs is suggested by distortion or an irregular interface between the tumor and myometrium, obliteration of tissue planes between the tumor and bladder or colon, less than 3-mm separation between the tumor and intrapelvic muscles, and displacement or encasement of pelvic blood vessels. Bowel involvement is evidenced by thickening of the bowel wall, matting together of bowel loops, and evidence of bowel obstruction.
- Peritoneal implants are seen as often subtle thickening or enhancement of the peritoneum, or as soft tissue nodules of variable size (see Figs. 9.4–9.6). Key areas to carefully examine include the undersurfaces of the diaphragm, the paracolic gutters, the cul-de-sac, and the surface of the bowel. The presence of ascites makes peritoneal implants more evident on CT. *Omental cake* refers to irregular, often marked, thickening of the greater omentum separating the bowel from the anterior abdominal wall. The greater omentum, normally of fat density, becomes of soft-tissue density when it is involved by tumor. Extensive peritoneal seeding when the tumor nodules are small (<5 mm) may not be evident.
- The presence of ascites usually indicates peritoneal spread even if peritoneal tumor nodules are not visualized.
- Lymphatic metastases usually follow gonadal lymphatics, skipping pelvic nodes, to involve lymph nodes at the renal hilum, a pattern similar to that of testicular cancers.
- Hematogenous spread of tumor occurs late in the course of the disease. Advanced disease or tumor recurrence may be seen as solid organ metastases in the liver and spleen.

Benign Adnexal Findings

Although ultrasonography is the primary imaging modality for female pelvic masses, adnexal masses may be discovered incidentally on CT. CT may also be used to further characterize unclear ultrasound diagnoses. Some conditions to consider include the following:

- *Normal ovaries* are seen as oval soft-tissue masses of approximately 4 × 3 × 2 cm in women of childbearing age. Follicles are best seen on postcontrast scans (Fig. 18.18). Visualization of follicles provides definitive identification of the ovary. Normal follicles are thin-walled low-attenuation cysts smaller than 3 cm. Postmenopausal ovaries are smaller and lack follicles, making them more difficult to identify. Ovaries may be confused with bowel, blood vessels, and lymph nodes.

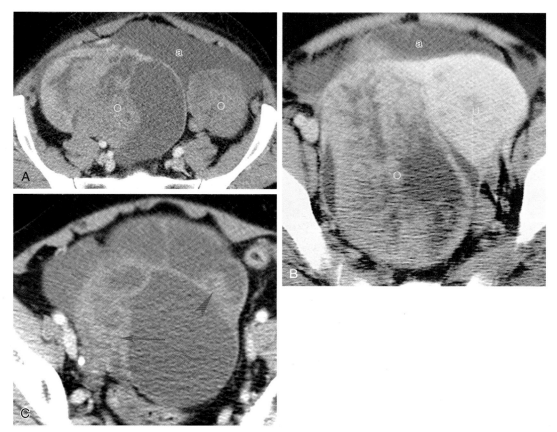

FIG. 18.17 **Ovarian carcinoma.** (A) Both ovaries *(O)* are replaced and enlarged by tumors with predominant solid components. Ascites *(a)* is present, providing strong evidence of tumor spread to the peritoneal cavity. An enhancing tumor nodule (arrow) is seen implanted on the parietal peritoneum. (B) A large mass *(O)* with predominant solid components arises from the right ovary and displaces the uterus *(U)* anteriorly and leftward. Ascites *(a)* is present. (C) A predominantly cystic mass arises from the right ovary. Nodular septations *(arrowhead)* and enhancing solid components *(arrow)* are evidence of malignancy. The tumor proved to be a serous cystadenocarcinoma.

- *Normal corpus luteum.* Following ovulation the corpus luteum is the highly vascular structure that identifies the location on the ovary of the ruptured dominant follicle. The normal corpus luteum is highly variable in appearance, seen as a collapsed cyst, a thick or thin-walled cyst, or a solid mass. A key feature is intense enhancement of the cyst wall or solid tissue (Fig. 18.19). Because patients may present with pelvic pain related to ovulation and undergo CT examination, this normal physiologic structure must be recognized. Recent ovulation may be further evidenced by a small volume of hemorrhagic fluid in dependent pelvic recesses. The normal corpus luteum resolves with menstruation.

- *Functional ovarian cysts.* Benign ovarian cysts, including follicular cysts, dominant follicles, and corpus luteum cysts, are common incidental findings. On CT they are well defined, are thin walled (<3 mm), have homogeneous internal density near that of water, and are larger than 3 cm (Fig. 18.20).

- *Hemorrhagic functional cysts* appear more complex, with internal attenuation above that of water. Fluid-fluid levels and clots outlined by lower-attenuation fluid may be present. The key features are that the walls of the cyst are uniform in thickness and enhancement, and that no enhancement is present internally within the cyst. Acute hemorrhage into a functional cyst may cause acute pelvic pain. The

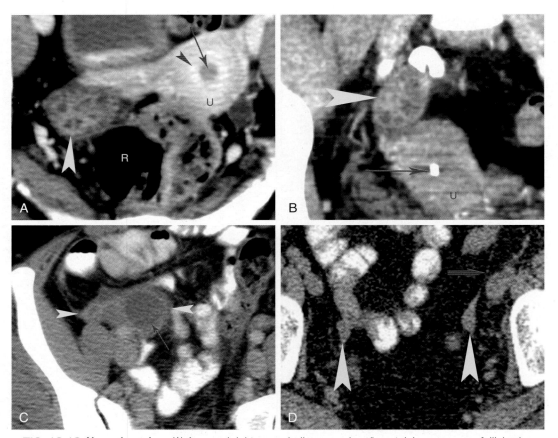

FIG. 18.18 Normal ovaries. (A) A normal right ovary *(yellow arrowhead)* containing numerous follicles is seen adjacent to the uterus *(U)* in a 32-year-old woman. Administration of intravenous contrast medium has enhanced the walls of the follicles, making them more visible than on noncontrast scans. The uterine cavity contains fluid *(red arrow)*, and the endometrium *(red arrowhead)* is enhances. (B) In another patient, aged 25 years, coronal CT demonstrates the variable position of the normal ovary *(yellow arrowhead)* cranial to the uterus *(U)*. An intrauterine device *(red arrow)* is partially visualized within the uterine cavity. (C) A thin-walled 2.5-cm cyst *(red arrow)* on the right ovary (between *yellow arrowheads*) is a dominant follicle in this 34-year-old woman. This is a normal physiologic structure. No further evaluation or follow-up is necessary. (D) Normal postmenopausal ovaries *(yellow arrowheads)* are identified bilaterally in this 68-year-old woman. A landmark confirming the identity of the small postmenopausal ovary is the suspensory ligament *(red arrow)* of the ovary, which extends in the broad ligament to the pelvic sidewall. *R*, Rectum.

cyst may rupture and hemorrhage into the peritoneal cavity (Fig. 18.21). Functional and hemorrhagic ovarian cysts can be reexamined with ultrasonography to determine if they resolve after one or two menstrual cycles.

- *Benign cystic teratoma.* The presence of fat-density fluid, teeth, bone, hair, or fat-fluid levels allows definitive CT diagnosis of benign cystic teratoma in most cases (Fig. 18.22). Dermoid plugs are conglomerations of tissue and hair seen as soft-tissue nodules inside the cysts.

- *Ovarian cystadenoma.* Benign ovarian tumors tend to have regular thin walls, fine septations, no solid components, and no associated ascites (Fig. 18.23). Definitive differentiation of benign cystic ovarian tumors from malignant cystic ovarian tumors is not possible with CT. If the lesion persists on follow-up ultrasonography performed after two menstrual cycles, a cystic tumor may be suspected and further evaluation is warranted.

- *Paraovarian cysts* arise from the broad ligament, are uniformly benign, and account for 10% to 20% of

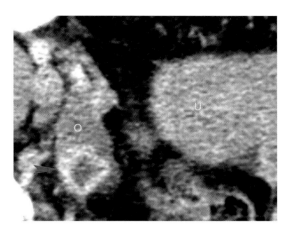

FIG. 18.19 **Normal corpus luteum.** A rim-enhancing mass *(red arrowhead)* on the right ovary *(O)* of a 28-year-old woman is characteristic of a normal corpus luteum, marking the site of ovulation. A small volume of fluid (not shown on this image) is often seen in the cul-de-sac in association with this normal finding. *U,* Uterus.

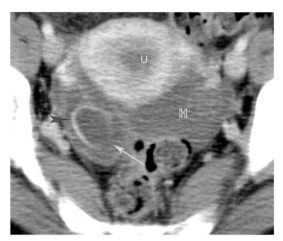

FIG. 18.21 **Hemorrhage functional cyst with rupture.** The thin enhancing wall *(red arrowhead)* of a functional ovarian cyst that has undergone spontaneous hemorrhage is discontinuous *(yellow arrow)* at the site of cyst rupture resulting in hemorrhage *(H)* into the peritoneal cavity. *U,* Uterus.

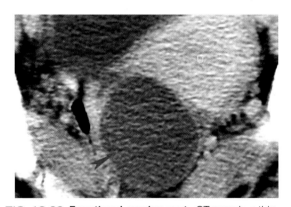

FIG. 18.20 **Functional ovarian cyst.** CT reveals a thin-walled 4.5-cm cyst *(arrowhead)* of uniformly low attenuation in the right adnexa adjacent to the uterus *(U)*. These characteristics are most indicative of a functional ovarian cyst. Follow-up with ultrasonography 10 weeks later confirmed complete resolution.

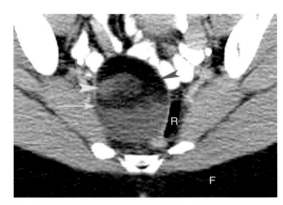

FIG. 18.22 **Benign cystic teratoma.** A mass impinging on the gas-filled rectum *(R)* is definitively characterized by CT to be a benign cystic teratoma arising from the right ovary. Fat-attenuation fluid *(red arrowhead)* representing sebum is characteristic. Compare the attenuation of the fluid with that of subcutaneous fat *(F)*. Suspended strands of hair within the sebum produces a fluid level *(yellow arrow)*, and a dermoid plug *(yellow arrowhead)* produces a soft-tissue nodule.

all adnexal masses. Most are thin-walled simple cysts that may be large (8 cm or greater) or small. Uncommonly they occur multiply or bilaterally. CT is diagnostic if the cyst can be accessed as being separate from the ovary.

- *Endometriomas* arise from deposits of endometrial glands and stroma on peritoneal surfaces. Most (80%) arise on the ovary. The wall is initially thin but may thicken and become irregular with time. Internal contents are of high attenuation, reflecting

blood (Fig. 18.24). Coexisting endometrial deposits on adjacent tissues may cause scarring and retraction, simulating malignant disease. Endometrial deposits often result in enhancement of the peritoneal surface. Endometriomas can be confirmed by MRI showing the characteristic finding of *"T2-shading."*

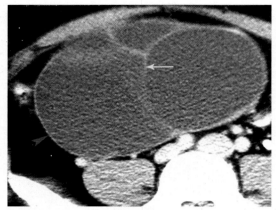

FIG. 18.23 **Benign mucinous ovarian cystadenoma.** A large cystic mass containing homogeneous low-attenuation fluid extends out of the pelvis. The outer walls *(red arrowhead)* and the internal septations *(yellow arrow)* are thin (<3 mm). Surgical removal and examination by pathology is needed to confirm a benign diagnosis.

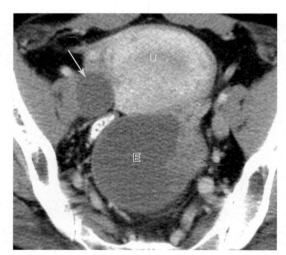

FIG. 18.24 **Endometrioma.** A well-defined thin-walled predominantly cystic mass *(E)* is shown in the cul-de-sac on post-contrast CT. The solid-appearing portion *(red arrowhead)* of the mass showed no enhancement. Serial CT images confirmed the mass as being separate from the ovaries. Subsequent MRI showed T2 shading characteristic of endometrioma. The solid portion of the lesion was confirmed as clotted blood. The right ovary contains a functional cyst *(yellow arrow)*. *U*, Uterus.

The fluid within endometriomas is of high intensity on T1-weighted images and show loss of signal intensity on T2-weighted images.

- *Peritoneal inclusion cysts* result from inflammation of the peritoneal lining that entraps a functioning

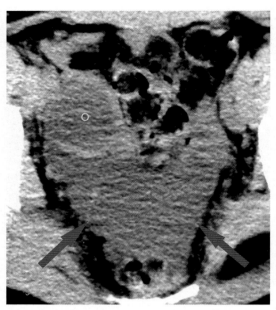

FIG. 18.25 **Peritoneal inclusion cyst.** CT image of the pelvis of a 41-year-old woman with chronic pelvic pain showing loculated fluid *(arrows)* distending the peritoneal recesses of the pelvis and incorporating the right ovary *(O)*.

ovary. The adhesions and inflammation impair absorption of peritoneal fluid and ovarian secretions. Patients present with periodic pelvic pain and swelling and frequently have a history of endometriosis or pelvic inflammatory disease. CT shows a unilocular or multilocular cystic mass expanding the contours of pelvic peritoneal recesses and entrapping an ovary (Fig. 18.25). Fluid extension into peritoneal recesses, rather than forming a rounded mass, is characteristic.

- *Hydrosalpinx* refers to a dilated fallopian tube filled with fluid caused by blockage of the tube at the fimbriated end. The causes include endometriosis, pelvic inflammatory disease, and scarring resulting from other infectious or inflammatory diseases of the pelvis. As the tube dilates, it becomes tortuous, folding back on itself, simulating a septate mass. Sagittal and coronal reformations are often helpful in recognizing the complex mass as a dilated tube (Fig. 18.26).

- *Spinal meningeal cyst,* also called a *perineural, arachnoid,* or *nerve root sheath cyst,* may mimic an ovarian or adnexal lesion. The cyst arises from and is intimately associated with the sacrum. It may be unilocular or multilocular, has thin walls, and contains fluid (cerebrospinal fluid) of water attenuation.

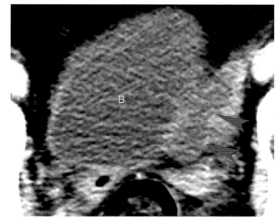

FIG. 18.26 **Hydrosalpinx.** Axial CT of the pelvis reveals an elongated fluid-filled tubular structure *(arrowheads)* with thick walls abutting the bladder.

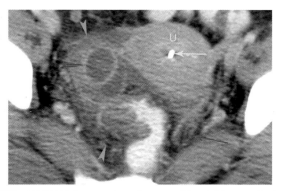

FIG. 18.27 **Tubo-ovarian abscess.** The right ovary *(red arrowhead)* is encased in purulent fluid (between *green arrowheads)* extending from the cul-de-sac. The left fallopian tube *(red arrow)* is filled with pus, with inflammatory thickening of its wall. An intrauterine device *(yellow arrow)* is present in the cavity of the uterus *(U)*.

Pelvic Inflammatory Disease

Pelvic inflammatory disease (PID) refers to infection and inflammation of the endometrium, fallopian tubes, and ovaries. Infection is caused by *Neisseria gonorrhoeae* or *Chlamydia trachomatis*, or is polymicrobial. CT is commonly the initial imaging study.

- Early findings include thickening of the fallopian tubes and enlargement (edema) and abnormal enhancement of the ovaries. Thickening of the wall of the fallopian tube is a highly specific CT finding of acute PID.
- More advanced PID presents with dilated fallopian tubes filled with high-attenuation fluid (pyosalpinx), and complex fluid collections with septa, debris, fluid-fluid levels, or gas in the adnexa. This inflammatory mass is called a *tubo-ovarian abscess* (Fig. 18.27).
- The inflammatory process may incorporate adjacent small bowel or large bowel, obstruct the ureters, and inflame and thicken the bladder wall.

Adnexal Torsion

With adnexal torsion the ovary, fallopian tube, or both structures twist on the vascular pedicle, causing vascular compromise. Torsion may be partial, impairing only venous drainage, complete, occluding arterial supply, or intermittent. Unrelieved torsion may result in hemorrhagic infarction of the ovary. Because patients often present with severe pain, CT may provide the initial images.

- Most cases of torsion involve a preexisting adnexal mass, most commonly a benign cystic teratoma, hydrosalpinx, or functional cyst. The wall of the mass thickens, and its contents may bleed with torsion.

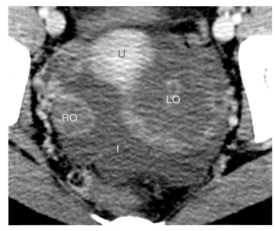

FIG. 18.28 **Left adnexal torsion.** CT of a 20-year-old woman with severe left pelvic pain shows complex enlargement of the cystic left ovary *(LO)* with wall thickening *(red arrowhead)*, fluid *(f)* in the cul-de-sac, and a normal right ovary *(RO)*. Acute left adnexal torsion was confirmed on surgery. *U,* Uterus.

- Major findings include thickening of the wall of the fallopian tube (>3 mm), tubal distension, smooth thickening of the wall of the mass, pelvic ascites, and deviation of the uterus to the affected side (Fig. 18.28).
- The twisted vascular pedicle may be visualized.
- Differential diagnosis of a complex adnexal mass includes tubo-ovarian abscess, ectopic pregnancy, and ruptured hemorrhagic ovarian cyst.

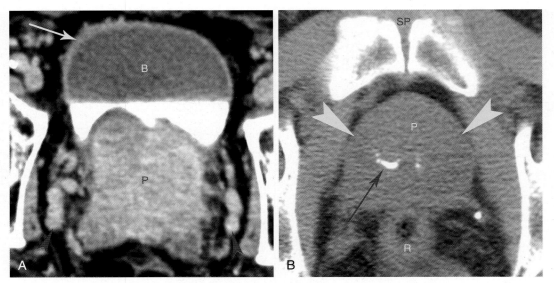

FIG. 18.29 Benign prostatic hypertrophy. (A) Axial plane delayed postcontrast CT reveals a large heterogeneous prostate *(P)* bulging into the base of the bladder *(B)*. The wall of the bladder *(yellow arrow)* shows mild hypertrophy reflecting outflow obstruction caused by prostatic enlargement. Prominent periprostatic vessels *(red arrowheads)* are evident. Prominent pelvic vessels are a common and benign finding confirmed by documenting contrast enhancement of the venous structures. (B) Noncontrast CT in another patient shows the characteristic coarse and linear calcifications *(red arrow)* associated with benign prostatic hypertrophy and chronic prostatitis. The prostate *(P)* is mildly enlarged *(yellow arrowheads)*. The symphysis pubis *(SP)* is the anatomic landmark for the normal location of the prostate. *R*, Rectum.

PROSTATE

Benign Prostatic Hypertrophy

Benign prostatic hypertrophy results in nodular enlargement of the prostate, with constriction of the urethra and obstruction of bladder emptying. It is indistinguishable from prostate carcinoma on CT.

- The prostate is enlarged and commonly has a lobulated contour (Fig. 18.29). Nodules may cause high- and low-attenuation regions within the prostate with variable enhancement.
- Cystic degeneration and coarse calcifications are common.
- The bladder base is elevated, and the prostate projects upward into the bladder lumen.
- Bladder wall thickening and trabeculation result from chronic bladder outlet obstruction. Diverticula may project through the bladder wall.

Prostate Cancer

Prostate cancer is the second most common malignancy in males. Prostate carcinoma spreads by direct extension to periprostatic tissues and the seminal vesicles. Lymphatic spread is similar to that in bladder cancer, with early involvement of internal iliac and obturator nodes and later involvement of para-aortic nodes. Hematogenous spread to the axial skeleton via vertebral veins is particularly characteristic. CT does not accurately demonstrate intraprostatic architecture and is poor at demonstrating intraprostatic tumor (Fig. 18.30). CT for regional staging of prostate cancer is neither sensitive nor specific enough to be clinically useful. CT may be used to detect distant metastases. Multiparametric MRI is now the imaging method of choice for detection and staging of prostate cancer. The Prostate Imaging and Reporting Data System, now in version 2, provides international consensus for a standardized reporting system based on multiparametric MRI.

- Enlargement of the prostate is common and may be as a result of benign prostatic hypertrophy and/or tumor growth. Nodules or stranding densities in the periprostatic fat are CT signs of tumor extension outside the prostate gland.
- Asymmetric size of the seminal vesicles and infiltration of fat between the bladder base, prostate, and seminal vesicles are CT evidence of tumor involvement. Bladder involvement is very difficult to detect accurately on CT. Rectal invasion is rare.
- Nodes larger than 10 mm on CT are usually involved with metastatic tumor.

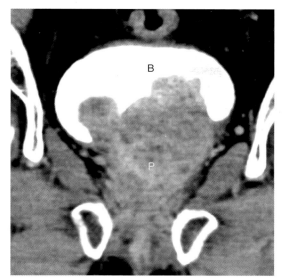

FIG. 18.30 **Prostate cancer.** Coronal CT image showing massive nodular enlargement of the prostate (P) elevating the base of the bladder (B) and projecting into the bladder lumen with prominent nodules. Transrectal prostate biopsy revealed predominantly benign prostatic hypertrophy with cancer in the right prostate lobe. The cancer is indistinguishable on CT from benign hypertrophy. Cystoscopy is indicated to exclude a uroepithelial tumor arising from the bladder mucosa.

Cystic Lesions of the Prostate

Cystic lesions of the prostate are uncommon but often prominent findings on CT of the male pelvis.

- *Prostate abscess* occurs as a complication of bacterial prostatitis. Patients present with pelvic pain, dysuria, fever, and tenderness on transrectal prostate examination. In patients with acute prostatitis, failure to improve with antibiotic treatment or development of sepsis suggests possible prostate abscess. CT shows a complex fluid collection within the prostate (Fig. 18.31). Periprostatic inflammatory changes and prominent vascularity may be present.
- *Prostatic utricle cysts* and *müllerian duct cysts* are congenital lesions of the prostate that are indistinguishable by CT. Both appear on CT as well-defined cysts in the midline in the upper half of the prostate (Fig. 18.32). Small cysts are usually incidental lesions, whereas large cysts may cause bladder outlet obstruction, pain, and hematuria.
- *Cysts associated with benign prostatic hypertrophy* are the cysts most commonly found in the prostate gland and are usually located laterally rather than in the midline of the gland.

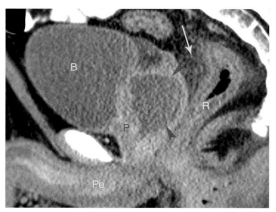

FIG. 18.31 **Prostate abscess.** Sagittal plane CT reveals a large fluid collection *(red arrowheads)* that expands and distorts the prostate gland (P) in this patient with pyuria, dysuria, and severe pelvic pain. The bladder (B) is distended, reflecting painful urination and acute bladder outlet obstruction. Inflammatory stranding *(yellow arrow)* is present in the fatty tissue between the prostate and the rectum (R). *Pe*, Penis.

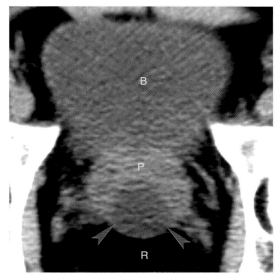

FIG. 18.32 **Utricle cyst of the prostate.** Axial CT without intravenous contrast medium shows a well-defined cyst *(red arrowheads)* in the midline of the prostate (P) in a 37-year-old man with bladder outlet obstruction symptoms. The prostate is not enlarged. Surgery confirmed a congenital utricle cyst of the prostate. *B*, Bladder; *R*, Gas-filled rectum.

- *Prostate retention cysts* occur with obstruction of prostate ductules usually in the lateral aspects of the gland.
- *Cystadenoma* of the prostate is a rare benign tumor consisting of cysts, glandular tissue, and fibrous stroma. Large lesions present with bladder outlet obstruction.
- *Cystic appearance of prostate carcinoma* is rare.

TESTES

Testicular Cancer

Testicular germ cell tumors can be separated into seminomas (55%) and nonseminomas (45%). Seminomas are treated with radical inguinal orchiectomy and radiation and generally do not require retroperitoneal node dissection for staging. Seminomas are highly curable even when disease is advanced. Nonseminomatous germ cell tumors include embryonal cell carcinoma, yolk sac tumors, teratoma, and choriocarcinoma. These tumors are radioresistant, are treated with orchiectomy and chemotherapy, and generally do require retroperitoneal node dissection for staging. Lymphatic spread of tumor is most common, with nodal involvement following an orderly ascending pattern. Initial spread is along gonadal lymphatics following testicular veins to renal hilar nodes. Alternatively, lymphatic metastases may follow the external iliac chain to the para-aortic nodes. Internal iliac and inguinal nodes are generally not involved. Lymphatic spread to the mediastinum and hematogenous spread to the lungs rarely occurs without para-aortic disease, except for choriocarcinoma, which spreads hematogenously early. CT remains the imaging method of choice for initial tumor staging.

- Pelvic and retroperitoneal adenopathy is most pronounced on the side of involvement. Nodal enlargement near the ipsilateral renal hilum is particularly characteristic (Fig. 18.33). Inguinal nodes are involved only when the scrotum is invaded by tumor. Bulky nodal metastases may have low attenuation internally as a result of tumor necrosis. Cystic changes and heterogeneity of lymph node attenuation are signs of tumor involvement. Use of 8-mm or larger short-axis dimension as the criterion for nodal involvement is highly specific but with low sensitivity. Up to 30% of patients may have metastatic nodal spread not detected by CT.
- Lymphoma may mimic germ cell tumors on CT. B-cell lymphoma is the most common testicular malignancy in men older than 60 years. It involves both testes in 30% of cases.
- Absence of the spermatic cord identifies the side of orchiectomy.

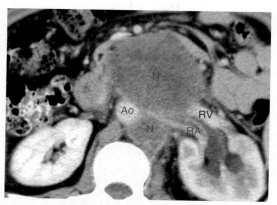

FIG. 18.33 Metastatic testicular cancer. In a patient with carcinoma of the left testis, CT at the level of the hilum of the left kidney shows massive confluent adenopathy *(N)* obstructing the left renal vein *(RV)* and enveloping the left renal artery *(RA)* and the aorta *(Ao)*. This is a typical location for metastatic spread of cancer from the left testis spreading along lymphatics, which parallel the course of the left testicular vein. Note delayed enhancement of the left kidney compared with the right kidney caused by renal vein obstruction.

Undescended Testes

Undescended testes may be located anywhere along the course of testicular descent from the lower pole of the kidney to the superficial inguinal ring. Undescended testes are at high risk of development of malignancy (48-fold risk) and of torsion (10-fold risk). CT is 95% sensitive for detection of ectopic testes.

- The undescended testis appears as an oval soft-tissue density of up to 4 cm. Undescended testes are usually atrophic. CT detection of intra-abdominal testes requires optimal bowel opacification and enhancement with intravenous contrast medium to opacify normal structures.
- Testes in the inguinal canal can be easily identified on CT as long as one knows where to look (Fig. 18.34). The inguinal canal runs an oblique, medially directed course through the flat muscles of the abdominal wall between the deep and superficial inguinal rings. The deep (internal) inguinal ring is located midway between the anterior superior iliac spine and the symphysis pubis. The superficial (external) inguinal ring is located just above the pubic crest.
- Undescended testes in adult men may be complicated by tumor.

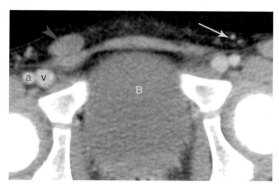

FIG. 18.34 **Undescended testis.** An undescended testis *(red arrowhead)* is seen in the right inguinal canal near the external inguinal ring in this 5-year-old boy with an undescended right testis. A normal spermatic cord *(yellow arrow)* in the inguinal canal is seen on the left. The left testis was in the normal location in the scrotum. *a*, Right common femoral artery; *B*, bladder; *v*, right common femoral vein.

SUGGESTED READING

Bladder

Lee, C. H., Tan, C. H., de Castro Faria, S., & Kundra, V. (2017). Role of imaging in the local staging of urothelial carcinoma of the bladder. *AJR. Am J Roentgenol, 208*, 1193–1205.

Raman, S. P., & Fishman, E. K. (2014). Bladder malignancies on CT: The underrated role of CT in diagnosis. *AJR. Am J Roentgenol, 203*, 347–354.

Wong-You–Cheong, J. J., Woodward, P. J., Manning, M. A., & Davis, C. J. (2006). Inflammatory and nonneoplastic bladder masses: Radiologic-pathologic correlation. *Radiographics, 26*, 1847–1868.

Uterus and Ovaries

Cohen, D. T., Oliva, E., Hahn, P. F., et al. (2007). Uterine smooth-muscle tumors with unusual growth patterns: Imaging with pathologic correlation. *AJR. Am J Roentgenol, 188*, 246–255.

Duigenan, S., Oliva, E., & Lee, S. I. (2012). Ovarian torsion: Diagnostic features on CT and MRI with pathologic correlation. *AJR. Am J Roentgenol, 198*, W122–W131.

Iraha, Y., Okada, M., Iraha, R., et al. (2017). CT and MR imaging of gynecologic emergencies. *Radiographics, 37*, 1569–1586.

Javadi, S., Ganeshan, D. M., Qayyum, A., et al. (2016). Ovarian cancer, the revised FIGO staging system, and the role of imaging. *AJR. Am J Roentgenol, 206*, 1351–1360.

Lalwani, N., Prasad, S. R., Vikram, R., et al. (2011). Histologic, molecular, and cytogenetic features of ovarian cancers: Implications for diagnosis and treatment. *Radiographics, 31*, 625–646.

Miccò, M., Sala, E., Lakhman, Y., et al. (2015). Imaging features of uncommon gynecologic cancers. *AJR. Am J Roentgenol, 205*, 1346–1359.

Raithantha, A., Papadopoulou, I., Stewart, V., et al. (2016). Cervical cancer staging: A resident's primer. *Radiographics, 36*, 933–934.

Revzin, M. V., Mathur, M., Dave, H. B., et al. (2016). Pelvic inflammatory disease: Multimodality imaging approach with clinical-pathologic correlation. *Radiographics, 36*, 1579–1596.

Prostate and Testes

Kreydin, E. I., Barrisford, G. W., Feldman, A. S., & Preston, M. A. (2013). Testicular cancer: What the radiologist needs to know. *AJR. Am J Roentgenol, 200*, 1215–1225.

Marko, J., Wolfman, D. J., Aubin, A. L., & Sesterhenn, I. A. (2017). Testicular seminoma and its mimics. *Radiographics, 37*, 1085–1098.

Moreno, C. C., Small, W. C., Camacho, J. C., et al. (2015). Testicular tumors: What radiologists need to know – differential diagnosis, staging, and management. *Radiographics, 35*, 400–415.

Rosenkrantz, A. B., Oto, A., Turkbey, B., & Westphalen, A. C. (2016). Prostate Imaging Reporting And Data System (PI-RADS), version 2: A critical look. *AJR. Am J Roentgenol, 206*, 117921183.

Tabatabaei, S., Saylor, P. J., Coen, J., & Dahl, D. M. (2011). Prostate cancer imaging: What surgeons, radiation oncologists, and medical oncologists want to know. *AJR. Am J Roentgenol, 196*, 1263–1266.

CHAPTER 19

CT in Musculoskeletal Trauma

NANCY M. MAJOR

INTRODUCTION

The advent of increasing numbers of rows of detectors has expanded the utility for CT technology. Multidetector CT (MDCT) has the ability to produce near-isotropic voxel images that allow multiplanar reformations and faster data acquisition. This technique is particularly valuable in the setting of trauma, for which conventional radiographs can be difficult to obtain because patients may be unable to comply with positioning requirements. Volume-rendered spiral CT can result in significant savings in terms of patient time spent in the radiology department. This technique also provides useful information for appropriate treatment and surgical planning by displaying three-dimensional spatial relationships in a two-dimensional image.

CT has two major roles in the evaluation of musculoskeletal trauma: (1) to define or exclude a fracture that was equivocal on conventional radiographs and (2) to determine the extent of a previously diagnosed fracture to assist in guiding therapy. In both trauma and nontrauma settings, spiral CT can provide information regarding soft-tissue abnormalities and demonstrate the osseous anatomy, particularly in anatomically complex areas such as the spine, pelvis, and scapula, for which conventional radiography may be limited.

Optimization of scanning techniques depends on the clinical question being addressed and the anatomic location to be examined. Small areas of interest combine narrow collimation (1–2 mm) and a pitch of 1 to 1.5 with small reconstructed increments (1 mm). Large areas of interest can be examined with wider collimation (3 mm) and a pitch of 1 to 2 with reconstruction every 2 to 3 mm.

There is considerable interest in CT dose reduction. In some circumstances, such as imaging of metallic prostheses, the exposure factors (peak kilovoltage and tube current) cannot be reduced without image quality being affected. The patient dose can be limited by careful positioning of the anatomic structure

and limiting the area to be scanned. Low-kilovoltage techniques have been described for extremity and pelvis imaging without significant degradation of images. The polytrauma patient dose can be decreased by making a single pass of the chest, abdomen, and pelvis rather than scouting and scanning each region separately.

In the setting of trauma, MDCT is used to assess other body regions, and studies have shown that the spine can be included as part of the scan. Because of the high-quality two- and three-dimensional images, adequate images of the thoracic and lumbar spine can be obtained from chest and abdominal CT data (Fig. 19.1).

Three-dimensional reconstructions are often performed for fractures of the acetabulum, scapula, and calcaneus and for complicated fractures of the pelvis to assist with surgical planning (Fig. 19.2).

According to the current American College of Radiology appropriateness criteria, the use of radiography in patients suspected of having a cervical spine injury should be reserved for adult patients when MDCT is not readily available, indicating that radiography should not be considered a substitute for CT. However, radiation exposure should always be minimized. Exposure during CT evaluations can be reduced by the use of automated exposure-control options according to the patient's body habitus. Many manufacturers of CT equipment have developed dose-reduction solutions.

CERVICAL SPINE TRAUMA

MDCT can detect 97% to 100% of cervical spine fractures, compared with 60% to 70% for conventional radiography. MDCT is widely used to complement conventional radiography for examination of the cervical spine following blunt trauma. Before helical scanning became available, conventional radiographs were the only radiologic means of imaging the cervical spine to exclude or diagnose injury following

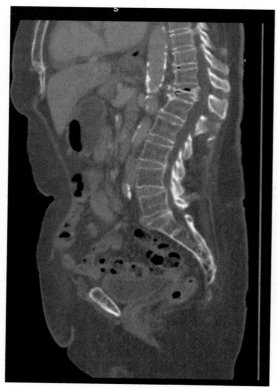

FIG. 19.1 Reformatted spine image. Sagittal reformatted image from chest-abdomen-pelvis CT demonstrating the marked compression fracture of T12.

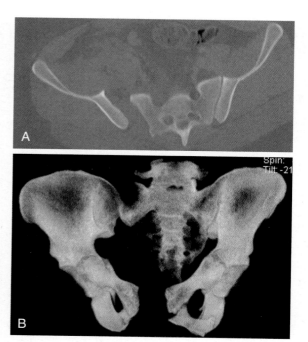

FIG. 19.2 Pelvic fracture. (A) Axial image through the pelvis during chest-abdomen-pelvis trauma CT revealing an open book pelvic fracture with marked diastasis of the right sacroiliac joint. (B) Three-dimensional reconstruction in a different polytrauma patient shows the complex fracture around the pelvic ring with diastasis of the pubic symphysis.

blunt trauma. The limitations of conventional radiography include poor visualization of areas with overlapping structures and the presence of other disease such as osteoarthrosis or rheumatoid arthritis or superimposed artifacts such as an endotracheal tube (Fig. 19.3). In addition, the lower cervical and upper thoracic spine can be difficult to image on conventional radiographs for similar reasons and is well visualized by MDCT (Fig. 19.4).

Importantly, in the clinical setting of spine fusion, either with hardware or secondary to ankylosis from ankylosing spondylitis or diffuse idiopathic skeletal hyperostosis, in a patient who presents with suspected injury after blunt trauma, a search for a fracture must include CT with reformatted images (Fig. 19.5).

The detection accuracy for ligamentous injury of MDCT is not clearly documented, and magnetic resonance imaging (MRI) is highly sensitive in detecting these injuries.

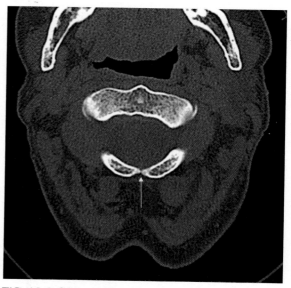

FIG. 19.3 C1 incomplete fusion. Axial CT image through C1 showing an incomplete fusion *(arrow)*. Because of bone overlap, the lucency on a conventional radiograph could not conclusively visualize this area.

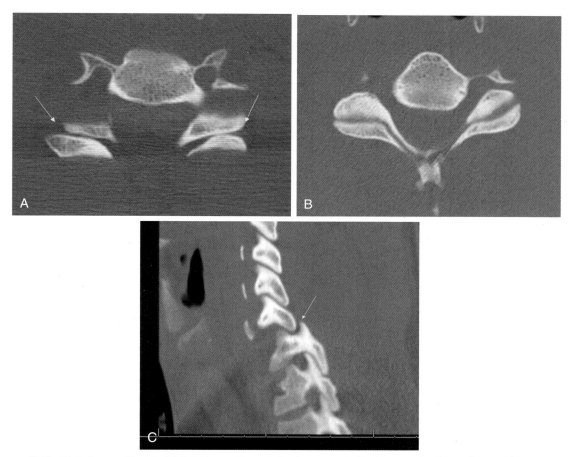

FIG. 19.4 **Jumped facet.** (A) Axial image through the lower cervical spine revealing jumped facets *(arrows)*. (B) Axial image showing normal facet joints for comparison. (C) Sagittal reformatted image revealing the malalignment of the facet joint *(arrow)*.

THORACIC SPINE

The thoracic spine is demonstrated nicely with reformatted images for chest-abdomen-pelvis CT in the setting of blunt trauma. CT can readily demonstrate a compression fracture (isolated to the vertebral body) from an unstable fracture involving the posterior elements, thus requiring surgical intervention (Fig. 19.1). An unstable fracture involving the posterior elements is seen on conventional radiographs as widening of the interpedicular distance. As stated earlier and worth reiterating, for a patient who has fusion of the thoracic spine and presents with back pain after blunt trauma, a fracture must be sought with use of CT with reformatted images. An additional utility of CT is assessment of

the presence of an underlying lesion that may not be appreciated with conventional radiography. A pathologic fracture can more readily be diagnosed and the extent of the pathologic process more accurately determined (Fig. 19.6).

LUMBAR SPINE

Compression deformities of the lumbar spine are regularly seen on routine spine evaluation with conventional radiographs. When such an observation is made in the setting of trauma, an acute fracture is difficult to exclude as a cause, particularly if the patient is experiencing pain referable to this area.

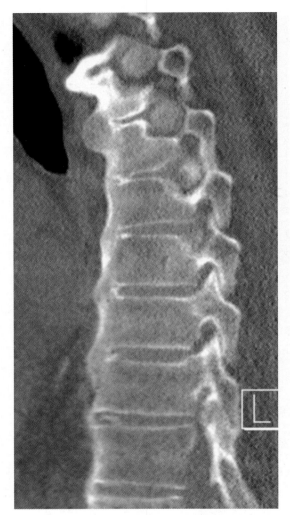

FIG. 19.5 Diffuse idiopathic skeletal hyperostosis.
Sagittal reformatted image coned to the upper and mid
thoracic spine in a patient with diffuse idiopathic skeletal
hyperostosis after a motor vehicle crash and upper back
pain. Note the osseous fusion anteriorly. In individuals
with spine fusion (osseous or postsurgical) with pain after
trauma, CT should be done to exclude a fracture.

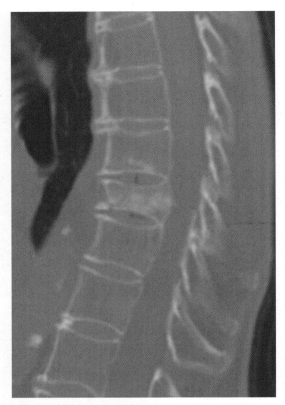

FIG. 19.6 Pathologic fracture of the thoracic spine.
Sagittal reformatted image through the thoracic and upper
lumbar spine revealing a compression fracture of the
vertebral body. The increased density within the vertebral
body is from a metastatic lesion. Note the convex posterior
margin seen with collapse of a vertebral body with metastatic disease.

Cross-sectional imaging can aid in diagnosing fractures of the vertebral body. If a fracture is suspected
on screening of the thoracolumbar spine during a CT
assessment of the chest and abdomen/pelvis for internal organ injury, a repeated scan for specific evaluation of thoracic or lumbar injury may be necessary
(Fig. 19.7).

CT examination provides accurate depiction of
the extension of fractures into the posterior elements
and of fracture fragments into the spinal canal. Volume rendering can provide additional assessment of
the extent of the fracture. If the patient has neurologic
symptoms, MRI can be performed as a complementary
examination.

In the lumbar spine, spondylolysis (pars interarticularis defect) is a posttraumatic entity that is clearly
shown by CT. A pars interarticularis defect can be a
result of an acute injury or secondary to repetitive stress
changes through the osseous pars. Pars defects can be
readily identified in an axial slice at the mid vertebral
body. Other structures present at this level include the
basivertebral plexus, identified in the posterior mid

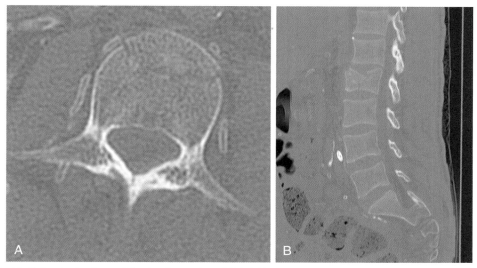

FIG. 19.7 **Acute fracture of the lumbar spine.** (A) Axial image through L2 demonstrating end plate fractures. The pedicles are not disrupted, and the fracture is confined to the vertebral body. (B) Sagittal reformatted representative image confirming the lack of posterior element involvement or compromise of the central canal.

vertebral body at the same level where the pedicles are also identified. The lamina should be a continuous bony ring at the midbody slice, and a defect in the osseous ring is a spondylolysis (Fig. 19.8). A pars interarticularis break can be overlooked, particularly if the defect is smooth along its margins and resembles facet joints. For this reason, any defect in the bony ring that occurs on a slice that includes the basivertebral plexus is a spondylolysis until proven otherwise. Another way to identify a pars interarticularis defect is to recognize that facet joints should not be present on every axial image obtained through the vertebral body. If facet joints are noted on each image through the vertebral body, a pars interarticularis defect is likely.

Imaging with CT can also assist in identifying the presence of a pathologic fracture. The presence of a superimposed lytic or blastic lesion in the setting of a collapsed vertebral body can be readily ascertained with cross-sectional imaging, and the pattern of the trabecular arrangement can help in identifying a pathologic fracture from multiple myeloma/plasmacytoma (Fig. 19.9). Patients with preexisting conditions such as a primary malignancy may also experience blunt trauma, and thus the pattern of the fracture and the appearance of the vertebral body and its trabeculae must be evaluated in all settings of trauma.

HIP AND PELVIS

After a fracture has been determined or is suspected on conventional radiography, or noted on chest-abdomen-pelvis trauma CT, dedicated CT through the pelvis is recommended for further characterization (Fig. 19.10). CT will assist in identifying other occult pelvic ring fractures not identified on the initial radiographs as well as detailing the appearance of the fracture about the hip. If a patient has sustained a hip dislocation, CT on reduction is recommended to exclude intra-articular fracture fragments or loose bodies and assist with surgical planning (Fig. 19.11). If intra-articular fracture fragments or loose bodies go undetected, they may lead to accelerated articular cartilage destruction as a result of irregular joint articulation. Multiplanar reconstruction capabilities reduce the need for additional radiographs, thus decreasing the radiation dose to the patient.

Sacral stress fractures and insufficiency fractures have a characteristic appearance on CT. Sacral stress fractures occur most often in the athletic population secondary to abnormal stresses across normal bone. This has been described in long-distance runners, for example. CT will demonstrate a fracture line parallel to the sacroiliac joint. Callus formation along the fracture may also be seen as linear sclerosis. It is important to

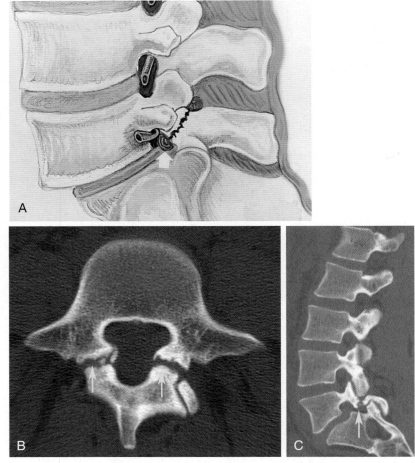

FIG. 19.8 Spondylolysis. (A) Artist rendering of a pars interarticularis break *(arrow)*. (B) Axial CT image demonstrating a bilateral spondylolysis *(arrows)*. (C) Reformatted sagittal CT image nicely depicting the pars interarticularis break *(arrow)*. No spondylolisthesis is present.

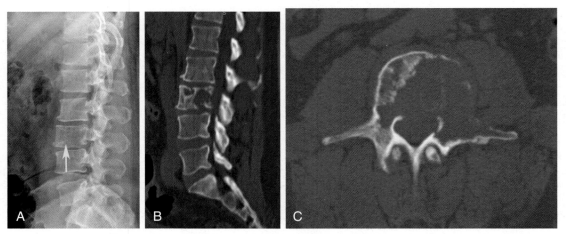

FIG. 19.9 Lytic lesion with pathologic fracture. (A) Lateral radiograph through the lumbar spine taken after acute onset of low back pain while the patient was riding in a car that went over a bump in the road demonstrating a lytic lesion through the L3 vertebral body *(arrow)*. (B) Sagittal reformatted CT image demonstrating a lytic lesion through the L3 vertebral body with a pathologic fracture. (C) Axial CT through the L3 vertebral body demonstrates a large lytic lesion. Cross-sectional imaging also allows identification of potential associated soft-tissue mass.

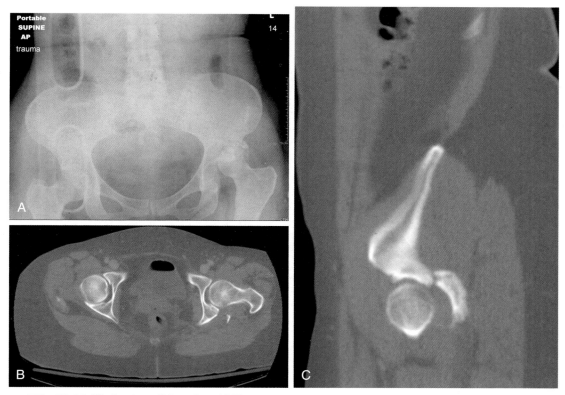

FIG. 19.10 Hip fracture dislocation. (A) Trauma, portable anteroposterior pelvis obtained in the emergency department demonstrates a fracture dislocation of the left hip. (B) Axial CT image after reduction demonstrating the fracture of the posterior acetabulum. (C) Sagittal reformatted CT image demonstrating the displacement of the posterior acetabulum. The reformatted images assist with surgical planning.

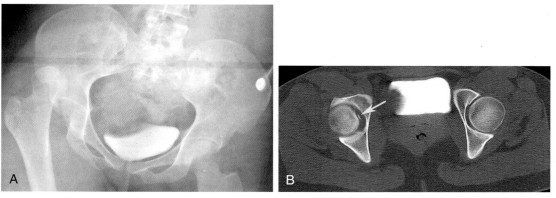

FIG. 19.11 Hip dislocation. (A) Conventional radiograph of the pelvis demonstrating a right hip dislocation. (B) Axial CT image after reduction showing an intra-articular body in the right hip joint *(arrow)*.

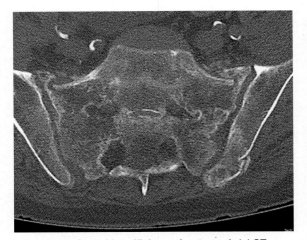

FIG. 19.12 Sacral insufficiency fracture. Axial CT image through the sacrum demonstrating bilateral sacral insufficiency fractures in this osteoporotic male patient. Note the fracture lines parallel the sacroiliac joint. The linearity of the fracture lines and the presence of intact sacral foramina indicates an insufficiency fracture and not metastatic disease.

assess the sacrum on lumbar spine CT in patients being imaged for low back pain. In this patient population, in particular, sacral stress fractures may mimic lumbar disk disease.

Sacral insufficiency fractures occur as a result of normal stresses through abnormal bone and are seen in osteoporotic patients and those who have had pelvic radiation therapy that included the sacrum in the radiated field. The fracture lines parallel the sacroiliac joint and can be bilateral. Recognition of the linear fracture line excludes metastatic disease as a cause of back pain in this patient population (Fig. 19.12).

Supra-acetabular insufficiency fractures are another type of fracture worth recognizing. They can be mistaken for metastatic lesions when imaged by MRI, and the curvilinear fracture line is not evident. CT will clearly depict the fracture line. Patients who have had pelvic radiation therapy in this location and those with osteoporosis can experience these painful insufficiency fractures (Fig. 19.13).

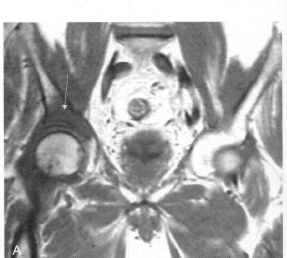
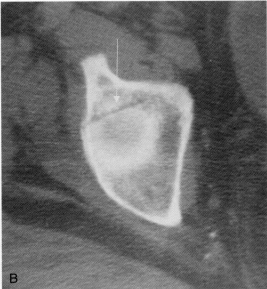

FIG. 19.13 Supra-acetabular insufficiency fracture. (A) Coronal T1-weighted image in a 60-year-old woman with right hip pain and a history of breast cancer demonstrating a focus of diffuse low signal in the right supra-acetabular region *(arrow)*. (B) Axial CT through the acetabulum reveals the linear fracture line *(arrow)*. Patients who are at risk of sacral insufficiency fractures are also at risk of supra-acetabular insufficiency fractures (post radiation and osteoporotic).

SCAPULA

Fractures of the scapula are a result of high-velocity injury and often accompany injuries to the shoulder, chest wall, and lungs. These fractures can be very difficult to identify by conventional radiography because of bone overlap, mediastinal structures, and associated rib fractures. CT with reformations will accurately depict the location and extent of scapular fractures, which will assist with operative intervention if the glenoid is involved or a fracture dislocation is present.

CT of the shoulder is recommended, as in the fracture dislocation of the hip, after reduction, if the joint remains distended or abnormal in appearance to exclude the possibility of an intra-articular fracture fragment or loose body.

Posterior shoulder dislocations can be difficult to identify on conventional radiographs. If all anteroposterior radiographs appear to be in internal rotation, this suggests the patient has limited mobility at the joint, and a posterior dislocation should be suspected and CT should be performed. The humeral head impaction and injury to the glenoid can be appreciated (Fig. 19.14).

RIBS

Rib and sternum trauma are an important topic. Sternal fractures are on the rise as a result of airbag deployment in motor vehicle crashes. Although a flail chest remains a clinical diagnosis, the pattern of rib involvement as demonstrated on CT can assist with appropriate management by the recognition of associated soft-tissue and organ injury. Similarly, trauma to the sternum suggests high-velocity blunt trauma, and suspicion for associated soft-tissue, vascular, pulmonary, or cardiac injury exists (Fig. 19.15).

Injuries to the *first through fourth ribs* require high-velocity trauma and may be associated with vascular or brachial plexus injury (Fig. 19.16). Evaluation of the aortic arch and subclavian and brachial arteries may be indicated particularly when a widened mediastinum

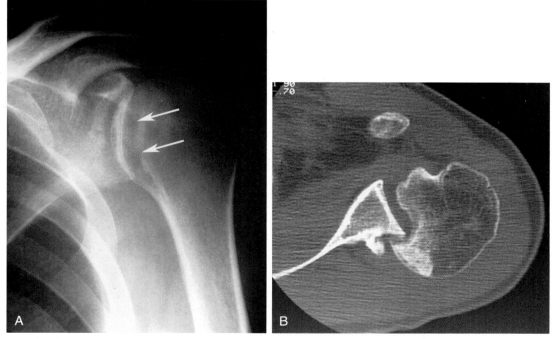

FIG. 19.14 **Posterior shoulder dislocation.** (A) Anteroposterior radiograph of the shoulder is in internal rotation. A vertical lucency in the humerus *(arrows)*, a trough sign, indicates an impaction from a posterior dislocation. (B) Axial CT image demonstrating an impacted, posteriorly dislocated humeral head and avulsion of the posterior glenoid.

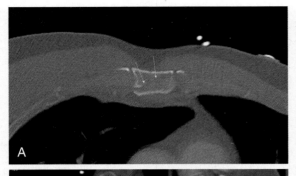

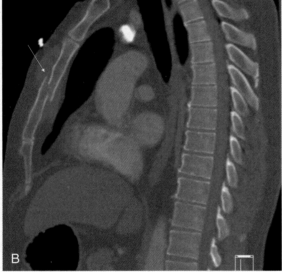

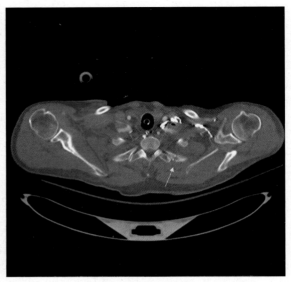

FIG. 19.16 **Upper rib injury.** Axial image through the chest demonstrating a posterior, nondisplaced rib fracture of the left second rib *(arrow)*. A fracture in this location warrants concern for additional soft-tissue/vascular injury.

FIG. 19.15 **Fracture of the sternum.** (A) Axial CT image through the chest demonstrating a minimally displaced fracture of the sternum *(arrows)*. (B) Sagittal reformatted image clearly depicting the fracture *(arrow)*. In the setting of a sternal fracture there should be an exhaustive search for associated injuries as this type of fracture indicates high-velocity blunt trauma.

is present. Injuries to the *fifth through ninth ribs* are more likely to be lateral or posterior. Rib fractures in this region can be associated with pulmonary laceration, contusion, hemothorax, and pneumothorax. Injuries to the lower ribs are considered markers for a solid organ injury such as liver and splenic injuries (Fig. 19.17).

The American College of Radiology has established an algorithm for the imaging evaluation of rib fractures. The first decision involves evaluation of the mechanism of injury. For blunt trauma with a high-energy mechanism, CT angiography or contrast-enhanced chest CT should be performed. In these situations the examination is tailored to investigate soft-tissue, vascular, or internal organ damage. Chest radiography is a complementary examination; however, studies have shown that injuries are underestimated on anteroposterior radiographs when compared with CT images. It is worth noting that the rib series radiation dose is similar to that of unenhanced chest CT.

Rib lesions can be incidentally noted, and these are discussed more in Chapter 20. However, potential confusion for a fracture may exist if there is a lack of knowledge of rib lesions. Although not an exhaustive list, chronic rib fractures with callus and fibrous dysplasia are the two most commonly encountered benign rib lesions (Fig. 19.18).

Up to 50% of rib fractures are missed on radiography even with dedicated oblique views. Dedicated views provide little, if any, additional information resulting in management change, and in the setting of trauma should be avoided unless documentation is necessary (legal requirement).

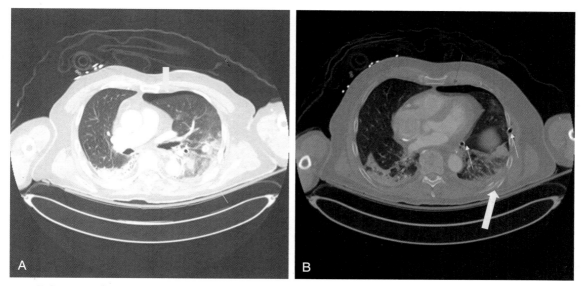

FIG. 19.17 **Acute posterior left fifth rib fracture.** (A) Evaluation of CT in lung windows demonstrates consolidation in the region of the posterior bilateral lungs with an anterior left pneumothorax *(fat yellow arrow)*. A minimally displaced posterior fifth rib fracture is present *(thin yellow arrow)*. (B) A chest tube has been placed *(thin yellow arrows)*, and the bone windows demonstrate the rib fracture to better advantage *(fat yellow arrow)*. The pneumothorax has decreased in size *(thin red arrow)*.

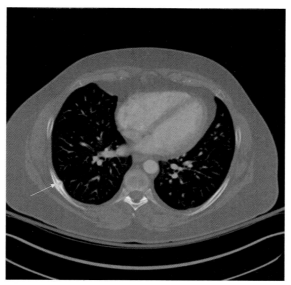

FIG. 19.18 **Benign rib lesions.** Subacute fracture with abundant callus formation should be easily recognized and not confused for a sclerotic metastatic lesion. In this example the fracture line is still evident *(arrow)*.

CONCLUSION

Imaging of the trauma patient should be fast, efficient, and accurate for timely diagnosis and management. MDCT with volume rendering achieves these goals and allows depiction of complex and difficult anatomic areas such as the spine, pelvis, shoulder girdle, and ribs. Knowledge of patterns of injury as detected on CT can assist with surgical and clinical management.

SUGGESTED READING

Buckwalter, K. A., Rydberg, J., Kopecky, K. K., Crow, K., & Yang, E. L. (2001). Musculoskeletal imaging with multislice CT. *AJR. Am J Roentgenol, 176*(4), 979–986.

Bush, L., Brookshire, R., Roche, B., et al. (2016). Evaluation of cervical spine clearance by computed tomographic scan alone in intoxicated patients with blunt trauma. *JAMA Surg, 151*(9), 807–813.

Inaba, K., Munera, F., McKenney, M., et al. (2006). Visceral torso computed tomography for clearance of the thoracolumbar spine in trauma: A review of the literature. *J Trauma, 60*(4), 915–920.

Klein, M. A. (2017). Lumbar spine evaluation: Accuracy on abdominal CT. *Br J Radiol, 90*(1079), 20170313.

Lee, S. H., Yun, S. J., Kim, D. H., Jo, H. H., Song, J. G., & Park, Y. S. (2017). Diagnostic usefulness of low-dose lumbar multi-detector CT with iterative reconstruction in trauma patients: A comparison with standard-dose CT. *Br J Radiol, 90*(1077), 20170181.

Munera, F., Rivas, L. A., Nunez, D. B., & Quencer, R. M. (2012). Imaging evaluation of adult spinal injuries: Emphasis on multidetector CT in cervical spine trauma. *Radiology, 263*(3), 645–660.

Talbot, B. S., Gange, C. P., Jr., Chaturvedi, A., Klionsky, N., Hobbs, S. K., & Chaturvedi, A. (2017). Traumatic rib injury: Patterns, imaging pitfalls, complications, and treatment— erratum. *Radiographics, 37*(3), 1004.

Verbeek, D. O., van der List, J. P., Villa, J. C., Wellman, D. S., & Helfet, D. L. (2017). Postoperative CT is superior for acetabular fracture reduction assessment and reliably predicts hip survivorship. *J Bone Joint Surg Am, 99*(20), 1745–1752.

Watura, R., Cobby, M., & Taylor, J. (2004). Multislice CT in imaging of trauma of the spine, pelvis and complex foot injuries. *Br J Radiol, 77*(Spec No 1), S46–S63.

CHAPTER 20

CT in Musculoskeletal Nontrauma

NANCY M. MAJOR

In this chapter entities such as disk disease and the osseous structures of the spinal canal will be discussed again, as well as postoperative spine changes. The appearances of the bones in the setting of some systemic diseases are additional descriptions in this chapter as are the incidentally encountered abnormalities in the axial skeleton and ribs when evaluation of chest-abdomen-pelvis imaging is performed. Metallic implants and the appearance of loosening, particle disease will also be demonstrated.

DISK DISEASE

The focus of this section is to demonstrate the utility of computed tomography (CT) in evaluating disk disease. Magnetic resonance imaging (MRI) has largely replaced CT for routine evaluation of disk disease and back pain. Because CT offers differences in density and the capability of multiplanar reformations and three-dimensional reconstruction, it is an excellent study and can easily be performed in patients who may not be a candidate for MRI. CT myelography is usually not necessary as disease can be readily depicted without the contrast from a myelogram.

The differences in density and the ability to image in bone as well as soft-tissue window allows the evaluation of disk disease and spinal canal and neuroforaminal narrowing, as well as assessment of nerve roots as they exit the thecal sac.

TECHNICAL CONSIDERATIONS

A proper imaging protocol for a diagnostic lumbar spine study is critical to reduce the chance of overlooking an abnormality. Patients should be scanned in a supine position with the knees slightly flexed over a cushion for comfort. Anteroposterior and lateral scout views are obtained. An anteroposterior scout view allows the radiologist to determine if transitional vertebrae are present. Recognition of transitional vertebrae and correct identification of vertebral body levels can prevent surgery at the wrong level. The lateral scout view is used to place cursors over the intended scan area. Contiguous slices,

no thicker than 5 mm, should be scanned from the midbody of L1 through the top of S1. The radiologist should protocol these studies to avoid performing angled gantry slices through the disk space alone. This "angled" approach leaves spaces or gaps in evaluation of the central canal, resulting in regions that are not imaged, allowing migrated free fragments of disk material and pars defects (spondylolysis) that occur at the mid vertebral body level to be missed if imaging is performed only through the disk spaces (Fig. 20.1). It is believed that angled images through the disk space more accurately

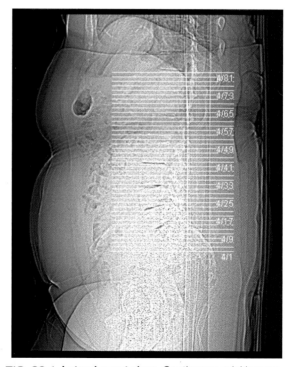

FIG. 20.1 **Lateral scout view.** Contiguous axial images, in this example, from the lower thoracic spine through the sacrum. There are no intervening gaps. This is the preferred protocol for evaluation of disk disease, spinal stenosis, and pars interarticularis defects.

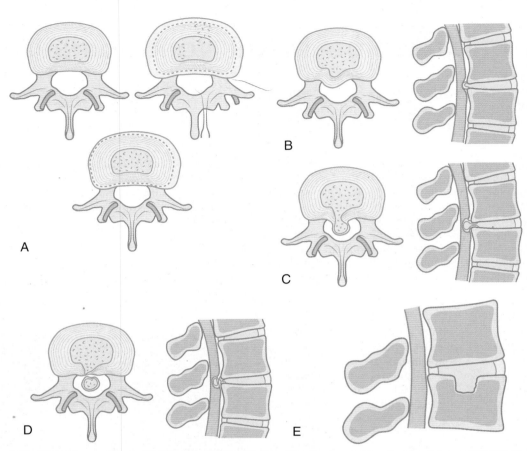

FIG. 20.2 **Nomenclature** (A) Disk bulge. Uniform bulge extending beyond the margins of the vertebral body throughout the circumference of the disk. (B) Protrusion. Disk material is displaced beyond less than 25% of the disk space with the greatest measure of displaced material less than the measure of the base of the displaced disk material at the disk space of origin. (C) Extrusion. Greatest measure of displaced disk material is greater than the measure of the base of the displaced disk material at the disk space of origin when measured in the same plane. (D) Sequestration. Disk material has lost continuity completely with the parent disk. (E) Schmorl node. Disks that move vertically through a gap in the vertebral body end plate. (Modified from Fardon, D. F., Williams, A. L., Dohring, E. J., Murtagh, F. R., Rothman, S. L., & Sze, G. K. (2014). Lumbar disc nomenclature: version 2.0: Recommendations of the combined task forces of the North American Spine Society, the American Society of Radiology and American Society of Neuroradiology. *Spine J*, *14*(11), 2525–2545.)

characterize disk protrusions than stacked, contiguous axial images particularly for surgeons at the time of surgery. However, changing the angle of the gantry will not falsely create nor eliminate disk protrusions that have a mass effect on the thecal sac. Thus contiguous imaging will identify disk disease, pars defects, and free fragments. If angled images are requested by the operating surgeon, one should be sure to also obtain contiguous images so as not to overlook potential disease contributing to the patient's symptoms.

Images should be obtained with a bone and soft-tissue algorithm. Images obtained with a soft-tissue algorithm are not suitable for accurate diagnosis of facet disease or other bone abnormalities. This technique can mimic hypertrophy of the normal anatomy. The combination of a soft-tissue algorithm to assess disk disease as well as nerve roots and ligamentum flavum and a bone algorithm to depict osseous abnormalities will accurately assess central canal and neuroforaminal narrowing. Sagittal and coronal reformatting is performed and will assist in the diagnosis of neuroforaminal narrowing, as well as bone fusion in the postoperative setting.

PATHOLOGY

Terminology is important in understanding and communicating the results of CT of the lumbar spine. The following terms are definitions accepted by American Society of Spine Radiology, the American Society of Neuroradiology, and the North American Spine Society and reflect changes in keeping with current concepts in radiologic and clinical care (Fig. 20.2).

A disk *bulge* is the presence of disk tissue extending beyond the edges of the vertebral body throughout the circumference of the disk. Disk bulges can be symmetric or asymmetric.

Disk *protrusion* is present when disk material is displaced beyond less than 25% of the disk space, with the greatest measure of displaced material less than the measure of the base of displaced disk material at the disk space of origin.

Extrusion is present when the greatest measure of displaced disk material is greater than the measure of the base of the displaced disk material at the disk space of origin when measured in the same plane. *Sequestration* is diagnosed when the disk material has lost continuity completely with the parent disk.

Disks that move vertically through a gap in the vertebral body end plate are referred to as *Schmorl nodes*. *Scheuermann disease* is a condition that can be seen incidentally when spine imaging is performed. This is a disease of childhood/adolescence that is a result of end plate osteochondrosis and multiple, sequential thoracic vertebral bodies that demonstrate multiple Schmorl nodes (Fig. 20.3). Adults are generally asymptomatic. When Scheuermann disease is severe, a kyphosis may occur.

Not surprisingly the CT images must correlate with the patient's symptoms. Disk material may demonstrate a mass effect on the thecal sac or a nerve root and may not be clinically symptomatic (Fig. 20.4).

The presence of a protrusion should prompt a search for a sequestration. Failure to recognize such an abnormality can lead to failed back surgery. A sequestration should be suggested when disk material (soft tissue higher in density than the thecal sac) is identified caudal or cephalad to the level of the disk space (Fig. 20.5). If the soft tissue is isodense to the thecal sac, it most likely represents a perineural cyst, Tarlov cyst, or conjoined nerve root. A Tarlov cyst is a perineural cyst and represents an enlarged nerve root sheath. It is a normal variant and rarely a cause of symptoms (Fig. 20.6).

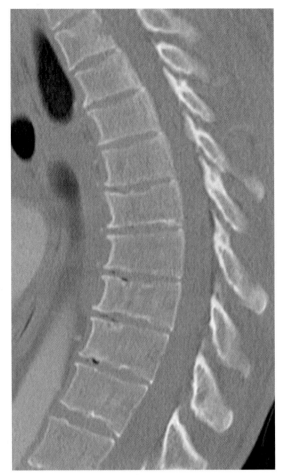

FIG. 20.3 **Scheuermann disease.** Multiple Schmorl nodes are incidentally found on the sagittal reformatted CT image. Note the end plate irregularities. This is an osteochondrosis that affects the maturing spine in childhood and adolescents.

Tarlov cysts can become large and erode bone as a result of cerebrospinal fluid (CSF) pulsations.

A conjoined nerve root is a congenital anomaly of two nerve roots exiting the thecal sac together instead of individually. The two nerve roots traverse the lateral recess together and appear as a density similar to that of the thecal sac on CT. A free fragment can have a similar appearance but will have higher attenuation compared with the thecal sac and conjoined nerve roots. The conjoined roots will invariably exit through their appropriate foramen (Fig. 20.7). An "empty" foramen is not encountered. Conjoined nerve roots are associated with a slightly wider

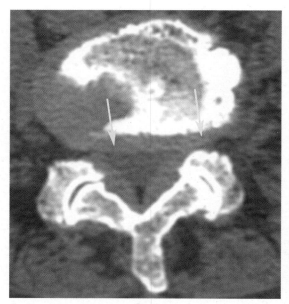

FIG. 20.4 **Broad-based disk bulge.** Axial CT image through the disk space demonstrating a broad-based disk bulge *(arrows)* demonstrating flattening of the anterior thecal sac.

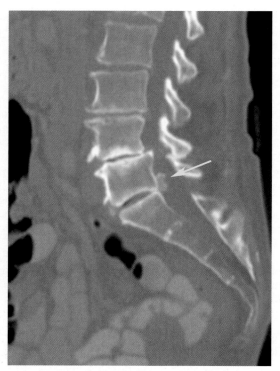

FIG. 20.5 **Sequestration.** Sagittal reformatted image demonstrating a calcified sequestered disk that has migrated cephalad from the parent disk at L5–S1 *(arrow)*. The presence of the calcification and increased density makes identification of this sequestered disk easier.

lateral recess than on the contralateral side. Conjoined roots occur in 1% to 3% of all patients and are incidental findings with no reported symptoms. The importance of their recognition is to avoid erroneous diagnosis of these normal variants as disk extrusions, which can result in explorations for free fragments and potential unfortunate neural damage during surgery. By noting density differences between conjoined roots and free fragments, the radiologist can avoid errors.

A *lateral disk* is a disk protrusion that occurs lateral to the neuroforamen and is one of the more commonly missed disk protrusions simply because it is overlooked. The search pattern should always include the region lateral to the neuroforamen. A lateral disk has huge implications for the surgeon. First, a lateral disk will irritate a nerve root that has already exited the neuroforamen and will therefore mimic a disk protrusion at a more cephalad level. For example, if a disk protrusion is present posteriorly at the level of L4–L5, it will usually have a mass effect on the L5 nerve root within the thecal sac. However, the L5 root can also be irritated by a lateral disk protrusion at the level of L5–S1. Therefore, if it is overlooked, such a disk protrusion can result in surgery at the level of the wrong disk space (in the example provided, incorrect surgery would be at the L4–L5 level) (Fig. 20.8). This situation is particularly

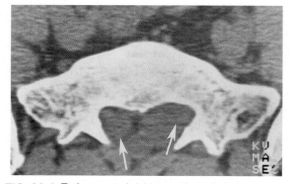

FIG. 20.6 **Tarlov cyst.** Axial image through the sacrum demonstrating dilatation of the nerve root sheaths *(arrows)*. Note that a perineural cyst is of the same density as the cerebrospinal fluid. This characteristic allows distinction between a perineural (Tarlov) cyst and a sequestered fragment (higher density). The cerebrospinal fluid pulsation can cause the Tarlov cyst to demonstrate well-defined smooth bone erosion as seen in this example.

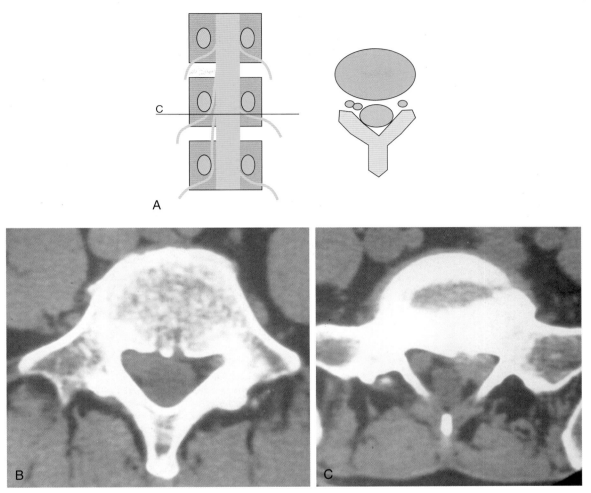

FIG. 20.7 **Conjoined nerve root.** (A) Two nerve roots arising from the thecal sac on the right in an asymmetric manner when compared with the left (C cursor level). (B) CT image obtained at the level of C in (A) demonstrating the two roots in the right lateral recess, not to be confused with a free fragment as the density of the conjoined root is similar to that of the thecal sac. Contrast that with (C), which demonstrates a free fragment (higher density) in the left lateral recess.

problematic in patients with multilevel disk abnormalities when one is attempting to determine the proper surgical level. Another important surgical implication for lateral disks is that a lateral disk does not require a laminectomy because it can be approached from outside the osseous central canal. The location of a lateral disk is not an area that a surgeon would normally explore. Lateral disks occur in less than 5% of patients but should be part of the search pattern in every patient at each disk level. The radiologist plays an enormous role in the ability to assess these findings and provide a necessary road map for surgical intervention.

SPINAL STENOSIS

Spinal stenosis has been classically divided into two types, congenital and acquired. Patients who experience congenital stenosis include achondroplastic dwarfs, patients with Morquio disease, and individuals born with a congenitally small thecal sac who have idiopathic spinal stenosis. Acquired stenosis includes osseous abnormalities that result in central canal narrowing such as degenerative joint (facet) disease with or without degenerative disk disease, posttraumatic stenosis, postsurgical stenosis, Paget disease, and calcification of the posterior longitudinal ligament.

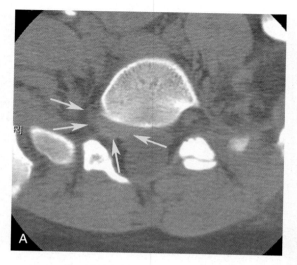

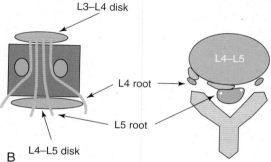

FIG. 20.8 **Lateral disk.** (A) Axial CT image through L5–S1 demonstrating a lesion of soft-tissue density on the right side just lateral to the right foramen (extraforaminal) *(arrows)*. (B) Drawing of a lateral disk demonstrating how a disk protrusion at L4–L5 would typically affect the L5 nerve root. However, a lateral disk at the same level affects the L4 nerve root. L4 nerve root abnormality most often is a result of a disk protrusion at L3–L4. An unrecognized lateral disk can result in surgery at the wrong level. Radiologists should include this region as part of the search pattern and recognize the presence of lateral disks.

A preferred classification for spinal stenosis is based on anatomic location. Stenosis can be described as *central canal stenosis, neuroforaminal stenosis,* or *lateral recess stenosis.* In each of these areas the most common cause of stenosis is osteoarthrosis of facet joints or disk disease as classified earlier.

Central Canal Stenosis

For decades, radiologists have been asked to measure the central canal to diagnose spinal stenosis.

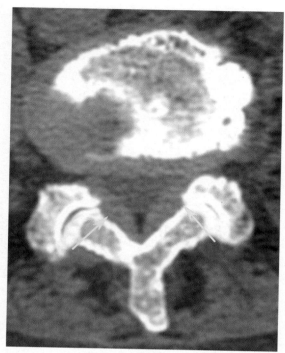

FIG. 20.9 **Central canal stenosis.** The central canal stenosis in this example is a result of the combination of broad-based disk bulge, facet arthrosis, and ligamentum flavum thickening *(arrows)*. The thecal sac is difficult to visualize as a separate and distinct structure because the epidural fat has been obliterated. When the epidural fat is no longer visualized, spinal stenosis should be suspected.

Discordance in the size of the bony canal and the thecal sac must be present for stenosis to be clinically manifest. A simple measurement of the central canal (without reference to the size of the bone canal) does not address the "fit" of the thecal sac within the canal, so such measurements are virtually meaningless. An exception to this situation may be the cervical spine, for which a narrow central canal has been correlated with increased risk of spinal cord injury in football players.

The most useful CT criteria for diagnosing central canal stenosis are obliteration of the epidural fat and flattening of the thecal sac. Both of these findings can be present without symptoms of spinal stenosis, and therefore stenosis can only be suggested by the radiologist, and clinical correlation is required.

The most common cause of central canal stenosis is secondary to facet arthrosis, which results in hypertrophy of the facet joints and encroachment of the central canal and lateral recess (Fig. 20.9). Another common cause of

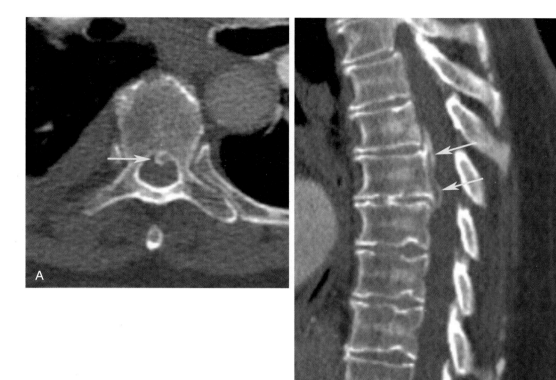

FIG. 20.10 Ossification of the posterior longitudinal ligament. (A) Axial image through the thoracic spine demonstrating central ossification *(arrow)*. A calcified central disk protrusion or a central osteophyte may have a similar appearance. Recognizing the ossification along the ligament is key to making this diagnosis as seen in (B). (B) Sagittal image demonstrating a long segment of ossification along the posterior longitudinal ligament *(arrows)* within the thoracic spine.

central canal stenosis is "hypertrophy" of the ligamentum flavum. The ligamentum flavum does not actually hypertrophy, but rather buckles inward because of facet slippage and associated narrowing of the disk space. Because this condition represents soft-tissue encroachment, measurements of the size of the bone canal would not reflect this process, which is another reason why measurements are not reliable indicators of spinal stenosis.

Paget disease affecting a vertebral body, which occurs less often now than in the past, involves enlargement of the vertebral body and can occasionally result in central canal stenosis, as can ossification of the posterior longitudinal ligament. It has been reported that up to 25% of patients with diffuse idiopathic skeletal hyperostosis, a common entity in individuals older than 50 years, have ossification of the posterior longitudinal ligament (Fig. 20.10). Other causes of central canal stenosis include trauma and postoperative changes.

Neuroforaminal Stenosis

The causes of neuroforaminal stenosis, similarly to those of central canal stenosis, can be diverse but are usually caused by osteophytes emanating from the vertebral body or from the superior articular facet. Disk protrusions and postoperative scarring can also occur in the foramen.

The nerve root exits the central canal in the superior aspect of the neuroforamen. Encroachment in the inferior aspect of the foramen, near the disk space, is an infrequent cause of clinical problems. The nerve root is immobile in the neuroforamen. Therefore even a small amount of stenosis in the superior aspect of the foramen can cause severe clinical symptoms, whereas severe stenosis of the inferior aspect of the foramen may result in no symptoms at all. For these reasons, the amount of narrowing of the neuroforamina often does not correlate with clinical findings.

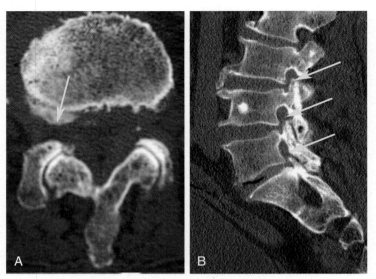

FIG. 20.11 Neuroforaminal stenosis. (A) An osteophyte arising from the posterior right margin of the vertebral body is extending into the right neuroforamen, resulting in neuroforaminal stenosis *(arrow)*. (B) Sagittal reformatted image showing an additional cause of neuroforaminal narrowing. Note the presence of facet arthropathy resulting in narrowing of the normal "keyhole" appearance of the foramen *(arrows)*.

Although many believe that sagittal reformatted images through the neuroforamen are adequate for identification of stenosis, axial images are by far more reliable in fully demonstrating the degree of neuroforaminal stenosis and its cause. The neuroforamen and the nerve root can be seen in their entirety with axial images, whereas a single reformatted sagittal image will show volume rendering of the axial slice (Fig. 20.11).

A cause of unsuccessful back surgery is failure to preoperatively identify neuroforaminal stenosis in a patient undergoing surgical diskectomy, which can result in the performance of an inadequate procedure. Disk disease and stenosis in any of its forms most often occur together and should be identified by the radiologist.

Lateral Recess Stenosis

The lateral recess is the bony portion of the central canal that is just caudad and cephalad to the neuroforamen. When the neuroforamen ends as one proceeds caudally, the lateral recess begins. This area has also been referred to as the *nerve root canal* because the nerve roots, after they exit the thecal sac and before they exit the central canal through the neuroforamen, run in this osseous triangular space. In the lateral recess the nerve roots are vulnerable to being impinged by osteophytes, disk fragments, and scar tissue from previous surgery (Fig. 20.12). As with the neuroforamen, the amount of

stenosis often does not correlate with the clinical presentation. Therefore it is best to note whether the lateral recess is or is not normal in appearance. Narrowing must be correlated clinically.

SPONDYLOLYSIS AND SPONDYLOLISTHESIS

Spondylolysis (pars interarticularis defect, discussed in Chapter 19) can cause low back pain and sciatica and can occasionally cause spinal stenosis. A fibrocartilaginous mass can develop around a pars fracture that can extend into the central canal and cause a mass effect on the thecal sac or nerve roots. The radiologist should search for the fibrocartilaginous proliferation in patients with a pars defect to avoid the unfortunate situation of spinal fusion being performed without removal of the offending soft-tissue mass within the central canal.

Spondylolisthesis is defined as anterior displacement of a cephalad vertebral body with respect to the caudad vertebral body, and is graded in the severity of displacement relative to the lower vertebral body. Grade 1 is defined as less than 25%, grade 2 as 25% to 50%, grade 3 as 50% to 75%, and grade 4 as 75% to 100% slip relative to the caudal vertebral body (Fig. 20.13). Spondylolisthesis can cause central canal stenosis, and a more advanced grade can cause neuroforaminal

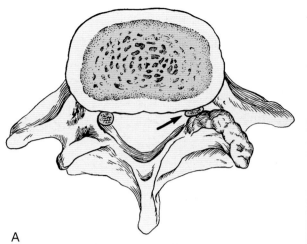

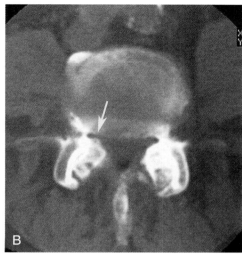

FIG. 20.12 **Lateral recess stenosis.** (A) A nerve root *(arrow)* under a mass affect in the lateral recess as a result of the bony overgrowth. (B) The right lateral recess is narrowed because of the bone overgrowth *(arrow)*. The nerve root lies in the lateral recess and can be impinged by this process. Recognizing the location of the abnormality can assist the surgeon with operative planning.

stenosis. Occasionally, the pars defect will extend into the neuroforamen and impinge on the nerve root. Spondylolisthesis may be a result of spondylolysis or spondylosis (facet joint arthrosis).

SACROILIAC JOINTS

Conventional radiographs of the sacroiliac joints can be extremely difficult to interpret secondary to anatomic obliquity of the joints themselves and the superimposed soft tissues. CT is a more reliable examination than conventional radiography and is also more reproducible, more sensitive, and more accurate than conventional radiography and results in less radiation exposure. Additional advantages of CT evaluation are that it can be performed rapidly by decreasing the number of slices necessary to evaluate the sacroiliac joints (compared with pelvis imaging), and it can be performed at relatively low cost and is therefore more cost-effective than conventional radiography.

Sacroiliac joint symptoms can occasionally be the cause of back pain. Sacroiliac joint abnormalities are part of the symptom complex of many arthritides, particularly the spondyloarthropathies.

Sacroiliac joint sclerosis and erosions can be identified with much more clarity on CT images than on conventional radiographs. Osteoarthrosis of the sacroiliac joints can cause erosions and can mimic a spondyloarthropathy or infection (Fig. 20.14).

Erosions and sclerosis in the sacroiliac joints increase with age, so patients older than 40 years often have sacroiliac joint abnormalities.

Osteitis condensans ilii is diagnosed when triangular foci of sclerosis are noted in the ilium abutting the sacroiliac joint. This is an incidental finding and is not associated with any symptoms.

STRESS CHANGES OF THE PUBIC SYMPHYSIS

This abnormality has been referred to as *osteitis pubis*, but there is rarely an inflammatory component associated with this entity. The relationship between changes in the sacroiliac joints and abnormal appearance of the pubic symphysis is a strong one. If sacroiliac joint changes are identified, then there should be a search for abnormalities in the pubic symphysis. Similarly, if bone changes within the pubic symphysis are identified, a careful search of the sacroiliac joints and sacral disease should be performed.

Osteitis pubis was historically defined as infection in the pubic symphysis, most often identified after bladder surgery. The name implies an inflammatory change in the joint space. However, any changes identified are not usually caused by an inflammatory process. Rather, stress changes, most often identified in athletes, lead to erosions and sclerosis within the pubic symphysis. Coexisting erosions and sclerosis are often seen in

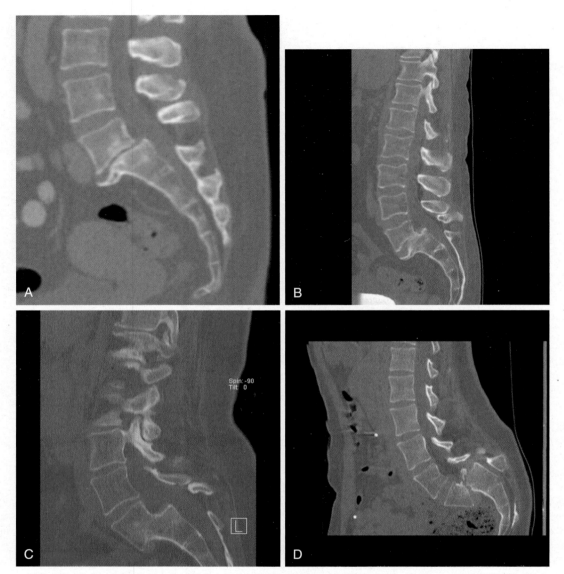

FIG. 20.13 **Spondylolisthesis.** (A) Grade 1 (<25%). (B) Grade 2 (25%–50%). (C) Grade 3 (50%–75%). (D) Grade 4 (75%–100%).

the sacroiliac joints in these individuals. Osteoarthrosis can also result in erosions and sclerosis at the pubic symphysis (Fig. 20.15).

TUMORS AND INFECTION

The use of CT in evaluating tumors and infection has largely been replaced by the use of MRI given its soft-tissue contrast as well as the multiplanar capabilities. CT can play an important role in evaluation of intraosseous lesions because of the ability to assess the presence of calcification, ossification, and cortical involvement. CT is more sensitive than conventional radiography, and CT is preferred over MRI to demonstrate peripheral or intraosseous calcifications. One example of this is myositis ossificans. If the pattern of ossification in myositis ossificans is not appreciated on imaging and a biopsy is performed because of suspicion of an aggressive lesion, the result may be devastating. Multiple

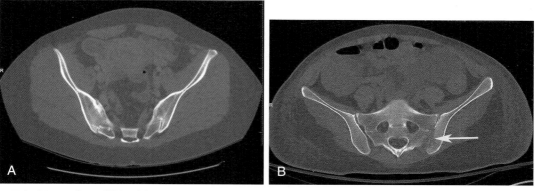

FIG. 20.14 **Sacroiliitis.** (A) Axial CT through the sacroiliac joints demonstrates bilateral ankylosis in this patient with ankylosing spondylitis. (B) Erosions are noted at the posterior margin of the left sacroiliac joint *(arrow)* in this patient with septic arthritis.

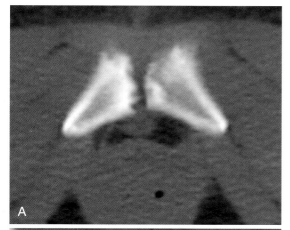

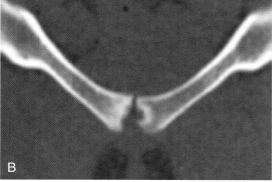

FIG. 20.15 **Stress changes of the pubic symphysis.** (A) Axial and (B) coronal reformatted images through the pubic symphysis showing the irregular cortical margin from stress changes. Recognition of the erosions should warrant an inspection of the sacroiliac joints. Often the stress changes in these joints can coexist.

mitotic figures in the biopsy specimen as a result of bone growth as the bone is ossifying and maturing can suggest an aggressive process, resulting in erroneous diagnosis and radical surgery. Myositis ossificans on MRI can mimic a sinister lesion because the pattern of ossification is not appreciated during evolution of the lesion, but it has a characteristic appearance on CT. The ossification remains in the periphery of the lesion (Fig. 20.16).

CT can be helpful in diagnosing bone involvement in multiple myeloma before such involvement becomes apparent on conventional radiographs. In particular, CT of the spine can show diffuse lytic lesions (Fig. 20.17). When myeloma has been more long-standing, the few remaining normal trabeculae within the vertebral body undergo compensatory hypertrophy, and the resulting appearance comprises thick, sclerotic bony struts with lytic areas between them (Fig. 20.18). A similar appearance of trabecular thickening within the vertebral body can be seen in plasmacytoma. This pattern for multiple myeloma and plasmacytoma can occasionally be confused with a spinal hemangioma. However, the latter reveals trabecular struts that are more ordered and symmetric (Fig. 20.19). Hemangiomas can be located anywhere within a vertebral body (or any bone for that matter) and are worth reporting despite their relatively common occurrence to allay concern that they reflect a more sinister process.

An increasing number of CT examinations are being performed to evaluate known or suspected musculoskeletal infections. This increase is likely caused by the prevalence of intravenous drug use and the growing population of immunocompromised patients, including those with human immunodeficiency virus, acquired

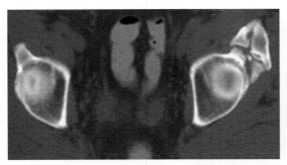

FIG. 20.16 **Myositis ossificans.** Ossification is noted in the region of the left rectus femoris origin. This is a result of a prior injury. It is important to recognize the presence of the ossification around the lesion as opposed to the central ossification as can be seen with a sinister lesion, parosteal osteosarcoma, and CT is the ideal examination for this assessment.

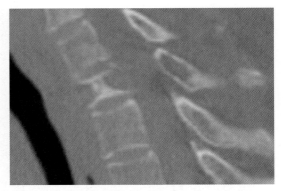

FIG. 20.18 **Plasmacytoma.** Sagittal reformatted image demonstrating a lytic lesion affecting a thoracic vertebral body. Note the thickening (increased density) of the remaining central trabeculae.

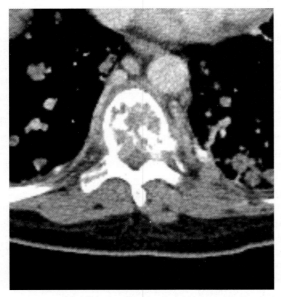

FIG. 20.17 **Multiple myeloma.** Axial image demonstrating multiple lytic foci within a thoracic vertebral body.

immunodeficiency syndrome, or an organ transplant, and renal dialysis patients. Helical CT with volume rendering is valuable in detecting infection, determining compartment involvement, and the extent of the process. This information is important for patient management (surgical versus medical) and for monitoring responses to treatment. CT with volume rendering can be used to evaluate cortical bone and associated soft-tissue masses

in suspected osteomyelitis. Multiplanar and three-dimensional images are useful in surgical planning, especially when the area of involvement is extensive. The administration of iodinated contrast medium is helpful in identifying rim enhancement of an abscess (Fig. 20.20).

CT can also play a role in identifying sequestrations in osteomyelitis. Identification of a sequestration has therapeutic significance as its presence usually requires surgical removal. Antibiotic therapy alone generally does not suffice because a sequestrum does not have a blood supply, and therefore antibiotics will have no effect in treatment.

If there is a clinical concern for a septic joint, arthrocentesis should be performed. Imaging is not helpful as the presence of a joint effusion does not indicate an infection. However, imaging can be helpful if a "dry tap" has occurred and the clinical concern remains high. Before taking the patient to the operating room to open the capsule and drain the fluid, confirmation can be helpful particularly in a clinical scenario that is confounded with other variables such as if the patient is obtunded or comorbidities (Fig. 20.21).

Necrotizing fasciitis requires a timely diagnosis. The rapidity of the spread and the subsequent deterioration in the patient's clinical condition require rapid diagnosis. Imaging studies should not delay surgical intervention. The CT characteristics of necrotizing fasciitis include soft-tissue gas associated with fluid collections within the deep fascia (Fig. 20.22). The potential advantages of CT include the ability to detect underlying infectious sources such as diverticulitis, osteomyelitis, and vascular rupture.

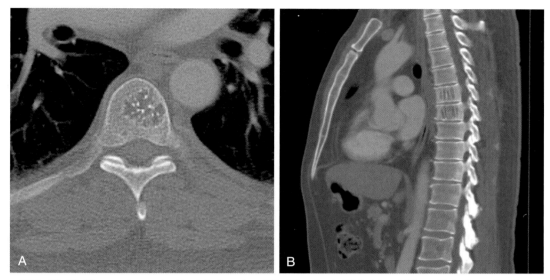

FIG. 20.19 **Hemangioma.** Incidentally found on CT of the chest. (A) Axial and (B) sagittal reformatted images revealing a typical appearance of dense, hypertrophied trabeculae arranged in a symmetric, columnar fashion unlike plasmacytoma.

INCIDENTAL FINDINGS

CT evaluation of the chest, abdomen, and pelvis may result in identification of nontraumatic bone abnormalities. A complete list of all possible incidental findings is beyond the scope of this chapter, but more commonly encountered abnormalities and examples of potentially confusing lesions are presented here.

Hemangiomas were mentioned earlier in the context of not being confused for multiple myeloma/plasmacytoma. They occur often enough for one to be comfortable with their appearance. The well-organized trabecular struts with the fatty elements within the lesion result in the characteristic appearance on CT (Fig. 20.19).

Schmorl nodes were introduced in the discussion of disk disease. These are not true "nodes," but are rather herniation of disk material through the end plate of a vertebral body (Fig. 20.23). Knowledge of the appearance and location of a Schmorl node is imperative so as not to mischaracterize and erroneously diagnosis a lytic lesion. A helpful observation in determining if a lesion is a Schmorl node is to recognize that the end plate must be involved. A Schmorl node can occur in any portion of the vertebral body as long as it involves the end plate, but is most often seen in the center of the vertebral body. A lateral scout view or a conventional radiograph may be helpful in determining the presence

of a Schmorl node. The intervertebral disk is avascular. Therefore after administration of contrast medium, there is no enhancement of a Schmorl node.

A Tarlov cyst was mentioned in the discussion of a sequestration. The discussion does not need to be reiterated, but what is worth emphasizing is the bone erosion that may occur as a result of the pressure effect of the pulsation of CSF (Fig. 20.6). The erosion results in well-defined margins, and the density of the lesion adjacent to the bone excavation is that of CSF. Recognition of this pattern of the process is important to avoid a biopsy. If concern exists for a soft-tissue mass resulting in erosion, the density of the soft-tissue mass would be higher than that of CSF. If CT is not diagnostic, MRI is strongly indicated before an attempted biopsy. MRI will show the fluid nature of the Tarlov cyst. There is no bone marrow edema associated with the perineural cysts on MRI. A pelvic mass or sacral tumor eroding into the bone may have an associated finding on MRI of bone marrow edema.

Paget disease can affect any bone in the body. Although the occurrence seems to be declining over time, it remains necessary to recognize this entity and its three different appearances. Knowledge of the different appearances is necessary not to mistakenly diagnose the lesion as a primary tumor of bone. The condition may be purely lytic, in which case it has a well-defined

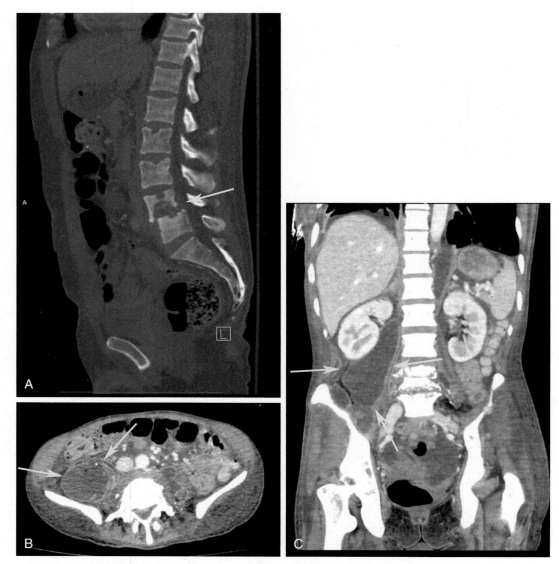

FIG. 20.20 Diskitis/osteomyelitis with abscess. (A) Sagittal reformatted CT image demonstrating destruction of the inferior and superior end plates of L4–L5 (arrow). Incidentally noted are Schmorl nodes at L2, L3, and the superior end plate of L4. (B) Axial and (C) coronal reformatted images demonstrating a large, peripherally enhanced, fluid-filled mass within the right psoas muscle representing a psoas abscess (arrows).

leading edge. The disease can also be purely sclerotic, or mixed lytic and sclerotic. Paget disease has associated findings of bone overgrowth, cortical thickening, and trabecular thickening. The trabecular thickening is not organized, as discussed previously for a hemangioma, making pagetic bone relatively easy to distinguish from a hemangioma. In addition, accompanying

cortical thickening is present, which is not seen with hemangiomas (Fig. 20.24). Paget disease can be distinguished from multiple myeloma by the cortical thickening and bone overgrowth, findings not seen in multiple myeloma. Additionally, for a potentially confusing case on CT, bone scintigraphy can make the distinction between Paget disease (marked increased

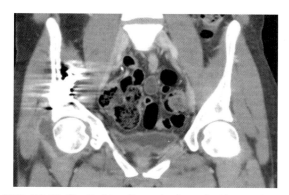

FIG. 20.21 **Septic hip.** Coronal reformatted image demonstrating a peripherally enhanced fluid collection within and adjacent to the right hip. Clinically, the patient was infected, but no fluid was obtained on initial aspiration. The findings confirmed a septic hip. Note the hardware artifact in the right supra-acetabular region.

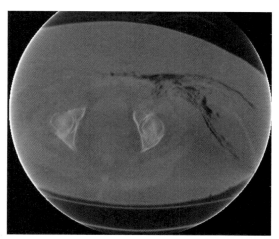

FIG. 20.22 **Necrotizing fasciitis.** Axial CT image obtained with lung windows demonstrating air within the subcutaneous and deep tissues of the left thigh. The appearance is characteristic of necrotizing fasciitis, although this should be a clinical diagnosis with timely surgical intervention as there is rapid deterioration of the patient's condition. A search for a potential source should be made, including abscess, diverticulitis, adjacent osteomyelitis, or vascular rupture. In this example the femoral neurovascular bundle is close to the problematic condition.

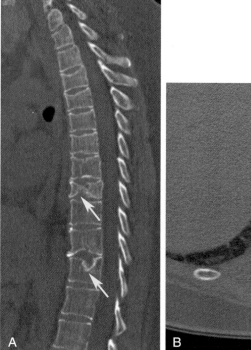
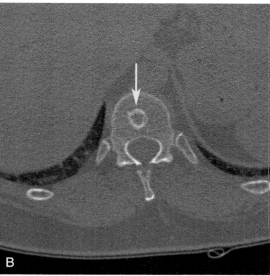

FIG. 20.23 (A) Sagittal reformatted CT image through the thoracic spine demonstrating several Schmorl nodes. Note the scalloped appearance with disk herniation into the end plate *(arrows)*. (B) Axial image through the end plate demonstrating the appearance of the "node" (herniated disk material) with a smooth sclerotic border *(arrow)*. This example demonstrates the herniated disk to be in the center of the vertebral body. The "nodes" may occur anywhere along the vertebral end plate but are most common centrally.

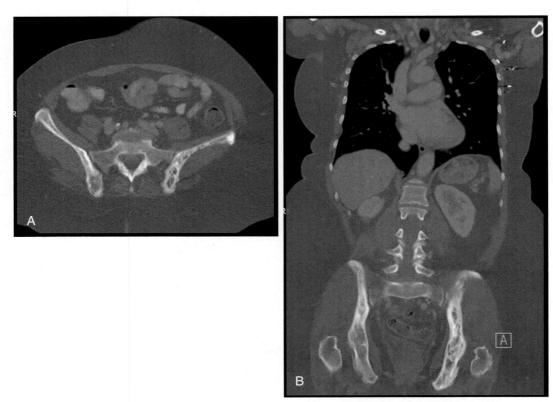

FIG. 20.24 Paget disease. (A) Axial image through the pelvis demonstrating the coarse trabeculae, thickened cortex, and enlargement of the left iliac bone and the right posterior ilium. This lesion should not be confused for an intraosseous hemangioma because of the disorganization of the trabecular thickening, presence of cortical thickening, and bone enlargement. (B) Coronal reformatted image demonstrating the bilateral involvement, left more than right.

in radionuclide uptake) and multiple myeloma (no uptake).

In long bones, Paget disease generally begins at one end of the bone at the articular surface and migrates to the other end (except the tibia). In the pelvis, a more common location of Paget disease, there may be thickening of the iliopectineal and or ilioischial lines, but this is not always the case. It seems that the greatest confusion arises when a patient is being imaged for prostate carcinoma and a blastic process is encountered in the pelvis. Assessment of additional findings such as cortical thickening, trabecular thickening, and bone enlargement may help to distinguish Paget disease from other blastic processes, including metastatic disease (Fig. 20.25).

Fibrous dysplasia (FD) is a congenital disorder of bone leading to the presence of fibrous and chondral tissues and even cysts within the lesion located within the bone marrow. Because of the presence of these different tissue types, FD can have a wide variety of appearances on CT. In general, FD is asymptomatic, can be found in any bone, and is therefore an incidental finding. FD is a well-defined lesion that is occasionally associated with thickened cortices but does not exhibit the trabecular thickening or bone enlargement of Paget disease (Fig. 20.26). Calcifications may be seen within the lesion, caused by the calcification of chondral elements reported in 10% to 30% of FD lesions. There may be associated endosteal scalloping given its medullary location, or there may be a sclerotic border, particularly if FD occurs in the intertrochanteric region. In summary, FD appears similar to many conditions on CT, but the lesion will not look aggressive. There will be no associated soft-tissue mass, permeative appearance, or periosteal reaction (unless a pathologic fracture is present). If a soft-tissue mass is encountered or periosteal reaction is present (without identification of a fracture) in association with a bone lesion, FD is not the diagnosis.

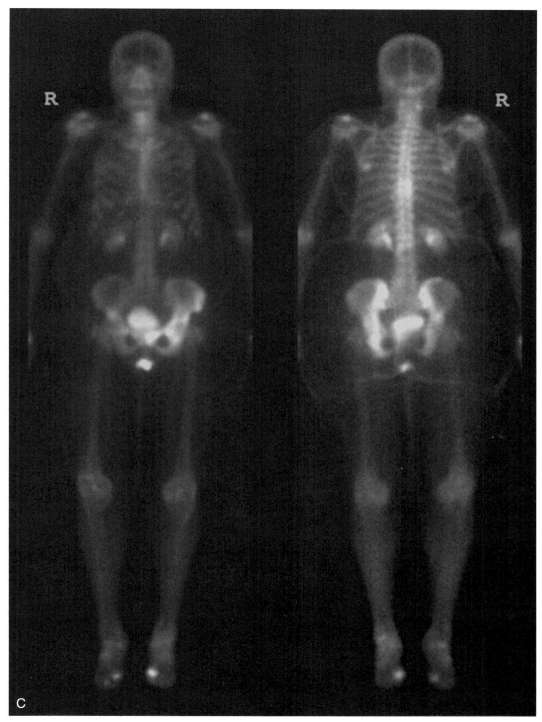

FIG. 20.24, cont'd (C) Bone scintigraphy demonstrates the bilateral nature and the intense radiotracer uptake characteristic of Paget disease. Multiple myeloma can have disorganized, thickened trabeculae that perhaps can be confusing for the lytic phase of Paget disease. Bone scintigraphy can be helpful if Paget disease cannot be easily distinguished from multiple myeloma on conventional x-ray.

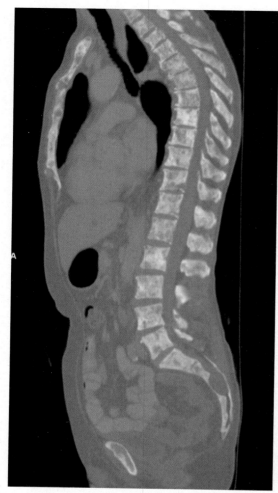

FIG. 20.25 Sclerotic bone metastasis. Sagittal reformatted image through the thoracic and lumbar spine demonstrating multiple sclerotic foci without characteristic bone enlargement seen with Paget disease.

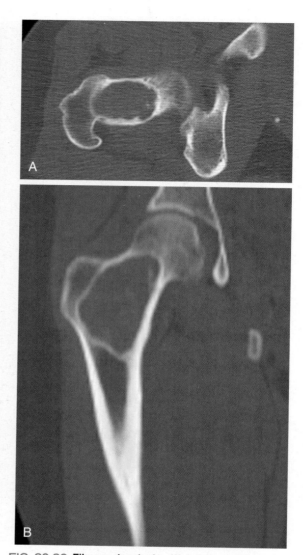

FIG. 20.26 Fibrous dysplasia. (A) Axial image through the right intertrochanteric region demonstrating a well-defined lesion with a sclerotic margin, indicating a benign entity. (B) Coronal reformatted image showing the well-defined extent of the lesion. The appearance in this location is characteristic of fibrous dysplasia.

An enchondroma is a centrally located, painless lesion that is incidentally found. Such lesions can be identified in any bone, and when they are identified within long and flat bones, they have a chondroid matrix. The typical appearance of a chondroid matrix comprises calcified arcs and circles resembling the letters *C* and *O* (Fig. 20.27). Endosteal scalloping may be present.

Avascular necrosis (AVN) and bone infarcts are a result of a progressive process leading to bone death. AVN is subarticular in location, whereas infarcts occur in diaphyseal locations. MRI and conventional radiography are used for staging and diagnosis of AVN. CT plays little role.

When AVN is identified on CT, curvilinear sclerosis in a subarticular location is pathognomonic (Fig. 20.28). Subchondral lucency is a late finding in AVN. MRI is sensitive and specific for this diagnosis and is recommended for evaluation and grading.

The increased utility of unenhanced CT in the trauma setting should encourage radiologists to be aware of the

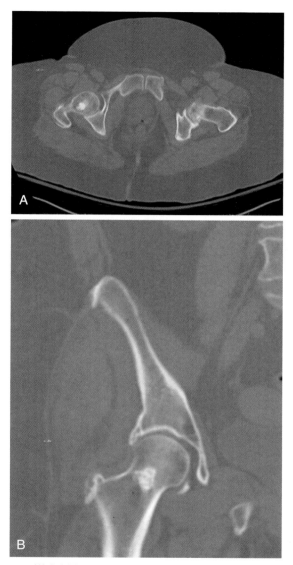

FIG. 20.27 **Enchondroma.** (A) Axial image through the hip joints demonstrating a calcified lesion noted incidentally. (B) Coronal reformatted image demonstrating to better advantage the characteristic arcs and circles of a chondroid lesion. The central location within the medullary space, the asymptomatic nature of the lesion, and the appearance of calcification in curvilinear orientation are characteristic of an enchondroma.

significance of rib fractures (see Chapter 19) and aware of the appearance and occurrence of incidentally encountered rib abnormalities. A not infrequently encountered rib lesion is that of FD. The appearance on CT is as a result of osseous replacement by immature woven bone. The presence of cyst-like changes and chondroid elements will result in a variety of appearances of FD.

Other benign lesions can have similar appearances to FD and include giant cell tumor, aneurysmal bone cyst, unicameral bone cyst, and other uncommon lesions. Bone metastases to ribs, similarly, may be encountered during the search for the primary lesion or follow-up disease assessment. Metastases may have a variety of appearances depending on the primary cancer (Fig. 20.29).

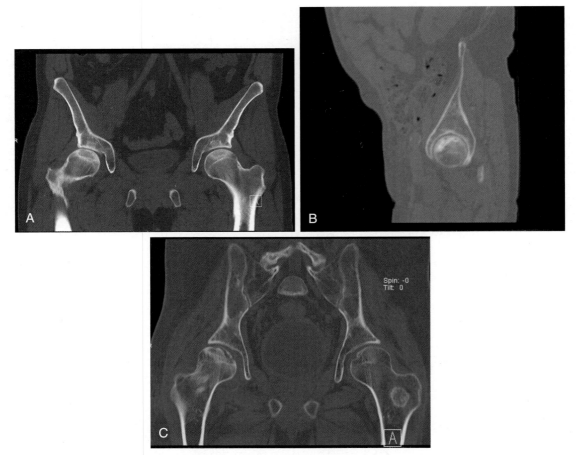

FIG. 20.28 **Progressive stages of avascular necrosis.** (A) Curvilinear sclerosis surrounds a relatively lucent center in the bilateral femoral epiphyses. This is characteristic of avascular necrosis. The bilaterality is seen in up to 40% of cases of avascular necrosis. (B) Sagittal reformatted image demonstrating focal subchondral sclerosis in the femoral head without evidence of collapse. (C) Coronal reformatted image showing subchondral collapse identified in the head of the right femor as evidenced by the presence of lucency and the irregularity of the articular surface of the femoral head. The left intertrochanteric region incidentally demonstrates a peripherally sclerotic, well-defined lucent lesion with focus of increased density in the inferior lesion. The location in the intertrochanteric region likely makes this fibrous dysplasia. However, the chondroid matrix within the lesion may make an enchondroma a differential consideration. However, the fact that both lesions are benign, and incidentally noted, makes the important diagnostic consideration that of a benign lesion.

Although all possible lesions cannot be reviewed in this chapter, some helpful tips have been provided for commonly encountered lesions. Primary lesions of bone are best characterized on conventional radiographs. If an incidental lesion is encountered on CT, the radiologist should assess the margins, density, and potential matrix and, if necessary, correlate the findings with conventional X-ray observations to avoid unnecessary biopsies.

METAL IMPLANTS

Imaging of postoperative patients with metallic implants may present a challenge. Metal causes artifacts such as beam hardening. These artifacts depend on the composition of the hardware and are lowest for titanium and highest for cobalt-chrome alloys. Artifacts also depend on the thickness and orientation of the implant and are severest in the direction of the thickest portion of the implant. When possible, the body part

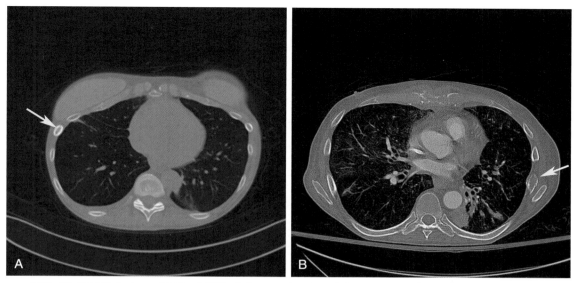

FIG. 20.29 **Rib lesions.** (A) Chest CT for follow-up of metastatic breast cancer demonstrates a sclerotic right rib lesion *(arrow)*. Recognition of this finding prompted additional imaging and altered patient management. (B) A minimally expansile, lytic lesion involving a left rib also demonstrates a pathologic fracture *(arrow)*.

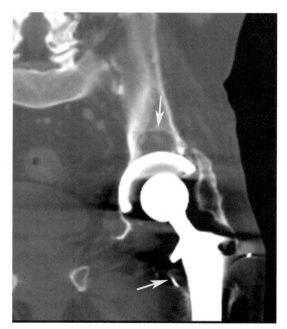

FIG. 20.30 **Hip prosthesis.** Coronal reformatted image demonstrating a left total hip arthroplasty without significant artifact allowing visualization of adjacent lytic, minimally expansile lesions in the acetabulum and proximal femur *(arrows)*. Heterotopic bone formation is noted lateral to the acetabulum.

should be positioned with the minimal cross-sectional area of the prosthesis presented to the X-ray beam. Metal artifacts also depend on the peak voltage, current, reconstruction algorithm, slice thickness, and orientation. A high peak voltage decreases artifacts by increasing the likelihood of X-ray penetration. An increase in current increases the photon flux striking the CT detectors and reduces artifacts, but this must be balanced against the increase in radiation dose. The use of bone or edge enhancement should be avoided because this increases hardware artifacts. It is recommended that standard bone or soft-tissue reconstruction algorithms be used when patients with dense metal implants are being imaged. Use of a thicker slice width also reduces metal artifacts by averaging the pixels (Fig. 20.30).

There is often a need to evaluate osseous fusion following fracture fixation, joint fusion, or complications of joint replacement surgery (loosening or periprosthetic fracture) (Fig. 20.31). Multidetector CT can also be used in preoperative assessment for revision prostheses to evaluate the bone stock quality and the potential need for bone grafting and reconstruction.

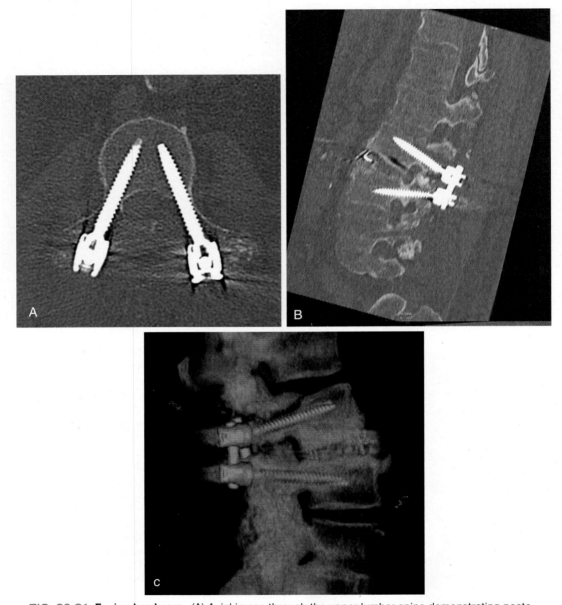

FIG. 20.31 **Fusion hardware.** (A) Axial image through the upper lumbar spine demonstrating posterior pedicle fixation without a hardware artifact. CT can be performed to assess patients for hardware complications such as loosening or fracture. (B) Sagittal reformation through the posterior fusion demonstrates incorporation of disk spacer graft and intact hardware without a hardware artifact. (C) Three-dimensional reconstruction demonstrates the intact hardware and graft incorporation, which can be viewed in multiple directions.

SUMMARY

This chapter has summarized the utility of CT for evaluating disk disease. Attention to density differences and the design of an appropriate protocol will allow more accurate diagnosis of disk disease. A well-designed protocol will also allow diagnosis of spondylolysis.

Although MRI has largely replaced CT for evaluation of sacroiliitis, erosions are readily identified with CT. Similarly, MRI is the primary modality for evaluating soft-tissue masses, but evaluation of differences in density and the administration of contrast medium can help with localization as well as in assisting with identification of an abscess and sequestration.

Awareness of commonly encountered osseous lesions and their appearance on CT can lead to appropriate diagnosis and eliminate an unnecessary biopsy.

Multidetector CT with volume rendering can compensate for streak artifacts and allows improved imaging of postoperative metal, enabling identification of nonunions, hardware failure, and bone stock in the setting of revision. Additionally, the decrease in streak artifacts allows evaluation of adjacent anatomy for more accurate diagnosis.

SUGGESTED READING

Boomsma, M. F., Edens, M. A., Van Lingen, C. P., et al. (2015). Development and first validation of a simplified CT-based classification system of soft tissue changes in large-head metal-on-metal total hip replacement: Intra- and interrater reliability and association with revision rates in a uniform cohort of 664 arthroplasties. *Skeletal Radiol*, *44*(8), 1141–1149.

Buckwalter, K. A., Rydberg, J., Kopecky, K. K., Crow, K., & Yang, E. L. (2001). Musculoskeletal imaging with multislice CT. *AJR. Am J Roentgenol*, *176*(4), 979–986.

Fardon, D. F., Williams, A. L., Dohring, E. J., Murtagh, F. R., Gabriel Rothman, S. L. & Sze, G. K. (2014). Lumbar disc nomenclature: Version 2.0: Recommendations of the combined task forces of the North American Spine Society, the American Society of Spine Radiology and the American Society of Neuroradiology. *Spine J*, *14*(11), 2525–2545.

Douglas-Akinwande, A. C., Buckwalter, K. A., Rydberg, J., Rankin, J. L., & Choplin, R. H. Multichannel CT: Evaluating the spine in postoperative patients with orthopedic hardware. *Radiographics*, 200;*26*(Suppl 1):S97–S110.

Gaudino, S., Martucci, M., Colantonio, R., et al. (2015). A systematic approach to vertebral hemangioma. *Skeletal Radiol*, *44*(1), 25–36.

Klein, M. A. (2017 Nov). Lumbar spine evaluation: Accuracy on abdominal CT. *Br J Radiol*, *90*(1079), 20170313.

Lee, M. J., Kim, S., Lee, S. A., et al. (2007). Overcoming artifacts from metallic orthopedic implants at high-field strength MR imaging and multi-detector CT. *Radiographics*, *27*(3), 791–803.

Park, J. S., Ryu, K. N., Hong, H. P., Park, Y. K., Chun, Y. S., & Yoo, M. C. (2004). Focal osteolysis in total hip replacement: CT findings. *Skeletal Radiol*, *33*(11), 632–640.

Subhas, N., Polster, J. M., Obuchowski, N. A., et al. (2016). Imaging of arthroplasties: improved image quality and lesion detection with iterative metal artifact reduction, a new CT metal artifact reduction technique. *AJR. Am J Roentgenol*, *207*(2), 378–385.

Index

Note: Page numbers followed by "f" indicate figures and "t" indicate tables.